Clinical Preventive Medicine

Health Promotion and Disease Prevention

Clinical Preventive Medicine

Health Promotion and Disease Prevention

Edited by

EDITOR-IN-CHIEF
T. Warner Hudson, M.D.
Assistant Clinical Professor, Department of Family Practice, University of California, Davis, School of Medicine; Medical Director, CableData, Rancho Cordova, California

PEDIATRIC SECTION EDITOR
Michael A. Reinhart, M.D., M.P.H.
Associate Clinical Professor, Department of Pediatrics, University of California, Davis, School of Medicine; Associate Clinical Professor, Department of Pediatrics, University of California, Davis, Medical Center, Sacramento, California

ADULT SECTION EDITOR
Steven D. Rose, M.D., M.S.
Assistant Clinical Professor, Department of Medicine, University of California, Davis, School of Medicine; Assistant Clinical Professor of Medicine, Department of Medicine, University of California, Davis, Medical Center and the Permanente Medical Group, Kaiser/Permanente Medical Center, Sacramento, California

PRENATAL SECTION EDITOR
Gary K. Stewart, M.D., M.P.H.
Assistant Professor, Department of Obstetrics and Gynecology, University of California, Davis, School of Medicine; Attending Obstetrician and Gynecologist, Sutter Community Hospitals, Sacramento, California

Foreword by
Robert S. Lawrence, M.D.
Director, Department of Medicine, Director, Division of Primary Care, and Charles S. Davidson Associate Professor of Medicine, Harvard Medical School, Boston, Massachusetts; Chairman, U.S. Preventive Services Task Force

Little, Brown and Company
Boston/Toronto

First Edition

Library of Congress Catalog Card No. 87-83684

ISBN 0-316-37909-3

Printed in the United States of America

DON (H)

To Anne

Contents

Foreword

The dramatic achievements of public health in the early decades of this century all but eliminated the major infectious diseases responsible for much of the morbidity and mortality in the industrialized world. Only polio remained to succumb to the achievements of post World War II biotechnology. A "new morbidity" emerged from the victory over epidemic contagions, characterized by chronic and degenerative diseases such as atherosclerotic cardiovascular disease, maturity-onset diabetes mellitus, and cancer, or by disorders of behavior such as alcoholism, drug abuse, smoking, obesity, unwanted teenage pregnancies, accidents, and homicide.

The biomedical revolution of the past 40 years greatly expanded our understanding of the basic mechanisms of disease and provided diagnostic and therapeutic technologies of dazzling sophistication. But as our ability to diagnose and treat the clinical manifestations of the new morbidity has improved, our knowledge of the root causes of the behaviors that produce it and our ability to intervene and modify these behaviors remain limited. Nowhere is this illustrated more strikingly than in the AIDS epidemic. In a few short years scientists have discovered and characterized the human immunodeficiency virus down to the molecular level, but we still search for answers to the behaviors that sustain the epidemic and for a public policy to provide appropriately for its victims.

A new paradigm is needed to help the clinician integrate health promotion and disease prevention with clinical medicine, to couple the public health successes of primary and secondary prevention with the medical management and tertiary prevention of the complications of chronic disease. *Clinical Preventive Medicine: Health Promotion and Disease Prevention* provides the paradigm and explicates the details of health promotion and disease prevention in a practical and clear way. The emphasis on case-finding rather than screening improves the predictive value of the tests recommended for each sex and age group. The integration of efforts to detect asymptomatic disease or risk factors and counseling for healthier behaviors with periodic health examinations triggered by symptomatic conditions or age-specific guidelines promises to close the gap between preventive medicine and curative services.

The authors of this text have captured a dynamic and evolving field of medicine to produce a useful guide for the primary care clinician. Application of the principles described in this text will enhance the knowledge and skills of the practitioner and the health of his or her patients.

Robert S. Lawrence, M.D.

Preface

This book grew out of a simple need. As residents, fellows, faculty, and clinicians, it became clear to us that there was no single source book to which one could refer with confidence for current health promotion or disease prevention recommendations, their justification, and details of performance. The United States Preventive Services Task Force, the American Cancer Society, the American Academy of Pediatrics, the American Heart Association, and the Centers for Disease Control—to name just a few—make excellent recommendations in their respective areas. They do not always agree, and recommendations, not to mention consensus, can be difficult to find in some areas, such as the role of tympanostomy tubes in preventing significant childhood conductive hearing loss or routine glaucoma testing in adults.

Clinical Preventive Medicine: Health Promotion and Disease Prevention has been written to fill this need: to be the book to which the clinician can turn to find out more about the problem to be prevented or the positive health behavior to be promoted and to find out what should be done, how it should be done, why it should be done, how often it should be done, and with whom it should be done. It is directed to practicing physicians in obstetrics and gynecology, pediatrics, internal medicine, family medicine, and general practice. The text is also relevant to the work of nurse practitioners, physician assistants, residents, and medical students.

The book is organized in multiple layers that enable the reader to find specific information simply and quickly. It is divided into three major areas of the life cycle: prenatal; infant, child, and adolescent; and adult. Within each of these areas are two groups of chapters: the health promotion chapters and the more numerous disease prevention chapters. Within each chapter type, similar organizational templates have been used to ensure coverage of the information and to facilitate its easy location by the reader.

The goal of the book is to be a primary source for the growing numbers of clinicians who, in addition to providing state-of-the-art downstream, "after-the-falls" injury or disease care, are also interested in providing state-of-the-art upstream, "before-the-falls" preventive care. The primary focus is the periodic health examination integrated into ongoing clinical practice, risk assessment, and case-finding rather than mass screening. Because of space and focus considerations we have not attempted to cover the broad areas of occupational or environmental health, public health, or health administration as these areas are well covered by existing books. There are certainly many unanswered questions and some uncovered areas, but it is our hope that this book will be a bridge to bring this increasingly important side of the health care equation to a higher level of proactive and systematic use, more fully understood and integrated into the daily practice of medicine.

T.W.H.
M.A.R.
S.D.R.
G.K.S.

Acknowledgments

We would like to acknowledge the following people who helped and supported us during the writing and production of this book:

Our families, especially Anne Hudson, Felicia Stewart, Debbie Rose, and Dorothy Yerxa Reinhart.

Olga Pshevlozky and Jane Anderson for their hard work and persistence in transcribing, and Barbara Claire, Sheila Stetson, and Karen Upcraft for their active, patient, and friendly assistance.

The entire staff of the University of California, Davis, School of Medicine Department of Family Practice, especially Edna Knopp, Wilhelmina Cottman, Carol Doyle, Kathleen J. Raygurt, Rebecca J. Tracy, and the others who offered valuable assistance and support, including Ollie Butler and Correne Treguboff.

Bob Davidson for believing in the project; Terri L. Malmgren and Dena P. Sehr of the Medical Library; Ken Niswander for saying it "could be done"; Bill Burnett and the California Health Manpower Commission for enabling the project to get started; Elizabeth Willingham of Little, Brown for keeping it moving; and CableData for enabling it to be completed.

Contributing Authors

Raymond Adelman, M.D.

Professor of Pediatrics, Section of Pediatric Nephrology, Department of Pediatrics, University of California, Davis, School of Medicine; Professor of Pediatrics, Section of Pediatric Nephrology, Department of Pediatrics, University of California, Davis Medical Center, Sacramento, California

Zvi Appelman, M.D.

Fellow, Reproductive Genetics, University of California, San Francisco, School of Medicine; Fellow, Reproductive Genetics, Department of Obstetrics and Gynecology, University of California, San Francisco General Hospital Medical Center, San Francisco, California

Jose Arevalo, M.D.

Assistant Professor, Department of Family Practice, University of California, Davis, School of Medicine; Assistant Professor, Department of Family Practice, University of California, Davis Medical Center, Sacramento, California

Daniel R. Benson, M.D.

Professor of Orthopaedic Surgery, Department of Orthopaedics, University of California, Davis, School of Medicine; Professor of Orthopaedic Surgery, Department of Orthopaedics, University of California, Davis Medical Center, Sacramento, California

Klea D. Bertakis, M.D., M.P.H.

Associate Professor, Department of Family Practice, University of California, Davis, School of Medicine; Associate Professor, Department of Family Practice, University of California, Davis Medical Center, Sacramento, California

Stephen M. Blain, D.D.S.

Associate Clinical Professor, Pediatric Dentistry, University of California, Los Angeles, School of Dentistry; Attending, Hospital Dentistry, UCLA Center for Health Sciences, Los Angeles, California

Debbie Bulger, M.S.

National Product Manager, Perinatal Services, Adventist Health System, Arlington, Texas

Doug Campos-Outcalt, M.D., M.P.A.

Medical Director, Preventive Services, Maricopa County Division of Public Health, Phoenix, Arizona

Willard Centerwall, M.D., M.S., M.P.H.	Clinical Professor and Consultant, Departments of Medical Genetics and Pediatrics, Oregon Health Sciences University School of Medicine, Portland, Oregon; Professor Emeritus of Medical Genetics and Pediatrics, Loma Linda University School of Medicine, Loma Linda, California, and University of California, Davis, School of Medicine, Davis, California
Albert Chang, M.D., M.P.H.	Associate Professor of Maternal and Child Health, Division of Population and Family Health, University of California, Los Angeles, School of Public Health; Associate Professor of Maternal Child Health, Division of Population and Family Health, UCLA Center for Health Sciences, Los Angeles, California
Robert S. Chang, M.D., D.Sc.	Professor of Medical Microbiology, University of California, Davis, School of Medicine, Davis, California
Richard Chole, M.D., Ph.D.	Professor, Department of Otolaryngology, Head and Neck Surgery, University of California, Davis, School of Medicine; Professor, Department of Otolaryngology, Head and Neck Surgery, University of California, Davis Medical Center, Sacramento, California
Christel Cranston, M.D.	Behavioral-Developmental Pediatrics, Department of Pediatrics, University of California, Davis, School of Medicine; Behavioral-Developmental Pediatrics, Department of Pediatrics, University of California, Davis Medical Center, Sacramento, California
James E. Crutcher, M.D.	Chairman and Associate Professor, Department of Family Medicine, University of Texas Health Science Center at Tyler, Tyler, Texas
Kathryn Dewey, Ph.D.	Associate Professor, Department of Nutrition, University of California, Davis, School of Medicine
Dan Ferrigno, M.D.	Associate Clinical Professor, Department of Medicine, University of California, Davis, School of Medicine; Associate Clinical Professor, Department of Medicine, University of California, Davis Medical Center, Sacramento, California; Associate Corporate Medical Director, CompCare Corporation, Newport Beach, California

Gary A. Fields, M.D.	Assistant Clinical Professor, Department of Obstetrics and Gynecology, University of California, Davis, School of Medicine; Assistant Clinical Professor, Department of Obstetrics and Gynecology, University of California, Davis Medical Center; Senior Attending Physician, Department of Obstetrics and Gynecology, Sutter Community Hospitals, Sacramento, California
Faith T. Fitzgerald, M.D.	Professor of Medicine and Chief, Division of General Medicine, Department of Internal Medicine, University of California, Davis, School of Medicine; Professor of Medicine and Chief, Division of General Medicine, Department of Internal Medicine, University of California, Davis Medical Center, Sacramento, California
Neil Flynn, M.D.	Associate Professor of Clinical Medicine, Divisions of General Medicine and Infectious Diseases, Department of Internal Medicine, University of California, Davis, School of Medicine; Associate Professor of Clinical Medicine and Director, Clinic for AIDS and Related Disorders, University of California, Davis Medical Center, Sacramento, California
Mitchell S. Golbus, M.D.	Professor, Department of Obstetrics, Gynecology and Reproductive Sciences, University of California, San Francisco, School of Medicine; Professor, Department of Obstetrics, Gynecology and Reproductive Sciences, University of California, San Francisco General Hospital Medical Center, San Francisco, California
Lynn R. Goldman, M.D.	Chief, Environmental Epidemiology Unit, Epidemiological Studies and Surveillance Section, California Department of Health Services, Berkeley, California
Marvin Goldman, M.D.	Professor of Radiobiology, University of California, Davis, School of Medicine; Professor of Radiobiology, University of California, Davis Medical Center, Sacramento, California
David Gordon, Ph.D.	Assistant Clinical Professor, Department of Family Practice, University of California, Davis, School of Medicine; Assistant Clinical Professor, University of California, Davis Medical Center, Sacramento, California

Jane Gray, M.D.	Associate Clinical Professor, Department of Pediatrics, University of Colorado Health Sciences Center School of Medicine; Associate Clinical Professor, Department of Pediatrics, The C. Henry Kempe National Center for the Prevention and Treatment of Child Abuse and Neglect, Denver, Colorado
Linda Greve, P.H.N.	Nurse Coordinator, Newborn Screening Program, Department of Pediatrics, University of California, Davis, School of Medicine; Genetics and PKU Clinic Nurse, Department of Pediatrics, University of California, Davis Medical Center, Sacramento, California
Hanns C. Haesslein, M.D.	Associate Clinical Professor, Department of Obstetrics and Gynecology, University of California, Davis, School of Medicine; Director, Division of Maternal-Fetal Medicine, The Perinatal Center, Sutter Community Hospitals, Sacramento, California
John Harris, M.D.	Chief, California Birth Defects Monitoring Program, California Department of Health Services, Berkeley, California
Robert A. Hatcher, M.D., M.P.H.	Professor, Department of Gynecology and Obstetrics, Emory University School of Medicine; Professor of Gynecology and Obstetrics, Grady Memorial Hospital, Atlanta, Georgia
T. Warner Hudson, M.D.	Assistant Clinical Professor, Department of Family Practice, University of California, Davis, School of Medicine; Medical Director, CableData, Rancho Cordova, California
Eric W. Jensen, M.D.	Associate Professor of Psychiatry and Medicine, University of North Carolina at Chapel Hill School of Medicine; Attending Physician and Director, MEDWELL: Health and Stress Management Program, North Carolina Memorial Hospital, Chapel Hill, North Carolina
Richard L. Jones	Assistant Professor of Pediatric and Adolescent Medicine, Georgetown University School of Medicine; Assistant Professor of Pediatric and Adolescent Medicine, Georgetown University Children's Medical Center, Washington, D.C.
Norman Kahn, M.D.	Assistant Professor, Department of Family Practice, University of California, Davis, School of Medicine; Director, Family Practice Residency Network, Department of Family Practice, University of California, Davis Medical Center, Sacramento, California

Michael Kan, M.D.	Assistant Clinical Professor, Department of Family Practice, University of California, Davis, School of Medicine; Assistant Clinical Professor, Department of Family Practice, University of California, Davis Medical Center, Sacramento, California
Kris Koski	Assistant Professor, School of Dietetics and Human Nutrition, MacDonald College of McGill University, Montreal, Canada; Assistant Professor, Department of Medicine, McGill University, Division of Experimental Medicine, Montreal General Hospital, Montreal, Canada
Elizabeth Kubiak, M.D.	Assistant Clinical Professor of Dermatology, University of California, Davis, School of Medicine; Chief of Dermatology, Kaiser/Permanente Medical Center-South Sacramento, Sacramento, California
Lindy Kumagai, M.D.	Professor of Medicine, Division of Endocrinology, Department of Internal Medicine, University of California, Davis, School of Medicine; Professor of Medicine, Division of Endocrinology, Department of Internal Medicine, University of California, Davis Medical Center, Sacramento, California
Chinh Le, M.D.	Associate Clinical Professor, Department of Pediatrics, University of California, Davis, School of Medicine; Chief, Pediatric Infectious Diseases, Kaiser/Permanente Medical Center, Sacramento, California
Rebecca Leonard, Ph.D.	Associate Adjunct Professor, Department of Otolaryngology, University of California, Davis, School of Medicine; Director of Speech Pathology, ENT Clinic, University of California, Davis Medical Center, Sacramento, California
Ernest L. Lewis, M.D.	Professor of Clinical Urology, University of California, Davis, School of Medicine; Attending Surgeon, University of California, Davis Medical Center, Sacramento, California
Mark Lipman, M.D.	Fellow, Department of Internal Medicine, University of California, Davis, School of Medicine; Fellow, Department of Internal Medicine, University of California, Davis Medical Center, Sacramento, California
F. L. Don McClurg, Jr., M.D.	Private Practice in Otolaryngology, Sacramento, California

Robert McConaughy, M.D.	Acting Instructor, Psychiatry and Behavioral Sciences, Division of Child Psychiatry and Behavioral Sciences, University of Washington School of Medicine; Acting Medical Director, Inpatient Psychiatry Unit, Division of Child Psychiatry and Behavioral Sciences, Children's Hospital and Medical Center, Seattle, Washington
James A. McGregor, M.D.	Associate Professor, Department of Obstetrics and Gynecology, University of Colorado Health Sciences Center School of Medicine; Associate Professor, Department of Obstetrics and Gynecology, University of Colorado Health Sciences Center, Denver, Colorado
Trent MacKay, M.D., M.P.H.	Assistant Clinical Professor, Department of Obstetrics and Gynecology, University of California, Davis, School of Medicine; Assistant Clinical Professor, Department of Obstetrics and Gynecology, University of California, Davis Medical Center, Sacramento, California
Frederick J. Meyers, M.D.	Assistant Professor of Medicine, Division of Hematology/Oncology, Department of Internal Medicine, University of California, Davis, School of Medicine; Assistant Professor of Medicine, Division of Hematology/Oncology, Department of Internal Medicine, University of California, Davis Medical Center, Sacramento, California
Mary Meyers, M.D.	Clinical Instructor, Department of Obstetrics and Gynecology, University of California, Davis, School of Medicine; Clinical Instructor, Department of Obstetrics and Gynecology, University of California, Davis Medical Center, Sacramento, California
Peter Michael Miller, M.D.	Assistant Health Officer, Child Health Services, California Department of Health and Human Services, San Rafael, California
Jay Milstein, M.D.	Associate Professor, Department of Pediatrics, Division of Neonatology, University of California, Davis, School of Medicine; Associate Professor, Department of Pediatrics, University of California, Davis Medical Center, Sacramento, California
William A. Norcross, M.D.	Associate Clinical Professor, Community and Family Medicine, University of California, San Diego, School of Medicine; Associate Clinical Professor, Community and Family Medicine, UCSD Medical Center, San Diego, California

Lois F. O'Grady, M.D.	Professor of Medicine, Division of Hematology/Oncology, Department of Internal Medicine, University of California, Davis, School of Medicine; Professor of Medicine, Division of Hematology/Oncology, Department of Internal Medicine, University of California, Davis Medical Center, Sacramento, California
Richard H. Oi, M.D.	Associate Professor, Obstetrics-Gynecology and Pathology, Department of Obstetrics and Gynecology, University of California, Davis, School of Medicine; Associate Professor, Obstetrics-Gynecology and Pathology, Department of Obstetrics and Gynecology, University of California, Davis Medical Center, Sacramento, California
Betty K. Patterson, M.D.	Assistant Clinical Professor, Department of Family Practice, University of California, Davis, School of Medicine; Woodland Memorial Hospital, Woodland, California, and Sutter Davis Hospital, Davis, California
Fran Pepitone-Rockwell, Ph.D.	Assistant Director, Developmental Programs, Undergraduate Admissions and Relations with Schools, University of California, Los Angeles, Los Angeles, California
Karen Poirier-Brode, M.D.	Assistant Clinical Professor, Department of Obstetrics and Gynecology, University of California, Davis, School of Medicine; Assistant Clinical Professor, Department of Obstetrics and Gynecology, University of California, Davis Medical Center, Sacramento, California
George Rab, M.D.	Associate Professor and Chief, Division of Children's Orthopedics, Department of Orthopedics, University of California, Davis, School of Medicine; Attending Surgeon, University of California, Davis Medical Center, Sacramento, California; Consulting Surgeon, Kaiser/Permanente Medical Center, Sacramento, California
Jean Ranc, M.A.	Therapist, MEDWELL: Health and Stress Management Program, Department of Psychiatry, University of North Carolina at Chapel Hill School of Medicine, Chapel Hill, North Carolina
Michael A. Reinhart, M.D., M.P.H.	Associate Clinical Professor, Department of Pediatrics, University of California, Davis, School of Medicine; Associate Clinical Professor, Department of Pediatrics, University of California, Davis Medical Center, Sacramento, California

Thomas A. Riemenschneider, M.D.	Professor of Pediatrics, Epidemiology, and Biostatistics, and Associate Dean, Case Western Reserve University School of Medicine; Associate Pediatrician, Division of Pediatric Cardiology, Rainbow Babies and Children's Hospital, Cleveland, Ohio
John Robbins, M.D.	Associate Professor of Clinical Medicine, Division of General Medicine, University of California, Davis, School of Medicine; Associate Professor of Clinical Medicine, Division of General Medicine, University of California, Davis Medical Center, Sacramento, California
Don Rockwell, M.D.	Professor, Department of Psychiatry, University of California, Los Angeles, UCLA School of Medicine; Director, Neuropsychiatric Hospital, Los Angeles, California
Peter Rogge, M.D.	Assistant Clinical Professor, Department of Obstetrics and Gynecology, University of California, Davis, School of Medicine; Assistant Clinical Professor, Department of Obstetrics and Gynecology, University of California, Davis Medical Center, Sacramento, California
Steven D. Rose, M.D., M.S.	Assistant Clinical Professor, Department of Medicine, University of California, Davis, School of Medicine; Assistant Clinical Professor, Department of Medicine, University of California, Davis Medical Center, and The Permanente Medical Group, Kaiser/Permanente Medical Center, Sacramento, California
Larry Saltzman, M.D.	Assistant Clinical Professor, Department of Family Practice, University of California, Davis, School of Medicine; Assistant Clinical Professor, Department of Family Practice, University of California, Davis Medical Center, Sacramento, California
Dewey Sandberg, M.D.	Chief Resident, Department of Family Practice, University of California, Davis, School of Medicine; Chief Resident, Department of Family Practice, University of California, Davis Medical Center, Sacramento, California
Jack M. Schneider, M.D.	Clinical Professor and Director, Division of Maternal-Fetal Medicine, Department of Obstetrics and Gynecology, University of California, Davis, School of Medicine; Director, Department of Perinatology and Medical Director, Perinatal Improvement Network, Sutter Community Hospitals and University of California, Davis Medical Center, Sacramento, California

Robert B. Shearin, M.D.	Professor of Pediatrics and Director, Pediatric Ambulatory Services and Division of Adolescent Medicine, Georgetown University School of Medicine; Professor of Pediatrics and Director, Pediatric Ambulatory Services and Division of Adolescent Medicine, Georgetown University Medical Center, Washington, D.C.
Gordon Smith, M.D.	Chief, Division of Ophthalmology, Children's Hospital Medical Center of Northern California, Walnut Creek, California
Felicia Stewart, M.D.	Clinical Lecturer, Department of Obstetrics and Gynecology, University of California, Davis, School of Medicine; Clinical Lecturer, Department of Obstetrics and Gynecology, University of California, Davis Medical Center, and Partner, Valley Center for Women's Health, Sacramento, California
Gary K. Stewart, M.D., M.P.H.	Assistant Professor, Department of Obstetrics and Gynecology, University of California, Davis, School of Medicine; Attending Obstetrician and Gynecologist, Department of Obstetrics and Gynecology, Sutter Community Hospitals, Sacramento, California
Jeff Tanji, M.D.	Assistant Professor, Department of Family Practice, University of California, Davis, School of Medicine; Assistant Professor, Department of Family Practice, University of California, Davis Medical Center, Sacramento, California
Duane Townsend, M.D.	Clinical Professor, Department of Obstetrics and Gynecology, University of California, Davis, School of Medicine; Clinical Professor, Department of Obstetrics and Gynecology, University of California, Davis Medical Center, Sacramento, California
Philip A. Trask, D.D.S.	Diplomate, American Board of Pediatric Dentistry; Staff, Department of Pediatrics, Santa Monica Hospital, and Dental Staff, Department of Surgery, Saint Johns Hospital, Santa Monica, California
James Trussell, Ph.D.	Professor of Economics and Public Affairs, Office of Population Research, Princeton University, Princeton, New Jersey
Lee Vogel, M.D.	Postdoctoral Geriatrics Fellow, Division of Family Medicine, University of California, San Diego, School of Medicine; Postdoctoral Geriatrics Fellow, UCSD Medical Center, San Diego, California

Sarah Woerner, M.D.	Clinical Faculty, Department of Pediatrics, University of California, Davis, School of Medicine; Clinical Faculty, Department of Pediatrics, University of California, Davis Medical Center, Sacramento, California
Israel Zelikovic, M.D.	Fellow, Division of Pediatric Nephrology, Department of Pediatrics, University of California, Davis, School of Medicine; Fellow, Division of Pediatric Nephrology, Department of Pediatrics, University of California, Davis Medical Center, Sacramento, California

Clinical Preventive Medicine

Health Promotion and Disease Prevention

1

Foundations of the Periodic Health Examination

T. Warner Hudson

The promotion of good health and the prevention of injuries and diseases are crucial components of good health care. The problem facing health care providers is separating well-intentioned enthusiasm embracing all sorts of unproved panaceas from decisions based on sound data. Measures that definitely are beneficial and that can be applied economically and practically must be incorporated into our practices, and we must omit the measures that are too difficult, costly, ineffective, or risky or will not be tolerated by our patients.

A growing number of factors have heightened the demands for and allure of prevention. The cost and complexity of disease care and cure have increased dramatically. Many diseases, like lung cancer and acquired immune deficiency syndrome (AIDS), remain virtually undaunted in their lethality. The widening malpractice crisis has witnessed greater awards for sins of omission, such as the failure to follow preventive service recommendations. Our society values individual well-being highly and seems not to tolerate a poor outcome if it was preventable. The primary care provider spends the majority of his or her time on well care. Fortunately, there have been significant advances in the effectiveness of health promotion and disease prevention services, which when carefully evaluated, selected, organized, and scheduled based on the risk assessment of individuals, provide a rational approach: the periodic health examination.

I. Historical perspective. The concept of the periodic health examination was first brought to the United States by Dr. G. M. Gould at the turn of the twentieth century[1]. Early screening efforts to identify physical defects were mistakenly equated with elimination of disease. Dr. E. L. Fisk worked with Metropolitan Life and other insurance companies to encourage policyholders to be examined at his Life Extension Institute, where he somewhat dubiously claimed that detection of minor abnormalities would lead to a reduction in mortality[2]. By 1922, the American Medical Association (AMA) endorsed these efforts, and in 1923 the National Health Council encouraged Americans to have an annual physical examination with the slogan "Have a Health Examination on Your Birthday." Enthusiasm languished during the Depression and World War II, but interest resumed with executive screening in the 1950s. Technology soon brought multiphasic screening, but closer scrutiny in the 1970s by the Kaiser and East London studies showed little or no overall benefit from such broad and unselective efforts (see Chap. 70).

In 1975, two family physicians, Frame and Carlson [3], reviewed periodic health screening using selective criteria. Frame recently updated these reviews [4]. Shortly after Frame and Carlson's original reviews, Breslow and Somers published their Lifetime Health Monitoring recommendations [5], followed by the Canadian Task Force [6], which issues periodic updates [7]. The Surgeon General's Report on Health Promotion and Disease Prevention [8] was released in 1979, and the American Cancer Society recommendations [9] were released in 1980. In 1981, the American College of Physicians stated that "in lieu of the traditional annual physical examination each internist [should] develop an **individualized** plan for preventive health care for each patient." They summarized the earlier recommendations, commended them, and reiterated that they are all minimal recommendations for low-risk, asymptomatic individuals [10]. In 1983, the AMA endorsed periodic health examination [11], and in 1984, the United States Office of Disease Prevention and Health Promotion, which was created by Public Law 94-317 in 1976, launched a new committee, the United States Preventive Services Task Force, to establish recommendations and to focus on their implementation for the American people. In 1987, the American Heart Association issued recommendations on risk factor evaluation of healthy adults [11a].

II. Definitions and concepts. The following definitions and concepts are described as they are used in this book:

A. Health. The World Health Organization charter broadly defines health as "a state of complete physical, mental, and social well-being and not merely the absence of disease" [8]. Some people would even add economic, intellectual, and spiritual well-being. This ideal state is certainly a difficult one to measure, if not achieve, and may in part explain the preoccupation that health care has had in coping with disease and dying and its focus on absence of disease as the goal of health care. Health then, is one end of a spectrum:

Health——Absence of disease——Disease——Death

It is determined by the dynamic interaction of three primary factors: behavior, environment, and heredity.

B. **Health promotion** [8, 12, 13]. Health promotion can be very broadly defined as any activity altering behavior, environment, or heredity in a positive direction. However, the narrower definition used in this book reflects that used by the Surgeon General's Report: Health promotion activities are individual-oriented activities (behaviors) that help people move their life-styles toward optimal health. There are a number of factors involved in adopting a new, healthier behavior or in discontinuing an unhealthy behavior. These include: knowledge, understanding, attitudes, beliefs, motivation, inertia, habit, addiction, reminders (cues), rewards, and penalties, to mention a few. Attention to some of these factors and not others may make changes in health behavior more difficult than it might otherwise be.

   Certain health promotion activities are applicable to everyone. These we have termed **general health promotion.** Others apply to at-risk individuals and are termed **specific health promotion.** Implicit in this terminology is the notion that some **risk assessment** has taken place.

C. **Health protection** includes environment-oriented activities [8], such as occupational and environmental health, nuclear war prevention, and environmental aspects of injury control. Although these are essential ingredients in the optimization of health, they are not the principal focus of this book's orientation to the busy clinician. Note that this definition is completely different from that used by the Canadian Task Force.

D. **Disease prevention** activities are designed to reduce the likelihood of the occurrence of a specific disease in an individual **(primary prevention)** or to detect its early symptomless stages when early intervention is more effective in interrupting or minimizing the progression of the disease than later intervention **(secondary prevention)**. Secondary prevention generally involves an **early detection** test that, if abnormal, is followed by **early intervention** to arrest or ameliorate disease progression. **Tertiary prevention** involves treatment of injury or disease to prevent more devastating effects than those that have already occurred. This is the focus of curative medicine and is outside the scope of this book.

E. **Periodic health examination (PHE)** is that prospective set of health promotion and disease prevention services based on age, sex, risk factors, and level of health that occur at appropriate intervals over the life cycle of the individual. It applies to asymptomatic or apparently well individuals and is probably best provided in a primary care setting. **Health maintenance, well-child care,** and **routine prenatal care** are often used synonymously with PHE. PHE may employ **case finding** strategies that seek to detect disease in individuals who are seeking care for other reasons, or it may be a principal reason for a health care visit. It may at times employ **mass screening** technologies on unselected individuals, such as phenylketonuria (PKU) screening but these screening technologies and the evaluation and follow-up of the abnormals are woven into the fabric of ongoing primary care.

F. **Health care provider** as used in this book refers to physicians, nurse practitioners, physician assistants, dentists, psychologists, nurses, health educators, and others who are involved in the delivery of health care. Some contributors to the book have used specific role labels when a more generic label, health care provider, may have done equally well.

G. **Epidemiologic terms and principles** [14]

   1. **Sensitivity:** The probability that a test result will be positive when the condition is present.

$$\frac{\text{True positives (TP)}}{\text{TP+False negatives (FN)}} \times 100 = \text{Sensitivity} = \text{TP rate.}$$

   2. **Specificity:** The probability that a test will be negative when the condition is absent.

$$\frac{\text{True negatives (TN)}}{\text{TN+False positives (FP)}} \times 100 = \text{Specificity} = \text{TN rate.}$$

Although a high sensitivity and specificity are important test characteristics, they do not establish a test's clinical usefulness.

3. **Prevalence:** The number of cases of a condition at a point in time.
4. **Incidence:** The number of new cases of a condition over a specified interval, often one year.
5. **Predictive value (PV)** or posterior probability is the probability that disease is present when the test is positive (PV ⊕). The PV ⊖ is the probability that disease is absent when the test is negative. Simply stated,

$$PV \oplus = \frac{TP}{TP+FP} \times 100 \text{ and } PV \ominus = \frac{TN}{TN+FN} \times 100.$$

PV is much more useful clinically than sensitivity and specificity. It is determined not only by the test characteristics but also by the prevalence of the disease in the population being tested (prior probability).

6. **Bayes' theorem** was described by an eighteenth-century English mathematician, the Rev. Thomas Bayes, and states that predictive value is proportional to prevalence. In other words, when the prevalence, or prior probability, is high, a positive test is more likely to be a true positive. Conversely, when the prevalence is low, a positive result is more likely to represent a false positive. For example, if the PKU prevalence is 1/10,000, then the results are as follows (assume sensitivity=100% and specificity=99.95%):

	Screening Test		
	⊕	⊖	Total
Disease			
PKU	10	–	10
No PKU	50	99,940	99,990
Total	60	99,940	100,000

$$\text{The PV} \oplus = \frac{10}{10+50} \times 100 = 16.67\%$$

Note that this also means that there is an 83.3% likelihood that a positive test is falsely positive.

If the PKU prevalence increases to 10/10,000, then the results are as follows:

	Screening Test		
	⊕	⊖	Total
Disease			
PKU	100	–	100
No PKU	50	99,850	99,990
Total	150	99,850	100,000

$$\text{The PV} \oplus = \frac{100}{100+50} \times 100 = 67\%$$

Note that in this case, there is now a 33% likelihood of a positive test being falsely positive. In these two examples, as prevalence increases 10 times, predictive value positive increases 4 times.

7. **Effectiveness** is a measure of the benefits of a health promotion or disease prevention service under usual clinical conditions, when circumstances of selection and compliance are not ideal. This is a more realistic measure of the clinical usefulness of a service than efficacy.
8. **Efficacy** is a measure of a service's potential benefits under idealized conditions, as in research situations.

III. Selecting services

A. Health promotion. Clearly, evaluation of health promotion services is a science in its infancy. Defining health is difficult, and measuring it is even more complex. However, a model for evaluation of health promotion services (programs) has recently been proposed by Lawrence Green, Dr.P.H. [15], from which the following criteria are derived:

1. The health promotion efforts should be relatively simple, safe, inexpensive, and acceptable to those involved.

2. The health promotion efforts must produce positive actions (behavior, life-style).
3. These actions (behavior, life-style) must produce positive outcomes, better health-related outcomes, lower health care costs, and lower absenteeism or higher productivity than in other people.

This book evaluates (justifies) health promotion services or activities on the basis of effectiveness or benefits, risks, costs, and acceptability.

B. Disease prevention. Evaluation criteria for disease prevention services have evolved further than those for health promotion. The following criteria are derived from earlier works [3, 6].

1. **The problem (the disease):**
   - a. Must have a definite effect on length or quality of life.
   - b. Must affect substantial numbers of people.
   - c. Must have a natural history that is well understood.
   - d. Must have an asymptomatic period during which early detection and intervention reduce morbidity and/or mortality more than with later intervention.
2. **Early detection test:**
   - a. Must be sensitive, specific, and predictive (test characteristics). Predictive value is probably the most important characteristic.
   - b. Must be safe. Since the test is applied to "everyone," small problems are magnified, and rare, untoward effects become significant.
   - c. Must be inexpensive. Follow-up costs for further evaluation should be considered.
   - d. Must be easy to administer. Adequate human and equipment resources should be available.
   - e. Must be acceptable to health care providers and patients.
3. **Early intervention (or primary prevention):**
   - a. Must be more effective than late intervention.
   - b. Must have benefits that outweigh risks. Again, small or rare risks are magnified, as are small gains.
   - c. Resources must be available for follow-up diagnostic or therapeutic intervention if required.
   - d. Must be acceptable to patients and health care providers.

These criteria provide the basis for the structure of the justification portion(s) in each disease prevention chapter of this book.

IV. Implementation

A. Research. The process of training health care providers to provide quality health promotion and disease prevention services will always be dependent on the research, which defines questions, tests them, provides answers, and examines how well solutions work in the world of medical practice.

B. Education. Evaluating information and transmitting the digested form to the practicing health care providers is the next step in this process. Efforts by those organizations and individuals previously mentioned and by the following organizations are particularly helpful: the American College of Physicians (ACP) Clinical Efficacy Assessment Project (CEAP), the Society of Teachers of Family Medicine, the Association of Teachers of Preventive Medicine, the United States Preventive Services Task Force, the Centers for Disease Control, the various specialty societies, the American Academy of Pediatrics, the American Academy of Family Physicians, the American Public Health Association, the American Cancer Society, the American Heart Association, the American Thoracic Society, and the American College of Preventive Medicine. However, the practicing health care provider is in an uncertain situation in numerous areas where data are incomplete, confusion and disagreement exist, recommendations often change, and information is not widely available. One of the intentions of this book is to bridge this gap.

Basic medical education on the undergraduate and graduate levels is beginning to offer better training in health promotion and disease prevention, as encouraged by the Association of American Medical Colleges (AAMC) General Professional Education of Physicians (GPEP) report [16]. Continuing medical education is beginning to offer more in this area, and greater knowledge, demands, and expectations on the part of consumers encourage health care providers to be more sophisticated in their understanding and provision of these services.

C. Behavior. Integrating the PHE into ongoing primary care requires a way of thinking and operating fundamentally different from that required to respond to illness, even if the basic knowledge, understanding, motivation, and other elements required to initiate the PHE exist. Instead of responding to a complaint, a headache, diabetes, or a backache, the health care provider must think and act prospectively and proactively.

Changing health care provider and patient behaviors is a complex, slow, and difficult task. Providers often disagree with published guidelines and exceed or fall short of them. More impressive is the wide discrepancy between their own recommendations and what they actually do, as they often exceed or fall short of their own recommendations [17]. Reminders in the form of PHE flow sheets [18], nursing reminders, or computer-generated reminders [19] all help with providers' compliance, particularly if the behavior is one that is already accepted by the provider.

Lawsuits and increased malpractice premiums resulting from failure to adhere to published screening guidelines can be expected to enhance compliance behavior among health care providers [20]. In fact, economics in general exerts a powerful influence on provider and patient behavior, as noted below.

Provider behavior is only part of the problem. For example, it is well known that the patients at highest risk for cervical cancer are those who have never been screened. Getting patients into health care settings, then, is also an important part of the process. Effecting new health behaviors in patients once they are seen in the health care setting is then possible, though far from guaranteed, as many of the chapters in this book describe.

D. **Economics** is certainly a critical variable in changing both health care provider and patient behavior. It has been argued that it should not have to be proved that the benefits of health promotion and disease prevention are economical. Treatment of illness should be thrifty, if possible, but costs are accepted. Louise Russell from the Brookings Institution [21] points out that prevention may be as costly as other medical programs, that these costs should be accepted, and that society should weigh the value of beneficial prevention programs against those of other programs: education, housing, agriculture, defense, and so forth.

Health care provider reimbursement for health promotion and disease prevention services has been an obstacle to widespread provider acceptance of these services. In the area of public reimbursement, current discussions to enhance the reimbursed value of cognitive services relative to procedural services may eventually have an impact on health care provider reimbursement for these services. In the private sector, a great deal has been happening as well. INSURE is a project initiated by a consortium of the largest health insurance companies to look at the acceptability, cost, and effectiveness of providing insurance coverage for selected preventive services [22]. The study is not yet completed, but initial results indicate that provider and patient acceptance is excellent and cost is much lower than anticipated. The effectiveness information is not yet in, but we may be able to make some inferences from another study. The Rand Corporation study of free health care found that in a young adult nondisabled population, patients receiving free health care had better visual acuity and lower blood pressure. However, the free care did not have any apparent effect on smoking, weight, or cholesterol levels [23]. As information like this accrues, other market forces are operating. As health care coverage through employer-offered insurance plans grows, the role of corporations of all sizes in affecting the provision of and coverage for health promotion and disease prevention services will be increasingly significant [24], and will undoubtedly affect health care provider behavior.

Equipment and health care provider resources are yet another important part of this equation. In some areas resources are quite limited. It has been said that we do not have enough radiologists or mammography machines available to meet the current American Cancer Society mammography recommendations if they were followed by providers and patients. In other areas, the resources required to meet recommendations may be quite small.

It is estimated that 50% of the mortality from the 10 leading causes of death is preventable by individual life-style changes [8], which on the surface appears to be inexpensive. Human and equipment resources, cost, and financing questions are the key variables that are just beginning to be thoroughly examined for health promotion and disease prevention services.

V. **Conclusion.** The principal focus of this book is to provide the busy primary care provider with information on what may or should be offered in a PHE, how the service should be performed, to whom it should be offered, and how often and why it should or should not be offered. The recommendations are based on the opinions of the contributors, who considered available data, standard practice, other authoritative recommendations, and legal, practical, and financial issues. Recommendations in these areas are imperfect, are constantly changing, and in some cases are controversial. They apply to asymptomatic individuals and must be modified to the realities of different settings. These recommendations are neither a minimum nor a maximum set. Together, they represent an important portion of primary care: the periodic health examination.

References

1. Gould, G. M. A system of personal biologic examination: The condition of adequate medical and scientific conduct of life. *J.A.M.A.* 35:134, 1900. *An eloquent speech to the AMA introducing the periodic health examination to the United States.*
2. Charap, M. H. The periodic health examination: Genesis of a myth. *Ann. Intern. Med.* 95(6):733, 1981. *Good historical review.*
3. Frame, P. S., and Carlson, S. J. A critical review of periodic health screening using specific screening criteria. *J. Fam. Pract.* 2:29, 1975. *A classic critical review.*
4. Frame, P. S. A critical review of adult health maintenance. Parts 1–4. *J. Fam. Pract.* 22:341, 417, 511; 23:29, 1986. *Recent update of a classic work.*
5. Breslow, L., and Somers, A. R. The lifetime health-monitoring program. A practical approach to preventive medicine. *N. Engl. J. Med.* 296(11):601, 1977. *Periodic health examination over the entire life-cycle introduced.*
6. Canadian Task Force on the Periodic Health Examination. The periodic health exam. *Can. Med. Assoc. J.* 121(9):1193, 1979. *Canadian Task Force report; a detailed paradigm.*
7. Canadian Task Force on the Periodic Health Examination. The periodic health examination: 2. 1984 update. *Can. Med. Assoc. J.* 130(10):1278, 1984. *One of ongoing series of updates to original recommendations.*
8. U.S. Public Health Service. *Healthy People: The Surgeon General's Report on Health Promotion and Disease Prevention, 1979.* Washington, D.C.: Government Printing Office, 1979. *Summary report and background papers.*
9. American Cancer Society. Guidelines for the cancer-related checkup. Recommendations and rationale. *CA* 30(4):194, 1980. *The original ACS guidelines.*
10. Medical Practice Committee, American College of Physicians. Periodic health examination: A guide for designing individualized preventive health care in the asymptomatic patient. *Ann. Intern. Med.* 95(6): 729, 1981. *ACP summary of Frame and Carlson, Breslow and Somers, Canadian Task Force, and American Cancer Society recommendations.*
11. Council on Scientific Affairs. Medical evaluation of healthy persons. *J.A.M.A.* 249(12):1626, 1983. *AMA policy statement on PHE.*

11a. Grundy, S. M., et al. Cardiovascular and risk factor evaluation of healthy American adults. A statement for physicians by an ad hoc committee appointed by the Steering Committee, American Heart Association. *Circulation* 75:1340A, 1987. *American Heart Association recommendations.*

12. O'Donnell, M. P. Definition of health promotion. *Am. J. Health Prom.* 1:4, 1986. *A simple definition of health promotion.*
13. Taylor, R. R., Ureda, J. R., and Denham, J. W. (eds.). *Health Promotion. Principles and Clinical Applications.* Norwalk, CT: Appleton-Century-Crofts, 1982. *Very practical, readable, and thorough textbook on health promotion.*
14. Griner, P. F., et al. Selection and interpretation of diagnostic tests and procedures. Principles and applications. *Ann. Intern. Med.* (4 Pt. 2):557, 1981. *Excellent and thorough review.*
15. Green, L. W. Research agenda: Building a consensus on research questions. *Am. J. Health Prom.* 1:70, 1986. *Proposed model for evaluation of health promotion programs by former director of United States Office of Health Promotion and Disease Prevention.*
16. *Physicians for the Twenty-First Century. Report of the Panel on the General Professional Education of the Physician and College Preparation for Medicine.* Washington, D.C.: Association of American Medical Colleges, 1984. *The GPEP report.*
17. Woo, B., et al. Screening procedures in the asymptomatic adult. Comparison of physicians' recommendations, patients' desires, published guidelines, and actual practice. *J.A.M.A.* 254(11):1480, 1985. *A fascinating study pointing out the disparity between physicians' recommendations for certain PHE services and their actual behaviors.*
18. Prislin, M. D., Vandenbark, M. S., and Clarkson, O. D. The impact of a health screening flow sheet on the performance and documentation of health screening procedures. *Fam. Med.* 18:290, 1986. *Study showing that PHE flow sheets serve as a cue to prompt health care providers to better comply with guidelines, but are not used for documentation of the services.*

19. McDonald, C. J., et al. Reminders to physicians from an introspective computer medical record: A two-year randomized trial. *Ann. Intern. Med.* 100(1):130, 1984. *Large study showing benefit from computer-generated reminders.*
20. Kornblum, A. Failure to diagnose breast cancer hot topic. *Amer. Med. News.* 3+, 1986. *As of January 1, 1986, COPIC Insurance Co. of Colorado, a physician-created liability insurance company, may levy up to a $25,000 surcharge and cancel policies for physicians involved in breast cancer malpractice claims who failed to observe ACS mammography guidelines.*
21. Russell, L. B. *Evaluating Preventive Medical Care as a Health Strategy.* Washington, D.C.: Brookings Institution, 1985. *A monograph on evaluating preventive services.*
22. Brook, R. H., et al. Does free care improve adults' health? Results from a randomized controlled trial. *N. Engl. J. Med.* 309(23):1426, 1983. *The Rand health insurance experiment.*
23. Rosen, M. A., and Logsdon, D. N. The INSURE Project on preventive health services. *Statistical Bulletin* 66(1):25. 1985. *A brief synopsis of progress in the project.*
24. Fielding, J. *Corporate Health Management.* Reading, MA: Addison-Wesley, 1984. *An excellent textbook that includes a chapter on health promotion and disease prevention.*

Prenatal Care

2

Risk Assessment

Betty K. Patterson

I. The need

A. Definition. Risk assessment in perinatal medicine is a way of identifying historic and clinical factors that are known to adversely affect neonatal outcome, in an attempt to identify pregnancies that might have an unfavorable outcome.

B. Identification of high-risk patients. Despite significant advances in prenatal care, we have still been unable to reduce perinatal mortality in North America much below 25–30 deaths/1000 live births. It is widely felt that one of the reasons for this is our inability to recognize the fetus at risk. In a systematic review of all the perinatal deaths in one county in 1973, it was seen that one-fourth of these deaths could have been prevented if various modalities of care that were known and available at the time had been properly used [1]. Twenty-two percent of the preventable deaths occurred in high-risk mothers who were either not identified as such or who were identified but improperly managed. In an effort to identify these high-risk situations in the antepartum period, several risk-scoring approaches have been studied [2–6]. These will be reviewed and evaluated in this section, and a comprehensive yet concise system will be presented.

C. Justification. Once these high-risk pregnancies have been identified, the obstetrician can formulate an individual plan of action to optimize the prenatal and intrapartum care. High-risk patients might benefit from procedures such as ultrasound examinations, amniocentesis, contraction stress testing, and intrapartum electronic fetal monitoring. Additionally, screening of women at risk is effective in predicting 50–60% of spontaneous premature labors, and these patients can be transferred to tertiary care centers for delivery [4, 7].

II. Evaluation of risk factors.

Requirements for an effective risk-scoring system include simplicity of use (especially regarding time and space constraints), and accurate identification of patients likely to have a poor outcome. Studies evaluating risk assessment in perinatal medicine can be grouped into two main categories: those involving the prenatal period only, and those that combine risks in the prenatal and intrapartum periods. Both of these types of scoring systems will be considered with their inherent advantages, disadvantages, and predictive values, when available.

A. Prenatal risk scoring

1. **Components.** There is no one uniform list of prenatal risk factors with which everyone agrees. Various reports list 26–67 different risk markers [3–6]. These range from the woman's occupation, socioeconomic status, and eating habits, to her medical history. There do appear to be certain minimum factors that all prenatal screening forms should include, such as age, previous stillbirth or low birth weight infant, medical disorders, Rh isoimmunization, gestational diabetes, multiple pregnancy, premature spontaneous rupture of membranes, prematurity, malpresentation, and bleeding after 20 weeks [8]. Additional studies need to be done to precisely define which individual factors are most predictive.
2. **Effectiveness.** Several studies have assessed risk scoring during the prenatal period and all have shown a correlation between increasing risk scores and increased perinatal mortality rates [2–6]. There has also been an association between increasing risk scores and low Apgar values. In a large prospective study by Morrison involving 16,733 deliveries, 70% of the perinatal deaths occurred in the group of patients with high risk scores [5]. However, **30% of perinatal deaths occurred in the so-called low-risk group and were not predicted by the scoring system.** Many of these deaths were random, unpredictable events, such as cord accidents or abruptions, but it is suggested that the sensitivity of this system might be improved by the addition of an intrapartum component.

I. Reproductive history

Item	Score	
Age <16	=1	
Age 16–35	=0	
Age >35	=2	___
Parity 0	=1	
Parity 1–4	=0	
Parity 5+	=2	___
Past obstetric history		
Habitual abortion infertility	=1	___
PPH/Manual removal	=1	___
Baby >9 lbs	=1	___
Baby <5 lbs	=1	___
Hypertension/ toxemia	=1	___
Previous cesarean	=2	___
Stillbirth or neonatal death	=3	___
Prolonged or difficult labor	=1	___
Incompetent cervix	=1	___
Other	=_	___
Category score ____		

II. Associated conditions

Item	Score	
Weight <100 lbs	=0	
or >200 lbs	=1	___
Smoking >1 pack/day	=1	___
Alcohol (moderate)	=1	___
Drug dependencies	=2	___
Previous gynosurgery	=1	___
Chronic renal disease	=2	___
Gestational diabetes	=1	___
Diabetes mellitus	=3	___
Cardiac disease	=3	___
Frequent urinary tract infection, pyelonephritis	=2	___
Other medical disorders (seizures, lupus, etc.) Score according to severity (1–3)	=_	___
DES daughter	=_	___
Other	=_	___
Category score ____		

III. Present pregnancy

Item	Score	1st visit	36 wks
Bleeding <20 wks	=1	___	___
Bleeding >20 wks	=3	___	___
Anemia <10 gm	=1	___	___
Hypertension	=2	___	___
Moderate to severe toxemia	=3	___	___
Premature ruptured membranes	=2	___	___
Intrauterine growth retardation	=3	___	___
Multiple pregnancy breech/mal-presentation	=3	___	___
Rh isoimmunization	=3	___	___
Sexually transmitted disease (including hepatitis B)	=1	___	___
Other	=	___	___
Category score ____			

TOTAL RISK SCORE 1st visit _____ 36 weeks _____

Fig. 2-1. Prenatal scoring form. Note that low risk=0–2, high risk=3–6, and extreme risk=7+.

Edwards, et al. [6] described an antenatal scoring system involving 67 factors that separate low-risk pregnancies from high-risk pregnancies. They found that 88.6% of the total perinatal deaths occurred in the high-risk group. The predictive value for high-risk cases was 42% and for low-risk cases was 87.5%.

B. Combined prenatal and intrapartum screening. The most widely used scoring form of this type is that of Hobel, et al [3]. It combines the use of 50 prenatal factors with 40 intrapartum factors and 35 neonatal factors. This study shows that **intrapartum events are in general more predictive than prenatal events.** The authors propose the use of a programmable calculator during the intrapartum period, which could quickly assess risk and probabilities in time to effect treatment [9]. The use of Hobel's system has been reported in over 5000 patients [10], with a predictive value of 93.5% in classifying the low-risk cases and a 35% predictive value in high-risk cases.

The principal advantage of this system is its slightly higher predictive value, which must be weighed against its complexity as well as the fact that identifying risk factors in the intrapartum period gives one less time to initiate preventive measures and to effect change.

III. Recommendations

A. When to assess. Ideally, risk assessment begins preconception and continues throughout pregnancy. Practically, formal risk assessment and scoring is done with the history and physical examination at the first prenatal visit and then again at 36 weeks. The early assessment is helpful in planning methods of surveillance during the pregnancy such as ultrasound, amniocentesis, and glucose monitoring. The second assessment at 36 weeks allows the health care provider to assess risks that have developed during the pregnancy, such as intrauterine growth retardation and hypertension, and to plan appropriate stress testing and intrapartum management.

B. What to assess. Many risk-scoring forms are available. Those described by Hobel [3, 9], Sokal [10], and Goodwin and Morrison (modified version) [5] (Fig. 2-1), as well as those commercially available from the Hollister Corporation, are all reasonable choices.

References

1. Harper, R. G., et al. The high-risk perinatal registry. A systematic approach for reducing perinatal mortality. *Obstet. Gynecol.* 50(3):264, 1977. *An interesting review of perinatal mortality.*
2. Goodwin, J. W., Dunne, J. T., and Thomas, B. W. Antepartum identification of the fetus at risk. *Can. Med. Assoc. J.* 101(8):57, 1969. *A simplified technique for identifying the high-risk pregnancy.*
3. Hobel, C. J., et al. Prenatal and intrapartum high-risk screening. I. Prediction of the high-risk neonate. *Am. J. Obstet. Gynecol.* 117(1):1, 1973. *An excellent study.*
4. Coopland, A. T., et al. A simplified antepartum high-risk pregnancy scoring form: Statistical analysis of 5459 cases. *Can. Med. Assoc. J.* 116(9):999, 1977. *Excellent format for scoring form presented.*
5. Morrison, I., and Olsen, J. Perinatal mortality and antepartum risk scoring. *Obstet. Gynecol.* 53(3):362, 1979. *Expands and confirms Goodwin's work.*
6. Edwards, L. E., et al. A simplified antepartum risk-scoring system. *Obstet. Gynecol.* 54(2):237, 1979. *Evaluates another risk-scoring system.*
7. Halliday, H. L., Jones, P. K., and Jones, S. L. Method of screening obstetric patients to prevent reproductive wastage. *Obstet. Gynecol.* 55(5):656, 1980. *Combines community hospital and university center to assess risk and examine outcomes.*
8. Cohen, L. Task force calls for uniform prenatal records. *Can. Med. Assoc. J.* 130(10):1377, 1984. *Highlights task force report on high-risk pregnancies.*
9. Hobel, C. J., et al. Prenatal and intrapartum high-risk screening II. Risk factors reassessed. *Am. J. Obstet. Gynecol.* 135:1051, 1979. *Uses a programmable calculator to predict probabilities of neonatal risk.*
10. Sokal, R. J., et al. Clinical application of high-risk scoring on an obstetric service. *Am. J. Obstet. Gynecol.* 128(6):652, 1977. *Demonstrates that risk-scoring can be used effectively in a clinical setting.*

Health Promotion

3 Nutrition

Larry Saltzman

Calories and Protein

I. The problem

A. Definition. Malnutrition in pregnancy refers to an inadequate or excessive consumption of a specific nutritional category.

B. Description. The role nutrition plays in reproductive outcome is complicated by genetic, social, cultural, economic, and many other factors. Given the limitations of research in this area, we are forced to rely on epidemiologic evidence. Such research has shown:

1. Poor nutrition in the mother is associated with low birth weight infants and poor reproductive performance [1].
2. Poorly nourished women who are provided supplemental foods during pregnancy have larger babies [2].
3. Women who were previously well nourished will have babies of reduced birth weight if their diets are severely limited during pregnancy [3, 4].

We do know that the lowest perinatal mortality rates occur among infants weighing 3501–4000 gm who have attained a gestational age of 40–41 weeks [5]. The best single predictor of initial neonatal health is birth weight.

C. Epidemiology. Intrauterine growth retardation (IUGR) is an abnormality of fetal growth and development affecting 3–10% of all pregnancies. Factors responsible for IUGR vary and may result from chronic uteroplacental insufficiency, early congenital infection, drug exposure, or fetal genetic abnormalities limiting growth potential (see Chap. 24). Statistics compiled by the World Health Organization indicate that in developed countries about one-third of low birth weight infants were in term pregnancies (therefore, were IUGRs), with maternal malnutrition a significant contributing factor.

Certain groups of women are **at high risk** for prenatal malnutrition and should be given close supervision and counseling. These include:

1. Adolescent women (within four years of menarche)
2. Women who have had three or more pregnancies during the past two years
3. Women with a history of poor obstetric or fetal performance
4. Economically deprived women
5. Food faddists ingesting a bizarre or nutritionally restrictive diet
6. Heavy smokers, drug addicts, and alcoholics
7. Women on a therapeutic diet for chronic systemic disease
8. Women with a prepartum weight at the first prenatal visit of less than 85% or greater than 120% of standard weight

II. General health promotion

A. Methods

1. Diet assessment and modification

a. Initial assessment at the first prenatal exam should include the following:

(1) General historical information. Previous obstetrical history, medical illness, social history, the need for food assistance programs, and personal history to elicit information on the use of cigarettes, drugs, alcohol, and caffeine.

(2) Personal background data. Living situation with emphasis on food budgeting, cooking facilities, and meal planning and preparation. Any cultural or ethnic food practices, cravings, pica, or special diets should be noted, in addition to any food allergies, intolerances, dietary supplements, or medications used. The ages and sexes of anyone eating with the family should be determined.

Table 3-1. Recommended dietary allowances for adult women (ages 23–50 years)

	Nonpregnant	Pregnant
Energy	2000	2300
Protein (g)	44	74
Vitamin A		
RE[a]	800	1000
IU	4000	5000
Vitamin D (IU)	400	400
Vitamin E (mg)	8	10
Vitamin C (ascorbic acid) (mg)	60	80
Folic acid (μg)	400	800
Niacin (mg)	13	15
Riboflavin (mg)	1.2	1.5
Thiamine (mg)	1.0	1.4
Vitamin B_6 (mg)	2.0	2.6
Vitamin B_{12} (μg)	3.0	4.0
Calcium (mg)	800	1200
Phosphorus (mg)	800	1200
Iodine (μg)	100	125
Iron (mg)	18	18[b]
Magnesium (mg)	300	450
Zinc (mg)	15	20

[a]RE (retinol equivalent) replaces IU (international unit) as the standard measure of vitamin A activity.

[b]The increased requirement during pregnancy cannot be met by the iron content of habitual American diets or by existing iron stores of many women; therefore, the use of 30–60 mg supplemental iron is recommended.

Source: Food and Nutrition Board, National Research Council. *Recommended Dietary Allowance* (8th ed.). Washington, D.C.: Government Printing Office, 1980, with the permission of the National Academy of Sciences.

(3) Diet history. The diet history, taken from a food record or nutritional interview, can be obtained in several ways. One way is to have the patient recall her food intake over the previous 24 hours. Alternatively, or in addition, the recall can be linked to the "activity-associated general day's food intake pattern." Using this tool, the interview can be structured with a series of focal points to enhance detail. The patient can also be requested to record a diet diary to include one week's intake to be reviewed at the next prenatal visit, and through this diary a specific food group analysis can be made. After these histories are obtained, they can be analyzed not only to match Recommended Daily Allowances (RDAs) for pregnancy, but also to assure consumption of adequate servings from all food groups.

(4) The physical exam must include anthropometric evaluations, a dental exam, and general physical inspection.

(5) Laboratory studies, including hemoglobin and hematocrit.

b. Follow-up prenatal visits should include:

(1) Evaluation of maternal weight to determine whether it represents inadequate, adequate, or excess weight gain.

(2) Evaluation of uterine size and estimation of fetal weight. Each visit should be charted, noting the relationship to the norm on the graph.

(3) Interval diet history with education on changing dietary requirements as the pregnancy progresses.

2. Caloric and protein intake. The average cumulative cost of a pregnancy is 75,000–80,000 kcals or about 300 kcals/day over prepregnancy needs. This is, however, a bit misleading as the fetus at 3 months only weighs approximately 6 gm and does not require the energy for its sustenance and growth that a term infant requires (see Table 3-1 for Recommended Daily Allowances). Average caloric requirements in the first trimester are 150 kcals/day, increasing to approximately 350 kcals/day in the third trimester. The RDAs state that the energy intake should not fall below 36 kcals/kg/day. For optimal protein utilization, a

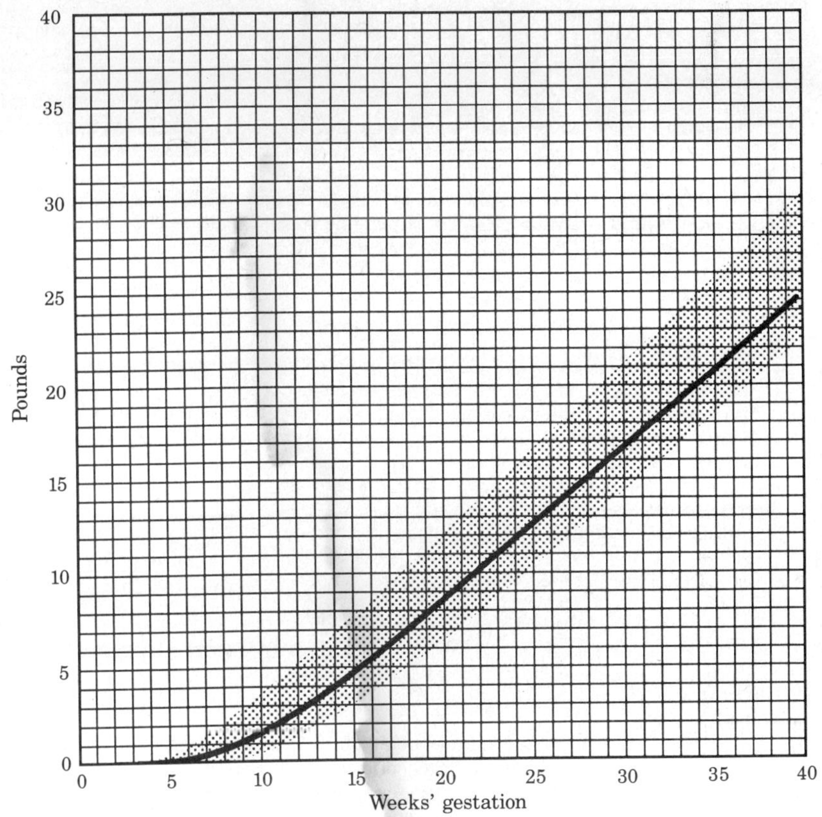

Fig. 3-1. Prenatal weight gain.

woman should consume 5 gm of carbohydrates for each 100 kcals (or the diet must be minimally 20% carbohydrates).

Recommended protein intake is 30 gm above prepregnancy needs or a minimum of 76 gm of protein/day, with a maximum thought to be 100 gm/day.

3. **Weight gain.** The pattern of weight accumulation is more important than the total weight gain. The ideal maternal weight gain for healthy women ranges from 22–30 lb. Maternal fat stores, which are promoted by progesterone, a lipogenic hormone, are included in this estimate. The pattern of gain should be approximately 2–4 lb in the first trimester, 4–6 more lb from 12–20 weeks, and then 1 lb/week up to delivery (Fig. 3-1). In the third trimester most of the weight gain is due to rapid growth of the fetus. A poor weight gain at this time should alert the clinician to possible IUGR. Key points regarding weight gain in pregnancy are as follows:
   - **a.** Inadequate weight gain is less than 1 kg/month in the second and third trimesters.
   - **b.** Excessive gain is greater than 3 kg/month.
   - **c.** Total weight gain of less than 11 kg tends to be associated with low birth weights and higher perinatal mortality. (Obese females should still gain a minimum of 15 lb in a pregnancy.)
   - **d.** Total weight gain of greater than 40 lb has been shown to increase maternal fat stores only and not newborn weight.
   - **e.** Edema fluid may account for increased body weight with possible accumulation of up to 9 liters (15 lb). A study by Thomson [6] reports that women with mild edema may have slightly larger babies and a lower rate of prematurity.

f. Women who are underweight at conception (i.e., 10% below ideal body weight for their height and age) should gain at a greater than average rate, while obese women (i.e., 20% above ideal body weight) should be kept at near average (9–11 kg) and follow a normal curve.

B. Justification

1. **Benefits.** Adequate calorie and protein intake promotes optimal weight gain, optimal birth weight, and therefore optimal neonatal outcome. Intervention during prenatal care when weight gain is inadequate has been shown to improve outcome [7].
2. **Risks.** The risks of promoting maternal weight gain relate more to future maternal weight control problems and possible obesity than to fetal health.
3. **Cost.** The daily cost of increasing the diet to meet caloric and protein intake is low.
4. **Acceptability.** Acceptability is high, with good compliance, especially when adequate time is given to nutritional counseling during prenatal visits.

III. Recommendations

A. Good nutritional habits and ideal weight should be encouraged prior to conception.

B. Comprehensive physical and nutritional assessments should be initiated at the first prenatal visit, and reevaluations should be done at each subsequent visit.

C. Special care should be given to women who are nutritionally at risk, and specific nutritional risk assessment should be made.

D. Caloric intake should increase by an average of 300 kcal/day over the nonpregnant state to promote appropriate weight gain.

E. Protein intake should rise 30 gm/day throughout pregnancy to average 75–100 gm/day.

Vitamins and Minerals

I. The problem

A. Description

1. **Iron.** The fetus does appear to be a "perfect parasite" with respect to iron, as the only cause of neonatal iron deficiency is prematurity. Because the infant does drain the maternal system, every effort should be made by the mother to consume adequate amounts of iron through iron-rich foods or supplements. Pregnancy does increase iron absorption, from 10% in nonpregnant women to 30% in pregnancy.
2. **Folic acid.** Folic acid is important in fetal DNA synthesis and maternal erythropoiesis. Levels are decreased in pregnancy by increased urinary excretion. Deficiencies may be associated with megaloblastic anemia, abruptio placentae, antepartum bleeding, spontaneous abortions, and fetal malformations. Folic acid is the vitamin for which intakes are most likely to fall short of recommendations during pregnancy.
3. **Calcium and vitamin D.** Calcium and vitamin D are needed for fetal skeletal development. The fetus uses active transport across the placenta to draw on maternal calcium stores in the third trimester, causing relative maternal hypocalcemia if supplements are not adequate.

   Vitamin D is needed to ensure calcium absorption, and deficiency can result in poor fetal skeletal mineralization.
4. **Vitamin A.** Vitamin A is needed for integrity of epithelial tissues.
5. **Water-soluble vitamins B complex and C.** These compounds are important because they function as coenzymes for energy production. They cross the placenta by active transport mechanisms (as do essential amino acids).

B. Epidemiology

1. **Iron.** Approximately one-third of pregnant women in the United States have virtually no detectable iron stores. A large but unknown proportion of pregnant women have very low iron intakes. Many women begin iron supplementation only after they have been pregnant for some time. Average prepregnancy stores are 0.3 gm among healthy, college-aged women; 18–21 mg of iron must be absorbed daily to meet pregnancy requirements and maintain maternal stores. A generally well-balanced diet will supply 6 mg of iron/1000 cal; therefore normal dietary sources cannot meet these requirements without overingestion of calories.
2. **Folic acid.** Decreased serum folate levels have been found in up to 60% of other-

wise normal pregnancies, with the incidence of folate-responsive megaloblastic anemia in middle class parous women estimated at 2.5–5.0%.

3. **Calcium and vitamin D.** Limited statistics on risk groups are available.
4. **Vitamin A.** Deficiency syndromes are seldom seen since vitamin A is available in a variety of foods. The serum levels decrease during the first trimester and then rise shortly before term.
5. **Water-soluble vitamins B and C.** Deficiency states are rare in the United States population, since water-soluble vitamins are easily found in adequate levels in a normal diet. Important points to note are:
   a. True vegetarians are at risk for inadequate dietary intake of vitamin B_{12}.
   b. Thiamine deficiency is largely due to decreased food intake in a diet consisting mainly of refined carbohydrates.
   c. Pyridoxine decline occurs in pregnancy to 25% of prepregnant levels due to increased urinary excretion.
   d. Vitamin C intake of less than 20 mg/day (one-third of RDA) is associated with low serum levels and possibly with an increase in prematurity and premature ruptures of membranes. Excessive ingestion of ascorbic acid is much more prevalent.

II. General health promotion

A. Methods

1. **Diet.** (See Table 3-1 for RDAs.)
   a. **Iron.** Sources of iron-rich foods to meet the requirement of 6 mg of iron/1000 kcal include meats, whole wheat (or fortified products), seafood, green leafy vegetables, nuts, and legumes.
   b. **Folic acid** is easily found in green leafy vegetables, but 80% is destroyed by cooking.
   c. **Calcium and vitamin D.** An intake of four servings of dairy foods or the equivalent of 28 oz of milk/day meets the requirements.
   d. **Vitamin A.** High levels exist in yellow vegetables.
   e. **Water-soluble vitamins B and C** are easily found in fruits and vegetables.
2. **Supplementation** is accomplished by using formulated prenatal vitamins to bring all intake to recommended levels. Over-the-counter compounds with slightly more folic acid are readily available. Vitamins should be specifically labeled for prenatal use and generally should include all vitamin and mineral compounds listed in Table 3-1.

B. Justification

1. **Benefits.** In recommended amounts, vitamin and mineral supplements are felt to prevent the deficiency states and problems outlined above.
2. **Risk and side effects.** Over-supplementation may cause the following:
   a. **Iron.** Gastric irritation with or without constipation, the latter of which can be relieved by stool softeners.
   b. **Folic acid.** No risks or side effects.
   c. **Calcium and vitamin D.** Excessive vitamin D has been associated with aortic stenosis, hypercalcemia, and craniofacial anomalies in the infant [8].
   d. **Vitamin A.** Excessive doses in amounts as low as 40,000 IU/day have been associated with neural tube defects in the infant [9].
   e. **Water-soluble vitamins B and C.** Infants exposed to a maternal diet of greater than 1000 mg of vitamin C/day are at risk of developing a "withdrawal" type of infantile scurvy [10]. Their systems are conditioned for higher quantities in utero, and without infant supplements, scurvy may occur.
3. **Cost.** The daily cost of a combined prenatal supplement to provide all recommended vitamins and minerals is approximately 12 cents/day.
4. **Acceptability** varies, depending on whether the patient is complying with a diet or is taking supplements, but is generally thought to be very good.

III. Recommendations

A. Iron. Diet or supplements should provide 60 mg of elemental iron. Options include ferrous sulfate (300 mg; 20% elemental iron) or preparations of ferrous gluconate (11% elemental iron) and ferrous fumarate (33% elemental iron).

B. Folic acid. Minimal supplementation is 300 μg above prepregnancy needs, with a total intake of 0.8–1.0 mg of folic acid/day. This is the only vitamin thought to absolutely require supplementation during pregnancy.

C. Calcium and vitamin D. Calcium is required in minimum levels of 1200 mg/day from dairy food or supplements. Adolescents (defined as within four years of menarche) require 1600 mg/day. Four hundred IU of vitamin D are needed/day.

D. Vitamin A. The RDA is 5000 IU/day.

E. Water-soluble vitamins B and C. Specific levels recommended are listed in Table 3-1. Although not absolutely required as supplements, they are routinely included in most prenatal vitamin preparations.

References

1. Bergner, L., and Susser, M. W. Low birthweight and prenatal nutrition: An interpretive review. *Pediatrics* 46:946, 1970. *Assesses the relationship between low birth weight outcomes and prenatal diet habits in a retrospective review.*
2. Lechtig, A., et al. Effect of food supplementation during pregnancy on birth weight. *Pediatrics* 56(4): 508, 1975. *Discusses increase in calories and its relation to increased maternal weight gain and an improved birth weight.*
3. Smith, C. A. Effects of maternal undernutrition upon the newborn infant in Holland (1944–1945). *J. Pediatr.* 30:299, 1947. *Study during acute starvation over an 18-month period and its conclusion, showing an increase in low birth weight infants and in fetal wastage.*
4. Antonov, A. N. Children born during the seige of Leningrad in 1942. *J. Pediatr.* 30:250, 1947. *Epidemiologic study of a natural experience of starvation during pregnancy and its outcomes.*
5. Hytten, F. E., and Leitch, I. *The Physiology of Human Pregnancy* (2nd ed.). Oxford: Blackwell, 1971. *Statistics to support the idea that higher birth weights lead to improved neonatal outcomes, and a look at ranges of weight gained in pregnancies.*
6. Thomson, A. M., Hytten, F. E., and Billewicz, W. Z. The epidemiology of oedema during pregnancy. *J. Obstet. Gynaec. Brit. Comm.* 74:1, 1967. *Discusses patterns of fluid accumulation during pregnancy and helps differentiate abnormal patterns, as in toxemia, versus normal fluid collection.*
7. Simpson, J. W., Lawless, R. W., and Mitchell, A. C. Responsibility of the obstetrician to the fetus. II. Influence of prepregnancy weight and pregnancy weight gain on birthweight. *Obstet. Gynecol.* 45(5):481, 1975. *Review to support counseling of good weight gain during pregnancy.*
8. Friedman, W. F., and Mills, L. F. The relationship between vitamin D and the craniofacial and dental anomalies of the supravalvular aortic stenosis syndrome. *Pediatrics* 43: 12–8, 1969. *Good study of toxic effects of megadose vitamin D therapy and specifics, describing various malformations seen.*
9. Gal, I., Sharman, I. M., and Pryse-Davies, J. Vitamin A in relation to human congenital malformation. In D. H. M. Woollam (ed.), *Advances in Teratology* Vol. 5. New York: Academic, 1972. Pp. 143–159. *Specific information on toxicity of vitamin A in the fetus, and malformations encountered.*
10. Cochrane, W. A. Overnutrition in prenatal and neonatal life: A problem? *Can. Med. Assoc. J.* 93:893, 1965. *Looks at several authorities and their specific problems in relation to toxicity in prenatal care.*

Suggested Readings

Bishop, P. A., et al. *Clinical Obstetrics.* C. B. Lull and R. A. Kimbrough (eds.). Philadelphia: Lippincott, 1953. *Complete text on obstetrical care prepared "by members of the Staff of the Pennsylvania Hospital." Illustrations give guidelines including standard deviations of expected weight gain in pregnancy, to alert health care providers to abnormal levels.*

Churchill, J. A., and Berendes, H. W. Intelligence of children whose mothers had acetonuria during pregnancy. *Sci. Publ. Pan Am. Health Org.* 185:30, 1969. *Long-term study following children who were exposed to ketosis during fetal life.*

Dwyer, J. Impact of maternal nutrition on infant health. *Med. Times* 111(7):30, 1983. *Good review of maternal nutrition and substance use in pregnancy.*

Giroud, A. *The Nutrition of the Embryo.* Springfield, IL: Thomas, 1970. *General text of nutrition for the embryo, including states of vitamin toxicity syndromes.*

Hillman, R. W., and Goodhart, R. S. Nutrition in Pregnancy. In R. S. Goodhart and M. E. Shils (eds.), *Modern Nutrition in Health and Disease: Dietotherapy* (5th ed.). Philadelphia: Lea & Febiger, 1973. Pp. 647–658. *General review of diet in pregnancy, including deficiency states.*

Leader, A. Maternal nutrition in pregnancy. *Curr. Probl. Obstet. Gynecol.* 6(7):3, 1983. *Extensive review of nutritional components in pregnancy.*

Naeye, R. L. Weight gain and the outcome of pregnancy. *Am. J. Obstet. Gynecol.* 135(1):3, 1979. *Looks at outcomes of pregnancies in women who were overweight, underweight, and at normal weight at the start of pregnancy, and the influence of different levels of gain.*

National Research Council. Committee on Maternal Nutrition. *Maternal Nutrition and the Course of Pregnancy.* Washington, D.C.: National Academy of Sciences, 1970. *Good review of the role of nutrition in weight gain and support of pregnancy.*

National Research Council. *Recommended Dietary Allowance* (8th ed.). Washington, D.C.: Government Printing Office, 1980. *See Table 3-1; reprinted with the permission of the National Academy of Sciences.*

Page, E. W., and Page, E. P. Leg cramps in pregnancy: Etiology and treatment. *Obstet. Gynecol.* 1:94, 1953. *Study to determine etiology of leg cramps and offers some ideas for therapy.*

Pitkin, R. M. Nutrition during Pregnancy: The Clinical Approach. In M. Winick (ed.), *Nutritional Disorders of American Women.* New York: Wiley, 1977. Pp. 27–36. *This volume gives good insight into the problems of nutrition in women of all age groups through the life-cycle.*

Seeds, J. W. Impaired fetal growth: Definition and clinical diagnosis. *Obstet. Gynecol.* 64(3):303, 1984. *Discussion of IUGR in relation to maternal nutrition and how one makes the diagnosis.*

Thomson, A. M. Diet in pregnancy. 3. Diet in relation to the course and outcome of pregnancy. *Brit. J. Nutr.* 13:509, 1959. *At the time, the conclusions of this study seemed significant. In retrospect, we now know these important assumptions are false.*

Worthington-Roberts, B. S., Vermeersch, J., and Williams, S. R. *Nutrition in Pregnancy and Lactation* (3rd ed.). St. Louis: Times Mirror/Mosby, 1985. *A thorough text on nutrition in pregnancy and lactation. A good tool for education of health care providers covering theories, problem cases, recommendations, and guidance in prenatal care. Should be required in the library of anyone interested in this subject.*

4 Drugs in Pregnancy

Larry Saltzman

I. The problem

A. Description. Drug use in pregnancy, including use of prescription drugs, alcohol, and cigarettes, may influence pregnancy outcome. Prenatal care providers and all other providers who may be caring for women are frequently confronted with questions concerning the safety of drugs and other substances in pregnancy. Important concepts in understanding drug effects in pregnancy include:

1. **Mechanisms and principles of placental transfer**
   - **a.** Simple diffusion, usually of nonionized lipid-soluble drugs (anesthetic gases).
   - **b.** Facilitated diffusion (water-soluble vitamins).
   - **c.** Active transport (endogenous substrates).
   - **d.** Greater lipid solubility means more diffusion.
   - **e.** Molecular size (drugs of molecular weight less than 600 diffuse freely across the placenta, while those over 1000 do not).
2. **Embryonic development periods during which drugs may affect the fetus (days from last menstrual period)**
   - **a. 1–31 days.** During fertilization and implantation, teratogenic agents have an all-or-none effect. Either the pregnancy is terminated due to toxic effects of drugs during this cycle of cell differentiation, or it continues without any morphologic damage to the organism. In general, the risk of adverse effects in this stage of pregnancy is small.
   - **b. 32–71 days.** The embryonic period and the classic teratogenic period is the time of organogenesis and is the period when teratogenic effects occur due to extreme sensitivity to toxic agents. Unfortunately, this period occurs just when a woman is one week late for her menses and may not be aware of a pregnancy. This is the most potentially dangerous period.
   - **c. 72–280 days.** During the fetal period, there is little effect by teratogens. However, exposure to toxins during this period can cause reduction in cell size and number in various organs.

B. Epidemiology

1. **General concepts.** Gross congenital anomalies are present in 2–3% of all infants and are the third leading cause of infant mortality in the United States, accounting for 15% of all deaths at less than one year of age. Twenty-five percent of congenital malformations are caused by genetic abnormalities. Sixty to 65% of anomalies have unidentified causes (most likely a combination of environment and genetic predispositions), which leaves an estimated 5–10% of birth defects as a direct result of teratogens. These 5–10% of birth defects representing one or two anomalies/2000 births are preventable by avoiding teratogens. Numerous studies have confirmed the widespread use of both prescription and nonprescription drugs by pregnant women. More than 20% of pregnant women receive more than five drugs; 80% of these are over-the-counter products, and 20% are prescribed by physicians. Approximately 97% of pregnant women use at least one over-the-counter preparation during pregnancy [1].
2. **Specific problem areas**
   - **a. Alcohol.** Fetal alcohol syndrome (FAS) [2, 3] occurs in about 1–2/1000 births, with partial expression in 3–5/1000 births (Table 4-1). Based on current estimates, FAS in the United States is a leading cause of mental retardation and birth defects with a prevalence similar to that of two other major birth defects: Down's syndrome and spina bifida.
   - **b. Smoking.** Estimates show that 22–28% of American women smoke during pregnancy. Associated risks to the pregnancy and fetus include low birth weight (average 250 gm or less), spontaneous abortion [4], abruptio placenta, and placenta previa.

Table 4-1. Principal features of the fetal alcohol syndrome (observed in 245 persons)

Feature	Manifestation
Central nervous system dysfunction	
Intellectual	Mild to moderate mental retardation[a]
Neurologic	Microcephaly[a]
	Poor coordination, hypotonia[b]
Behavioral	Irritability in infancy[a]
	Hyperactivity in childhood[b]
Growth deficiency	
Prenatal	<2SD for length and weight[a]
Postnatal	<2SD for length and weight[a]
	Disproportionately diminished adipose tissue[b]
Facial characteristics	
Eyes	Short palpebral fissures[a]
Nose	Short, upturned[b]
	Hypoplastic philtrum[a]
Maxilla	Hypoplastic[b]
Mouth	Thinned upper vermilion[a]
	Retrognathia in infancy[a]
	Micrognathia or relative prognathia in adolescence[b]

[a]Seen in >80% of patients
[b]Seen in >50% of patients
Source: S. K. Clarren and D. W. Smith. The fetal alcohol syndrome. Reprinted by permission of *The New England Journal of Medicine* (298:1063, 1978).

c. **Narcotic addiction.** Pregnancies involving maternal narcotic addiction are high-risk. Maternal addiction causes increases in IUGR and neonatal and perinatal mortality by 1.5 to 6 fold. In addition, vertical transmission of human immunodeficiency virus (HIV) is more likely in infected parenteral drug abusers. Postnatal growth, behavior, and learning may be adversely affected in the offspring of addicted mothers.

C. **Risk groups** (Tables 4-2, 4-3, 4-4, 4-5). Risk groups can be broken down into two components: the risk of medications or substances themselves, and a pregnant patient's habits in using common drugs that are risky to the fetus.

1. **Medication classes.** In 1980, the Federal Drug Administration (FDA) defined risk factors for all drugs based on the level of risk the drug poses to the fetus, as follows (with examples):
    a. **Category A** (potassium chloride): Controlled studies in women fail to demonstrate a risk to the fetus in the first trimester, and there is no evidence of risk in later trimesters. The possibility of fetal harm appears remote.
    b. **Category B** (insulin): Research has yielded two sets of findings: (1) Animal reproduction studies have not demonstrated a fetal risk, and there are no controlled studies in pregnant women, or (2) animal reproduction studies have shown an adverse effect (other than a decrease in fertility) that was not confirmed in controlled studies in women in the first trimester. (There is no evidence of a risk in later trimesters.)
    c. **Category C** (isoniazid): Research has yielded two sets of findings: (1) Studies in animals have revealed adverse effects on the fetus (teratogenic or embryocidal or other), and there are no controlled studies in women, or (2) studies in women and animals are not available. Drugs should be given only if the potential benefit justifies the potential risk to the fetus.
    d. **Category D** (diazepam): There is positive evidence of human fetal risk, but the benefits from use in pregnant women may be acceptable despite the risk (e.g., if the drug is needed in a life-threatening situation or for a serious disease for which safer drugs cannot be used or are ineffective).
    e. **Category X** (diethylstilbestrol): Studies in animals or human beings have demonstrated fetal abnormalities, or there is evidence of fetal risk based on human experience, or both. The risk of the use of the drug in pregnant women clearly outweighs any possible benefit. The drug is contraindicated in women who are or may become pregnant.

Table 4-2. Drug risks outweighing benefits in first trimester

Drug	Effects
Cytotoxic drugs (methotrexate)	Multiple anomalies
Antibiotics	
Streptomycin	Eighth nerve damage, micromelia, multiple skeletal anomalies
Tetracycline	Inhibition of bone growth, micromelia, syndactyly, discoloration of teeth
Chloroquine	Retinal damage, eighth nerve damage
Sex steroids	VACTERL syndrome
Diethylstilbestrol	Clear cell adenocarcinoma of vagina and cervix, genital tract abnormalities
Thalidomide	Limb, auricle, eye, visceral malformations
Abused substances	
Ethanol	Fetal alcohol syndrome
Cigarettes	Increased first trimester abortion, intrauterine growth retardation
Amphetamines	Transposition of great vessels, cleft palate
LSD	Chromosomal abnormalities
Caffeine	Spontaneous abortion, stillbirth
Narcotics	Increased neonatal morbidity
Anticonvulsants	Cardiac anomalies, cleft palate, minor skeletal defects
Diphenylhydantoin	
Trimethadione	
Paramethadione	
Oral anticoagulants	Skeletal and facial anomalies, mental retardation
Bishydroxycoumarin	
Sodium warfarin	
Oral hypoglycemics	Increase of anomalies
Chlorpropamide	
Tolbutamide	
Podophyllin (in laxatives)	Multiple anomalies (safe in topical treatment of condyloma)
Radiation	Increase of malformations, blood disorders
Acutane	Increase of malformations

Table 4-3. Drug risks versus benefits uncertain in the first trimester

Drug	Effects
Antibiotics	
Gentamycin	Eighth nerve damage
Kanamycin	Eighth nerve damage
Trimethoprim/sulfa	Cleft palate
Metronidazole	None
Abused substances	
Barbiturates	Increase of anomalies
Cannabis	Increase of anomalies
Psychotropic substances	
Benzodiazepine	Cardiac defects
Lithium	Goiter, eye anomalies, cleft palate
Anti-thyroid medications	Goiter, hypothyroidism, mental retardation
Thiouracil	
Propylthiouracil	

Table 4-4. Drug benefits outweighing risks in first trimester

Drug	Effects
Antibiotics	
Sulfonamides	Cleft palate, facial and skeletal defects
Rifampin	Spina bifida, cleft palate
Isoniazid	Increase of anomalies
D-penicillamine	Connective tissue defects
Chloramphenicol	None
Penicillins	None
Steroids	
Clomiphene	Increase of anomalies, neural tube defects, Down's syndrome
Glucocorticoids	Cleft palate, cardiac defects
Psychotropic drugs	
Tricyclic antidepressants	Central nervous system and limb malformations
Haloperidol	Limb malformations
Phenothiazines	None
Imipramine	Central nervous system and limb malformations
Asthma medications	
Isoproterenol	None
Terbutaline	None
Theophylline	None
Antihistamines	None
Heparin	None
Insulin	None
Antiemetics	(off the market)
General anesthesia	Increase of anomalies
Over-the-counter medications	
Salicylates	Central nervous systems, visceral and skeletal malformations
Acetominophen	None
Antacids	Increase of anomalies

2. Patient's habits

a. Alcohol consumption. The relationship between amount of consumption and risk of FAS is as follows, defined in volumes of 1 oz of absolute alcohol (i.e., two mixed drinks, 8 oz of wine, or two 12-oz cans of beer).

(1) One oz daily of absolute alcohol has been linked to lower birth weight.

(2) One to 2 oz daily in the month prior to recognition of pregnancy has resulted in infants with recognizable signs of altered growth and morphogenesis.

(3) Greater than 3 oz daily is definitely a risk level.

(4) Binge drinking may result in structural abnormalities of the fetal brain.

(5) Alcohol consumption is associated with other nutritional risk factors such as hypoglycemia, alcoholic ketoacidosis, vitamin deficiencies (thiamine, folic acid, magnesium), and poor caloric intake.

(6) Lesser levels of alcohol intake and more intermittent consumption may carry a fetal risk, but this has not been documented.

b. Smoking. As few as five cigarettes/day have been associated with smoking-related problems in the fetus [5].

c. Narcotic or illicit drug use. Chronic use of narcotics to the point of addiction can affect the fetus with consequent IUGR and possible neonatal symptoms after birth.

d. Chronic medication use for disease states (e.g., seizure control). Use of certain medications deemed necessary for the health of the mother may affect the fetus. Antiseizure medications are known teratogens, but risks-benefits may require their continued use during pregnancy. Oral hypoglycemics for diabetes mellitus should be replaced by insulin usage.

Table 4-5. Drug effects in the second and third trimesters

Drug	Effects
Amphetamines	Fetal thrombocytopenia
Aspirin	Fetal bleeding Premature closure of ductus arteriosus Prolonged gestation Increased duration of labor Increased maternal bleeding with labor and delivery
Indomethacin	Premature closure of ductus arteriosus
Barbiturates	Neonatal bleeding Neonatal withdrawal syndrome ? Decreased neonatal jaundice
Diphenylhydantoin	Fetal or neonatal hemorrhage
Primidone	Fetal or neonatal hemorrhage
Benzodiazepines	Neonatal withdrawal syndrome
Chloramphenicol	Gray baby syndrome and death
Nitrofurantoin	Hyperbilirubinemia Hemolytic anemia
Sulfonamides	Hyperbilirubinemia
Tetracyclines	Discoloration of infant's teeth Depression of bone growth
Chlorpropamide	Neonatal hypoglycemia
Tolbutamide	?
Curare	Fetal curarization
Local anesthetics	Large doses may cause fetal methemoglobinemia Hypotension as regionals
Halothane	Uterine relaxation Decreased response to oxytocics and ergot
Cytotoxic drugs	IUGR Hypoplastic gonads Increased susceptibility to infection
Corticosteroids	Placental insufficiency Increased perinatal mortality
Diazoxide	Neonatal hyperglycemia Neonatal alopecia Prolonged beta-adrenergic blockage
Propranolol	Decreased fetal cardiac output
Methyldopa	Neonatal meconium ileus
Reserpine	Increased neonatal respiratory secretions, nasal congestion, cyanosis, and anorexia Neonatal thermal instability Neonatal depression Neonatal galactorrhea
Thiazides	Fetal or neonatal jaundice Thrombocytopenia
Ganglionic blockers	Paralytic ileus in newborn
Lithium	Neonatal goiter Electrolyte imbalances
Placidyl	Neonatal central nervous system depression Neonatal withdrawal syndrome
Narcotics	Respiratory depression
Narcotic addiction	Respiratory depression Low birth weight Neonatal death Neonatal withdrawal syndrome

Table 4-5 *continued*

Thiouracils	Neonatal goiter Hypothyroidism
Iodides	Neonatal goiter Hypothyroidism
Quinine	Deafness Thrombocytopenia
Warfarin	Fetal hemorrhage Increased stillbirth Increased maternal bleeding

II. Health promotion

A. Methods

1. **History.** Initial health assessment must record answers to specific questions relating to drug use, alcohol intake, smoking habits, chronic medications, medications in the home for occasional use, and a review of medical and social history for related clues. Quantitation, duration of use, timing during pregnancy, and other specifics should be obtained.
2. **Lab tests**
   a. Toxicology screens to confirm drug use and possible toxic levels should be performed where indicated.
   b. Carboxyhemoglobin levels may be drawn on smokers to show mothers that their level of consumption does get into their system.
3. **Evaluation of prenatal nutrition and fetal growth.** See Chap. 3 for guidelines concerning adequate prenatal growth progress.
4. **Choice of medications.** When medications are required for maternal health, consideration should be given to using those that provide the greatest benefit for the least risk (see Table 4-2).

B. Justification

1. **Benefits.** Avoidance of drugs, alcohol, and tobacco improves perinatal outcomes with less congenital anomalies, mental impairment, and fetal wastage. Studies have shown that physicians can be effective in improving outcomes by decreasing patient alcohol and cigarette use during pregnancy.
2. **Risks.** There are few risks to provider intervention to reduce a patient's unhealthy habits. It is worthwhile noting that efforts to alter substance abuse behavior in pregnant women through induction of guilt are unlikely to succeed. Risks of ongoing drug use are discussed above. Risks of using specific medications are found in Tables 4-2, 4-3, 4-4, and 4-5.
3. **Cost.** Health promotion in this area is an integral part of prenatal care and generates minimal additional costs. There are costs for brochures, referrals, counseling, and detoxification programs, but the numbers and means to express the costs are not clear cut.
4. **Acceptability.** Successful avoidance of potential teratogens and counseling to decrease or eliminate use of social drugs is very difficult to assess. Pregnancy seems to be a motivator for smoking cessation in 35% of women, with long-term cessation less common. Widespread knowledge of potential problems with drug intake, smoking, and alcohol consumption undoubtedly is having a significant impact on the current generation.

III. Recommendations

A. Pregnant women should be informed that no drug should be considered to be without risk.

B. Patients need to be educated concerning the risks of legal drugs (alcohol, cigarettes) and advised about the hazards of illegal substances.
   1. Over-the-counter drugs are, in general, contraindicated in pregnancy. Risk-benefit considerations may lead to their use, but only after medical consultation.
   2. Alcohol consumption should be avoided [6, 7].
   3. Cigarette use should cease. In cases where that cannot be achieved, the least number of cigarettes/day should be smoked [8, 9].
   4. Caffeine intake should be as low a quantity as possible [10, 11].
   5. Drug, alcohol, or tobacco addicts should be considered for withdrawal programs prior to or during prenatal care.

- **C.** Pregnant women should take only medications that have been approved by their physician.
- **D.** When considering drug use, the potential benefits of the drug to the mother and fetus must be weighed against possible adverse effects on the fetus.
- **E.** Each drug a pregnant woman takes must be documented in the antepartum chart.

References

1. Hill, R. M., et al. Utilization of over-the-counter drugs during pregnancy. *Clin. Obstet. Gynecol.* 20(2):381, 1977. *Discusses use and overuse of over-the-counter drugs and possible implications in pregnancy.*
2. Clarren S. K., and Smith, D. W. The fetal alcohol syndrome. *N. Engl. J. Med.* 298(19):1063, 1978. *Review on the effects of alcohol. Describes in detail morphologic changes and diagnosis of this syndrome.*
3. California Department of Health Services. *Dangers of Drinking Alcohol During Pregnancy.* Maternal-Child Health Branch, California Department of Health Services, 1980. *This paper represents an excellent review of current findings regarding the effects of alcohol intake on the fetus, as well as recommendations and guidelines for counseling and treatment of the drinking woman during the childbearing years.*
4. Kline, J., et al. Smoking: A risk factor for spontaneous abortion. *N. Engl. J. Med.* 297(15):793, 1977. *Retrospective study concluding that smoking during pregnancy is a risk factor for spontaneous abortion.*
5. Russell, C. S., Taylor, R., and Maddison, R. N. Some effects of smoking in pregnancy. *J. Obstet. Gynaec. Brit. Comm.* 73:742, 1966. *Observations of the effects of smoking on neonatal outcome and potential problems for infants.*
6. Surgeon general's advisory on alcohol and pregnancy. *FDA Drug Bull.* 11(2):9, 1981. *Brief summary of effects on pregnancies from alcohol and guidelines for counseling.*
7. Rosett, H. L., Weiner, L., and Edelin, K. C. Treatment experience with pregnant problem drinkers. *J.A.M.A.* 249(15):2029, 1983. *Discussion of intervention on alcohol abuse and successful effects of counseling.*
8. Hickner, J., Westenberg, C., and Dittenbir, M. Effect of pregnancy on smoking behavior: A baseline study. *J. Fam. Pract.* 18(2):241, 1984. *Discussion of effect of positive intervention on smoking cessation during pregnancy.*
9. Fielding, J. E. Smoking and pregnancy. *N. Engl. J. Med.* 298(6):337, 1978. *Brief review on effects of smoking on pregnancies, and recommendations to help reduce smoking among pregnant women.*
10. Weathersbee, P. S., Olsen, L. K., and Lodge, J. R. Caffeine: Its direct and indirect influence on reproduction. *J. Reprod. Med.* 19(2):55, 1977. *Review of biochemical effects of caffeine on reproductive systems.*
11. Weathersbee, P. S., Olsen, L. K., and Lodge, J. R. Caffeine and pregnancy. *Postgrad. Med.* 62(3):64, 1977. *A retrospective study comparing caffeine consumption in a general population with a Mormon community. Results show increased fetal wastage with consumption of greater than 600 mg of caffeine/day.*

Suggested Readings

Beeley, L. Adverse effects of drugs in the first trimester of pregnancy. *Clin. Obstet. Gynaecol.* 8(2):261, 1981. *Current review on drug effects in pregnancy. Very good references. Looks at effects of drug groups in general versus individual drugs.*

Chasnoff, I. J., et al. Cocaine use in pregnancy. *N. Engl. J. Med.* 313(11):666, 1985. *Discussion of link between cocaine use and pregnancy outcome.*

Danis, R. P., Newton, N., and Keith, L. Pregnancy and alcohol. *Curr. Probl. Obstet. Gynecol.* 4(6):2, 1981. *Thorough review of effects of alcohol on pregnancy covering theoretical animal models of injury, prospective human studies, risk to the fetus, and prevention. Large number of articles included as references.*

Gordis, E., and Kreek, M. J. Alcoholism and drug addiction in pregnancy. *Curr. Probl. Obstet. Gynecol.* 1(3):5, 1977. *Very complete review on effects of alcohol, narcotics, barbiturates, and sedatives. Includes discussion on diagnosis, effects on reproductive physiology, pregnancy management, and therapies for the fetus and neonate.*

Hill, L. M., and Kleinberg, F. Effects of drugs and chemicals on the fetus and newborn. Parts 1 and 2. *Mayo Clin. Proc.* 59(10):707, 1984, and 59(11):755, 1984 (respectively). *Thorough review of all classes of drugs and their effects on pregnancy.*

Hill, W. Fetal and neonatal hazards of drugs during pregnancy. *Obstet. Gynecol. Grand Rounds.* University of California, Davis Medical Center. September 26, 1984. *A thorough discussion of mechanisms of drug effects on pregnancy, with tables of specific agents and effects.*

Howard, F. M., and Hill, J. M. Drugs in pregnancy. *Obstet. Gynecol. Surv.* 34(9):643, 1979. *Very complete review on the effects of drugs in pregnancy. Good references for the original studies on each drug group.*

Linn, S., et al. The association of marijuana use with outcome of pregnancy. *Am. J. Public Health* 73(10):1161, 1983. *Attempt to link effects of marijuana to poor prenatal outcome. No strong relationship was found.*

5 Exercise in Pregnancy

Gary A. Fields

I. The problem

A. Description

1. Physiology of pregnancy. The state of pregnancy increases cardiac output so that by the end of the second trimester, the average woman will have a 30–50% increase over nonpregnant levels. There is a slight decrease to approximately 10% above nonpregnant levels in the third trimester. The increase in cardiac output is a function of increases in stroke volume and heart rate. Changes in heart rate are evident from very early in pregnancy, and hormonal as well as vascular mechanisms have been proposed to explain this phenomenon. The overall average increase of 16 beats per minute plateaus at approximately 32 weeks. The changes in cardiac output are paralleled by similar changes in blood volume [1, 2].

In humans, the 40–50% elevation in blood volume is secondary to a 30–60% increase in plasma volume, and a 20–30% increase in red cell mass. This net hemodilution is responsible for the characteristic drop in hematocrit seen in late pregnancy [1]. The pregnant woman's minute ventilation increases by approximately 50%, secondary to progesterone effects on the respiratory center. This is caused by an increased tidal volume as respiratory frequency remains unchanged. There is a resultant drop in PCO_2 of about 10 mm Hg; however, blood pH remains normal as there is a compensatory increased renal excretion of bicarbonate. The work of breathing increases throughout pregnancy, for as the uterus enlarges, the diaphragm functions at a mechanical disadvantage [2].

The basal temperature rise of approximately 0.5 °C seen at ovulation persists to midgestation, when it begins to approach normal values. Since heat expenditure is a major consideration in exercise, this elevation must represent a disadvantage in pregnancy [3].

Resting oxygen consumption rises throughout pregnancy with the major elevation occurring when the feto-placental unit is growing and enlarging most rapidly. At term, this reaches 16–32% over nonpregnant levels. Maximal oxygen consumption in pregnancy has not been studied in great detail. It has been estimated that a maximal work level during pregnancy would require approximately a 10% higher Vo_2 [1, 2, 4].

The accumulation of body fat represents a major metabolic adaptation during pregnancy. Both circulating free fatty acids and plasma triglycerides increase approximately threefold by the third trimester. Insulin sensitivity is markedly reduced as pregnancy advances; this, and other hormonal and metabolic effects, lead to the so-called diabetogenic effects of pregnancy. However, in spite of reduced glucose tolerance, the pregnant woman cannot tolerate even brief periods of fasting without a series of metabolic events called "accelerated starvation" resulting in hypoglycemia, hypoinsulinemia, hyperketonemia, and hypoalaninemia. Utilization of glucose and amino acids by the fetus seems to be the cause of this response [1, 2].

2. Response to exercise. Much of the information on the effects of exercise in pregnancy has been drawn from animal studies. Studies with humans have led to conflicting results due to differing controls and types of exercises employed. Despite these shortcomings, certain facts have emerged from this vast array of data that seem applicable to clinical and pragmatic concerns. Depending on the exercise in question, the absolute cardiac output achieved during exercise is slightly increased compared with nonpregnant exercise, probably secondary to the increase in resting cardiac output seen in pregnancy. Maintaining adequate venous return is often the limiting factor, but taking this into consideration, the pregnant woman is able to increase cardiac output in response to the demands of exercise as well as a nonpregnant woman.

Any change in the distribution of the cardiac output that occurs during exercise is a major consideration when assessing the effects of exercise on the fetoplacental unit. As pregnancy advances, an increasing percentage of the cardiac output supplies the uterus. The cotyledonous proportion of the uterine blood flow increases with the size of the fetus, while the myometrial flow remains relatively constant. Many studies have shown a decreasing uterine blood flow in response to exercise. The magnitude of the change depends on the duration and intensity of the exercise. The myometrial flow appears to be sacrificed to maintain cotyledonous flow, thus blunting the effects of exercise on the fetus. The fetal heart rate has been studied extensively as a measure of fetal well-being. There have been no predictable changes noted during exercise; thus, in a healthy pregnancy, placental blood flow seems to be adequately maintained during exercise. In pregnancies complicated by conditions known to compromise placental transfer, several studies have demonstrated decelerations and reflex tachycardias in response to the stimulation of exercise. Some authors have even suggested that exercise testing be employed as a test of placental insufficiency [1, 4–8].

When considering oxygen consumption during exercise, one must separate weight-bearing work from cycling exercise. The oxygen consumption during running and walking per kilogram of body weight is no different in pregnancy. The extra work required is directly related to the increases in body weight. There seems to be little difference in energy expended during cycle exercise in pregnancy as opposed to the postpartum state. Thus, the added work of exercise during pregnancy can be directly attributed to the increased weight of the pregnancy [1, 2, 8].

Fasting glucose levels are reduced during pregnancy, and even with short exercise, blood glucose values fall. The responses of other substrates are similar to that seen in nonpregnant women.

Early animal work has clearly demonstrated the teratogenicity of hyperthermia during pregnancy. Exposures to temperatures in excess of 39°C were often associated with neural tube defects. Studies of humans have been less convincing, and despite increases in mean resting skin temperature, thermal balance can be maintained during exercise throughout pregnancy. Again, consideration must be given to ambient temperature and the intensity and duration of the exercise, as elevation of core temperature is potentially teratogenic. This is especially a concern as dehydration often accompanies body heat accumulation, a combination that could be devastating to the fetus [1, 3].

B. Epidemiology. From the preceding review, one can appreciate how uniquely adapted the pregnant state is to meeting the added metabolic demands of the growing fetus. It is more difficult to fully assess the extent to which exercise can affect the progress and outcome of any specific pregnancy. The ability to maintain oxygenation, nutritional substrate levels, and body temperature must be assured. It has been known for some time that babies born to working mothers weigh less than comparable babies born to nonworking mothers. In addition, the level of work determines the amount of growth reduction noted. These observations have been confirmed in laboratory animals where smaller offspring have been consistently observed in animals subjected to strenuous exercise. Human research has been less convincing, but one recent study demonstrated that continual endurance exercise during the course of pregnancy was consistently associated with lower birth weights (by approximately 500 gm) and gestations shortened by an average of eight days. However, it is interesting to note that the mothers who exercised the most strenuously had the lowest preconceptional weight and gained the least amount during pregnancy, as compared to a moderate or minimally exercising control. Therefore, maternal weight factors, as well as the degree of stress associated with the exercise, must be considered before firm conclusions can be drawn [9].

II. General health promotion

A. Methods

1. **Description and performance.** There are some physical activities that seem to be more readily adapted to the pregnant state. Cycling, swimming, and walking, as opposed to running or sports associated with rapid motions, are better tolerated. Each program must be individualized with consideration given to prior conditioning, physical disabilities, time, and facilities available. The program must be satisfying and enjoyable. Each woman should progress at her own pace

without feeling pressure to compete. It is hoped that the program will be continued or expanded postpartum so that the cardiovascular fitness achieved will persist. The progress of pregnancy and fetal growth must be carefully monitored, and any deviation from the norm should be reason to reassess the exercise prescription. In this way, exercise can be utilized during pregnancy to promote both aerobic fitness and maternal well-being without jeopardizing the developing fetus.

2. **Pregnancy prescription.** The following guidelines have been developed by a task force of the American College of Obstetricians and Gynecologists [10] and are based on the unique physical and physiologic conditions that exist during pregnancy and the postpartum period. They can be used as a reference for the initiation and maintenance of a safe exercise program. **During pregnancy and postpartum:**
   - **a.** It is preferable to continue an ongoing exercise program into pregnancy than to initiate a new program, keeping the following guidelines in mind.
   - **b.** Regular exercise (at least three times/week) is preferable to intermittent activity. Competitive activities should be discouraged.
   - **c.** Vigorous exercise should not be performed in hot, humid weather or during a period of febrile illness.
   - **d.** Ballistic movements (jerky, bouncy motions) should be avoided. Exercise should be done on a wooden floor or a tightly carpeted surface to reduce shock and provide sure footing.
   - **e.** Deep flexion or extension of joints should be avoided because of connective tissue laxity. Activities that require jumping, jarring motions, or rapid changes in direction should be avoided because of joint instability.
   - **f.** Vigorous exercise should be preceded by a five-minute period of muscle warm-up. This can be accomplished by slow walking or stationary cycling with low resistance.
   - **g.** Vigorous exercise should be followed by a period of gradually declining activity that includes gentle stationary stretching. Because connective tissue laxity increases the risk of joint injury, stretches should not be taken to the point of maximum resistance.
   - **h.** Heart rate should be measured at times of peak activity. Target heart rates and limits established in consultation with the physician should not be exceeded.
   - **i.** Care should be taken to gradually rise from the floor to avoid orthostatic hypotension. Some form of activity involving the legs should be continued for a brief period.
   - **j.** Liquids should be taken liberally before and after exercise to prevent dehydration. If necessary, activity should be interrupted to replenish fluids.
   - **k.** Women who have led sedentary life-styles should begin with physical activity of very low intensity and advance activity levels very gradually.
   - **l.** If any unusual symptoms appear, activity should be stopped and the physician consulted.

   During pregnancy only:
   - **a.** Maternal heart rate should not exceed 140 beats/minute.
   - **b.** Strenuous activities should not exceed 15 minutes in duration.
   - **c.** No exercise should be performed in the supine position after the fourth month of gestation is completed.
   - **d.** Exercises that employ the Valsalva maneuver should be avoided.
   - **e.** Caloric intake should be adequate to meet not only the extra energy needs of pregnancy, but also of the exercise performed.
   - **f.** Maternal core temperature should not exceed 38°C.

B. Justification

1. **Effectiveness or benefits.** Although exercise improves flexibility, strength, and endurance, there is no good evidence that exercise programs during pregnancy lead to shorter labors or better neonatal outcomes. A sedentary life-style during pregnancy should not be viewed as a risk factor. Again, it cannot be overemphasized that women should be encouraged to lead normal lives during pregnancy. If exercise has been previously incorporated into her life, she should be encouraged to continue exercising while pregnant. As a way to improve self-image and energy levels, exercise programs may be offered during pregnancy. However, exercise may not be either necessary or beneficial for every pregnant woman.

2. **Risks and side effects.** The American College of Obstetricians and Gynecologists (ACOG) has outlined both relative and absolute contraindications to exercise during pregnancy [10]. Two recent studies have found no significant risks to exercise for pregnant women and one found some benefit [11, 12]. It is obvious that specific medical complications that would contraindicate exercise in a nonpregnant state would similarly be contraindicated during pregnancy. In addition, any of the medical or surgical complications of pregnancy are relative contraindications to the initiation or maintenance of exercise programs during pregnancy. Each physician must individualize the pregnant women's exercise program with respect to the specific risk factor(s) present. Women with diabetes have been maintained quite successfully in exercise programs and illustrate how these programs can be utilized to aid in the management of these complicated patients.
3. **Costs.** Cost considerations for most exercise programs are modest and, utilizing the ACOG guidelines, home programs can be safely entertained.

III. Recommendations

A. Exercise programs can be safely continued or initiated during pregnancy.

B. Nonweight-bearing activities are better tolerated and subject the gravid woman to fewer injuries.

C. Any complications of pregnancy are reason to reassess the exercise prescription.

D. The specific recommendations established by the American College of Obstetricians and Gynecologists should be followed as guidelines for all exercising pregnant women.

References

1. Artal, R., and Wiswell, R. A. (eds.). *Exercise in Pregnancy.* Baltimore: Williams & Wilkins, 1986. *A comprehensive text on all aspects of exercise and reproduction. Especially useful as a reference source for basic physiologic information on the subject.*
2. Gorski, J. Exercise during pregnancy: Maternal and fetal responses. A brief review. *Med. Sci. Sports Exerc.* 17(4):407, 1985. *A wonderful overview of exercise physiology and its effects on pregnancy and the fetus. Remarkably succinct and readable.*
3. Jones, R. L., et al. Thermoregulation during aerobic exercise in pregnancy. *Obstet. Gynecol.* 65(3): 340, 1985. *Investigative report addressing the issue of hyperthermia and heat effects of exercise during pregnancy.*
4. Jovanovic, L., Kessler, A., and Peterson, C. M. Human maternal and fetal response to graded exercise. *J. Appl. Physiol.* 58(5):1719, 1985. *A carefully designed study documenting the varying fetal and maternal changes to different exercise durations and intensities.*
5. Botti, J. J., and Jones, R. L. Aerobic conditioning, nutrition, and pregnancy. *Clin. Nutr.* 4(1):14, 1985. *A good review on the effects of exercise on pregnancy, with a discussion of the potential benefits and risks.*
6. Collings, C. A., Curet, L. B., and Mullin, J. P. Maternal and fetal responses to a maternal aerobic exercise program. *Am. J. Obstet. Gynecol.* 145(6): 702, 1983. *A well-done study on the effects of submaximal exercise on absolute and functional aerobic capacity during pregnancy. Also discusses effects of physical training on fetal growth and labor.*
7. Collings, C., and Curet, L. B. Fetal heart rate response to maternal exercise. *Am. J. Obstet. Gynecol.* 151(4):498, 1985. *A specific study concerned with fetal heart rate changes during pregnancy, especially in relation to gestational age.*
8. Morton, M. J., et al. Exercise dynamics in late gestation: Effects of physical training. *Am. J. Obstet. Gynecol.* 152(1):91, 1985. *The specific characteristics of late gestation are highlighted in this article, which measures heart rate and stroke volume changes in response to exercise.*
9. Clapp, J. F. 3d, and Dickstein, S. Endurance exercise and pregnancy outcome. *Med. Sci. Sports Exerc.* 16(6): 556, 1984. *An interesting study documenting the effects of endurance exercise (and hard physical labor) on the outcome of pregnancy.*
10. American College of Obstetricians and Gynecologists. *Exercise in Pregnancy.* ACOG Technical Bulletin. Chicago: 1985. *The ACOG bulletin—a necessary reference.*
11. Kulpa, P. J., White, B. M., and Visscher, R. Aerobic exercise and pregnancy. *Am. J. Obstet. Gynecol.* 156:1395, 1987. *Randomized controlled study of exercise in pregnancy looking at obstetric and neonatal outcome.*
12. Hall, D. C., and Kaufmann, D. A. Effects of aerobic and strength conditioning on pregnancy outcomes. *Am. J. Obstet. Gynecol.* 157:1199, 1987. *Retrospective study of different exercise levels and pregnancy outcomes.*

6 Radiation and Ultrasound

Marvin Goldman

I. The problem

A. Risks of ultrasound and ionizing radiation in pregnancy

The use of ionizing radiation and ultrasound as diagnostic tools is of immeasurable utility during the prenatal period. However, in both of these tools, energy is transmitted to and deposited within fetal tissues, and abuse of these technologies can be detrimental both to the fetus and to the pregnant mother.

1. **Diagnostic ultrasound.** In the case of ultrasonic exposure of the fetus, the potential effects on health are quite minimal, provided that the exposure does not introduce a sufficient amount of vibrational energy to thermally increase the temperature of the fetus by more than 1° C. Simply stated, the risk from ultrasonic scanning of the fetus is that of a potential thermal denaturation, whereas the risk from ionizing radiation is associated with cell killing and the induction of latent health effects [1].

   Studies in experimental animals have shown that exposures in excess of 50–80 mW/cm² have resulted in fetal weight reduction in rodents, and that in addition to acoustic intensity, the pulse repetition rate may contribute to the biological risk [2].

   To date, there have been no reported adverse health effects in fetuses exposed to diagnostic ultrasound. One report, however, in analyzing the birth weight of some 2135 children, indicated a possibility of reduction of fetal weight [2]. The absence of any large-scale, major, control studies does not prevent us from conclusively linking this finding to ultrasound; and, at this time, the bulk of medical literature suggests no adverse risk to the fetus when exposed to diagnostic ultrasound [2].

2. **Ionizing radiation.** Overexposure of the mammalian embryo or fetus to high doses of ionizing radiation can result in embryonic death, gross congenital malformations, and intrauterine growth retardation [2]. In addition, ionizing radiation exposure of children in utero can increase the risk of leukemia or other types of fatal cancers for a period that can persist for up to 10 years from birth [3]. Most of our information on the effects of prenatal irradiation in humans comes from studies of the survivors of the atomic explosions on Hiroshima and Nagasaki, particularly those who were exposed while still in utero, and from retrospective surveys of children exposed in utero supplemented by extensive studies of prenatal exposure in experimental mammals [2]. The level of risk and the health consequences are highly dependent not only on the radiation dose, but also on the stage of development at the time of irradiation [3].

B. Epidemiology.

Over half of all pregnant women have at least one ultrasound exam during their pregnancy. This implies that in time about one half of the population will have been exposed to ultrasound prior to birth. "Epidemiologic studies and surveys of clinical experience have yielded no firm evidence of any adverse effects from diagnostic ultrasound, in spite of large clinical usage" [2].

X-ray pelvimetry procedures have been declining, largely due to the efficacy of ultrasound and the possible deleterious effects on the fetus. In 1980, about 1 in 13 births were accompanied by pelvic x-ray exam, i.e., 250,000 exams for 3.6 million live births. In utero irradiation is associated with an increased risk for childhood cancer and leukemia. The risk is measurable but quite small and is about 5 in 10 million/rad of exposure. It is probably closer to 1 in 10 million/rad for exposure during the third trimester [3].

II. Health promotion: Safe use of ultrasound and ionizing radiation in pregnancy

A. Description of ultrasound.

Most diagnostic applications of ultrasound employ a frequency range of 1–10 mHz. Ultrasonic radiation is either a continuous wave or is in the form of pulse fields. Continuous wave instruments are useful in the identification of moving structures and blood flow velocity, whereas pulse fields have their application for pulse echo imaging to detect reflections from anatomical structures. Ultrasonic accessibility is impaired to some extent by bone and to a greater extent by air spaces; a gaseous bowel or an inflated lung is a practically impenetrable barrier. Diagnostic ultrasound is now available to almost all pregnant women in the United States. The following is a list of diagnostic applications of ultrasound in pregnancy.

1. Estimation of fetal age.
2. Diagnosis of multiple pregnancy.
3. Placental localization.
4. Amniotic cavity.
5. Fetal heart monitoring.
6. Fetal growth rate, molar pregnancy, ectopic pregnancy.
7. Congenital anomalies.

During pregnancy, diagnostic ultrasound has a clear-cut practical utility. In the diagnostic range of energy, ultrasonic scanning provides an exceptionally safe and useful tool. As with any technology, excessive ultrasonic energy may cause injury, but within the range of energies and intensities used in prenatal diagnosis, the overwhelming weight of evidence supports the conclusion that this is a technology with minimal and negligible health risks.

B. **Ultrasound methods.** Based on currently available information, prenatal health care providers should:

1. Perform diagnostic ultrasound exams for specific medical indications.
2. Not use ultrasound for routine screening at the present time.
3. Supply patients with exposure time and intensity, if requested.
4. Try to keep patient exposures to less than 10 mW/cm^2 (temporal-spatial average).
5. Strive to obtain the most medically significant information with the least ultrasonic exposure (i.e., minimal dwell times, minimal total exposure time, and, where adjustable, minimal intensity).
6. Not use ultrasound exposure conditions where significant fetal temperature elevations ($>1°$ C) might be produced [2].

C. **Description of ionizing radiation.** The use of ionizing radiation in the diagnosis and therapy of the embryo or fetus is rare. The major consideration relates to radiation used in diagnosis and therapy of the pregnant mother.

Ionizing radiation exposure of the embryo and fetus acts primarily on cell nuclei, and simply put, poses the risk of inducing chromosomal aberrations. At high doses, these lesions will cause cell death and possible loss of the embryo and fetus. Furthermore, cell destruction during critical developmental phases can result in malformations. At lower doses, injury to cellular DNA can put the irradiated tissues at risk for subsequent development of malignancy. The risk to the embryo or fetus is a function of both the amount of radiation absorbed and the stage of development of the embryo or fetus (Table 6-1). Typical radiation doses for diagnostic procedures are shown in Table 6-2.

The basic tenet of radiation protection is at all times to keep radiation exposures to a level that is "as low as reasonably achievable," consistent with the benefit to be derived from the radiation exposure. Scientific debate over the precise quantitative nature of the dose-response relationship for the induction of health effects from low levels of ionizing radiation has at times resulted in an exaggerated fear of the consequences of exposure. While current thinking assumes that there is a quantifiable radiation risk that is proportional to every radiation exposure, one must keep in perspective the relatively small value of risk when weighing the need for any diagnostic radiation procedure. Although fetal tissues are more sensitive to the deleterious effects of ionizing radiation than adult tissues, the difference is less than a factor of ten. Thus, even one of the highest radiation doses, that is, an abdominal obstetric examination delivering approximately 1000 mrad to the fetus, would carry an associated additional cancer risk of approximately 5 in 10,000, while a routine radiographic chest examination would carry an associated fetal cancer risk of about 1 in 10 million (see Table 6-3).

D. **Ionizing radiation methods**

1. As a general principle, no radiologic examination should ever be carried out unless there is significant medical need for the examination at that time.
2. The National Council on Radiation in Pregnancy (NCRP) also notes "that no radiological examination for which there is significant medical need should be denied a patient, even if she is pregnant, for the risk to the patient of not hav-

Table 6-1. Lethal dose estimates of ionizing radiation for the human fetus

Time post-conception	Median lethal dose (D_{50}, rad)	1% lethal risk (D_{01}, rad)
Day 1	26–37	10
Day 14	52	15
Day 18	56	20
Day 28	82	25
Day 50	96	30
Late fetus to term	110–150	35

Source: J. S. Evans, D. W. Moeller, and D. W. Cooper. *Health Effects Model for Nuclear Power Plant Accident Consequence Analysis.* NUREG/CR-4214. Washington, D.C.: U.S. Nuclear Regulatory Commission, 1985.

Table 6-2. Estimated dose of ionizing radiation to ovaries by examination type

Type of x-ray examination	Mean dose (mrad/exam)	Reported range
Low dose group		
Dental	0.06	0.03–0.1
Head, cervical spine	0.5	<0.5–3
Extremities	0.5	<0.5–18
Shoulder	0.5	<0.5–3
Thoracic spine	11	<10.0–55
Chest (radiographic)	1	0.2–43
Chest (photofluorographic)	3	0.9–40
Mammography	<10	–––
Moderate dose group		
Upper gastrointestinal series	170	5–1230
Cholecystography, Cholangiography	80	14–1600
Femur (distal)	<50	1–50
High dose group*		
Lumbar spine	700	20–2900
Lumbosacral spine	–––	73–1780
Pelvis	220	40–1600
Hip and femur (proximal)	125	53–1000
Urography, IV or retrograde pyelogram	600	85–4000 200–3000
Lower gastrointestinal tract (barium enema)	900	20–9200
Abdomen	220	18–1400
Abdomen (obstetric)	1000 (fetal)	110–1600
Pelvimetry	4000	160–4000
Hysterosalpingography	1200	200–6700

*Embryo (uterus) dose in high dose group is generally 25–50% greater than the ovarian dose. Does not include fluoroscopy, which could further increase embryo dose appreciably.
Source: National Council on Radiation Protection and Measurements. *Medical Radiation Exposure of Pregnant and Potentially Pregnant Women: Recommendations of the National Council on Radiation Protection and Measurements.* (NCRP report no. 54). Washington, D.C.: The Council, 1977.

Table 6-3. Prenatal radiation risk to fetus

Effect		Risk (per 1000 mrad)
Mental retardation		
0–7 wks' gestation		0
8–15 wks' gestation		0.004
16–25 wks' gestation		0.001
Induced malformations		
2–8 wks' gestation		0.005
Overall weighted summary (integration of the following effects)		
Mortality Inductions of malformations Mental retardation Tumors Leukemia	weighed over period of pregnancy where effective	0.002
Natural incidence of malformations		0.06

Source: Adapted from United Nations. Scientific Committee on the Effects of Atomic Radiation. General Assembly Document, 35 Session, Biological Effects of Prenatal Irradiation. (A.AC. 82/R.448). Vienna: United Nations, 1986.

Table 6-4. In utero radiation risks

*Absolute cancer risks**
25×10^{-6}/year/rad for leukemia till age 12
plus 28×10^{-6}/year/rad for cancers till age 10
(i.e., 5 in a 100,000/year/rad
or 5 in 10,000 overall/rad)

Relative cancer risks
5.0 for first trimester exposure
1.5 for second and third trimester exposure

*Upper limit from National Research Council. *The Effects on Populations of Exposure to Low Levels of Ionizing Radiation.* Committee on the Biological Effects of Ionizing Radiations, Division of Medical Sciences, Assembly of Life Sciences, National Research Council. Washington, D.C.: National Academy, 1980.

ing an indicated examination is also an indirect health risk to the embryo-fetus" [4]. To further put this in perspective, "the risk of any radiation injury from a radiological examination (such as a routine chest x-ray) is so small that it would be offset by any slight medical benefit" [4].

3. "There is also a level, presumably, above which the risk of the radiological procedure is so great that it should not be carried out except to counteract a life-threatening situation (such as radiation treatment of cancer)" [4].
4. When embryo/fetal doses are kept to levels below 1000 mrad, the probability of inducing any measurable effect is so small as to be outweighed by any significant benefit of examination.
5. At doses higher than 1000 mrad, most of our information is derived from the study of children who were in utero at the time of the atomic bombings of Hiroshima and Nagasaki and from animal experimentation. The data now suggest no practical threshold for the induction of effects such as congenital malformations or mental retardation.

   Epidemiologic studies also show that prenatally irradiated children will manifest an excess risk of between 1 in 1000 to 1 in 10,000/1000 mrad during the first decade of life for the development of leukemia and other cancers. The risk appears greatest during the second and third trimesters of pregnancy (Table 6-4).
6. Whatever the risks, women should be counseled regarding the potential risks and benefits, as well as all the other options.

Table 6-5. Guide for physicians regarding radiologic considerations of women of childbearing capacity

1. Every diagnostic x-ray exam or nuclear medical procedure involving the abdomen or pelvis area of women of reproduction potential should carry a notation that the consultation is being requested only after consideration of the possibility or knowledge of pregnancy.
2. In cases of known pregnancy, the attending physician should consult with the radiologist in determining the extent of the exam, since the radiation exposure can often be reduced if only a specific question needs answering, as compared to a thorough and detailed procedure designated to deliver maximum information. Judgment should be used in decisions regarding needed procedures.
3. Where pregnancy is not suspected, the patient should be advised to defer the risk of pregnancy for at least two months after the abdominal or pelvic examination.

The following information should be obtained for abdominal or pelvic radiologic exams (complete for all females age 12–55):

___ Potential for pregnancy.

___ Pregnancy not suspected. Patient has been advised not to run a risk of pregnancy until 2 months after examination has been performed.

___ Potential for pregnancy, but postponement is not indicated.

___ Pregnant; postponement to term is not indicated.

___ Consider possibility of minimal examination.

Source: National Council on Radiation Protection and Measurements. *Medical Radiation Exposure of Pregnant and Potentially Pregnant Women: Recommendations of the National Council on Radiation Protection and Measurements.* (NCRP report no. 54). Washington, D.C.: The Council, 1977.

Table 6-6. NCRP decision guides for scheduling or postponing elective examination of the abdomen or pelvis in women of childbearing capacity*

I. Is the exam of the abdomen or pelvis an elective procedure for the patient?
   A. No. ___ Go to II.
   B. Yes. ___ Go to IV.

II. Is patient pregnant?
   A. No. There is no chance of unsuspected pregnancy. ___ Proceed with the exam. Advise patient to avoid risk of pregnancy until 2 months after exam.
   B. Yes, or pregnancy cannot be ruled out. ___ Advise patient that medical judgment indicates that the need for the exam outweighs the possible slight risk to the embryo or fetus. Go to III.

III. Can the exam be modified to reduce the dose to the uterus (embryo or fetus, if present)?
   A. No. ___ Proceed with the exam.
   B. Yes. ___ Proceed with the modified exam.

IV. How many days after the onset of the last menses would exam be performed?
   A. 0–14 days. ___ Proceed with exam. Advise patient to avoid pregnancy for 2 months.
   B. 15 days or more. ___ Postpone exam until menstruation ensues. If patient proves to be pregnant, postpone exam until term.

*For elective examinations, i.e., those not of immediate importance to patient's health, and those that could be postponed to term if patient is proven pregnant without significant risk to the health of patient or her conceptus (see high dose group of Table 6-2).

Source: National Council on Radiation Protection and Measurements. *Medical Radiation Exposure of Pregnant and Potentially Pregnant Women: Recommendations of the National Council on Radiation Protection and Measurements.* (NCRP report no. 54). Washington, D.C.: The Council, 1977.

III. Recommendations

A. Diagnostic ultrasound. Based on currently available information, prenatal health care providers should:

1. Use diagnostic ultrasound for specific medical reasons.
2. Not use diagnostic ultrasound for routine screening at the present time.
3. Supply patients with exposure time and intensity, if requested.
4. Try to keep patient exposures to less than 10 mW/cm².
5. Strive to obtain the most medically significant information with the least ultrasonic exposure.
6. Not use ultrasound exposure conditions where significant fetal temperature elevations (>1° C) might be produced [2].

B. Ionizing radiation. Based on currently available information, prenatal health care providers should:

1. Use diagnostic x-rays in pregnant women only if there is a significant medical need for the examination that cannot be met by an alternative, safer mode, e.g., ultrasound.
2. Consider all reproductive-age women as potentially pregnant and take necessary precautions (Tables 6-5 and 6-6).
3. Not withhold needed diagnostic x-rays if clearly medically indicated.
4. Keep the radiation dose as low as reasonably achievable.
5. Consider therapeutic radiation only when the mother's life is threatened, e.g., invasive carcinoma.
6. Know that when embryo/fetal doses are below 1000 mrad, any significant medical benefit outweighs the risks.
7. Know that doses above 1000 mrad to the fetus, risks of leukemia increase, and above 10,000 mrad, the risk of congenital malformation or mental retardation increases.
8. Consult with the radiologist, whenever possible and advisable, before undertaking any significant radiologic procedures in women who are or may be pregnant.
9. Offer counseling when significant risks are present. At some very high level of risk, abortion may become an option.

References

1. Goldman, M. Ionizing radiation and its risks. *West. J. Med.* 137(6):540, 1982. *Good overview—tutorial summary of basic and practical radiobiology.*
2. National Council on Radiation Protection and Measurements. *Biological Effects of Ultrasound: Mechanism and Clinical Implications: Recommendations of the National Council on Radiation Protection and Measurements.* (NCRP report no. 74). Bethesda, MD: The Council, 1983. *In-depth overview of basics, data base, and recommendations on dosage limitations.*
3. National Research Council. *The Effects on Populations of Exposure to Low Levels of Ionizing Radiation.* Committee on the Biological Effects of Ionizing Radiations, Division of Medical Sciences, Assembly of Life Sciences, National Research Council. Washington, D.C.: National Academy, 1980. *Quantitation methods and up-to-date information on radiation risks.*
4. National Council on Radiation Protection and Measurements. *Medical Radiation Exposure of Pregnant and Potentially Pregnant Women: Recommendations of the National Council on Radiation Protection and Measurements.* (NCRP report no. 54). Washington, D.C.: The Council, 1977. *Recommendation for limiting radiation exposure to embryo and fetus.*

Suggested Readings

Evans, J. S., Moeller, D. W., and Cooper, D. W. *Health Effects Model for Nuclear Power Plant Accident Consequence Analysis.* NUREG/CR-4214. Washington, D.C.: U.S. Nuclear Regulatory Commission, 1985. *Up-to-date assessment of radiation risks.*

Hussey, M. *Basic Physics and Technology of Medical Diagnostic Ultrasound.* New York: Elsevier, 1985. *Emphasis on technology.*

National Council on Radiation Protection and Measurements. *Radiation Protection in Pediatric Radiology: Recommendations of the National Council on Radiation Protection and Measurements.* (NCRP report no. 68). Washington, D.C.: The Council, 1981. *Good on methods and recommendations to limit child exposures.*

National Council on Radiation Protection and Measurements. *Protection in Nuclear Medicine and Ultrasound Diagnostic Procedures in Children: Recommendations of the National Council on Radiation Protection and Measurements.* (NCRP report no. 73). Washington, D.C.: The Council, 1983. *Emphasis on risk-benefit and improved techniques.*

Sanders, R. C., and James, A. E., Jr. (eds.). *The Principles and Practice of Ultrasonography in Obstetrics and Gynecology.* New York: Appleton-Century-Crofts, 1977. *Practical technical overview.*

Stewart, H. F., and M. E. Stratmeyer (eds.). *An Overview of Ultrasound: Theory, Measurement, Medical Applications, and Biological Effects.* Rockville, MD: U.S. Dept. of Health and Human Services, Public Health Service, Food and Drug Administration, Bureau of Radiological Health, 1982. *Good review of theory and practice.*

White, D. N. (ed.). *Recent Advances in Perinatal Pathology and Physiology. (Ultrasound in Biomedicine Research Series.) Vol. 4.* Chichester, England: Research Studies, 1980. *Overview of research emphasizing physiology.*

Williams, A. R. *Ultrasound: Biological Effects and Potential Hazards.* (Series title: *Medical Physics Series.*) London: Academic, 1983. *Good on basics and theory.*

World Health Organization. *Ultrasound. Environmental Health Criteria No. 22.* Geneva: WHO, 1982. *Good review.*

United Nations. Scientific Committee on the Effects of Atomic Radiation. *General Assembly Document, 35 Session, Biological Effects of Prenatal Irradiation.* (A.AC.82/R.448). Vienna: United Nations, 1986. *Encyclopedic compendium and analysis of current data.*

7 Perinatal Education

Debbie Bulger

I. The problem

A. Description. The predominant focus of perinatal education has been preparation for labor and delivery. Classes in hospitals, schools, and community agencies and through private sources often deal with discussions of hospital practices, delivery style, pain relief, and labor rehearsal using relaxation and breathing techniques. Less attention has been paid to the full spectrum of educational experiences designed to meet the varying needs of prospective and new parents at each stage of the childbearing year. Ideally, resources should be available to address the needs of prepregnancy, early pregnancy, the intrapartum period, early postpartum adjustment, and parenting and baby care (Table 7-1). Many opportunities for perinatal education occur outside the classroom environment. Integration of education into routine caregiving allows sustained, meaningful parent education [1, 2]. Effective parent education is a crucial function of perinatal medical practice.

B. Goals. Recommendations for access to prenatal and parenting education have come from many sources. The Surgeon General's Workshop on Maternal and Infant Health recommended that each state develop a plan to ensure access to such education for all families, whether urban or rural. The American College of Obstetricians and Gynecologists (ACOG), the Nurses Association of the American College of Obstetricians and Gynecologists (NAACOG), the American Academy of Pediatrics (AAP), the American College of Nurse-Midwives (ACNM), and the American Nurses Association (ANA) jointly support preparation for childbirth classes with the following goals [3] (Table 7-2):

1. To increase the community's awareness of its responsibility toward ensuring a healthy outcome for mother and child.
2. To serve as opportunities for the community and health care providers to match their expectations and achieve mutual goals from the childbirth experience.
3. To assist the community in becoming eligible for participation in the full family-centered program.
4. To include a tour of the hospital's maternity and newborn units.

Although specific goals for various types of education classes differ, the following four interdependent goals are frequently proffered:

1. To impart information that allows the woman and family to make informed choices and to increase their ability to participate more fully in their own care.
2. To provide pain relief during labor and delivery.
3. To allay anxiety of the unknown.
4. To heighten the enjoyment of the birthing experience.

The concepts of preconception counseling are gaining wider acceptance, and certainly antenatal preparation for new roles as parents and for care and development of the anticipated family addition is also an important goal of perinatal education. Starting with a prenatal visit in the third trimester, the American Academy of Pediatrics has detailed and arranged in time sequence specific topics for counseling and anticipatory guidance [1]. Issues that the family physician or pediatrician can help with before the baby's birth include the following:

1. Parenting
2. Breast- versus bottle-feeding
3. Breast-feeding support
4. Circumcision
5. Infant car seat selection

II. Techniques

A. Methods. Whatever the specific benefits of perinatal education in particular, health

Table 7-1. Types of classes for the childbearing year

Class	Content focus
Prepregnancy fairs/classes	Assist family in decisionmaking about pregnancy.
Early pregnancy	Nutrition, physiology, emotional adjustment to pregnancy.
Preparation for birthing (Lamaze, Bradley, etc.)	Breathing and relaxation techniques for labor and delivery—consideration of choices in childbirth.
Cesarean birth preparation	Physiology, operative procedures, and emotions associated with cesarean birth.
Sibling preparation	Play activities directed toward having a new baby in the family.
Children at birth	Preparation for being present at labor and delivery.
Hospital tours	Familiarization with the hospital environment.
Early discharge preparation	Instruction for early home care for both mother and baby. When to call health care provider.
Postpartum instruction	Infant feeding, caretaking, family planning.
Mother/father/parent support groups	Peer support with trained facilitator.
Infant care	Postdischarge instruction in growth and development, signs of illness, infant safety, infant nutrition.

Special needs:
Pregnant adolescents
Single parents
Adoptive parents
Parents of high-risk or chronically ill infants
Perinatal death support groups
Grandparents class
Preterm labor (for high-risk pregnancies)

education in general provides learning experiences leading to responsible decisionmaking and voluntary adoption of healthful practices.

1. **Behavior change** can best be reached through joint decisionmaking by the health care provider and parents. Taking an active role in one's own health care enhances self-confidence and self-esteem, and may positively affect compliance. Assistance in planning for structured perinatal education should be an integral part of the care a family receives from its health care providers.
2. Ideally, **preparation for pregnancy,** childbirth, and parenting should begin before conception.
3. **The critical period** surrounding the birth of a child may constitute a window during which education is particularly effective. Caplan's pioneering work in crisis theory described the disequilibrium that occurs during role transition and the resultant increased receptivity to new coping responses. LeMaster [4] applied Caplan's work to the crisis of becoming a parent for the first time. In the inpatient setting, the practitioner can take an active role, either personally or through department representatives, in the development and review of standardized teaching protocols that safeguard program consistency. Multidisciplinary instruction allows efficient utilization of resources. Examples of inpatient perinatal education programs include dietary instruction for women with pregnancy-induced glucose intolerance, preoperative cesarean teaching, postpartum breast- or bottle-feeding assistance, and infant car-passenger safety instruction. The trend toward shortened postpartum stays increases the importance of effective communication to ensure continuity of care. Traditional techniques such as printed information about signs of illness, when to call the physician, and home visits by a nurse practitioner, as well as innovative methods such as home video programs, have been used successfully.
4. An excellent opportunity for **the family physician or pediatrician to instruct**

Table 7-2. Resource organizations

ACOG/NAACOG 600 Maryland Avenue, SW Washington, DC 20024-2588	
American Academy of Pediatrics 141 Northwest Point Road P.O. Box 927 Elk Grove Village, IL 60007	
American Academy of Husband Coached Childbirth (Bradley) P.O. Box 5224 Sherman Oaks, CA 91413	Trains and certifies instructors to teach Bradley method of prepared childbirth
American Society for Psychoprophylaxis in Obstetrics (ASPO) 1411 K Street, NW Washington, DC 20005	Trains and certifies instructors to teach Lamaze method of prepared childbirth
C/Sec, Inc. Cesarean/Support, Education and Concern 300 Sheafe Street Chestnut Hill, MA 02167	Information and assistance with cesarean birth—local chapters
International Childbirth Education Association (ICEA) P.O. Box 20852 Milwaukee, WI 53220	Resources and clearinghouse for enhancement of birthing and parent/child relationships
La Leche League 9161 Minneapolis Avenue Franklin Park, IL 60131	Information and assistance with breast-feeding—local chapters

parents is to conduct the newborn examination in the parent's presence. Demonstrating the newborn's amazing capabilities, normal reflexes, behaviors, and individual temperament can strengthen the new parents' knowledge of their infant. In addition, the physician's handling of the baby serves as a role model for the parents [5].

5. **The following principles** are helpful in selecting appropriate prenatal and postdischarge classes:
   a. Objectives of courses should be clearly stated and outlines available on request.
   b. Instructors should have appropriate qualifications.
   c. Classes should stress preventive measures and should encourage women to assume responsibility in health care.
   d. Information should be presented through several media (printed, audio, visual, models, etc.) to appeal to all the senses.
   e. Education should include participation of those in the woman's support system to ensure support in following recommended practices.
   f. Individual preferences should be respected, including life-styles and role definitions.
6. **The relationship** of the childbirth educator to other health care professionals is outlined in detail in **Guidelines for Childbirth Education,** published by NAACOG [6]. Good communication among all members of the health care team is essential for optimal functioning. Mechanisms such as monthly meetings among hospital staff, educators, and physician representatives are useful for exchanging information and providing feedback. It is important that whatever "brand" of classes is attended, principles of adult education be followed and instructors be adequately qualified.
7. **Perinatal education programs** are available from many sources, including hospitals, colleges and universities, private instructors, public schools (especially programs for pregnant minors), public health departments, and the American Red

Table 7-3. Early pregnancy course outline (three 2-hour classes in series)

Class I: Normal changes and nutrition
- A. Introductions/outline of class
- B. Fetal development
- C. Common physical and emotional changes
- D. Distribute 3-day diet assessment
- E. Film (nutrition, exercise, prenatal care, fetal development)

Class II: Nutrition and complications of pregnancy
- A. Review
- B. Complications of pregnancy/antepartum tests
- C. Nutrition during pregnancy
- D. Evaluation of 3-day diet intake
- E. Weight gain
- F. Smoking, alcohol, and drugs
- G. Exercise/stress reduction (floor exercises)
- H. Relaxation

Class III:
- A. Review
- B. How a child will influence lives
- C. Activities during pregnancy
- D. Childbirth choices
- E. Parenting choices, film
- F. Exercise/stress reduction (floor exercises)
- G. Evaluation

Source: The Perinatal Center, Sutter Memorial Hospital, Sacramento, California, 1986.

Cross. Community instructors often teach in several programs and may meet informally to exchange ideas. Those who have credentials from associations such as the American Society for Psychoprophylaxis in Obstetrics (ASPO, commonly referred to as Lamaze) and the American Academy of Husband Coached Childbirth (Bradley method) often meet on a regular basis and may communicate through a newsletter.

8. **Hospital education coordinators** and childbirth education associations are good sources to use to learn which classes are available in a community. For the practitioner who has never attended childbirth education programs, it is a worthwhile investment of time to participate in a series. Such attendance enhances one's ability to counsel clients and encourages good communication with instructors. A list of resource organizations is included in Table 7-2. Health care providers who wish to offer their own class series will find especially useful the program content outlined by trimester in the NAACOG booklet **Guidelines for Childbirth Education.** A sample outline for a three-class series for the first trimester is included in Table 7-3.
9. **Evaluation of any program** should be ongoing. The purpose of the evaluation is to provide information about the effectiveness of a program and to maintain quality over time. Evaluation techniques include feedback forms and questionnaires filled out by parents, return demonstrations, "posttests" during program development, interviews with class participants, and observed behavior changes. Continual evaluation enables adjustments in program content to be made on the basis of the needs and desires of the particular client population.

B. Justification

1. **Effectiveness.** Although research supporting the advantages of perinatal education is plentiful, much of it does not stand up to careful scrutiny because of inherent methodological limitations. Research shortcomings have included the fact that most control and experimental groups are self-selected, control groups receiving attention/placebo treatment are not included, and obstetricians utilized have been aware of the type of preparation of specific clients. Additionally, human behavior is so complex and the number of variables involved are so numerous that attempts to ascribe behavioral outcomes solely to a specific educational program are dubious.

   Enkin [7] compared parents who participated in childbirth preparation classes with parents who wanted to participate but could not enroll due to a limited number of spaces. Women who had taken the classes used significantly less analgesia and anesthesia, required less use of forceps, and reported a more favorable experience in labor and delivery than women who had not been able to take the classes. Likewise, Scott and Rose [8], and Huttel, et al. [9] found statistically significant fewer drugs used and more favorable experiences reported among mothers who had taken Lamaze training.

The role of classes in allaying anxiety may be significant. Knowledge of hospital procedures gained from class participation, as well as inclusion of a support person, may increase a family's ability to make decisions and to remain in control during the birthing experience.

The animal experiments of Morishima [10] and others demonstrated a reduced uterine blood flow resulting in a decreased fetal heart rate and fetal oxygenation brought on by experiment-imposed stress and pain. In human research, Lederman and colleagues [11] found that physiologic elevations of plasma epinephrine are significantly associated with decreased uterine activity, longer labors, and self-reported anxiety.

Sosa's [12] introduction of an **untrained** companion who provided emotional support to a woman from the time of hospital admission until delivery resulted in labors 2½ times shorter than those experienced by unaccompanied women in the group. Both groups had little, if any, prenatal preparation.

Although several studies reported less pain felt by trained parturients, it is of note that Charles, et al. [13] observed that pleasure and pain scores were not highly correlated. Trained women reported significantly less pain and more enjoyment, but it was possible to score highly in both pain and enjoyment. In their own words, the women remained "in control of themselves."

Loss of control can generate intense anxiety. The hospital environment is generally not conducive to feelings of individuality and partnership in decisionmaking on the part of those perceived as "patients." Many hospital routines exist solely for the convenience and sense of security of the staff. In one extreme example, Norman Cousins relates how he moved out of the hospital and into a hotel room in order to escape being awakened for meals, medication, and baths—in other words, to regain control [14]. Skills learned in the class environment may enable women and their support persons to "beat the system."

In a rare, randomized, prospectively controlled trial, Casey [15] and others found that parents who received education about fever management demonstrated fewer inappropriate calls to the physician and reduced medication errors.

Future research in perinatal education will assist health care providers in answering questions regarding the timing, duration, and method of instruction used. Evidence suggests that understanding infant capabilities, having a positive self-image, and having access to a support system may be more important to successful birthing and parenting than academic knowledge.

2. **Risks.** The principal risk is that misinformation may be given, or that the education, although well-intended, does not address important areas. It is of note that Pridham and Schutz [16] could find no significant differences between primiparous and multiparous parents in the extent to which they perceived themselves to be prepared for infant care. The areas in which parents felt preparation was inadequate included cesarean birth (both from parents who had had vaginal deliveries as well as parents who had had abdominal deliveries), adjustment to changes in the marriage caused by the pregnancy and birth, sibling preparation, sexuality, and preparation of the father for parenthood.
3. **Costs.** Costs of classes vary widely depending on the local market, number of classes in a series, and pricing strategy of the class sponsor. It is not unusual for a hospital to offer classes at no charge or at below-market value to encourage consumers to select the sponsoring facility for the birth of their baby. Charges for a six-class preparation for childbirth series typically range from $35–70. Single sessions such as a sibling class may range from $5–15. Many instructors have special arrangements for women or couples unable to pay the full price.
4. **Acceptability.** Market research has shown that consumers desire information and education about childbirth and seek these services when selecting health care providers and facilities.

III. Recommendations

A. Encourage women and families to assume responsibility in health care.
B. Begin counseling regarding childbirth preconception.
C. Utilize multidisciplinary instruction for efficient allocation of resources.

D. Refer parents to classes taught by credentialed instructors who employ adult education principles and a class evaluation mechanism.
E. Utilize newborn examinations as opportunities for parent education.

References

1. American Academy of Pediatrics. *Guidelines for Health Supervision.* Elk Grove Village, IL: AAP, 1985. *Guide to integrating pediatric care and parent education.*
2. Fulginiti, V. A., et al. Pediatric patient education: Challenge for the '80s. *Pediatrics* 74(5 Pt.2):913, 1984. *Analysis of pediatrician's role as educator.*
3. Interprofessional Task Force on Health Care of Women and Children. *Joint Position Statement on the Development of Family-centered Maternity/Newborn Care in Hospitals.* Chicago: The Task Force, 1978. *Position statement on family-centered maternity care.*
4. LeMaster, E. E. Parenthood as Crisis. In H. J. Parad (ed.), *Crisis Intervention: Selected Readings.* New York: Family Service Assn. Of America, 1965. Pp.111–117. *Classic work on crisis of becoming a parent.*
5. Charney, E. Counseling of parents around the birth of a baby. *Pediatr. Rev.* 4(6):167, 1982. *The pediatrician as role model.*
6. The Nurses Association of the American College of Obstetricians and Gynecologists. *Guidelines for Childbirth Education.* Washington, D.C.: NAACOG, 1981. *Role of childbirth educator; curriculum content for childbirth classes.*
7. Enkin, M. W., et al. An Adequately Controlled Study of the Effectiveness of PPM Training. In N. Morris (ed.), *Psychosomatic Medicine in Obstetrics and Gynaecology.* Basel, Switzerland: Karger, 1972. Pp.62–67. *Better childbirth experiences through education.*
8. Scott, J. R., and Rose, N. B. Effect of psychoprophylaxis (Lamaze preparation) on labor and delivery in primiparas. *N. Engl. J. Med.* 294(22):1205, 1976. *Positive effect of Lamaze classes.*
9. Huttel, F.A., et al. A quantitative evaluation of psychoprophylaxis in childbirth. *J. Psychosom. Res.* 16(2):81, 1972. *Positive effect of Lamaze classes.*
10. Morishima, H. O., Yeh, M. N., and James, L. S. Reduced uterine blood flow and fetal hypoxemia with acute maternal stress: Experimental observations in the pregnant baboon. *Am. J. Obstet. Gynecol.* 134(3):270, 1979. *Stress reduces uterine blood flow in animals.*
11. Lederman, R. P., et al. The relationship of maternal anxiety, plasma catecholamines, and plasma cortisol to progress in labor. *Am. J. Obstet. Gynecol.* 132(5):495, 1978. *In humans, decreased uterine blood flow and larger babies found under stress.*
12. Sosa, R., et al. The effect of a supportive companion on perinatal problems, length of labor, and mother-infant interaction. *N. Engl. J. Med.* 303(11):597, 1980. *Landmark study that demonstrated that the presence of an untrained companion shortened labor.*
13. Charles, A. G., et al. Obstetric and psychological effects of psychoprophylactic preparation for childbirth. *Am. J. Obstet. Gynecol.* 131(1):44, 1978. *Analysis of perceived pain and enjoyment levels during childbirth.*
14. Cousins, N. Anatomy of an illness as perceived by the patient. *N. Engl. J. Med.* 295(26):1458, 1976. *A powerful and insightful article about the challenges of being ill. The response of health care providers and one person's striving to get well.*
15. Casey, R., et al. Fever therapy: An educational intervention for parents. *Pediatrics* 73(5):600, 1984. *Well-designed study on effect of education on behavior.*
16. Pridham, K. F., and Schutz, M. E. Preparation of parents for birthing and infant care. *J. Fam. Pract.* 13(2):181, 1981. *The physician as counselor.*

II Disease Prevention

8 Hypertension in Pregnancy

Hanns C. Haesslein

Chronic Hypertension

I. The problem

A. Definition. The definition of hypertension in pregnancy is the same as that in the nonpregnant woman: a diastolic blood pressure greater than 90 mm Hg (on two occasions), or a systolic blood pressure greater than 140 mm Hg, either antedating the pregnancy or in the first trimester, without significant proteinuria [1].

B. Epidemiology. Approximately 4% of white and 8% of black gravidas present at their first trimester prenatal visit with elevated blood pressures. This level of blood pressure is never normal in a gravida, no matter what her age. The large majority of hypertensive pregnant women are ultimately classified as essential hypertensives—but renal, arterial, connective tissue, diabetic, and other causes comprise about 10–20% of the total. The impact of the hypertension is not only the increased risk (5.7%) of superimposed pregnancy-induced hypertension (PIH) (see PIH portion of this chapter), but also the risk of fetal disease due to intrauterine growth retardation and abruptio placenta. These combined problems lead to a perinatal mortality of about 2.6% [2].

C. Risk factors for hypertension in pregnancy are a strong familial history of hypertension, a history of previous renal disease, a known history of diabetes with vascular disease, or connective tissue disease. At any age, black women are also at higher risk than whites.

II. Primary prevention. Every effort should be made to attend to optimal weight, exercise, and diet while avoiding drugs and alcohol, which may produce hypertension. These efforts may prevent the occurrence of some hypertension, and ideally these efforts should be ongoing in all individuals, i.e., preconception (see Chap. 72).

III. Secondary prevention

A. Early detection

1. Methods

a. Blood pressure measurement. In pregnancy, detection of chronic hypertension depends on accurate serial blood pressure measurements in the sitting or left lateral recumbent position. It is most important to realize that there is a physiologic **decrease** in blood pressure in the middle trimester of pregnancy, so that any blood pressure greater than 135 mm Hg systolic or 85 mm Hg diastolic during that time should be considered potentially problematic. This physiologic decrease may mask mild hypertension in the patient or may make early pregnancy-elevated blood pressures actually improve with or without treatment. This frequently lulls the health care provider into believing that the initial mild hypertension was an artifactual "first-visit hypertension," or that a given therapy is wonderfully effective. Unfortunately, in the third trimester, the hypertension reappears and may worsen severely, especially if PIH superimposes itself (a 20% risk in this situation).

b. Evaluation. Unless the specific etiology of the hypertension is known, cost-effective evaluation of hypertension includes a blood urea nitrogen (BUN) test (>10 mg/dl is abnormal in pregnancy), an antinuclear antibody test (ANA), and a urinalysis. Proteinuria in association with hypertension at less than 20 weeks indicates probable renal disease, whereas after 20 weeks the onset of PIH is more likely. Palpation of all peripheral pulses for coarctation, funduscopic examination for hemorrhages and exudates, and auscultation for renal artery stenosis are also indicated.

2. **Justification.** Blood pressure measurement is accurate, predictive, safe, inexpensive, and well accepted (see Chap. 72). The cost of the laboratory tests described above is generally less than $40. The test battery is usually well accepted by patients since it requires only phlebotomy.

B. Early intervention

1. **Methods**

a. **Drug regimens used in pregnancy** [3]

(1) **Alphamethyldopa** (750–2000 mg/day) taken orally has been used for an extended period of time in pregnancy without known risk to the fetus, although it does cross the placenta readily. The usual side effect is depression, though usually mild, and, rarely, a positive Coombs' reaction after prolonged use. Hemolysis and liver enzyme elevation rarely occur.

(2) **Hydralazine** (40–160 mg/day) is much less commonly used due to some problems with side effects such as headaches, tachycardia, and nausea, but it does appear to be relatively safe for the fetus.

(3) **Beta blockers,** usually propranolol (40–160 mg/day), have also been used. It is still controversial whether propranolol itself leads to possible increased risk of fetal growth retardation [4].

For outpatient management, the patient should be taught the use of a home blood pressure monitor, with twice daily pressure recording. She should report any blood pressure greater than 95 mm Hg diastolic. Increased rest and possibly cessation of employment may be useful but have been poorly quantified. She should be warned to report immediately any hand or facial edema, epigastric or hepatic pain, headaches, or scotomata as possible signs of superimposed PIH.

b. **Fetal surveillance,** although not a direct treatment, is a concomitant necessity. Fetal ultrasonography should be performed every 4 weeks starting at 26 weeks' gestation, since it is highly sensitive in recognizing intrauterine growth retardation. It is important to understand that reasonable maternal blood pressure control **does not** ensure normal fetal growth. Indeed, severe growth retardation can occur even with well-controlled hypertension.

To ensure an adequate fetal health status, weekly use of contraction stress testing (CST), biweekly nonstress testing (NST), or, more recently, the biophysical profile (BPP) is indicated. These tests should start at 30–36 weeks' gestation, depending on the severity of the hypertension or evidence of fetal growth retardation; the more severe, the earlier surveillance is started. If beta blocker therapy is used, especially in high doses, fetal cardiac rate should also be observed at each office visit, since fetal bradycardia has been reported and may be deleterious to the fetus by decreasing fetal perfusion.

2. **Justification**

a. **Effectiveness.** Interestingly, there is no evidence that treatment of chronic hypertension with diastolic blood pressure of less than 95 mm Hg improves maternal or perinatal outcome. With a diastolic pressure of 95–100 mm Hg, the use of drug therapy is controversial. Above 100 mm Hg diastolic, use of antihypertensive medication appears to be of some benefit to the mother (decreased risk of stroke) and arguably to the fetus [5]. A diastolic blood pressure greater than 110 mm Hg is considered a semi-emergency requiring immediate antihypertensive treatment, and greater than 120 mm Hg diastolic requires hospitalization immediately.

b. **Costs.** The costs of the above surveillance methods vary.

(1) **Home monitoring blood pressure cuff.** A manual cuff at $35, or a digital cuff at about $65, is relatively inexpensive and can be used by the patient for a lifetime of blood pressure monitoring.

(2) **Fetal surveillance.** Specific costs include: the nonstress test, currently costing about $65–80; the contraction stress test, $125–150; and biophysical profiles, costing approximately $250 since they involve utilization of ultrasound for up to 30 minutes each time. In general, the nonstress test is most easily accepted by patients since it is entirely noninvasive and requires only passive recording of the fetal heart rate. The contraction stress test, if done by nipple stimulation, is again relatively well tolerated, whereas if pitocin infusion is needed, an IV must be started. A fetal

biophysical profile (ultrasound scoring of fetal movements, breathing, and amniotic fluid volume, plus a nonstress test) appears to be well tolerated by the patient, who finds it extremely interesting to watch her fetus on the monitoring screen. In general, the biophysical profile currently should be used as a backup to the previous two tests, except in circumstances where external fetal heart rate tracings cannot be adequately obtained.

IV. Recommendations

A. Primary prevention. Counsel all women about diet, exercise, weight control, and drug and alcohol avoidance.

B. Secondary prevention

1. Early detection. The following preventive measures are recommended:

a. Blood pressure measurement in both arms at the first prenatal visit and then at each subsequent prenatal visit, in either the sitting or left lateral recumbent position. Any blood pressure of greater than 135/85 is of concern.

b. Careful funduscopic examination looking for evidence of chronic hypertensive disease, palpation of peripheral pulses, and abdominal auscultation for bruits.

c. Screening urinalysis, especially for proteinuria or casts.

d. If diastolic blood pressure is greater than 90 mm Hg, perform an ANA, BUN, and repeat urinalysis. (If **proteinuria** is present, perform the **PIH pregnancy blood screen tests** and follow as a PIH patient.) (See PIH section of this chapter.)

2. Early intervention

a. Diastolic blood pressure between 80 and 90 mm Hg and no proteinuria. Patient should do serial blood pressure observations daily at home, with routine prenatal visit intervals.

b. Diastolic blood pressure greater than 90 mm Hg, less than 100 mm Hg. Requires home blood pressure monitoring, increased rest in a lateral position, and possible cessation of work. Also, counsel the patient to avoid cofactors, such as smoking and extreme exercise.

c. Diastolic blood pressure greater than 100 mm Hg. Requires immediate antihypertensive therapy and initiation of fetal surveillance when the patient is over 26 weeks' gestation. A baseline ultrasound should be performed and repeated monthly.

d. Drug therapy. If blood pressure is above 95 mm Hg diastolic, the first choice drug would be methyldopa (Aldomet), 250–500 mg, tid–qid. We do not advocate the use of diuretics, due to the problems with inhibition of plasma volume expansion and possible fetal side effects. If methyldopa is not sufficient, hydralazine may be added as the second drug, 10–40 mg q6h.

e. Some authorities feel that propranolol can be safely used in pregnancy, in its usual dose of 40 mg bid and increased as necessary up to 160 mg/day. If a patient is already well controlled on a beta blocker before pregnancy, it may be reasonable to keep her on it throughout the pregnancy with careful fetal surveillance [4].

f. Fetal surveillance. Initial ultrasonography should be performed, with a repeat at 32 weeks to check for head circumference-to-abdominal circumference ratios, fluid volume, and placental grading to anticipate possible intrauterine growth retardation. If the patient is on antihypertensive therapy, contraction stress tests starting at 30–36 weeks and continued on a weekly basis should be initiated. Should the patient have severe hypertension and earlier evidence of intrauterine growth retardation, fetal surveillance should be initiated earlier.

Pregnancy-Induced Hypertension

I. The problem

A. Definition. Hypertension whose initial onset is after the twentieth week of pregnancy usually represents a unique disease that, although occasionally devastating to the gravida and her fetus, is completely cured by delivery and rarely recurs. This disease is called pregnancy-induced hypertension (PIH) in the United States (or toxemia or preeclampsia), and EPH gestosis (edema, proteinuria, and hypertension of pregnancy) in the rest of the world [3].

B. Description. It is currently thought that PIH is caused by vascular-immunologic malfunctions involving platelet and fibrin deposition in the microcirculation, increasing capillary permeability, inability of the intravascular volume to expand, and a marked sensitivity to pressor agents. Thromboxane A_2 and prostacyclin are thought to be mediators of this process. It is a well-studied fact that PIH is a disease that can be detected by such methods as angiotensin II infusion up to 6–8 weeks before clinical evidence of the disease occurs. Failure to adequately expand the plasma volume (as measured by direct and indirect means) is another early indicator of potential PIH. The **major target** organs in PIH are the kidney, liver, brain, and placenta [1].

C. Epidemiology. PIH occurs in up to 7% of deliveries in the United States and contributes substantially to maternal mortality and perinatal mortality (38/1000 deliveries), while neonatal mortality is mainly related to the consequences of prematurity and rarely to problems that mirror the maternal disease [6].

D. Risk groups. Primigravidas are much more frequently affected than multigravidas. Women with multiple gestations, fetal hydrops, molar pregnancy, diabetes mellitus, or chronic hypertension, or women whose mothers had eclampsia are all at increased risk. Any multigravida with PIH should be carefully evaluated for possible underlying chronic hypertension, for having a pregnancy by a different partner, for connective tissue disease, and for diabetes mellitus.

II. Secondary prevention

A. Early detection

1. Methods

a. Blood pressure measurement. Currently, the most common and standardized method for detecting PIH is the careful observation of increases in the diastolic blood pressure (by > 15 mm Hg) or the systolic blood pressure (by > 30 mm Hg) in two observational periods, more than 6 hours apart, occurring after 20 weeks of pregnancy.

b. Proteinuria. If proteinuria on urine dipstick occurs in greater than trace quantity, further testing is also indicated.

c. Weight gain. A weight gain of more than 5 lb in a week, especially if associated with hand and facial edema, is worrisome.

d. Roll-over test. Although it has been well established that the physiologic changes of pregnancy-induced hypertension can start up to 8 weeks before the clinical disease becomes obvious to the clinician (as measured by an increase in blood pressure), the easiest method of early detection of underlying PIH, the "roll-over" test, first described over 10 years ago, is rarely used [7].

(1) Description. At 24–35 weeks' gestation, the patient is told to rest on her left side, recumbent. The blood pressure is taken and recorded every 5 minutes until the diastolic blood pressure is stable. The patient is then rolled onto her back, the blood pressure is immediately taken, and the diastolic is recorded and repeated in 5 minutes.

(2) Interpretation. If the diastolic blood pressure rises more than 20 mm Hg, the patient has a markedly increased risk of developing hypertension before delivery. If the test is equivocal, repeat it in 1–2 weeks. The cost of the test is the salary of the test person, usually a nurse, who performs the test.

2. Justification. Assessment of blood pressure and weight gain and checking for proteinuria are a medical standard of care; they are safe, inexpensive, and well accepted by providers and patients.

Although not entirely predictive (75–90% accurate), the "roll-over" test's simplicity warrants utilization especially in primigravidas, or in women with prior PIH histories, connective tissue disease, or diabetes mellitus.

B. Early intervention

1. Methods

a. Further evaluation

(1) History. Once suspicion of PIH arises, careful questioning about poor prognostic signs must be done. Ask carefully about headaches or blurry vision (indications of cerebral disturbance), right upper quadrant pain (liver involvement), epigastric pain (this may sound just like typical heartburn but is presumably due to gastric involvement), and swelling of the face (especially the periorbital areas) and the hands as evidence of increased extravascular fluid. If any of these symptoms are noted (in conjunction with an elevated blood pressure), hospitalization is indicated [8].

(2) **Physical exam.** Physical examination at the time of first detection of changes in the blood pressure should include a funduscopic examination, looking for retinal sheen, arterial vasospasm, or blunting of the optic disc margins. Auscultation of the lungs for pulmonary edema is necessary. Cardiac examination to exclude a gallop rhythm frequently shows lack of the systolic flow murmur of pregnancy, presumably due to severe decrease in the intravascular volume. Palpation of the liver and abdomen must be performed to rule out organ tenderness. Reflexes should be less than 3+ and no clonus should be present.

(3) **Lab** (PIH screening tests). A complete blood count (CBC) would show no evidence of hemoconcentration (hematocrit should be at least 10% lower than in early pregnancy). Platelet count should be above 150,000. The BUN should be low normal (< 10 mg/dl); serum creatinine, serum glutamic oxaloacetic transaminase (SGOT), and uric acid values should all be normal. If any of these tests are abnormal, daily repeat values are necessary.

b. **Management.** Management on an outpatient basis may be attempted if the patient has a blood pressure of less than 160/95, less than 2+ proteinuria, none of the poor prognostic signs of PIH listed above, and a pregnancy of less than 36 weeks' gestation. This will require a health care provider system that is responsive 24 hours a day, a reliable patient, and an initial and weekly **PIH screening tests** battery. If this is not available, hospitalization is required [9].

If all these tests show no evidence of severe PIH, the patient should be taught home blood pressure monitoring, instructed to dipstick her urine for protein twice daily, and warned to call the health care provider immediately if:

(1) Blood pressure is greater than 160/100.
(2) Proteinuria is 2+ or greater.
(3) There are any symptoms other than edema.
(4) There is decreased fetal movement.

The patient should also be seen weekly in the office, be scheduled for a weekly fetal surveillance method (currently we recommend contraction stress testing), as well as an ultrasound examination to rule out intrauterine growth retardation and oligohydramnios, and have weekly **PIH screening tests** (CBC, SGOT, uric acid, and BUN). **Delivery** should occur if:

(1) There is evidence of fetal lung maturity, as determined by amniocentesis after 36 weeks' gestation.
(2) There are any symptoms of worsening PIH.
(3) There is any evidence of fetal compromise, such as nonreassuring contraction stress testing, oligohydramnios, or moderate-to-severe growth retardation on ultrasound.

Whenever there is doubt as to the patient's capability or reliability, or the responsiveness of the health care provider support system, **hospitalization** should occur.

2. **Justification**

a. **Effectiveness.** This early intervention regimen, if strictly adhered to, defines a group of women that are relatively mildly affected by PIH. It can usually prolong their pregnancy more than 7 days, and rarely, if ever, will eclampsia occur.

b. **Risks.** The major risks are patient noncompliance and unevenness of physician response to status change.

c. **Costs.** The cost of an outpatient home monitoring system is basically the cost of the home blood pressure cuff, which is approximately $35 for a manual sphygmomanometer, or $65 for an automatic, digital system. Urine protein sticks cost approximately $16/bottle of 100.

d. **Acceptability.** Once patients understand the use of a blood pressure cuff, they enjoy being able to observe their own health, while avoiding or delaying hospitalization, in order to obtain total lung maturity in the fetus.

III. Recommendations

A. Early detection

1. If time and cost permit, screen all primigravidas and all high-risk multigravidas who have new partners with a "roll-over" test at 28–30 weeks' gestation.
2. Order repeat hemoglobin/hematocrit at 28–32 weeks to be sure that it has decreased by at least 10% from the initial value early in the pregnancy.
3. Whenever diastolic blood pressure increases more than 15 mm Hg over the previous values, or the systolic increases more than 30 mm Hg, perform PIH screening tests and then decide to either hospitalize or manage as an outpatient.

B. Early intervention

1. If the patient's blood pressure is less than 160/95 and she has less than 2+ proteinuria, normal PIH blood test, and no poor prognostic signs at less than 36 weeks' gestation, the following are indicated:
   a. Home blood pressure self-assessment and graph for recording blood pressures.
   b. Urine protein sticks, twice daily.
   c. Contraction stress test, weekly.
   d. Ultrasound every 3–4 weeks after 26 weeks' gestation to detect growth retardation and oligohydramnios and for placental grading. If indicated by abnormal contraction stress testing, a biophysical profile may also be useful.
   e. Bed rest, with the patient confined to home and resting in the lateral, recumbent position more than 18 hours a day, may be useful.
2. If the blood pressure is greater than 160/95, the patient has more than 2+ proteinuria, any of the poor diagnostic signs of PIH, or is more than 36 weeks' gestation, then hospitalization with the goal of stabilization and delivery is immediately indicated.

References

1. Gant, N. F., and Worley, R. J. *Hypertension in Pregnancy—Concepts and Management.* New York: Appleton-Century-Crofts, 1980. *Good review of concepts of PIH and standard therapeutic approaches.*
2. Page, E. W., and Christianson, R. Influence of blood pressure changes with and without proteinuria upon outcome of pregnancy. *Am. J. Obstet. Gynecol.* 126(7):821, 1976. *Studies clearly the influence of mean arterial pressure and proteinuria on ultimate fetal health.*
3. Sullivan, J. M. *Hypertension and Pregnancy.* Chicago: Yearbook, 1986. *Very good section on theory and management of both chronic hypertension and PIH; concise.*
4. Rubin, P. C. Current concepts: Beta blockers in pregnancy. *N. Engl. J. Med.* 305(22):1323, 1981. *Good review, with detailed analysis of drug versus disease effects.*
5. Ounsted, M. K., et al. Hypertension during pregnancy with and without specific treatment; the development of the children at the age of four years. *Br. J. Obstet. Gynaecol.* 87(1):19, 1980. *Study of methyldopa versus placebo indicating prognosis is slightly better for treatment group.*
6. Chesley, L. C. Hypertension in pregnancy: Definitions, familial factor, and remote prognosis. *Kidney Int.* 18(2):234, 1980. *A synopsis that is a classic; based on the author's long-term follow-up on 270 eclamptic patients, and other studies, to give the clinician some guidance regarding remote prognosis.*
7. Gant, N. F., et al. A clinical test useful for predicting the development of acute hypertension in pregnancy. *Am. J. Obstet. Gynecol.* 120:1, 1974. *The original description of the "roll-over" test.*
8. Goodlin, R. C. Severe pre-eclampsia: Another great imitator. *Am. J. Obstet. Gynecol.* 125(6):747, 1976. *An excellent article reviewing the symptoms of preeclampsia and the diseases they are mistaken for.*
9. *Management of Preeclampsia.* ACOG Technical Bulletin #91. Washington, D.C.: ACOG, February 1986. *The current standard of care for preeclampsia.*

9 Diabetes Mellitus and Pregnancy

Jack M. Schneider

I. The problem

A. Definition. The definition of clinically significant abnormal glucose tolerance complicating pregnancy is confusing. Different classifications have been suggested. Furthermore, some have been incorrectly interchanged (Table 9-1). White's Class A diabetes is **not** synonymous with gestational diabetes, as the former denotes preconception detection of glucose intolerance while gestational diabetes denotes postconception detection. Gestational diabetes and pregnancy-induced glucose intolerance are synonymous.

The author prefers the term *pregnancy-induced glucose intolerance* (PIGI) to avoid the negative connotations of the word *diabetes*, as most gestational diabetics normalize their glucose intolerance during pregnancy with appropriate nutritional intervention, and very few develop insulin-requiring diabetes later in life, particularly if ideal body weight is attained.

Women with abnormal glucose tolerance that is first detected in pregnancy represent a heterogeneous population including those with unrecognized glucose intolerance antedating conception as well as those with glucose intolerance postdating conception. The latter group includes cases of manifest diabetes presenting coincident with the pregnancy as well as cases of glucose intolerance restricted to the pregnant state. As no classification approach can differentiate this heterogeneity once conception has occurred, **prepregnancy** screening for abnormal glucose intolerance is a reasonable approach.

B. Description. Adverse pregnancy outcome is related first to the presence and severity of glucose intolerance and second to the presence of vasculopathy.

Women with glucose intolerance (glycohemoglobin >9%) manifest during the first 8 weeks of conception have an associated increased risk of producing progeny with congenital abnormalities. The abnormalities are highly variable in expression and may be multiple. After completed embryogenesis, abnormal maternal glucose tolerance (undetected or established, but not normalized) may be associated with perinatal mortality, macrosomia (with birth trauma and increased cesarean section risks), preterm birth, and neonatal complications including hypoglycemia, respiratory distress syndrome, hypocalcemia, and hyperbilirubinemia. Maternal complications include urinary and genital infections, exacerbation of vascular or neural complications, and pregnancy-induced hypertension.

Normalization of glucose homeostasis in the absence of vasculopathy reduces maternal and perinatal risks to the level seen in nondiabetic pregnant women. When the woman has diabetes-associated vasculopathy, particularly with severe renal involvement (serum creatinine ≥ 1.5 mg/dl), intrauterine growth retardation, preterm birth, and perinatal death are significantly increased.

C. Epidemiology. As many as 10% of pregnancies are complicated by abnormal glucose metabolism [1]. While in approximately 0.3% of pregnancies the woman is already administering insulin, the remainder of the at-risk group usually remain undetected until after pregnancy is initiated [2]. Pregnant women at increased risk for abnormal glucose tolerance include those with risk factors described in Table 9-2, particularly the following:

1. Age ≥ 25 years.
2. Positive family history of diabetes (grandparents, parents, siblings, children).
3. Previous obstetric history of:
   a. Abnormal glucose tolerance during pregnancy.
   b. Unexplained stillborn.
   c. Presence of fetal or neonatal malformation(s).
   d. Macrosomia (≥4000 gm birth weight).

Table 9-1. Classifications of glucose intolerance

National Diabetes Data Group (NDDG)
- Clinical
  - Diabetes Mellitus
    - Type I: insulin-dependent diabetes mellitus (IDDM)
    - Type II: noninsulin-dependent diabetes mellitus (NIDDM)
    - Other types: diabetes mellitus associated with other conditions
  - Impaired glucose tolerance: plasma glucose levels intermediate between values considered diabetic or unusual
  - Gestational diabetes: glucose intolerance diagnosed *during* pregnancy
- Statistical risk
  - Previous abnormality of glucose tolerance
  - Potential abnormality of glucose tolerance

White's classification (modified)
- Class A: chemical diabetes diagnosed *prior* to pregnancy; non-insulin requiring
- Class B: insulin-requiring diabetes diagnosed *prior* to pregnancy; onset after age 20, duration less than 10 years
- Class C: diabetes onset at age 10–19 or diabetes manifest for 10–19 years
- Class D: diabetes onset at age under 10 or diabetes manifest for 20 or more years
- Class F: renal disease complicating diabetes
- Class H: coronary artery disease complicating diabetes
- Class R: proliferative retinopathy complicating diabetes
- Class T: renal transplant complicating diabetes

Schneider's classification (pregnancy-related)
- Class I: noninsulin-requiring glucose intolerance responsive to nutritional management (pregnancy-induced glucose intolerance [PIGI])
- Class II: insulin-requiring glucose intolerance without vasculopathy
- Class III: insulin-requiring glucose intolerance with vasculopathy

Table 9-2. Historical risk factors for abnormal glucose tolerance in pregnancy

- Maternal age ≥25 years
- Positive family history
- Obesity (≥120% of ideal body weight), particularly if combined with positive family history
- Glycosuria (fasting or repetitive postprandial)
- Previous perinatal death
- Hydramnios
- Pregnancy-induced hypertension (preeclampsia)
- Previous overweight baby (≥4000 gm)
- Fetal congenital abnormalities (present or previous pregnancy)
- Previous unexplained low birth weight baby
- Recurrent infections (general, urinary tract, monilial)
- Repeated spontaneous abortion

It must be emphasized, however, that this list (Table 9-2) lacks adequate sensitivity (≅65%) and specificity (≅55%) to identify all women with pregnancy-induced glucose intolerance (gestational diabetes).

II. Secondary prevention

A. Early detection

1. **Methods.** Women not known to have normal blood glucose levels when first seen in pregnancy should be screened for abnormal glucose tolerance.
   a. **Risk factors.** Assessing only those women with risk factors other than maternal age fails to detect about one-half of the cases of abnormal glucose tolerance.
   b. **Fasting blood glucose and glucosuria.** Even in the nonpregnant state, it is noteworthy that neither the fasting blood glucose (FBG) nor assessment

Table 9-3. Two-hour postprandial capillary blood glucose (PPBG) test results and interventions

Blood glucose (mg/dl)	Action
≤120	No further testing necessary.
121–140	Diet; repeat 2-hour PPBG every 4–6 wk; if repeat PPBG <140 mg/dl at 34 or more weeks' gestation, discontinue PPBG testing and manage as uncomplicated pregnancy.
141–169	Diet; repeat fasting blood glucose and 2-hour PPBG every 2 wk; deliver at term if FBG ≤105 mg/dl *and* 2-hour PPBG values remain <170 mg/dl and no other complications of pregnancy exist.
≥170	Diet; insulin as necessary to keep fasting blood glucose 60–100 mg/dl and 1-hour PPBG <140 mg/dl; delivery timing dependent on presence or absence of other complications and fetal maturity; follow with fasting and PPBG after each of three main meals at 1–4 day/wk, if insulin therapy is required.

for glucosuria is as sensitive as a 2-hour postprandial blood glucose for detection of glucose tolerance abnormality [3]. This fact is even more significant in pregnancy wherein physiologic alterations tend to lower the FBG while increasing the occurrence of glycosuria, particularly postprandial [4, 5].

c. **Glycosylated hemoglobin (HbA_1).** This test is not useful in pregnancy to detect abnormal glucose tolerance per se.

d. **Blood glucose screening (24–28 weeks' gestation)**

(1) **50-gm oral glucose load** [6]. The woman ingests a 50-gm glucose solution in a 10-minute period. After no further eating (or smoking) for a period of 1 hour, a venous blood sample is obtained. The time of day or preingestion fasting period is not considered critical. A venous plasma glucose level of 140 mg/dl is recommended as the threshold level requiring a 100-gm oral glucose tolerance test.

(2) **100-gm oral carbohydrate meal** [7]. Following a 100-gm carbohydrate meal that reflects the woman's dietary preferences, a postprandial blood glucose (PPBG) obtained 2 hours after the start of the meal is determined either in the office on capillary whole blood utilizing a reflectance colorimeter, or in a laboratory on plasma. While venous plasma has a higher glucose value than a capillary sample, these differences are not significant over the usual range of results of 100–200 mg/dl. A meal is advised rather than a liquid glucose load to mimic the woman's dietary habits. Further, particularly early in the pregnancy, foodstuffs are better tolerated by the woman in the morning than a liquid glucose load because of the tendency for pregnant women to have morning nausea. Routine early morning testing minimizes effects of circadian alterations in glucose tolerance and of physical exercise, while enhancing comparability of data among patients, as well as in the individual patient tested serially. It is noteworthy that the previously recommended ingestion of high amounts of carbohydrates for 2–3 days prior to the test is not required except in instances of nutritional deprivation [3].

A normal (≤120 mg/dl) 2-hour postprandial glucose value at the initial encounter necessitates **no** further assessments for glucose intolerance during the present pregnancy. If the glucose value is greater than 120 mg/dl, a diet identical to that defined for a woman with insulin-requiring diabetes is initiated. Subsequent 2-hour postprandial glucose determinations are obtained after a meal representative of the prescribed diet, with further assessments and interventions as outlined in Table 9-3 [7].

e. **Glucose tolerance testing (GTT).** An oral glucose tolerance test is **not** recommended by this author. Although the GTT has been advocated to select pregnancies that are at potential perinatal risk because of abnormal glucose tolerance [6, 8], a single GTT in pregnancy is neither highly sensitive nor specific [9]. Two-hour postprandial blood glucose testing can accomplish this risk selection for the clinician and usually at a much lower expenditure of the woman's time and money. As glucose tolerance tends to decrease (i.e., an increase in PPBG) in the latter half of pregnancy, the cost for the GTT is more appropriately spread over serial 2-hour PPBG tests in those cases requiring follow-up [7].

2. **Justification.** Because of the tendency for pregnancy-induced glucose intolerance to be asymptomatic and because of the grave risks for mother and baby if undetected, all women should be screened for abnormal glucose metabolism. Some authorities have advised selective screening of patients: those who are 25 years of age or older, or those with one or more risk factors (see Table 9-2). Limited and late pregnancy screening approaches, however, do not address the issue of the prevention of fetal malformations, the leading cause of perinatal mortality in pregnancies complicated by abnormal glucose tolerance.

   Perinatal morbidity is also increased in undetected glucose intolerance. The financial costs of detection programs are far outweighed by the special care costs for the compromised newborn.

   An office-based test has a cost, including labor and materials, of approximately $3.

   Recommendations for uniform screening are relatively new, and acceptance by both health care providers and clients alike will remain low until the reward-inconvenience ratio is well promulgated.

B. Early intervention/treatment

1. **Methods.** The essentials of obtaining a good perinatal outcome include normalization of maternal blood glucose during the entire pregnancy, assessment of fetal well-being throughout pregnancy, and assurance of fetal maturity prior to delivery.

   a. Known diabetes prior to pregnancy

   (1) Preconception counseling. Counseling must be included for all women being managed for diabetes to ensure understanding of maternal and perinatal risks as well as to normalize blood glucose levels in the early weeks of pregnancy.

   (2) Diabetes management. Women at risk for pregnancy who are being managed with an oral hypoglycemic agent should be switched to insulin therapy and diet appropriate for pregnancy prior to conception to minimize risks to the fetus. While the issue of teratogenesis with oral drugs remains debatable, the quality of blood glucose control that is required in pregnancy is not obtainable with oral agents. Furthermore, neonatal hypoglycemia has been reported with some of these agents.

   The diabetic woman should receive essential education and should accomplish nutritional, psychosocial, and therapeutic milestones **prior** to initiation of pregnancy. A team approach to prepregnancy and intrapregnancy patient care improves pregnancy outcome.

   Hospitalization for blood glucose normalization is rarely necessary today when the pregnant woman is knowledgeable regarding diabetes and pregnancy. Adequate nutrition (a high-protein, relatively low-fat, high-fiber diet containing 1800–2200 cal with four or more feedings/day), split-dose insulin schedules, and self-assessments of blood glucose in the home utilizing a reflectance meter are the mainstays of maternal management.

   Ambulatory self-monitoring of blood glucose, compared to laboratory-based assessments with frequent hospitalizations, has an average cost savings/pregnancy of approximately $80,000. The desirable blood glucose values are a fasting level of 60–100 mg/dl and a 1-hour postprandial level of $\leq$140 mg/dl. While a glycosolated hemoglobin (HbA_1) value may be obtained to assess the quality of recent blood glucose level, once normal blood glucose values are demonstrated by self-assessed blood samplings, no further HbA_1 determinations are warranted.

   Fetal assessments for anomalies (maternal serum alpha-fetoprotein screen at 16 weeks' gestation, serial ultrasonography), well-being (ultrasonography for growth and development, and fetal heart rhythm testing for placental insufficiency), and maturity (prior to elective delivery) should follow the recommendations of obstetric perinatal consultants. If local resources are lacking, consultation and referral should be sought.

b. Glucose intolerance discovered during prenatal care. Glucose intolerance responsive to initial nutritional intervention alone is followed as outlined in Table 9-3. When insulin therapy is required maternal and fetal assessments are the same as for the woman requiring insulin prior to conception.

2. Justification

a. Effectiveness. Appropriate management of women with glucose intolerance throughout the pregnancy can result in perinatal mortality rates no greater than presently pertain for all pregnancies in the United States [6, 10, 11]. Morbidity is also significantly decreased. For this to be accomplished, early (ideally prepregnancy) detection and appropriate consumer-provider actions are essential.

(1) Diabetes known prior to pregnancy. Counseling of women known to have abnormal blood glucose homeostasis in order to effect normal blood glucose homeostasis before conception has a remarkably favorable influence on the quality of pregnancy outcome. A normal HbA_1 value in the first 8 weeks of pregnancy is associated with the same perinatal outcomes as expected in normal pregnancies. Elevated HbA_1 levels, however, as still typically encountered in most insulin-requiring women in early pregnancy because of inappropriate preconceptual management, have an associated fivefold or greater increased risk for congenital abnormalities [12, 13].

Most of the complications attributable to diabetes later in gestation are also avoided when near euglycemic maternal blood glucose levels prevail.

(2) Pregnancy-induced glucose intolerance (gestational diabetes). The entire gamut of maternal and perinatal complications that occur in the pregnancy with PIGI is avoidable if the abnormal glucose tolerance is discovered and then appropriately managed. Unfortunately, 50–75% of pregnant women with this disorder go undetected because a screening procedure for glucose intolerance is not in place.

b. Risks. The risks of glucose control with nutritional intervention alone (PIGI, gestational diabetes) are negligible. The risk of using insulin for insulin-requiring diabetic women in the main is hypoglycemia for the mother and fetus. Although this complication is significant, the complication rates are low and are outweighed by the serious untoward perinatal sequelae of inadequately treated insulin-requiring diabetes in pregnancy.

c. Costs. Assuming a 75% savings of neonatal intensive care costs associated with diabetes-related perinatal complications when normalization of blood glucose homeostasis pertains throughout pregnancy, national savings are approximately $375 million/year [14].

III. Recommendations

A. Early detection

1. Women in the reproductive years with intact potential for pregnancy should be screened for abnormal glucose tolerance before pregnancy is initiated.
2. All pregnant women **not** known to be diabetic prior to pregnancy should have a 100-gm, 2-hour PPBG done at the time of initial prenatal screening.
3. Repeat 2-hour PPBG assessments should be done (see Table 9-3) in the woman having a plasma (or capillary blood) glucose value greater than 120 mg/dl at initial testing.
4. Pregnant women not known to be diabetic and not able to be screened as described above should have a 50-gm oral 1-hour PPBG determined, with the threshold for abnormal set at 140 mg/dl at 24–28 weeks' gestation.

B. Early intervention/treatment

1. Women discovered by screening to have abnormal glucose tolerance should be managed by initiation of appropriate diet and serial blood glucose testing (see Table 9-3).
2. Insulin-dependent women should be managed as follows:

a. With a diagnosis of diabetes mellitus comes the responsibility for a health care provider to impart to the woman the knowledge that normal blood glucose levels before initiation of pregnancy and during the first 8 weeks of the pregnancy significantly decrease the risk for congenital abnormalities in progeny.

b. Oral hypoglycemic agents should be avoided in women who may possibly become pregnant.
c. Blood glucose homeostasis should be normalized throughout the entire pregnancy employing appropriate diet and exercise regimens, split-dose insulin, and self-assessment of capillary blood glucose.
d. Fetal well-being and fetal maturity assessments are required in the group of women with abnormal glucose tolerance who require insulin therapy.

References

1. Mestman, J. H., Anderson, G. V., and Barton, P. Carbohydrate metabolism in pregnancy. A study of 658 patients with the use of the oral glucose tolerance test and the prednisolone glucose tolerance test. *Am. J. Obstet. Gynecol.* 109(1):41, 1971. *General review of carbohydrate metabolism in pregnancy.*
2. U.S. National Commission on Diabetes. *Report of the National Commission on Diabetes to the Congress of the United States.* Bethesda, MD: Dept. of Health, Education, and Welfare, 1976. *Definition of the risks of undetected glucose intolerance.*
3. Classification and diagnosis of diabetes mellitus and other categories of glucose intolerance. National Diabetes Data Group. *Diabetes* 28(12):1039, 1979. *Definitions of glucose intolerance, and testing guidelines and parameters.*
4. Lind, T. Metabolic changes in pregnancy relevant to diabetes mellitus. *Postgrad. Med. J.* 55(643): 353, 1979. *Metabolism, pregnancy, and diabetes.*
5. Fine, J. Glycosuria of pregnancy. *Br. J. Med.* 1(534):205, 1967. *Renal function in pregnancy related to glucose.*
6. Public health guidelines for enhancing diabetes control through maternal- and child-health programs. *M.M.W.R.* 35(13):201, 1986. *Good overview of public health prevention and complication issues.*
7. Schneider, J. M., and Curet, L. B. Obstetrical management of the pregnant diabetic. In J. W. Sciarra (ed.), *Gynecology and Obstetrics.* Philadelphia: Harper and Row, 1982. Pp. 1–32. *Practitioner review.*
8. Freinkel, N., et al. Gestational diabetes mellitus. *Diabetes* 34 (Suppl 2):1, 1985. *Advocacy for GTT.*
9. Barden, T. P., and Knowles, H. C. Jr. Diagnosis of diabetes in pregnancy. *Clin. Obstet. Gynecol.* 24(1):3, 1981. *Review of specificity and sensitivity of diagnostic procedures for diagnosis of diabetes in pregnancy.*
10. Schneider, J. M., et al. Ambulatory care of the pregnant diabetic. *Obstet. Gynecol.* 56(2):144, 1980. *Primer for ambulatory care of the insulin-dependent diabetic pregnant woman.*
11. Gabbe, S. F., et al. Management and outcome of pregnancy in diabetes mellitus, classes B to R. *Am. J. Obstet. Gynecol.* 129(7):723, 1977. *Practitioner review.*
12. Miller, E., et al. Elevated maternal hemoglobin A_{1C} in early pregnancy and major congenital anomalies in infants of diabetic mothers. *N. Engl. J. Med.* 304(22):1331, 1981. *Demonstrates the association between major congenital anomalies in infants of insulin-dependent diabetics with higher HbA_{1C} levels in the first trimester.*
13. Fuhrmann, K., et al. Prevention of congenital malformations in infants of insulin-dependent diabetic mothers. *Diabetes Care* 6(3):219, 1983. *Documentation of embryopathy with abnormal maternal blood glucose levels in early pregnancy.*
14. Scheffler, R., and Feuchtbaum, L. *Payment Issues and Options: California's Diabetes and Pregnancy Program.* Berkeley: Health Policy and Administration Program, University of California, 1986. (Supported by MCH Grant #85-86732, March 1986). *Cost-benefit analysis.*

Suggested Readings

Freinkel, N., Dooley, S. L., and Metzger, B. E. Care of the pregnant woman with insulin-dependent diabetes mellitus. *N. Engl. J. Med.* 313(2):96, 1985. *Practitioner review.*

Gabbe, S. G. Diabetes in pregnancy. *Clin. Obstet. Gynecol.* 28(3):455, 1985. *Practitioner review.*

Kivelowitz, T. S. *Diabetes: A Guide to Self-Management for Patients and their Families.* Englewood Cliffs, NJ: Prentice-Hall, 1981. *Client handbook.*

10 Urinary Tract Infections in Pregnancy

Gary K. Stewart

I. The problem

A. Definition. Urinary tract infection (UTI) in asymptomatic pregnant women was defined by Kass in 1960 as greater than 10^5 colonies of bacteria/ml of urine [1–4].

B. Description. Anatomic changes occur during pregnancy that contribute to the problem of urinary tract infections. Progesterone causes dilation of the ureters, while the enlarging uterus compresses them. Reflux and stasis increase the likelihood that asymptomatic bacteriuria (ABU) will become a symptomatic upper urinary tract infection. Because of the potential seriousness of UTI in pregnancy, early diagnosis and intervention are important. UTI in pregnancy can result in:

1. **Acute pyelonephritis.** One or two percent of all pregnant women develop acute pyelonephritis, which is a more serious illness in pregnancy than in the nonpregnant state because of the increased potential for developing septic shock (Schwartzman reaction). Long-term damage to renal function can result from these infections, and perhaps more important, treatment of asymptomatic bacteriuria in pregnancy will prevent acute pyelonephritis 70–80% of the time [5].
2. **Prematurity, low birth weight, fetal death, and infant mortality.** Nearly all investigators have found at least twice the risk of premature delivery in mothers who have bacteriuria; however, some have found the increase largely confined to those in whom infections are asymptomatic [2, 6, 7]. Additional maternal factors associated with urinary tract infection that might contribute to an increased risk of prematurity include elevated blood pressure, lowered plasma volume, and low body weight. In several series, the rate of prematurity could be effectively reduced by treatment of the bacteriuric woman but never to the level of the uninfected control group [2]. Bacteriuria tends to occur early rather than late in pregnancy, but this does not appear to be a finding of sufficient magnitude to skew statistics on prematurity.

   Infant mortality was increased threefold among bacteriuria mothers [6] while the fetal mortality rate was increased 2.4 times [6]. Low birth weight as another independent variable has been seen to be increasing among pregnant UTI patients [3, 4, 7, 8].

   Since there is a relatively low incidence of both bacteriuria and these adverse fetal effects, significant results require a large number of patients in any study. No such ideal study exists. Even so, it seems unlikely that asymptomatic bacteriuria contributes greatly to these problems, although any such contribution is amenable to preventive measures.
3. **Anemia.** Some studies have shown an association between bacteriuria and maternal anemia [9]. Treating the bacteriuric patients with antibiotics early in pregnancy prevented the development of anemia.
4. **Chronic renal disease.** The effect of bacteriuria during pregnancy on subsequent renal function has not been clarified. One study reported a high incidence of recurrent UTIs (20–50%) 2–4 years later, with higher rates in those with antibiotic-resistant organisms [5, 10, 11, 12]. Thirty-seven percent had abnormal intravenous pyelograms, and 10–15% of bacteriuric pregnant women are destined to have evidence of chronic pyelonephritis 10 years after delivery [12]. Certainly, this group of patients is at higher risk for infections in subsequent pregnancies.
5. **Hypertension.** In one study there was a twofold to fourfold increase in the incidence of hypertension in women with bacteriuria as compared to women without bacteriuria [2]. Some of the hypertension seemed to be reversible with antibiotic treatment. But, does treatment of bacteriuria prevent development of

increased blood pressure and its associated morbidity? There is presently no definite answer to that question.

6. **Hyperthermia.** Animal studies have shown heat to be an antimitotic teratogenic factor. The impact on morphogenesis is greater in the central nervous system during the early stages of development. A number of articles have appeared relating these findings to humans [13, 14]. Pyelonephritis is often associated with a significant temperature elevation, and although there are no studies to clarify the impact of lowering the temperature on maternal and infant morbidity and mortality, preventing febrile UTIs seems prudent.

C. **Epidemiology.** There is a 2.5–11% prevalence of asymptomatic bacteriuria in pregnant women, depending on parity, age, and socioeconomic status [1–4, 8]. Twenty to 30% of these women will develop pyelonephritis later in pregnancy if not treated. Early diagnosis and treatment can reduce this rate to 2–5% [2–4, 8, 9]. Women at higher risk for developing ABU and UTI during pregnancy include those with:

1. Advanced age.
2. Increased parity.
3. Lower socioeconomic status.
4. History of previous UTI.
5. Increased frequency of sexual intercourse.
6. Sickle trait.

II. **Secondary prevention.** It seems clear that urinary tract infections can be related to medical problems for the woman, for the pregnancy, and for the newborn. Prevention of many of these problems is possible.

A. **Early detection**

1. **Methods and test characteristics.** A carefully obtained (perineal antiseptic washing by patient with labia spread) midstream urine collection is recommended for screening purposes. Ideally, the urine should be evaluated and cultured immediately. Either prompt evaluation (within 30 minutes) or refrigeration at 4° C until it can be cultured is important to avoid a false or spurious high colony count.

   a. **Pour plate culture.** The standard against which all UTI screening tests must be measured is the pour plate culture. It is generally accepted that a count of greater than 100,000 bacteria/ml in a clean catch urine is diagnostic of UTI in an asymptomatic individual. Although the original work by Kass required two positive cultures to confirm the diagnosis of infection, current clinical application requires only one. If a count lies between 10,000 and 100,000, infection may be present, particularly in a symptomatic woman. Infections definitely exist with bacterial counts under 10,000, but these constitute a small minority and do not lend themselves to detection by screening. Since the ordinary pour plate culture seems too cumbersome and costly for screening, the following methods are evaluated [15, 16, 17]:

   b. **Proteinuria.** Determination of urinary protein correlates poorly with bacteriuria.

   c. **Pyuria.** Although the number of white cells in the urine commonly increases in the presence of infection, this is not uniformly true [15, 17]. False positives numbered 8–15% in one series [18], and 18% in another [19]. False negatives seem to depend on the severity of the infection but may approach 50%. Hence, pyuria alone is a particularly poor criterion for screening asymptomatic individuals. Using combinations of pyuria screening and miniature cultures is recommended by some but seems most likely to be useful in the **symptomatic,** nonpregnant patient.

   d. **Bacteriuria.** Gram's stain, methylene blue, and unstained examination of unspun urine have the advantage of utilizing existing supplies and personnel; when other methods are not available, these can be very helpful. False negatives are found in up to 10%, and false positives amount to about 25%, necessitating reexamination.

   e. **Miniature cultures.** Many investigators have felt that there is no substitute for actual culture of urine specimens, and several commercialized methods have been marketed to simplify these. All rely on small cultures of a small quantity of urine, such as might be absorbed on a length of filter paper. Colony counts are made and the specimen designated as positive, negative, or doubtful, depending on the number of colonies. Excellent results have been reported from most investigators.

   f. **Other.** A number of other tests have been developed and marketed in an attempt to simplify the screening procedures. These include the **Greiss nitrate test, catalase disc flotation, triphenyl tetrazolium test,** and the **quantitative glucose** test. They lack the reliability of the **miniature culture** tests, and therefore need not be considered here.

2. **Justification.** Based on this review, the miniculture tests are reliable and of acceptable cost. There are three components to the expense involved: personnel, permanent equipment, and expendable supplies. Reported estimates are, respectively, $0.75, $0.25, and $0.50 per individual test. Obviously, the cost of personnel is not only the largest cost but also the one most subject to variation, depending on the size of the group studied and the manner in which the screening can be integrated with other services. The cost-benefit ratio of preventing acute pyelonephritis in pregnancy by screening for bacteria shows it is highly beneficial.

B. Early intervention

1. **Methods.** Ideally, antibiotic treatment should be tailored to the specific organism causing the infection. In some of the simpler screening tests, specific organism identification may not be done, and in other cases treatment needs to be initiated before culture results are finalized.

   One must remember that all antibiotics cannot and should not be used during pregnancy. Suggested oral antimicrobial agents for initiating treatment of **asymptomatic** bacteriuria before specific cultures are available include:

   a. Amoxicillin/ampicillin 250–500 mg q6h.
   b. Nitrofurantoin 50–100 mg q6h.
   c. Sulfisoxazole 1–2 gm/day q6h (not recommended in third trimester).
   d. Cephalexin 500 mg q6h.

   These are consensus recommendations, but none of the medications are unequivocally authorized for use in pregnancy by the Food and Drug Administration. All medications are recommended to be given for 5–10 days. Although prolonged treatment has been advocated by some, control studies have not demonstrated any significant benefit beyond the conventional course of 10 days. Some recent reports have found that single-dose antibiotic treatment may be desirable in the nonpregnant woman; however, the failure rate during pregnancy is unacceptably high. Only about 20–30% of patients with chronic [4, 6, 8] infections remain free from significant bacteriuria after cessation of treatment, regardless of the type or duration of therapy. Some recurrences are due to the same species and strain of the microorganism that was present before treatment (relapse), whereas in others a new pathogen appears (reinfection). Any patient with recurrent or resistant UTI should have a thorough urologic investigation. Eleven percent of women will acquire bacteriuria after the initial prenatal screening, giving rise to the possible value of obtaining a second culture.

   If the patient has acute pyelonephritis, she should be hospitalized and treated with parenteral antibiotics and other supportive measures.

2. **Justification**

   a. **Effectiveness.** Treatment of ABU in pregnancy will prevent its progression to acute pyelonephritis 70–80% of the time.
   b. **Risk and side effects.** The treatment of a pregnant woman with the aforementioned group of drugs would appear to be without any fetal risks. Certainly, there **are** risks to **not** treating UTIs, as already noted. The possibility of maternal drug effects is always present—from gastritis to allergic reactions—but at no greater risk than in the nonpregnant state.
   c. **Costs and acceptability.** Various cost-benefit studies have been done using numbers based on others' experience, with nearly universal acceptance of the value of this approach. Cost and acceptability will vary with volume and with the efficiency of the system. In general, patients can easily provide the specimen, and in a well-organized lab the screening can be cheaply performed. Clearly, the most difficult task is setting up the protocols for **treatment** and follow-up.

III. Recommendations. Because of the documented seriousness of untreated ABU and the effectiveness of early detection and intervention, the following is advised:

A. Early detection

1. A clean catch midstream urine specimen is obtained on all prenatal patients as soon as pregnancy is identified.
2. A simple miniculture estimation of colony count is obtained. This can be organized in the office setting. Those cultures with greater than 100,000 colonies/ml should have a specific organism identified, if possible.

B. Early intervention

1. Those patients with a positive culture are treated with one of the previously noted antibiotics for 10 days.
2. Two weeks following treatment of bacteriuria, another culture is obtained.
    a. Positive cultures are again treated according to the culture results.
    b. Negative cultures are repeated again in the third trimester.
3. Those patients with an infection during pregnancy should have a repeat culture at one month postpartum.
4. After being treated for acute pyelonephritis, suppressive therapy should be instituted for the remainder of the pregnancy.
5. Those patients with recurrent bacteriuria should have an intravenous pyelogram (IVP) 3–6 months after delivery.

References

1. Kass, E. H. (ed.). *Progress in Pyelonephritis.* Philadelphia: Davis, 1965. *Many contributors, including E. H. Kass, K. L. Stuart, P. Kincaid-Smith, C. W. Norden, W. H. Kilpatric, M. Henderson, and P. Whalley; discussions on bacteriuria in pregnancy, pyelonephritis in pregnancy, and prematurity.*
2. Kass, E. H. Bacteriuria and pyelonephritis of pregnancy. *Arch. Intern. Med.* 105:194, 1960. *Original classic study showing relationship.*
3. Sweet, R. L. Bacteriuria and pyelonephritis during pregnancy. *Semin. Perinatal.* 1(1):25, 1977. *Excellent review and bibliography (122 references) with recommendations.*
4. Norden, C. W., and Kass, E. H. Bacteriuria of pregnancy—a critical appraisal. *Annu. Rev. Med.* 19:431, 1968. *A comprehensive review with bibliography.*
5. Zinner, S. H., and Kass, E. H. Long-term (10–14 years) follow-up of bacteriuria of pregnancy. *N. Engl. J. Med.* 285(15):820, 1971. *Good documentation and follow-up of a number of maternal abnormalities associated with bacteriuria.*
6. McGrady, G. A., Daling, J. R., and Peterson, D. R. Maternal urinary tract infections and adverse fetal outcomes. *Am. J. Epidemiol.* 121(3):377, 1985. *Review of birth certificate data from the state of Washington, 1981–1982. Good statistical study.*
7. Naeye, R. L. Causes of the excessive rates of perinatal mortality and prematurity in pregnancies complicated by maternal urinary tract infections. *N. Engl. J. Med.* 300(15):819, 1979. *This epidemiologic review of perinatal mortality confirmed a positive relationship with maternal urinary tract infection and indicated that the accompanying metabolic and other medical conditions were the direct causes of death.*
8. Kass, E. H. The role of asymptomatic bacteriuria in the pathogenesis of pyelonephritis. In E. L. Quinn and E. H. Kass (eds.), *Biology of Pyelonephritis.* Boston: Little, Brown, 1960. Pp. 399–412. *An outline of the evidence for Kass's observations of a maternal and fetal abnormality among patients with bacteriuria, and evidence of the value of prevention.*
9. Giles, C., and Brown, J. A. H. Urinary infection and anemia in pregnancy. *Br. Med. J.* 2(Suppl 5296):10, 1962. *Bacteriuria identified in a group of anemia patients whose hemoglobin improved after treatment of bacteriuria.*
10. Williams, J. D., et al. The treatment of bacteriuria in pregnant women with sulfamethazole and trimethoprion: A biological, clinical and toxicological study. *Postgrad. Med. J.* (Suppl) 45:71, 1969. *Treatment and follow-up of a group of antenatal patients looking at persistent infection and pregnancy outcome.*
11. Leigh, D. A., Gruneberg, R. N., and Brumfitt, W. Long-term follow-up of bacteriuria in pregnancy. *Lancet* 1(7543):603, 1968. *Confirmed that there was a significant persistence of bacteriuria after treatment, as well as correlated with other long-term maternal effects.*
12. Gruneberg, R. N., Leigh, D. A., and Brumfitt, W. Relationship of bacteriuria in pregnancy to acute pyelonephritis, prematurity, and fetal mortality. *Lancet* 2:7610, 1969. *Epidemiologic review of follow-up of 8907 antenatal patients.*
13. Smith, D. W., Clarren, S. K., and Harvey, M. A. S. Hyperthermia as a possible teratogenic agent. *J. Pediatr.* 92(6):878, 1978. *Review of a small number of cases with a defined syndrome was related to early prenatal hyperthermia.*
14. Miller, P., Smith, D. W., and Shepard, T. H. Maternal hyperthermia as a possible cause of anencephaly. *Lancet* 1(8063):519, 1978. *Implications of fever interfering with anterior neural-groove closure was given in a significant number of cases of anencephalic mothers.*
15. Latham, R. H., et al. Laboratory diagnosis of urinary tract infection in ambulatory women. *J.A.M.A.* 254(23):3333, 1985. *Excellent review of laboratory screening methods and estimates of cost effectiveness in screening.*

16. Stamey, T. A., and Pfau, A. Urinary infections: A selective review and some observations. *Cal. Med.* 113(6):16, 1970. *Good general review.*
17. Brumfitt, W., and Reeves, D. S. Screening procedures for urinary infection. In C. L. E. H. Sharp and H. Keen (eds.). *Presymptomatic Detection and Early Diagnosis: An Initial Appraisal.* Baltimore: Williams & Wilkins, 1968. *As described.*
18. Lam, C. N., et al. Pyuria and bacteriuria. *Arch. Dis. Child.* 42:275, 1967. *As described.*
19. Pryles, C. V., and Eliot, C. R. Pyuria and bacteriuria in infants and children. *Am. J. Dis. Child.* 110:628, 1965. *As described.*

11 Anemia in Pregnancy

Gary K. Stewart

I. The problem

A. Definition. As seen in Table 11-1, there is a variation in the mean hemoglobin/hematocrit (Hgb/Hct) in pregnancy, and thus a meaningful, precise definition of anemia in pregnancy is difficult. Most physicians would agree that a pregnant woman with a Hgb below 10 gm% or a Hct less than 30% would be considered anemic.

B. Description. The risks associated with anemia have been markedly diminished with the improvement of medical care and advancement in technologies. Anemia and the problems associated with it occur less frequently now in the developed world because of routine supplementation with iron and folic acid, the availability of food supplements for the poor, the availability of blood, the effectiveness of antibiotics, and the advent of perinatal and neonatal experts. Anemia in pregnancy is still a major problem in third world countries.

Anemia increases the mortality of pregnant women, particularly at delivery when the reserve against blood loss is decreased and in the postpartum period when the likelihood and severity of postpartum infection is increased. Although the risk to the fetus is harder to prove, increased risk of premature labor, fetal distress, perinatal death, and an association with certain speech, learning, and behavioral problems in children have been implicated [1].

There are a host of hematologic disorders—some very rare—that the pregnant woman may develop or already have. Table 11-2 lists some of the more common types of anemia and classifies them into subgroups based on the anemia's amenability to primary prevention.

The principal anemias of pregnancy are iron-deficiency anemia, folate deficiency, and sickle cell anemia. These first two types will be discussed in this chapter. The reader is referred to Chap. 14 for a discussion of sickle cell anemia.

Pregnancy produces increased stress on the transport and production of hemoglobin in the pregnant woman (see Table 11-1). In addition, there is a marked increase in blood volume, which is the result of a number of factors, including:

1. The A-V shunt phenomenon occurring secondary to the placental action.
2. Response to aldosterone and placental lactogen.
3. Increased erythropoietin activity.

To meet these demands, the pregnant woman is required to have a well-functioning hemopoietic system with adequate nutritive supplies (see Chap. 3). There is also general agreement in the United States that supplemental iron and folic acid are needed for optimal pregnancy management.

Iron-Deficiency Anemia

I. The problem

A. Definition. The most common type of anemia occurring in pregnancy (and certainly the most well known) is characterized by hypochromic microcytic red blood cells, low or absent iron stores, low serum iron concentration, low transferrin saturation, elevated serum transferrin, and low serum ferritin.

B. Description and epidemiology. Iron is an important element in the human body. About two-thirds of the body's iron is incorporated into hemoglobin.

The normal woman has a substantial loss of iron each month through menstruation, so her body stores must be constantly replaced by dietary intake. The absorption of iron by the intestinal epithelium is poorly understood, but it is clear that iron clearance is limited to a 10-20% of the amount of iron intake.

Table 11-1. Changes in blood volume during pregnancy

	Pre-pregnancy	First trimester	Second trimester	Third trimester	Postpartum (30 days)	Postpartum (31–70 days)
Total blood volume (ml)	3945	4038	4731	5210	4200	4062
Plasma volume (ml)	2474	2671	3186	3569	2659	2601
Red cell mass (ml)	1488	1408	1410	1716	1395	1486
Hematocrit (%)	39.3	36.1	33.4	33.8	35.5	37.6

Source: R. D. Lange and R. Dynesius. Blood volume changes during pregnancy. *Clin. Haematol.* 2(3): 433, 1973.

Table 11-2. Classification and causes of anemia during pregnancy

Acquired/preventable	Acquired/not preventable	Hereditary
Iron deficiency	Physiologic dilution	Thalassemia
Folate deficiency	Aplastic anemia	Sickle cell anemia
Infection	Systemic disease	Sickle cell—hemoglobin C
Hemolytic anemia		Sickle cell—thalassemia
		Homologous hemoglobin C
		Other hemoglobinopathies
		Hemolytic anemias without hemoglobinopathies

Table 11-3. Iron need with pregnancy

	Average need (mg)
Fetal iron (75 mg/kg body wt)	280
Placenta and cord	75
Expansion of red cell mass (1 mg/ml of red cells)	300
Total additional iron requirements during pregnancy	655 (subtotal)
Blood loss due to delivery (0.5 mg/ml of blood)	250
Lactation (6 mo)	150
Total iron loss following pregnancy	400 (subtotal)
Total pregnancy-related iron requirement	1055

The average American diet contains 6 mg of iron/1000 cal consumed. An average woman takes in approximately 2000 cal/day—12 mg of iron—but absorbs only 10% of that, or 1.2 mg. Combined with the amount of iron lost daily through the skin and mucous membranes (1 mg), this provides very little iron to meet the needs of pregnancy. As shown in Table 11-3 (excluding the requirements of delivery and lactation), the daily average iron requirement for pregnancy is approximately 2.5 mg, and when combined with the body's ongoing nonpregnant requirements for iron, this figure amounts to 4.0 mg/day. This demand varies with the duration of the pregnancy, increasing as gestation advances to reach approximately 6 mg/day in the third trimester.

This picture is painted with the knowledge that many women begin pregnancy with very low or totally absent stores of iron. Iron-deficiency anemia is also common in nonpregnant women, primarily because of the iron loss associated with menstru-

Table 11-4. Iron preparations

Oral preparation	Salt	Elemental iron
Ferrous sulphate* (tablets) (20% elemental Fe)	195 mg 300 mg 325 mg	39 mg 60 mg 65 mg
Ferrous sulphate syrup	40 mg/ml	8 mg/ml
Ferrous sulphate oral solution	125 mg/ml	25 mg/ml
Ferrous fumarate (35% elemental Fe)	200 mg	66 mg
Ferrous gluconate (12% elemental Fe)	320 mg	60 mg

*Ferrous sulphate elixir also available.

ation (approximately 30 mg/menses). Ten percent or more of the nonpregnant female population may be iron deficient. Scott and Pritchard [2] found that as much as 24% of the nonpregnant population have no iron stores. It is not surprising, then, that 90-95% of anemias in pregnancy originate from iron deficiency.

II. Primary prevention

A. Methods

1. **Pregnancy screening, health education, and nutritional counseling and assessment** are key elements in assisting women to arrive for prenatal care with adequate iron stores and good nutritional habits and information.
2. **Iron prophylaxis.** To prevent iron-deficiency anemia in pregnancy, the recommended prophylactic dose is 60 mg elemental iron daily [3], which may be given bid in smaller amounts to decrease gastrointestinal symptoms. Available oral iron preparations are noted in Table 11-4.

   It is essential that the coating of the iron tablet dissolves quickly in the stomach; therefore, enteric-coated tablets are not useful. Ascorbic acid may increase the absorption of iron as much as 30%, but this increased absorption is associated with a significant increase in side effects of the iron. Therefore, the usefulness of this practice may be limited. When taken on an empty stomach, iron absorption is increased.

B. Justification/costs/risks/acceptability. See Chap. 3.

III. Secondary prevention

A. Early detection

1. **Methods**
   - **a.** An initial hemoglobin or hematocrit is performed on all prenatal patients. Those with a hemoglobin of less than 10% or a hematocrit of less than 30% require further evaluation.
   - **b.** An evaluation of red blood cell indices is recommended for all patients with a hemoglobin of less than 10 gm% or a hematocrit of less than 30% in the first trimester. Iron-deficiency patients have red blood cell indices showing a hypochromic microcytic picture.
   - **c.** A reticulocyte count is ordered on all anemic patients and is usually normal (not elevated) in patients with iron deficiency.
   - **d.** Serum iron may be decreased and the total iron binding capacity (TIBC) is increased (% saturation—Fe/TIBC $<16\%$).
   - **e.** Serum ferritin levels are decreased (<10 mg/ml).
   - **f.** Bone marrow iron stores are markedly diminished.
2. **Justification**
   - **a.** Initial hemoglobin screening by either hemoglobin or hematocrit is a standard prenatal procedure that has long been recognized as a simple, inexpensive (approximately $5), and reproducible test that is well accepted by patients. Hemoglobin screening is usually accomplished at the time phlebotomy is done for other prenatal laboratory procedures and has minimal risks that are associated primarily with pain, discomfort, and minor infection.
   - **b.** Red blood cell indices offer a simple, objective, mechanical interpretation of the size and density of the red blood cell. It is a standard hematologic measurement used to assist in determining the type and cause of anemia, is in-

expensive (usually part of the cost of the complete blood count test), requires little time (most often done by computerized lab counting chambers), and is acceptable to patients, because once the blood is drawn, it requires no further interaction on their part. It has limitations in terms of interpretation inasmuch as there are occasional other diagnoses that may also be hypochromic microcytic, such as anemias associated with chronic disease (e.g., rheumatoid arthritis) or thalassemia.

c. The reticulocyte count assists in determining if there is an increased production of red blood cells. Although usually normal in iron-deficiency anemia the reticulocyte count will increase once iron therapy is undertaken and absorption occurs. This test is inexpensive ($5–10) and well accepted (it can be done with venipuncture and has few complications associated with its use).

d. The serum iron is determined from blood obtained from a venipuncture (cost is $16–20) and is a standard test to diagnose iron-deficiency anemia. It is nearly always accompanied by the TIBC, which gives further objective evidence of iron deficiency.

e. Serum ferritin levels are generally diminished in patients with iron-deficiency anemia. This measurement parallels the measurement of body iron stores, otherwise accessible only by more invasive techniques (i.e., bone marrow aspiration). Serum ferritin levels are measured from blood collection, thus necessitating phlebotomy (but can be obtained when taking some of the above tests), and is not very expensive ($38–40).

f. Bone marrow studies are rarely needed to diagnose and manage patients with iron-deficiency anemia. The cost ($90–100) and the potential complications of bleeding, hematoma formations, and pain and discomfort, make it a procedure that should be used only in unusual circumstances for patients with iron-deficiency anemia.

B. Early intervention

1. Methods

a. **Oral iron therapy.** If iron deficiency is established, a therapeutic dose of a simple iron salt is recommended—typically 300 mg of ferrous sulphate or ferrous gluconate tid (see Table 11-4).

b. **Parenteral iron therapy.** Intramuscular and intravenous iron preparations are available for instances where oral therapy is contraindicated, or when oral therapy fails and the anemia is moderate to severe.

c. **Dietary adjustments** may assist patients in increasing the total amount of iron presented to the gastrointestinal tract for absorption.

d. **Medical or surgical treatment** may be necessary for other disease processes that may be causing iron deficiency, i.e. chronic blood loss from parasitic or other intestinal loss or nonabsorption of iron.

2. Justification

a. **Oral iron therapy** is very effective. Although the amount absorbed will be less if taken with or after meals, doing so will significantly increase compliance. The principal side effect is maternal gastrointestinal irritation. Constipation also can be bothersome and may require use of a stool softener. The cost of ferrous sulphate ($FeSO_4$) is $1–3/100 tablets. Incidentally, slow-release iron preparations are often marketed to decrease gastrointestinal irritability but seem to vary greatly in their absorption and are quite costly.

Of particular note, fatal childhood poisoning secondary to ingestion of iron is well known and should be made clear to patients.

b. **Parenteral iron therapy** is very effective in restoring body iron stores, and if normal gastrointestinal absorption is available, it is as fast and effective in restoring hemoglobin levels. Parenteral therapy carries a definite, although low, risk of anaphylaxis and death, as well as a number of unpleasant side effects from skin discoloration and nausea and vomiting to pain and discomfort. Because this therapy may require hematologist supervision and intravenous administration, a course of therapy may cost as much as $200.

c. **Dietary adjustments** are effective in assisting certain patients but are almost always inadequate to meet full iron replacement needs. Because there is little risk or cost, and nutritional education is acceptable and desirable from a patient's perspective, this recommendation is easy to implement.

d. Clearly, if there is excess iron loss **or** inadequate iron absorption, identification and treatment is needed to discover whether the iron deficiency is a symptom of something significant requiring medical or surgical intervention, or if it is related to a less substantial disorder, such as hookworms, which is simple and inexpensive to diagnose and treat. More sophisticated evaluation may be required to diagnose an intestinal polyp, a bleeding ulcer, or other disorders. The cost and acceptability, therefore, will vary [4].

IV. Recommendations

A. Primary prevention

1. All patients should have prepregnancy education and screening to ensure adequate iron stores when pregnancy occurs.
2. Every prenatal patient should receive at least 60 mg of elemental iron daily throughout the pregnancy.

B. Secondary prevention

1. A Hgb or Hct should be performed at the first prenatal visit.
2. Those patients who are anemic should have their type of anemia diagnosed.
3. If a patient is suspected of having iron-deficiency anemia, 300 mg of ferrous sulphate tid should be provided.
4. A reticulocyte count should be obtained 2 weeks later, or a repeat Hgb/Hct 1 month later.
5. If no response is noted, further evaluation is required.

Anemia Secondary to Folic Acid Deficiency

I. The problem

A. Definition. Folic acid deficiency causes a macrocytic, megaloblastic anemia.

B. Description. Pregnancy exerts an increased demand for folic acid, which is required for all normal cellular metabolism. Folic acid comes from external sources such as leafy green vegetables, fruit, muscle, and liver, to name a few. The body's ability to store folate is limited to a small amount (sufficient for only a few months). Of some note is the fact that some drugs (diphenylhydantoin, oral contraceptives, and pyrimethamine) can interfere with folate metabolism and facilitate the development of this type of anemia.

C. Epidemiology. Folic acid deficiency in pregnancy varies from 0.5%–1.5% in the United States [5] and is the second most common cause of anemia in pregnancy. Fifty percent of these anemias are diagnosed during the pregnancy and 50% are diagnosed during the puerperium. Etiology may be traced to defects in ingestion and absorption, defects in utilization and metabolism, increased demand, and inadequate ingestion. Although caloric intake may be adequate in pregnancy, the substandard quality of foodstuffs may be the primary reason for folic acid deficiency (see Chap. 3).

II. Primary prevention

A. Methods

1. Prepregnancy screening, health education, and nutritional counseling and assessment are key elements in assisting women to arrive for prenatal care with adequate folate stores and good nutritional habits and information. Supplemental feeding and early nutrition also assist in this effort.
2. Folic acid prophylaxis (300–400 IU of folic acid) taken daily through at least 6 weeks postpartum will prevent this problem from occurring.

B. Justification (see Chap. 3). Folic acid supplementation costs approximately $4 for each pregnancy—or at a 1% deficiency rate in pregnancy, approximately $400 to prevent one episode of folic acid deficiency. If tests to determine serum folate levels would identify one in approximately five patients as folic acid deficient, at $20 per test, the cost of supplementation would be $100, excluding the expense of the routine prophylactic use of iron to which the folic acid-deficient patient would not respond. In spite of considerable support recommending routine folic acid supplementation in the United States, the cost-benefit of this practice is questionable.

III. Secondary prevention

A. Methods of early detection. Folic acid deficiency in pregnancy may be diagnosed by:

1. Symptoms of anorexia, nausea, vomiting, edema, and occasionally, jaundice and proteinuria.
2. Blood smear showing hypersegmentation of neutrophil nuclei and macrocytosis.
3. Decreased serum folate levels.
4. Bone marrow smear showing confirmation of megaloblastic anemia.

B. Justification for early detection

1. Signs and symptoms are unreliable in detecting folate deficiency anemia but can assist in pointing out those patients who might require evaluation. There is no risk in the review except that it has little specificity. There are few costs beyond those of routine assessment.
2. The blood smear in megaloblastic anemia will present a different diagnosis with B_{12} deficiency that is easily resolved with a serum folate level (see sec. **III.B. 3**) or a serum B_{12} determination. The blood smear has been a key for grouping patients into diagnostic categories. It is inexpensive ($10), easy to perform, and requires only a venipuncture; therefore, it has minimal risks and is very acceptable.
3. Serum folate levels are simple tests that cost $37–51, are easy to perform, and provide a specific, accurate result. A venipuncture is required with attendant minimal risks—the only negative item regarding the test's acceptability.
4. Bone marrow aspirates are rarely required to establish a diagnosis of folic acid deficiency or to confirm the specific etiology of a megaloblastic anemia. Because of the cost, pain, and risk, a bone marrow study is not a very acceptable procedure.

IV. Recommendations

A. Primary prevention

1. All patients should have prepregnancy education and screening to ensure adequate folate stores when pregnancy occurs.
2. Every prenatal patient should receive at least 400 mg of folic acid daily during pregnancy and for at least 6 weeks postpartum.

B. Secondary prevention

1. A Hgb or Hct should be performed at the first prenatal visit.
2. Those patients who are anemic should have their type of anemia diagnosed.
3. A suspicion of folic acid deficiency should be confirmed by a serum folate level.
4. Treatment consists of at least 1 mg/day of folic acid—either parenterally or orally.
5. Response to treatment should be followed. If no response is noted, further hematologic evaluation is required.

Overall Recommendations

Two of the more common anemias encountered in pregnancy have been discussed here. There are clearly many other types of anemia. Although there is a general assumption made here that anemia is bad, this assumption must be tempered with the following facts.

The marked change in plasma volume may make the use of Hgb and Hct somewhat limited as an indicator of maternal or fetal outcome in pregnancy. While the measurement of blood volume is a **better indicator** of potential problems, the risk/benefit ratio does not justify its routine use at this time, due to the cost and difficulty of such analysis.

Most important for clinicians to note when evaluating the hemoglobin-hematocrit value is whether or not it is **high**. A decreased plasma volume (which may be reflected in an elevated Hgb-Hct) has a high association with high-risk pregnancies, e.g., preeclampsia and eclampsia, fetal growth retardation, fetal death, and diabetes. Standards for the upper limits of Hgb measurement have not been established, so relative guidelines will have to be established individually.

I. Primary prevention

A. Prepregnancy screening, health education, and nutritional counseling and assessment are key elements in assisting women to arrive for prenatal care with adequate folic acid and iron stores and with good nutritional habits and information.

B. Supplemental feeding and early nutrition will also assist in this effort:

1. Folic acid supplementation: 400 mg daily through the pregnancy until at least 6 weeks postpartum.
2. Iron supplementation: 60 mg of elemental iron daily throughout the pregnancy until 6 weeks postpartum.

C. Obtain hemoglobin (or hematocrit) routinely.

1. First trimester: at first prenatal visit (to detect existing anemia).
2. Twenty-eight weeks' gestation (to detect anemia developing in pregnancy).
3. Thirty-six weeks' gestation (to verify adequate predelivery hemoglobin).
4. Two days' postpartum (to determine blood loss).
5. Six weeks' postpartum (to verify return to normal Hgb status).

D. Obtain history of familial anemias.
E. Perform laboratory screening hemoglobin electrophoresis for hemoglobinopathies, where family history indicates.
F. When anemias are detected, determine the type of anemia and treat as indicated.

References

1. McFee, J. G. Anemia in pregnancy—a reappraisal. *Obstet. Gynecol. Surv.* 28(11):769, 1973. *Excellent general review.*
2. Scott, D. E., and Pritchard, J. A. Iron deficiency in healthy young college women. *J.A.M.A.* 199(12):897, 1967. *Classic study evaluating iron stores in women.*
3. American College of Obstetricians and Gynecologists. *Assessment of Maternal Nutrition.* Washington, DC: ACOG, 1978 (revised 1982). *Recommendations for dietary and supplementary nutrition during antepartum, postpartum, lactating, and interconceptual periods.*
4. Goodlin, R. C. Why treat "physiologic" anemias of pregnancy. *J. Reprod. Med.* 27(10):639, 1982. *Provocative review arguing against aggressive treatment of "physiologic mid-trimester anemia."*
5. Kitay, D. Z. Folic acid deficiency in pregnancy. *Am. J. Obstet. Gynecol.* 104(7):1067, 1969. *Extensive review of subject, particularly emphasizing pathophysiology.*
6. Lange, R. D., and Dynesius, R. Blood volume changes during pregnancy. *Clin. Haematol.* 2(3):433, 1973. *This review of many studies is an excellent source of basic work on this subject.*

12 Isoimmunization

Hanns C. Haesslein

ABO Isoimmunization

I. The problem

A. Description. In blood group (ABO) incompatibility, the mother produces complement-binding anti-A or anti-B antibody, which causes fetal red cell hemolysis, is never severe enough to cause hydrops, and usually results in mild fetal anemia at birth. The reasons for this mild effect are: (1) the small number of A or B antigenic sites on fetal red cells, (2) the multitude of A and B antigen sites in the fetus that are not on the red cell (other tissues, secretions), and (3) the majority of anti-A and anti-B is IgM and does not cross the placenta.

The baby of an ABO incompatible couple (35% of the population) has a 25–30% risk that its cord blood sample will be direct antiglobulin positive (positive direct Coombs' test). Many of these infants will require phototherapy, but they will rarely require exchange transfusions. However, failure to detect and treat ABO incompatibility-caused hyperbilirubinemia can lead to kernicterus.

B. Epidemiology. Approximately 35% of marriages are ABO incompatible (wife O and husband A or B, or wife A or B with husband AB). About 25–30% of their children will have evidence of isoimmunization, with a positive direct Coombs' test.

II. Secondary prevention

A. Early detection

1. Methods

a. Direct Coombs' testing. All pregnant women should have blood type, Rh, and antibodies determined at the first prenatal visit. The blood type should be determined on the infant's cord blood immediately after birth, and direct Coombs' testing should be done when ABO incompatibility exists or if the infant has a type O mother.

b. Serum bilirubin. After obtaining a weakly positive or positive direct antiglobulin test (direct Coombs' test), serum bilirubin should be obtained from the newborn infant and repeated in 24 hours. If levels greater than 12–14 mg/dl are reached with a rapid rise, phototherapy may need to be initiated, with total bilirubin levels repeated q8h.

It should be noted that elevated cord blood bilirubin levels do not accurately predict high ultimate serum levels. Usually severe hyperbilirubinemia does **not** occur, but levels of 18–20 mg/dl can be reached in the second day of life. These levels warrant repeating testing in an otherwise healthy infant in 6–8 hours. If levels above 20 mg/dl are reached, exchange transfusion may be indicated.

2. Justification. Blood group, antibody, and bilirubin testing are routine practices in prenatal and newborn care. They are relatively inexpensive tests with good reliability and are easy to perform.

B. Early intervention

1. Methods. Phototherapy and exchange transfusions are indicated in infants with serum bilirubin levels greater than 12–14 mg/dl and 20 mg/dl, respectively. Exact protocols based on infant well-being, sex, gestational age, albumin levels and bilirubin binding studies should be consulted. The protocols determine thresholds for initiating and discontinuing these modalities [1].

2. Justification. Exchange transfusions are highly effective but may need to be done multiple times. The risk of severe complications is approximately 1%, with side effects of arrhythmias, sepsis, and emboli being most common. Cost per exchange is approximately $700.

III. Recommendations

A. Early detection

1. All pregnant women should have blood type, Rh, and antibodies determined at the first prenatal visit, and all newborns should have the same studies performed on cord blood immediately after birth.
2. Infants ABO-incompatible with their mothers or born to type O mothers should have direct Coombs' testing performed on cord blood immediately after delivery.
3. Infants with weakly positive or positive direct Coombs' tests should have serum bilirubin determined and repeated in 24 hours.

B. Early intervention. Phototherapy and exchange transfusion are reserved for those infants in whom bilirubin and known risk factors for kernicterus exceed established thresholds [1].

Anti-D Isoimmunization

I. The problem

A. Description. Women who have no Rh antigen in their red blood cells are called Rh-negative (D-negative). If they become exposed to as little as 0.25 ml of Rh-positive blood, they may develop anti-Rh (anti-D) antibody. A second exposure causes an anamnestic response resulting in rapid and strong antibody development.

An Rh- (or D-) negative woman carrying an Rh-positive fetus has a 14–17% chance of having detectable anti-Rh (anti-D) antibody at the beginning of her second pregnancy, placing her second Rh-positive fetus at risk for hemolytic disease of the newborn.

It is of primary importance to note that an Rh-negative woman can become sensitized not only by fetomaternal bleeding from an Rh-positive fetus at any time during pregnancy, but also from first trimester abortion (the D antigen is present at 32 days' postconception) [2]. In addition, known causes of isoimmunization include: abortion, both spontaneous and induced (3.5%); ectopic pregnancy (1%); amniocentesis in the second and third trimesters (1–3%); and incompatible blood transfusion (90–95%).

Whenever these women carry an Rh-positive fetus, they are at risk of developing an anti-D IgG immunoglobulin capable of crossing the placenta and causing fetal red cell destruction. This leads to anemia, overload of the erythropoietin system with hepatosplenomegaly and portal hypertension, and in severe cases, massive anasarca and heart failure. This clinical picture of an extremely edematous, very ill newborn is called hydrops fetalis.

B. Epidemiology. The risk of a gravida being sensitized by her first Rh-incompatible ABO-compatible pregnancy within 6 months of delivery is about 8%, with an additional risk of 8% with her second Rh-positive pregnancy [3], provided she is not protected by Rh immunoglobulin.

The risk in a second Rh-positive pregnancy occurs from "sensibilization," a concept whereby the primary immune response is too weak to detect the incompatibility but primes the mother for rapid antibody production in the face of a very small amount of Rh-positive cells in a subsequent pregnancy [4].

It should be noted that if the mother and fetus are ABO-incompatible at birth, the rate of sensitization to D is reduced by 80–90%, i.e. the risk of isoimmunization is about 2%.

Currently, rates for isoimmunization are approximately 2–3/1000 births. The perinatal mortality of these affected babies can be as low as 15/1000 [4].

C. Risk groups. The white population of the United States has a 15% incidence of Rh(D)-negative women, while those of pure Asian extraction are entirely Rh-positive, with blacks having a 2–8% incidence of Rh-negative genotype.

II. Methods of prevention. The current mainstay of prevention of Rh isoimmunization is the administration of anti-D immunoglobulin (Rh immune globulin [RhIg]). The globulin inhibits the maternal immune system from forming anti-D antibody by an uncertain mechanism; presumably antibody-mediated immune suppression (AMIS) works by the IgG molecule binding to the foreign red blood cells, which allows it to be trapped in the spleen and lymph nodes where T and B lymphocytes augment IgM and suppress the IgG response [5].

A. Testing. Tests routinely performed to determine who is a candidate for Rh immune globulin include [6]:

1. Initial prenatal visit: determine blood type, Rh, indirect Coombs'.

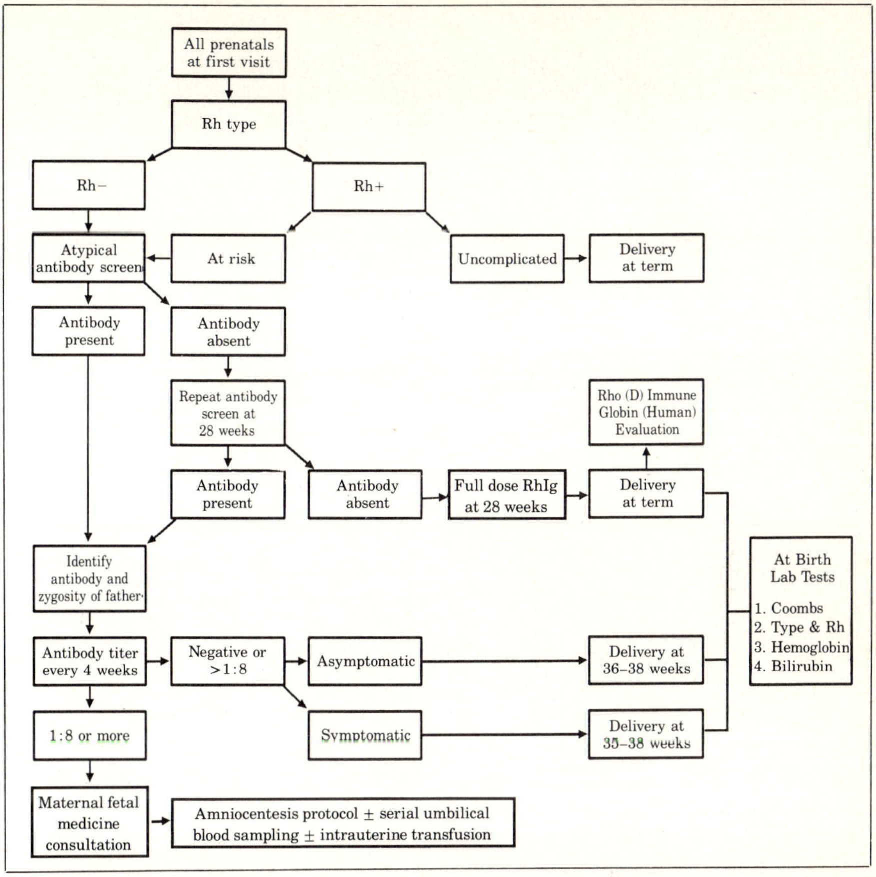

Fig. 12-1. Testing and management protocol for mild Rh sensitization. (Updated from E. H. Bishop and R. E. Brown. Management of Erythroblastosis. Chicago: *ACOG Technical Bulletin* No. 17, July 1972.)

2. If patient is Rh-negative, repeat indirect Coombs' at 28 weeks' gestation, and if negative, give Rh immune globulin (300 μg).
3. After delivery: check infant's Rh; if positive, give the nonsensitized mother Rh immune globulin (300 μg).
4. Occasionally, if only the maternal blood specimen for Rh type is obtained at delivery, a weakly positive indirect Coombs' test may be interpreted as meaning the mother is D-negative D^u-positive (D^u is an incomplete D antigen). If suspected, it should be easy to determine whether the mother really is D^u-positive, or if the test has resulted from a significant fetal-maternal hemorrhage. It is commonly recommended that the D-negative D^u-positive gravida not receive Rh immune globulin since the chance that she will develop anti-D antibody is extremely low.
5. If the mother's indirect Coombs' is positive initially or before Rh immune globulin administration, the testing and management protocol outlined in Fig. 12-1 should be followed.

   Fetal-maternal bleeding is detected with high sensitivity by the erythrocyte rosette test. If this qualitative test is positive, then a Kleihauer-Betke stain test quantitates the amount of bleed. This data easily determines the amount of Rh immune globulin to be administered.

B. Administration of Rh immune globulin [7, 8] (RhIg) to Rh-negative gravida with Rh-positive mate

1. After **any** abortion (the D antigen is present by 32 days' gestation).

2. After genetic amniocentesis, with repeat at 28 weeks (and at term, if infant is D-positive).
3. To all Rh-negative women at 28 weeks' gestation.
4. After third trimester amniocentesis.
5. Any time an Rh-incompatible transfusion is administered.
6. If there is suspicion of a large fetal-maternal bleed by Kleihauer-Betke test or enzyme-linked anti-globulin test (ELAT).
7. After delivery, if infant is D-positive.

C. Dosage. There are currently 50 μg and 300 μg doses of RhIg available at a cost of approximately $20–25, respectively. The smaller dose can neutralize approximately 2.5 ml of D-positive red cells, and the larger dose neutralizes 15 ml of D-positive red cells. Considering an average half-life of 23 days for the immunoglobulin, the following amounts seem to be logical with respect to anticipated risks:

1. Abortion or ectopic pregnancy of less than 12 weeks—50 μg.
2. Abortion or ectopic pregnancy of more than 12 weeks—300 μg.
3. Amniocentesis: genetic at 16 weeks—300 μg; and **repeat** at 28 weeks—300 μg.
4. Diagnostic amniocentesis, third trimester—300 μg.
5. Antepartum prophylaxis at 28 weeks—300 μg.
6. Postpartum—300 μg (more if evidence of greater than 15 ml fetal red blood cell bleed) usually given within 3 days of delivery, but later date may still decrease risk of sensitization. In multiple gestations or with antepartum bleeding, no extra RhIg is given unless the Kleihauer-Betke test indicates necessity for such.

III. Management of Rh isoimmunized pregnancy [9]

A. Methods

1. When a gravida is found to have an isoimmune antibody to either D or any of the antigens known to cause fetal disease, the management depends initially on the antibody level. In general, if the antibody titer is less than 1:8, monthly antibody titers are indicated.
2. When the titer reaches 1:8 or greater, the severity of fetal involvement is better approximated by serial amniocentesis at a frequency shown in Fig. 12-2. No further maternal antibody testing is then indicated. The amniocentesis determines the ΔOD_{450} (absorption of light passed through amniotic fluid at 450 mμ, the point at which bilirubin peaks). This value correlates fairly well with the severity of fetal erythroblastosis.
3. Amniocentesis should be initiated at 24–26 weeks' gestation, unless the mother has had a prior severely affected or stillborn infant, in which case the first amniocentesis should be done at 22 weeks' gestation, and the amniocentesis should be repeated according to Fig. 12-2.
4. If the ΔOD 450 is in zone 1, delivery by 37 weeks is indicated, when fetal lung maturity is present.
5. In zone 2, the fetal lung profile (L/S ratio, percent disaturated lecithin, and the presence of phosophatidyl glycerol) should be obtained at 35 weeks. Once fetal lung maturity has been reached or there is evidence of early hydrops by ultrasound, the fetus should be delivered.
6. In zone 3, the fetus is severely jeopardized and usually requires either intrauterine transfusion or close serial evaluation with ultrasound, fetal blood sampling, and contraction stress testing if less than 30 weeks' gestation. This should only be done at a properly equipped tertiary referral center [10].
7. Of greatest importance in interpreting serial ΔOD 450 values is the fact that values should always have a downward trend; should they stay the same or rise, repeat amniocentesis in 1 week is necessary, and fetal blood sampling for hemoglobin level may be necessary.
8. There are three newer techniques of treatment for severely Rh-sensitized gravida that are not yet widely accepted or utilized but deserve careful evaluation to determine their effectiveness and applicability.
   a. Desensitization by ingestion of a human erythrocyte membrane preparation to suppress preexisting antibodies [11].
   b. Using repeated small volume (1000 ml) plasmapheresis to decrease the circulating antibodies [12].
   c. Administration of promethazine to ameliorate the antibody response [13].

B. Justification

1. **Effectiveness**
   a. **Rh testing and RhIg.** Of major concern currently is the lack of complete postpartum immunization (only 90%) with Rh immune globulin, and the fact that

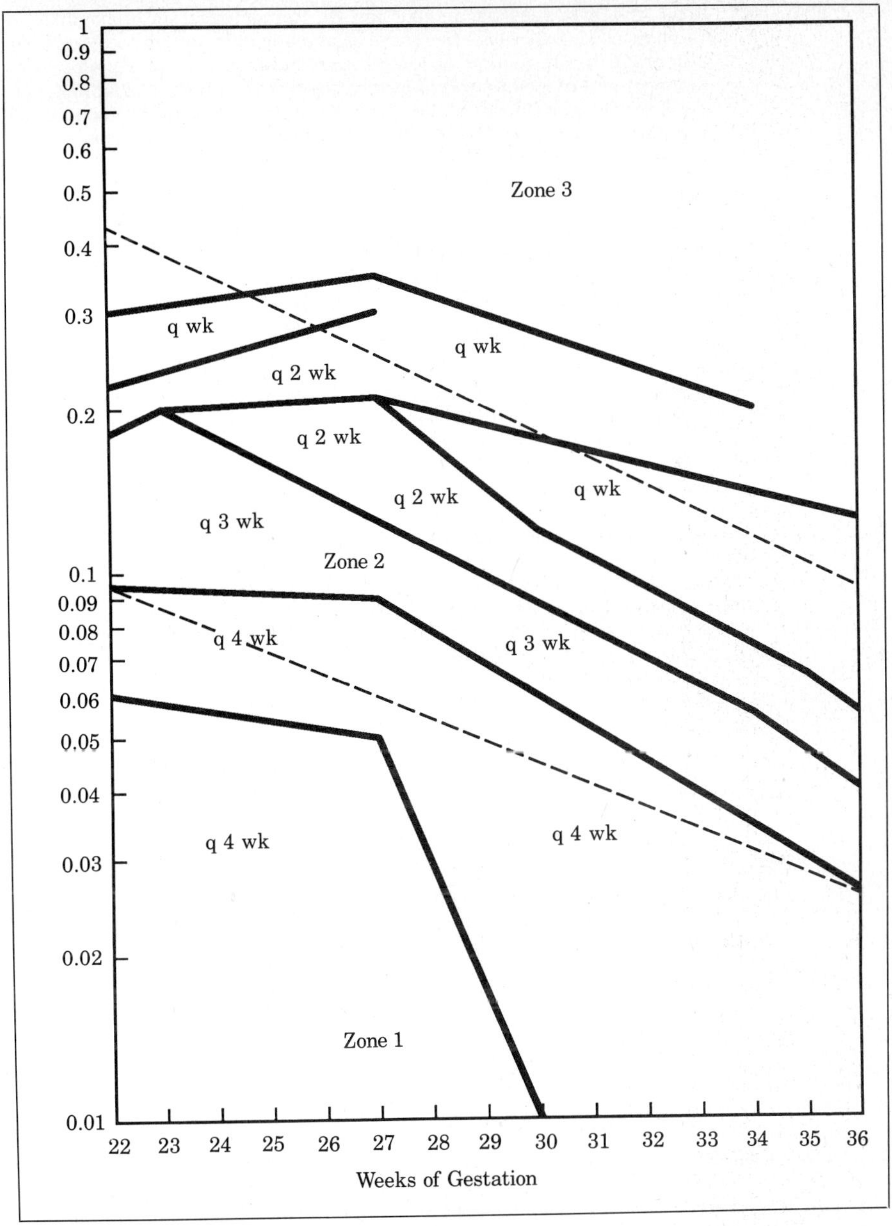

Fig. 12-2. Frequency of amniocentesis for sensitized gravida. (Modified from E. G. Hamilton. Intrauterine transfusion safeguard or peril? *Obstet. Gynecol.* 50:255, 1977.)

postpartum immunization will not prevent the approximately 1.5% isoimmunization occurring **before** delivery.

If one considers that about 210,000 D-negative women in the United States give birth annually to D-positive ABO compatible infants, and if one assumes only a 5% postpartum Rh immunization failure rate (of which 13–16% become sensitized ultimately), then a total of 1400 women/year become sensitized, despite postpartum Rh immune globulin. In addition, 3500 women who should be given Rh immune globulin are not; this means about 5000 women yearly become sensitized postpartum, plus around 500 more from abortions. For these reasons, antepartum Rh isoimmunization prophylaxis is recommended. Experience has shown that using both antepartum and postpartum RhIg can reduce the rate of isoimmunization to nearly zero.

b. **Management of isoimmunized pregnancy.** The combination of amniocentesis and intrauterine transfusion under 32 weeks' gestation has reduced the perinatal mortality to 15/1000. Morbidity from respiratory distress and exchange transfusion is still significant.

2. **Risks and side effects**

a. **Rh testing and RhIg.** There is only a very rare report of reaction to RhIg. Even giving RhIg to a D-positive woman results in no harm.

b. **Management of isoimmunized pregnancy.** The discomfort of amniocentesis is low, with a risk of problems to the fetus of about 1/1000 using ultrasound guidance. Intrauterine transfusion, however, carries a 1–2% risk of fetal death with each transfusion. Risk from fetal vascular sampling appears to be low.

3. **Costs**

a. **Rh testing and RhIg.** The major argument against combined antepartum/postpartum prophylaxis has been cost-effectiveness. Since the antepartum RhIg administration prevents 94% of sensitization before delivery, each prevented case costs about $3000, a cost-effective figure.

b. **Management of Rh isoimmunized pregnancy.** Each amniocentesis costs approximately $200. Intrauterine exchange transfusion costs $1000–2000. Neonatal intensive care costs $1000–2000/day. Total costs for severe cases can be more than $100,000.

4. **Acceptability.** In general, women with Rh sensitization rarely accept donor insemination by Rh-negative donors. They prefer to accept the risk of serial amniocentesis (low) and premature delivery (higher) unless intrauterine transfusion occurred in a previous pregnancy, at which time combined fetal and neonatal risk increases dramatically.

IV. **Recommendations**

A. All gravida should have a blood type, Rh type, and indirect Coombs' test done on the first pregnancy visit.

B. Those gravida that are D-negative should have a repeated indirect Coombs' test at 28 weeks, and administration of 300 μg of Rh isoimmune globulin. If the neonate is D-positive, another 300 μg should be administered after delivery.

C. D-negative women who abort under 12 weeks' gestation should receive 50 μg RhIg. Others, such as recipients of D-positive blood transfusion, amniocentesis, or antepartum bleeding, require 300 μg RhIg prophylaxis and careful follow-up.

D. For those gravida who are isoimmunized at the initial screening by the indirect Coombs' test, serial indirect Coombs' testing at monthly intervals is appropriate until the titer is 1:8 or greater.

E. Once a titer of 1:8 or greater has been reached, serial amniocentesis must be performed, with the timing of delivery dependent on evidence for the severity of erythroblastosis elicited from standard management graphs (see Fig. 12-2).

Non-D Isoimmunization

I. **The problem**

A. **Description.** Approximately 2% of all hemolytic disease of the newborn is caused by IgG antibodies other than A, B, or D. These antibodies can cause as severe and fatal a hemolysis as anti-D. The most common non-D antibodies, however, are anti-C, E, c, and e, which are all in the Rh system [14].

B. **Epidemiology.** Approximately 1.3% of all gravidas screened will have irregular antibodies (not Rh system). Many of these patients are sensitized through blood transfusions.

C. **Risk groups.** Any woman who has received blood products is at increased risk of irregular antibody sensitization. White women have a 10-fold higher rate of non-Rh isoimmunization than black women.

II. **Prevention.** There is basically no prevention known to isoimmunization by other than D antigen. No prevention is possible for C, E, c, e, and the irregular antibodies.

III. **Management**

A. The management of non-D Rh isoimmunization and irregular antibody isoimmunization is the same as for anti-D sensitization. Frequently forgotten is the need to determine the paternal phenotype of the antigen. For example, if a gravida is anti-Kell sensitized, which means she must be Kell-negative, fetal disease can only occur if the father is Kell-positive. If he is Kell-negative, the fetus must be Kell-negative (since the mother has to be), and erythroblastosis cannot occur.

B. The management of the non-D sensitized gravida is done according to the same scheme as anti-D isoimmunization. The potential severity of the fetal disease is described in Table 12-1.

IV. Recommendations

A. All gravidas should be screened at the first visit with a blood type, Rh type, and indirect Coombs' test.

B. Any Rh antibody or irregular antibody detected should be titrated and the follow-up performed as outlined in Fig. 12-1 under "Antibody present."

C. The father's phenotype for the antigen should be tested to make sure that he is antigen-positive. If he is negative, no further maternal surveillance is necessary.

Table 12-1. Irregular antibodies causing hemolytic disease of the newborn

Blood group system	Antigens related to hemolytic disease	Severity of hemolytic disease	Proposed management
Lewis*			
Kell	K	Mild to severe with hydrops fetalis	Amniotic fluid bilirubin studies
	k	Mild only	Expectant
	k_o	Mild only	Expectant
	Kp^a	Mild only	Expectant
	Kp^b	Mild only	Expectant
	Js^a	Mild only	Expectant
	Js^b	Mild only	Expectant
Duffy	Fy^a	Mild to severe with hydrops fetalis	Amniotic fluid bilirubin studies
	Fy^b†		
Kidd	Jk^a	Mild to severe	Amniotic fluid bilirubin studies
	Jk^b	Mild to severe	Amniotic fluid bilirubin studies
MNSs	M	Mild to severe	Amniotic fluid bilirubin studies
	N†		
	S	Mild to severe	Amniotic fluid bilirubin studies
	s	Mild to severe	Amniotic fluid bilirubin studies
	U	Mild to severe	Amniotic fluid bilirubin studies
	Mi^a	Moderate	Amniotic fluid bilirubin studies
	Mt^a	Moderate	Amniotic fluid bilirubin studies
	Vw	Mild only	Expectant
Lutheran	Lu^a	Mild only	Expectant
	Lu^b	Mild only	Expectant
Diego	Di^a	Mild to severe	Amniotic fluid bilirubin studies
	Di^b	Mild to severe	Amniotic fluid bilirubin studies
Xg	Xg^a	Mild only	Expectant
Public antigens	Yt^a	Moderate to severe	Amniotic fluid bilirubin studies
	Lan	Mild only	Expectant
	Ge	Mild only	Expectant
	Co^a	Severe	Amniotic fluid bilirubin studies

Table 12-1 (continued)

Blood group system	Antigens related to hemolytic disease	Severity of hemolytic disease	Proposed management
Private antigens	Batty	Mild only	Expectant
	Becker	Mild only	Expectant
	Berrens	Mild only	Expectant
	Biles	Moderate	Amniotic fluid bilirubin studies
	Evans	Mild only	Expectant
	Gonzales	Mild only	Expectant
	Good	Severe	Amniotic fluid bilirubin studies
	Heibel	Moderate	Amniotic fluid bilirubin studies
	Hunt	Mild only	Expectant
	Jobbins	Mild only	Expectant
	Radin	Moderate	Amniotic fluid bilirubin studies
	Rm	Mild only	Expectant
	Ven	Mild only	Expectant
	Wright	Severe	Amniotic fluid bilirubin studies
	Zd	Moderate	Amniotic fluid bilirubin studies

*Not a proven cause of hemolytic disease
†Not a cause of hemolytic disease
Source: Modified from L. Weinstein. Irregular antibodies causing hemolytic disease of the newborn. *Clin. Obstet. Gynecol.* 25(2):321, 1982.

References

1. Linderkamp, O., and Riegel, K. P. Exchange Transfusion. In N. M. Nelson (ed.), *Current Therapy in Neonatal-Perinatal Medicine.* St. Louis: Mosby, 1985. Pp. 335–42. *Good description of criteria for neonatal exchange transfusion.*
2. Chown, B. On the search for rhesus antibodies in very young foetuses. *Arch. Dis. Child.* 30:232, 1955. *Earliest formation of antibodies.*
3. Queenan, J. T. *Modern Management of the Rh Problem* (2d ed.). New York: Harper & Row, 1977. *An excellent review of the Rh problem in pregnancy by an obstetrician. Not current on prophylaxis, however.*
4. Nevanlinna, H. R. Factors affecting maternal Rh isoimmunization. *Ann. Med. Exper. et Biol. Fenniae* 31 (Suppl 2):1, 1953. *Early work describing concepts of second pregnancy sensitization.*
5. Bowman, J. M. Controversies in Rh prophylaxis. *Am. J. Obstet. Gynecol.* 151(3):289, 1985. *Superb review of the entire area of Rh prophylaxis.*
6. Pollack, W., Gorman, J. G., and Freda, V. J. Rh Immune Suppression: Past, Present, and Future. In F. D. Frigoletto Jr., J. F. Jewett, and A. A. Konugres (eds.), *Rh Hemolytic Disease—New Strategies for Eradication.* Boston: Hall, 1982. Pp. 9–70. *Outstanding review; comprehensive prevention analysis.*
7. Scott, J. R. Antenatal Prophylaxis: Experience at Utah. In F. D. Frigoletto Jr., J. F. Jewett, and A. A. Konugres (eds.), *Rh Hemolytic Disease—New Strategies for Eradication.* Boston: Hall, 1982. Pp. 191–8. *Shows effectiveness of antepartum prophylaxis.*
8. Prevention of RHO(D) Isoimmunization. Chicago: *ACOG Technical Bulletin* No. 79, 1984. *Standard-of-care information for Rh prophylaxis.*
9. Bishop, E. H., and Brown, R. E. Management of Erythroblastosis. Chicago: *ACOG Technical Bulletin* No. 17, July 1972. *Standard of care for assessment and follow-up of all Rh-negative gravida.*
10. Hamilton, E. G. Intrauterine transfusion—safeguard or peril? *Obstet. Gynecol.* 50(3):255, 1977. *Describes management of amniotic fluid delta OD 450 findings.*

11. Bierme, S. J., et al. Oral Rh treatment for severely immunised mothers (letter). *Lancet* 1(8116):604, 1979. *Fascinating research concept using ingested red cell membranes.*
12. Rubinstein, P. Repeated Small Volume Plasmapheresis in the Management of Hemolytic Disease of the Newborn. In F. D. Frigoletto, Jr., J. F. Jewett, and A. A. Konugres (eds.), *Rh Hemolytic Disease—New Strategies for Eradication.* Boston: Hall, 1982. Pp. 211–20. *Research paper describing an expensive and unproven approach to treatment of Rh-immunized gravidas.*
13. Gusdon, J. P. Jr., and Witherow, C. Possible ameliorating effects of erythroblastosis by promethazine hydrochloride. *Am. J. Obstet. Gynecol.* 117:1101, 1973. *This paper was followed by much controversy regarding risk and benefit.*
14. Weinstein, L. Irregular antibodies causing hemolytic disease of the newborn. *Clin. Obstet. Gynecol.* 25(2):321, 1982. *Definitive review of irregular (non-CDE) antibodies and what is known about their effects on the fetus.*

13 Genetic Disease and Pregnancy

Mitchell S. Golbus
and Zvi Appelman

I. The problem

A. Description. Genetic disease can be divided into three major groups:

1. Single gene disorders.
2. Chromosomal aberrations.
3. Multifactorial disorders.

These three groups of hereditary diseases affect about 2–3% of the newborns in the United States. Many of these genetic diseases are brought to the attention of health care providers during pregnancy when families suddenly realize that they might have an urgent problem and need consultation regarding a genetic disease. The variety of problems is almost endless: (1) A relative with a chromosomal disorder such as Down's syndrome, or an X-linked disorder such as hemophilia; (2) A carrier state in both parents for a recessive disease such as Tay-Sachs or sickle cell anemia that was found in a screening program; or (3) A multifactorial disease such as a neural tube defect.

B. Epidemiology. The epidemiology and incidence of the most common genetic diseases are listed in Tables 13-1 and 13-2.

II. Prevention

A. Early detection

1. Methods

a. Risk assessment. At some point during preconception or prenatal care, risk assessment should be done and should include factors such as maternal age, the woman's history, the father's history, and the family history of both parents. Environmental factors should be assessed by direct questions; some programs have special forms that cover these points.

b. Genetic counseling

(1) Description. Genetic counseling has been defined by an ad hoc committee of the American Society of Human Genetics. The definition refers to genetic counseling as a communication process dealing with the occurrence, or risk of recurrence, of a genetic disorder. This process includes helping the individual or family to: (1) understand the medical facts, including diagnosis, prognosis, and therapy; (2) understand the role of genetics in the disorder and the risk of recurrence; (3) understand the reproductive options; (4) choose a course of action appropriate for them; and (5) make the best possible adjustment to the disorder or to the risk of recurrence of that disorder. Basically, then, genetic counseling should be viewed as a specific type of instruction and advice given by a physician to a patient.

(2) Population. The unit of clinical genetic practice should be considered to be the family, not the individual. This represents an extension of the physician-patient relationship to a physician-family relationship. There are a number of situations in which genetic counseling is appropriate. Among the families that warrant genetic counseling are those in which: (1) there is a child affected with an autosomal recessive disorder, or the parents are both found to be carriers of the same deleterious recessive allele; (2) there is an autosomal dominant trait; (3) there is a sporadic instance of a dominantly inherited condition; (4) there are males affected with an X-linked disorder; (5) there is a family member with a congenital malformation; and (6) there is a family member with a known chromosomal aberration.

Table 13-1. Estimated frequency of hereditary disorders (per 100 liveborn)[a]

Genic[b]		
Autosomal recessive		
Mental retardation, severe	0.08	
Cystic fibrosis	0.05	
Deafness, severe (several forms)	0.05	
Blindness, severe (several forms)	0.02	
Adrenogénital syndrome	0.01	
Albinism	0.01	
Phenylketonuria	0.01	
Other aminoacidurias (several forms)	0.01	
Mucopolysaccharidoses, all forms	0.005	
Tay-Sachs disease	0.001	
Galactosemia	0.0005	
	0.25	
X-linked		
Duchenne muscular dystrophy	0.02	
Hemophilias A & B	0.01	
Other	0.02	
	0.05	
Autosomal dominants		
Blindness (several forms)	0.010	
Deafness (several forms)	0.010	
Marfan's syndrome	0.005	
Achondroplasia	0.005	
Neurofibromatosis	0.005	
Myotonic dystrophy	0.005	
Tuberous sclerosis	0.005	
All others	0.015	
	0.06	
Total genic disorders	0.36	
Chromosomal		
Autosomal		
Trisomy 21	0.13	
Trisomy 18	0.03	
Trisomy 13	0.02	
Translocations (familial)	0.01	
Deletions	0.01	
	0.20	
Sex chromosomes		
XO and X deletions	0.02	
Other severe sex chromosome defects	0.01	
XXY	0.10	
XXX	0.10	
XYY	0.10	
Others	0.015	
	0.35	
Total chromosomal	0.55	
Polygenic/multifactorial disorders		
Congenital malformations	English population	Estimate in United States newborns
Spina bifida and anencephaly	0.45	0.14
Congenital heart defects	0.40	0.25
Pyloric stenosis	0.30	
Talipes equinovarus	0.30	0.12
Cleft lip and cleft palate	0.10	0.08
Dislocated hips	0.10	0.07
	1.65	0.66

Table 13-1 (continued)

Total frequency of hereditary diseases	
Genic	0.36%
Chromosomal	0.55%
Polygenic/multifactorial malformations	1.65%
"Common diseases"	??
Total	2.56%+

[a]Figures based on English population.
[b]These figures represent a tally of **clinically apparent** disorders in newborns. Since some of these defects (for example, congenital heart disease) might not be apparent at birth, these figures must be considered as minimum ones. The spina bifida/anencephaly figures **are** certainly lower in the United States than in England, with an incidence of approximately 0.1% now being commonly found.

Table 13-2. Incidence of the most common biochemical disorders of metabolism

Disorder	Incidence
Cystinuria	1:7,000
Phenylketonuria	1:15,000 (California)
Histidinemia	1:24,000
Hartnup disease	1:26,000
Galactosemia	1:75,000
Maple syrup urine disease	1:200,000
Homocystinuria	1:220,000
Tay-Sachs disease	1:5,000 (Ashkenazi Jewish)
Tay-Sachs disease	1:400,000 (general population)

Source: H. L. Levy. Genetic screening. *Adv. Hum. Genet.* 4:1, 1973.

(3) Procedure. The process of genetic counseling can be divided into three major components: (1) obtaining and presenting relevant medical and genetic information; (2) helping in the formation of a plan, considering all options, that is appropriate to the patients' circumstances; and (3) dealing with psychological issues.

(a) Information. The first component of genetic counseling is obtaining and presenting the relevant medical and genetic information. Appropriate counseling requires accurate facts, starting with the diagnosis of the affected member(s) of the family. The counselor must be sure of the accuracy of the diagnosis before proceeding further.

Estimating the risk of occurrence or recurrence involves the use of three types of information. First, there is modular information arrived at by the rational use of Mendelian principles. Second, there is empirical information obtained from the analysis of data from population surveys. The third source is particular information derived from analysis of the family's pedigree. Laboratory information and age of onset relevant to the genetic condition also can be incorporated into the risk estimate using Bayesian calculations. Once obtained, the medical and genetic information must be presented to the family in a comprehensible manner. Curiously, the techniques and methods of medical counseling are not included in most medical school curricula.

(b) Formulating a plan. The second component is aiding the family to consider the information in light of the reproductive options available and to formulate a course of action appropriate to their individual circumstances. To allow a rational choice, a variety of viewpoints must be presented without any attempt at coercion. The extent to which positive guidance toward a particular decision is given varies greatly among counselors. It is virtually impossible to present information in a totally neutral fashion. To illustrate, quoting a 10%

risk of abnormality does not have the same psychological impact as quoting a 9 : 1 probability of a normal outcome. There may be no solution to this problem, but it is one that the counselor should be aware of, so that the choice of words can be made consciously rather than randomly.

The major concerns weighed by families considering their reproductive options are the risk of occurrence of a disorder and the burden of the disorder in terms of its severity and duration (survival time of the affected individual). However, there are many other considerations in parental genetic decisionmaking, including the couple's capacity to withstand adversity, the status of their marital relationship, their perceived impact of an affected child on existing or prospective children, their financial status, and the couple's individual and joint moral commitments.

(c) **Psychological issues.** The third component of genetic counseling is psychological. It is important to gain insight into the family's emotional state. The family is often anxious, hostile, and depressed about the situation that is bringing them to the genetic counselor. The educational aspects of counseling will be ineffective unless these feelings are dispelled or reduced. There are feelings of guilt, denial, grief, and mourning associated with giving birth to a child with a genetic disorder, and these feelings must be brought to the surface and dealt with.

In spite of the specialized nature of genetic counseling, it is neither desirable nor possible that it be carried out only by medical geneticists. For many problems, the ideal counselor is the family physician who knows the family's physical, emotional, and financial resources. For physicians who feel unsure of the area, or in situations where specialized diagnostic, risk ascertainment, or counseling skills are required, a referral can be made to a medical genetics service.

c. **Genetic screening.** There are several forms of genetic screening, each appropriate to the conditions for which screening is performed.

(1) **Chromosomal disorders in utero.**

(a) **Description.** One of the most common forms of genetic screening is **in utero** detection of chromosomal disorders. Advanced maternal age is the most common indication for prenatal diagnostic studies.

(b) **Population.** The relationship between the incidence of chromosomal trisomy and maternal age is well known. There is no absolute point above which maternal age should be considered "advanced," but most centers use 35 years as their criterion. Over 300,000 pregnancies have been monitored for this indication, and approximately 2.5% of the fetuses were found to be aneuploid. The age-specific risk of the fetus having trisomy rises from 0.9% at 35–36 years of age, to 7.8% at 43–44 years. These figures are approximately twice the maternal age-specific incidence of neonatal trisomy. The difference appears to be the result of late abortions and stillbirths of aneuploid fetuses.

Women who previously have borne a trisomic child have been considered to be at increased risk for having another. This was determined on the basis of a report of 1–2% recurrence risk, irrespective of maternal age. The prenatal diagnosis program data on recurrent trisomy 21 indicates a recurrence risk of 0.2% (4/1976) for women less than 35, and a recurrence risk equal to the age-specific risk for women over 35 years old. The cumulative experience has been that 1.3% of such at-risk fetuses are chromosomally abnormal. This includes anomalies other than trisomies and includes fetuses that would be late abortions and stillbirths. Thus, women with a prior trisomic child do **not** appear to be at a significantly increased risk in subsequent gestations. Justification of offering prenatal diagnosis to these families is on the basis of their manifesting great anxiety about fetal well-being.

The greatest risk of producing a chromosomally abnormal fetus exists for those individuals who are carriers of a balanced translocation. The magnitude of the risk is different for each specific translocation. For all examples for which data is available, the risk of trisomy is greater if the female rather than the male is the translocation carrier. Considering this heterogeneous group as a whole, 10% of the fetuses studied were aneuploid.

(c) **Procedure.** Prenatal diagnosis of chromosomal disorders is available by either **amniocentesis,** usually done at 16 menstrual weeks, or **chorionic villus sampling** (CVS), done at 9–12 menstrual weeks. CVS is a newer technique, probably with a slightly higher risk of pregnancy loss, and each couple will have to decide for themselves if they want prenatal diagnosis and, if so, by which technique.

CVS is done in the first trimester, preferably around the ninth week of gestation. Currently it is done by transcervical aspiration of trophoblastic tissue under ultrasonic guidance. It is done without anesthesia and usually with only minimal discomfort to the patient.

The villi are identified and may be processed by two methods. One involves culturing for 1–2 weeks, harvesting and giving out results in 2–3 weeks. The second method is direct in the sense that the villi are processed almost immediately and results are given out in days. The major disadvantage of the direct method is inferior resolution of chromosomal banding when compared to the first method. This problem may be overcome in the near future.

Amniocentesis, on the other hand, is done around the sixteenth week. A 22-gauge needle is inserted into the amniotic sac under ultrasonic guidance and 24 ml of fluid is withdrawn. The amniocytes are cultured for about 2 weeks, similar to the first method that was described for CVS. The turnaround time is also similar—about 2–3 weeks on average. The amniotic fluid is also studied for its α-fetoprotein level. The patients in the CVS program are screened for neural tube defects by their maternal serum α-fetoprotein (AFP) level, which is done at about the sixteenth week of gestation (Table 13-3).

The decision between CVS and amniocentesis is entirely individual. Some patients prefer early diagnosis by CVS and some prefer the relative safety of amniocentesis. Health care providers must try to help patients in their decision by supplying the most accurate data available.

(2) **The prenatal diagnosis of X-linked disorders.** Three approaches to the prenatal detection of X-linked disorders are possible.

(a) If the specific abnormality is known and detectable in utero at a gestation of less than 20 weeks, a specific diagnosis can be made. Fetal sex determination is generally done concurrently. This approach can now be used for the abnormalities listed in Table 13-4.

(b) If the genetic defect is not known but a useful linked restriction fragment length polymorphism **(RFLP)** is identified, determination of the DNA restriction pattern of the parents and fetus can be employed.

(c) If there is neither a specific test nor RFLP, then **fetal sex** can be determined, and the risk of a male fetus being affected is calculated as: (probability mother is carrier)$\times$0.5.

(3) **Mass screening: Maternal serum AFP screening**

(a) **Description.** Another type of genetic screening is to test the entire pregnant population to identify a subset of patients at high risk for a genetic problem. The concept of maternal serum AFP screening arose from the fact that amniotic fluid AFP reflected so accurately the presence of a neural tube defect (NTD) in the fetus.

(b) **Population.** Of newborns with neural tube defects, 90% are the first affected individuals in a family. Therefore, even if amniocentesis were employed in all families with a previously affected child, the disease incidence would be decreased by only 10%. Because AFP in the amniotic sac may cross to the maternal circulation, the concept of measuring maternal serum AFP to predict which fetuses might have an NTD arose. Serial measurements of maternal serum in normal gestations indicate that AFP levels rise to a peak of about 250 ng/ml at 32 weeks and then slowly decline. Because the maternal serum AFP concentration increases rapidly from 15–24 menstrual

Table 13-3. Comparison of chorionic villus sampling (CVS) and amniocentesis

	CVS	Amniocentesis
First trimester diagnosis	yes	no
Risk for miscarriage	1–2%[a]	0.5%
α-fetoprotein level	no[b]	yes
Patient discomfort	minimal	minimal
Option of first trimester abortion	yes	no
Maternal risk during termination	very low	low

[a] Probable.
[b] Can be done through maternal serum α-fetoprotein test.

Table 13-4. Specific diagnosis of abnormalities

Diagnosis	Approach
Adrenoleukodystrophy	Determination of very long chain fatty acids
Chronic granulomatous disease	Chemiluminescence and NBT reduction by fetal leukocytes
Fabry disease	Assay of ceramide trihexosidase
Fragile X/mental retardation	Cytogenic
Hemophilia A	RFLP; direct demonstration of mutation; factor VIII assays (fetal blood)
Hemophilia B	RFLP; direct demonstration of mutation; factor IX assays (fetal blood)
Hunter syndrome	Assay of iduronate sulfatase
Lesch-Nyhan syndrome	Assay of HGPRT; direct gene analysis
Menkes kinky hair syndrome	^{64}Cu uptake and retention
Ornithine transcarbamylase deficiency	RFLP; direct gene analysis; activity in fetal liver
Placental sulfatase deficiency	Enzyme assay

Key: NBT=nitrogen blue tetrazoladine; RFLP=restriction fragment length polymorphism; HGPRT=hypoxanthine guanine phosphoribosyl tranferase.

weeks, a correct determination of gestational age is crucial for diagnostic purposes.

(c) **Procedure.** Maternal blood is drawn between the fifteenth and eighteenth week of gestation. The patient's physician is responsible for drawing and shipping the blood sample to the local lab.

(4) **Carrier identification.** Currently most of the heterozygotes for recessive disease are identified by an affected offspring. The exceptions are carriers that are detected through a mass screening program. There are screening programs for Tay-Sachs disease and for hemoglobinopathies.

(a) **Description.** One type of genetic screening is identification of couples who are both heterozygotes (carriers) of the same autosomal recessive deleterious trait. These couples will be healthy themselves, but each offspring will have a 25% chance of being a homozygote affected with the particular disorder. Heterozygote screening is done to offer reproductive choices to carrier-carrier couples.

(b) **Populations.** Our current method of identifying heterozygotes for the autosomal recessive disorders is by the birth of the affected child. Even widespread application of prenatal diagnosis will provide only a small reduction in disease incidence. We are now entering an era

Table 13-5. Carrier detection of thalassemia

Test	α-thalassemia minor	β-thalassemia minor	Iron deficiency
Serum iron	>50 mg/dl	>50 mg/dl	<50 mg/dl
Iron saturation	>15%	>15%	<15%
$HbA_2(\alpha_2\delta_2)$	<3.5%	>3.5%	<3.5%

of mass screening for heterozygote detection. The criteria for such a program are: (1) a defined population group at risk; (2) an accurate, reliable, inexpensive method of carrier detection; and (3) the ability to provide prenatal diagnosis of the entity in question. Tay-Sachs disease is the first disorder to meet these criteria, and the Baltimore-Washington screening established the practicality of such an approach. Since then, a number of cities have embarked on Tay-Sachs heterozygote detection programs, and California has established the first statewide legislatively supported program. In California alone, there are 33,000 carriers of the Tay-Sachs gene, and 350 at risk couples in which both are carriers with a 25% risk of Tay-Sachs disease for each offspring. Identification of these couples will allow the use of prenatal diagnosis without the index case being born. The availability of prenatal diagnosis of the hemoglobinopathies has allowed these disorders to be tackled with similar mass screening efforts.

(c) Procedure

(i) Tay-Sachs screening. The parents' blood is tested for hexosaminidase A activity. In case of heterozygosity, only about 50% of the normal control activity will be found. The test should be done preferably before pregnancy or early in the first trimester.

(ii) Screening for hemoglobinopathies should be done prior to pregnancy or early in the first trimester. Simple, inexpensive, accurate screening tests for sickle hemoglobin are available.

The screening procedure for detection of thalassemia carriers is summarized in Table 13-5 and is based on the detection of microcytic anemia in the presence of normal serum iron levels. Mean corpuscular volume (MCV) of less than 80 requires further investigation as outlined in Table 13-5.

2. Justification

a. Test characteristics. The basic concept of heterozygote screening is to find carriers before they reproduce and thereby reduce the frequency of the disease. For such a program to be successful, the gene frequency should be high in a delineated population, there should be an inexpensive and accurate carrier detection test, and prenatal diagnosis should be available. Furthermore, because heterozygote testing programs are **voluntary,** educational efforts must be initiated or incorporated into existing community forums.

(1) Chromosomal, X-linked, and metabolic disorders. The predictive value of each test is variable and different from one test to another.

In mass screening tests, high sensitivity is required and therefore low specificity is anticipated. The false-positive cases are identified by further, more specific tests.

Some tests, such as chromosomal studies, are very accurate and have very high specificity and sensitivity; but even then mistakes can occur due to maternal contamination, mislabeling of specimens, or misinterpretation.

DNA studies including RFLPs are usually done in a way that provides accuracy greater than 95%, but there are limitations to the use of this technique because of meiotic recombination.

Other tests may provide probabilities but not a definite answer. It should be stressed that there is no test that is 100% sensitive and 100% specific, and correct interpretation of every test is of the utmost importance.

Table 13-6. Risks of mass screening program for elevated maternal serum α-fetoprotein level

Labeling	0–1%
False-positive[a]	4–5%
False-negative[b]	20%
Inherent risk of test	minimal

[a]False-positive maternal AFP results may be obtained in maternal serum by underestimation of the true gestational age or multiple gestations.
[b]False-negative results may be due to overestimation of the gestational age.

Table 13-7. Estimated costs of early detection of genetic disease

Test	Cost
Maternal serum α-fetoprotein screening	<$40
Tay-Sachs screening	<$25
Sickle cell disease screening	<$25
Thalassemia screening	<$40
Amniocentesis[a]	$850
Chorionic villus sampling[a]	$850
Ultrasound (level II)	$225
DNA workshop (nuclear family)[b]	$700

[a]Includes genetic counseling, physician's fees, and laboratory processing.
[b]Laboratory fees only.

(2) Mass screening (maternal AFP). After it was demonstrated that NTD could be identified from maternal serum screening, a collaborative study was initiated in the United Kingdom. Over 18,000 singleton and 150 twin pregnancies were monitored at 16–18 menstrual weeks, and maternal serum AFP levels of 2.5 times the median for gestational age were considered abnormal. Similar data are now available from a number of American pilot studies. Nearly 4.5% of the sera tested gave levels at or greater than the cutoff level and required a repeat serum assay and an ultrasound examination. The second serum level was normal or the sonography identified twins, a missed abortion, or misdating of the pregnancy in over one-half of these cases; thus, approximately 2% of the women in the serum screening study had amniocentesis. With the prevalence of NTD in the United States, 3.5% of these amniocenteses will identify an affected fetus.

Serum AFP measurement is a screening procedure that could potentially identify 90% of anencephalics and 75% of spina bifidas. If the serum level calling for intervention is high, there will be fewer amniocenteses but more NTD missed. If the level for intervention is low, there will be more amniocenteses but less NTD will be missed.

A number of statewide (California) or area-wide (New England states) maternal serum AFP screening programs are now operating.

b. Risks of mass screening program for elevated maternal AFP. See Table 13-6.

c. Costs. See Table 13-7.

d. Acceptability is very high for noninvasive tests and high for other tests. Most patients overcome their fears and hesitation due to a desire for the best possible outcome from a pregnancy.

B. Early intervention

1. Methods. First a nonintervention option is generally offered in all cases, and the decision of whether to intervene is left entirely to the patient.

a. For chromosomal aberrations, there is the option of pregnancy termination.

b. Gene disorders

(1) Option of termination.

Table 13-8. Risks, costs, and acceptability of first- and second-trimester abortion and of fetal surgery

	Risks	Costs	Acceptability
First-semester abortion	Perforation (0.5–1%) Infection (low) Bleeding (very low) Future infertility (low) Patient discomfort (minimal)	$150–500	Very high[a]
Second-semester abortion	Perforation/rupture (low) Infection (low) Bleeding (low) Future infertility (low) Patient discomfort (moderate–high)	$500–1500	High[a]
Fetal surgery	Experimental; all risk parameters unknown at present	$5000–10,000[b]	Unknown[c]

[a]It should be noted that some patients will not abort affected fetuses because of moral, ethical, and emotional considerations.
[b]An estimate that includes necessary tests done prior to surgery such as second level sonography, chromosomal studies, and fees for surgery, anesthesiology, medication, and one week of hospitalization.
[c]The data are limited, but at the present it seems that the acceptability of this procedure is not high, and many families reject this option because of its inherent risks and unproven results.

(2) Rarely, fetal treatment by specific medications is indicated and this option is offered in those rare disorders.

c. Multifactorial (anatomic defects)

(1) Option of termination.

(2) After careful evaluation and with specific anatomic defects (e.g., posterior urethral obstruction, diaphragmatic hernias), an option of a fetal surgical procedure may be offered on an experimental basis.

d. For multiple gestation when one fetus has any of the above-mentioned problems, selective termination may be offered.

2. Justification. The effectiveness of medical intervention is measured by reducing the burden to families and also to society. Each family makes its choice according to the family's needs, moral attitude, ethics, and emotions. A decision that is made by one family may be totally unacceptable to another family. However, most families when they come to a decision feel relief, and the burden is reduced substantially. Table 13-8 summarizes the risks, costs, and acceptability for first and second trimester abortions and for fetal surgery.

III. Recommendations.

A. Early detection

1. Whenever possible, carrier detection should be done prior to conception.
2. During pregnancy, tests should be done as early as possible.
3. Mass screening tests should be done when available.
4. Risk assessment should be done on each patient using family history, relevant medical history, and screening tests.
5. Specific diagnostic tests should be offered whenever indicated.

B. Early intervention

1. First trimester abortion has a very low risk and is preferred to second trimester abortion.
2. Second trimester abortion has a low risk but involves substantial patient discomfort.
3. Some fetuses can benefit from medical treatment during pregnancy.
4. Intrauterine procedures and fetal surgery are in the experimental stage and are offered only with rigorous controls.
5. The final decision for any intervention is made by the patient.

Selected Readings

Childs, B., et al. Tay-Sachs screening: Social and psychological impact. *Am. J. Hum. Genet.* 28:550, 1976. *An early attempt to measure the effect of carrier testing on the subjects.*

Evers-Kiebooms, G., and Van der Berghe, H. Impact of genetic counseling: A review of published follow-up studies. *Clin. Genet.* 15:465, 1979. *An important look at the influence of genetic counseling on the patients' subsequent decisionmaking.*

Golbus, M. S., et al. Prenatal genetic diagnosis in 3000 amniocenteses. *N. Engl. J. Med.* 300: 157, 1979. *The largest single series of genetic amniocenteses in the literature.*

Harrison, M. R., Golbus, M. S., and Filly, R. A. Management of the fetus with a correctable congenital defect. *J.A.M.A.* 246:774, 1981. *An early attempt to start thinking of the fetus as a patient in need of medical care.*

Hogge, W. A., Schonberg, S. A., and Golbus, M. S. Chorionic villus sampling: Experience of the first 1000 cases. *Am. J. Obstet. Gynecol.* 154: 1249, 1986. *The first of the large series of CVS cases reported.*

Holmes, L. B. Prospective Counseling for Hereditary Malformations in Newborns. In H. A. Lubs and F. de la Cruz (eds.), *Genetic Counseling.* New York: Raven, 1977. Pp. 241–248. *A good general statement on the problems of counseling patients about neonates with malformations.*

Jacobs, P. A. Epidemiology of chromosome abnormalities in man. *Am. J. Epidemiol.* 105:180, 1977. *An outstanding summary of knowledge about chromosome abnormalities.*

Levy, H. L. Genetic screening. *Adv. Hum. Genet.* 4:1, 1973. *A survey of the status of newborn screening—good factual information.*

Moore, K. L. *The Developing Human: Clinically Oriented Embryology.* Philadelphia: Saunders, 1973. *The best embryology text for the clinician.*

Simpson, J. L. Genes, chromosomes, and reproductive failure. *Fertil. Steril.* 33:107, 1980. *A good summary of the influence of genetics on reproduction.*

14 Sickle Cell Disease in Pregnancy

Karen Poirier-Brode

I. The problem

A. Definition. Sickle cell anemia is caused by the inheritance of a gene for sickle cell hemoglobin without a gene for the normal beta chain of adult hemoglobin. If two sickle cell genes are present in each cell, severe anemia and frequent attacks of bone pain and other crises occur. If one sickle hemoglobin gene and one hemoglobin C gene are inherited, a less severe anemia occurs. Other combinations such as hemoglobin S and D, S and G, S and beta-thalassemia, also cause varying degrees of anemia and clinical illness.

B. Description. Sickle cell hemoglobin differs from normal hemoglobin by the substitution of one amino acid (valine for glutamic acid) in each of the two beta chains of the hemoglobin molecule. This small chemical change alone is responsible for the clinical manifestations of hemolytic anemia, jaundice, and crises with bone pain and vascular obstruction. These occur because situations of low oxygen tension cause the altered hemoglobin molecules to gather and form rod-like masses. These, in turn, distort the erythrocytes into sickle shapes.

Patients with hemoglobin SS disease probably will have been identified prior to pregnancy. However, these patients may have their first crisis in pregnancy. Patients with hemoglobin SC disease may experience no problems until pregnancy. These patients then may have many crises, particularly during the last trimester and the puerperium.

The mating of two individuals with the sickling trait leads to a risk of development of sickle cell in their child. The pattern of inheritance is autosomal codominant. Theoretically, one of four offspring will have the disease and half will have the trait.

C. Epidemiology. The sickle cell trait is found in 8.4% of the United States black population. Sickle cell disease is found in 0.1% of American blacks, and sickle cell-hemoglobin C disease is observed in only about 0.05% of the black population. The frequency is higher in some areas of Africa.

II. Secondary prevention

A. Early detection

1. Methods

a. Description and performance. The Sickledex screen is a blood test used to screen for the presence of hemoglobin S. This test will not discriminate between those persons having only the trait and those having the other sickling hemoglobinopathies.

Hemoglobin electrophoresis is another test specific for the types of hemoglobin present in an individual's blood. The routine hemoglobin, peripheral smear and blood count evaluation may lead to a preliminary diagnosis as well.

b. Interpretation. Individuals with a positive Sickledex screen should have a hemoglobin electrophoresis performed to identify the specific hemoglobinopathy.

c. Timing. Prepregnancy screening is optimal. However, if this has not been done, screening should be done as early in pregnancy as possible. The test may be ordered during family planning visits or with routine prenatal laboratory tests. Prepregnancy screening should be a part of family planning and primary care health assessment and maintenance. Patients' rubella status, nutrition status, drug use, and personal habits (e.g., smoking) should be assessed, as should the presence of sickle disease. Such patients can be adequately prepared for pregnancy if they are carriers or have the disease.

d. Population. Patients at risk include individuals of black ancestry because of the high incidence of sickle cell trait (8.4%) in this population, and any patient with a picture of hemolytic anemia or morphologic abnormality of the erythrocytes (target cells, reticulocytes, or sickle cells).

2. **Justification**

a. **Value.** Screening for sickling tendency in indicated patients is a part of the routine standards and recommendations for prenatal care, providing they have not been previously screened. If the person is identified as a carrier or has the disease, these standards and recommendations call for special referral to a prenatal diagnostic center for genetic counseling prior to the fifteenth week of pregnancy. This recommendation applies to all situations where both parents are carriers for, or have a family history of, an autosomal recessive disorder that can be diagnosed prenatally.

In addition, it is important to identify those pregnant individuals with sickle cell disease because of the risk of more frequent crises during pregnancy requiring medical intervention.

The sickle cell trait may lead to an increase in bacteriuria and pyelonephritis in the antenatal period. These patients are susceptible to anoxia should general anesthesia be required. Anesthesiologists and anesthetists should therefore be aware of this condition.

b. **Risks.** Both the Sickledex screen and hemoglobin electrophoresis require phlebotomy. The most common problem is patient discomfort. Occasionally, individuals may experience bruising at the puncture site, and, rarely, local infection or septicemia may occur.

c. **Costs.** Prices in 1986 in Sacramento, California, are as follows: Sickledex, \$5.50; Hemoglobin electrophoresis, \$21; Blood count with peripheral smear, \$6.

d. **Acceptability.** The Sickledex screen and hemoglobin electrophoresis are generally very acceptable tests with good patient compliance and wide use by health care providers.

B. **Early intervention**

1. **Methods**

a. **Counseling.** Patients with hemoglobin SS or hemoglobin SC disease should be counseled that they will be prone to frequent crises during pregnancy and that partial exchange transfusions or erythrocytophoresis may be necessary to manage their situation during pregnancy and the puerperium. In addition to the maternal risks of a painful sickling crisis, these patients should be informed of the increased risk of infection, congestive heart failure, pulmonary complications, high fetal wastage with crisis, and the risk of anoxic brain damage in live-born infants. With good patient compliance and current recommended management, the outcomes approach those of the normal population.

When both parents of the fetus are determined to have sickling trait, they should be offered genetic counseling and the option of abortion if they are unwilling to give birth to an affected infant. Pregnant patients with sickle cell trait should be advised of their increased risk of urinary tract infection and risk of anoxia if general anesthesia is necessary.

Patients unwilling to accept the additional risks of pregnancy in the face of their sickling hemoglobinopathy can and should be offered the option of abortion.

b. **Genetic amniocentesis.** This is accomplished at about 15 weeks' gestation by aspiration of a small amount of amniotic fluid via a needle inserted into the uterine cavity under ultrasonic guidance. The cells from the fluid are cultured and then prepared for chromosome analysis.

c. **Abortion.** Pregnancy termination may be accomplished by a variety of procedures. Frequently the procedure chosen will depend on the gestational age of the pregnancy. Dilation and evacuation procedures, intraamniotic installation of prostaglandin or hysterotomy may be used.

d. **Consultation.** Patients with sickle cell problems should be followed by an obstetrician who is well acquainted with the problem of sickle cell disease or in consultation with an experienced hematologist.

e. **Urinalysis.** Frequent urinalysis should be performed to detect bacteriuria or urinary tract infection. If positive for significant bacteria, urine culture and sensitivity should be done and appropriate antibiotic therapy given.

f. **Prenatal supplements.** Folic acid supplementation of 1 mg/day is given. There is an increased demand (over the usual increase in pregnancy) because of accelerated red cell turnover in hemolysis. The necessity for iron supplementation may be determined by a combination of a complete blood count and differential with either a measurement of serum iron and total iron binding capacity, or serum ferritin and transferrin concentration. The iron stores may be high because of the hemolysis, and, in addition, the erythroid hyperplasia increases the absorption of iron. Although toxicity from usual prenatal doses would not occur, excess iron should not be given without indication.

The goal of the protocol is to maintain a hemoglobin A concentration of no less than 25% and a hematocrit of 25–30%.

g. **Partial exchange transfusion.** Pregnant women who have sickling hemoglobinopathies may require partial exchange transfusions or automated erythrocytophoresis starting near the end of the second trimester to achieve the desired hemoglobin and hematocrit concentrations.

h. **Sickle crisis management.** Generous fluid replacement using hypotonic solutions (i.e., ½ normal saline) may help to decrease the intracorpuscular concentration of hemoglobin and therefore to reduce sickling. Attention to fluid overload (particularly if transfusions are also occurring) and treatment of pain with standard narcotics form the basis for management. These patients should be managed by perinatal specialists and hematologists who are familiar with this disease.

j. **Antepartum fetal surveillance.** Serial ultrasounds and nonstress test electronic fetal heart rate monitoring should be used during the third trimester to help determine intrauterine fetal growth and fetal well-being (see Chap. 24).

2. **Justification**

a. **Effectiveness.** By following the above screening and management recommendations, patients will know the risk of sickle disease prior to pregnancy and can have a planned pregnancy; and health care providers will be able to diagnose the disease early and intervene early to minimize maternal morbidity and fetal wastage.

b. **Risks and side effects.** The effectiveness of early intervention in the management of pregnancies complicated by sickle cell disease clearly outweighs the risks. However, risks and side effects are not trivial.

(1) **Genetic amniocentesis,** done with a small-gauge needle placed with ultrasonic guidance, has a very low incidence of complications (<1%). The complications that can occur include leakage of amniotic fluid, vaginal bleeding, spontaneous abortion, premature labor pains, amnionitis, injury to the fetus, "bloody" taps, fetal maternal transfusion and Rh sensitization, abruptio placenta, and maternal peritonitis.

(2) **Abortion.** Second trimester abortions are associated with a low incidence of complications. The complication rate increases as gestational age advances. By technique, complication rates are lowest for dilation and evacuation done prior to 17 weeks' gestational age, followed by prostaglandin abortion, late dilation and evacuation, and hysterotomy. The major complications are those of hemorrhage, infection, retained products of conception, and uterine trauma. Systemic reactions to prostaglandins may occur. Late dilation and evacuation, and hysterotomy require major anesthesia.

(3) **Urinalysis.** Antibiotic therapy of urinary tract infections may result in the development of infection with resistant organisms. Allergic reactions to medications used are not infrequent occurrences.

(4) **Prenatal supplements.** Iron supplementation may cause gastritis with nausea and vomiting and may contribute to increased constipation.

(5) **Partial exchange transfusion.** Partial exchange transfusion and erythrocytophoresis share small risks of bleeding or infection at the phlebotomy site, septicemia, transfusion reaction, and transmission of viral illness such as hepatitis and acquired immune deficiency syndrome (AIDS). These procedures are uncomfortable and require time to accomplish.

(6) **Sickle crisis management.** Exchange transfusion carries the same risks outlined in sec. **II.B.2.b.(5)** above.

Narcotic administration may cause respiratory depression, and prolonged use may result in habituation.

Table 14-1. Costs of early intervention in sickle cell disease

Service	Cost
Genetic amniocentesis and counseling	$ 965
Second trimester abortion	$1500
Urinalysis	$ 11
Antibiotic treatment of bacteriuria or urinary tract infection	$ 7
Folic acid supplementation (1 mg/day)	$ 5/100 tablets
Iron studies	
Complete blood count with differential	$ 15
Serum iron	$ 16
Total iron binding capacity	$ 29
Serum ferritin level	$ 38
Transferritin saturation	$ 38
Iron supplementation ($FeSO_4$, 600 mg/day)	$ 1.25/100 tablets
Automated erythrocytophoresis	$ 400
Partial or complete exchange transfusion	$1400
Narcotic analgesia (hydromorphone hydrochloride [Dilaudid] 1–2 mg/4 hr or methadone 5–20 mg/8 hr)	$ 3/dose
Oxygen by nasal prongs	$ 30.50/setup (5.50/hour)
Ultrasound	$ 155
Nonstress test electronic fetal monitoring	$ 60

(7) **Antepartum fetal surveillance.** No risks to mother or fetus have been established for ultrasound as used in the clinical obstetric setting. The advantages of the technique in this situation would clearly outweigh any theoretical disadvantages.

c. **Costs.** Table 14-1 is a summary of costs for the procedures discussed.

d. **Acceptability**

(1) **Counseling.** Genetic counseling has a favorable reception by both patients and health care providers.

(2) **Genetic amniocentesis** is a procedure that is met by intense patient apprehension; however, in most cases patients find it acceptable. In the case of genetic determination of a fetus affected by sickle cell, it has not been readily accepted. This is probably secondary to some cultural factors—lower acceptability of abortion as an option may be one factor, and the close relationship to an affected individual who is coping with the disease may be another. Health care providers generally have good acceptance of this procedure.

(3) **Abortion.** Second trimester abortion for genetic reasons is usually associated with patient distress: The pregnancy may have been planned, and there may be little family or friend support for the pregnancy's termination. The patients are usually anxious to have termination effected as soon as possible after learning of an unacceptable fetal problem. Patients often elect to have a dilation and evacuation or hysterotomy rather than a prostaglandin abortion in order to be unaware of the event. Prolonged depression may follow the abortion. Health care providers will have varied attitudes on abortion, although acceptance of abortion for genetic reasons has wide acceptability. While patients find hysterotomy and dilation and evacuation procedures more psychologically acceptable than prostaglandin abortion, the reverse is true for health care providers.

(4) **Consultation.** Most patients recognize the value of expert consultation in complex medical situations.

(5) **Urinalysis.** Urinalysis and urine culture are acceptable to both patients and health care providers. However, antibiotic regimens for the treatment of bacteriuria and infection often do not have complete patient compliance.

(6) **Prenatal supplements.** Folic acid supplementation is usually met with

good compliance. Iron supplementation, because of frequent gastrointestinal upset, does not receive as much acceptance.

(7) **Partial exchange transfusion.** Partial exchange transfusions involve some patient discomfort, are time-consuming, and require close monitoring of intravascular volume. Automated erythrocytophoresis requires less time, and intravascular volume remains stable. This increases acceptability to patients and health care providers.

(8) **Sickle crisis management.** The methods used to manage a sickle cell crisis have good patient acceptability. All methods except for the frequent administration of narcotic analgesia have good acceptance by health care providers.

(9) **Antepartum fetal surveillance.** These tests are generally acceptable to patients and clinicians.

III. Recommendations

A. Patients of black ancestry or patients with a history of sickle cell disease in the family should be screened for the presence of sickle cell hemoglobin. A Sickledex screen or hemoglobin electrophoresis may be used. Ideally, this should be done prior to pregnancy.

B. All prenatal patients of black ancestry who were not previously screened should have the Sickledex screen or hemoglobin electrophoresis ordered at their first prenatal appointment.

C. All patients whose prenatal panel reveals abnormal erythrocytes on a peripheral blood smear should likewise be screened.

D. Prenatal patients who are positive for sickle cell trait or disease should request that the father of their fetus be tested for sickle cell.

E. All pregnant women with sickle cell trait or disease should be advised of their pregnancy risks.

F. When both parents of the fetus are found to carry the sickle gene, they should be referred for genetic counseling.

G. Appropriate consultation should be obtained for pregnant patients with sickle cell trait or disease. Urinalyses, antibiotics, prenatal supplements, partial exchange transfusion, antepartum fetal surveillance, and prompt management of all sickle cell crises should be used as necessary.

Suggested Readings

Chang, J. C., and Kan, Y. W. Antenatal diagnosis of sickle cell anaemia by direct analysis of the sickle cell mutation. *Lancet* 2(8256):1127, 1981. *Discussion of direct analysis for sickle cell, a technique that avoids the delay of cell culture.*

Levin, J., and Algazy, K. Hematologic Disorders. In G. Burrow and T. Ferris (eds.), *Medical Complications During Pregnancy* (2nd ed.). Philadelphia: Saunders, 1982. *Very good review of complications of sickle cell disease in pregnancy, with summary of treatment.*

Pastorek, J. G. II, and Seiler, B. Maternal death associated with sickle cell trait. *Am. J. Obstet. Gynecol.* 151(3):295, 1985. *Case report dealing with maternal mortality in sickle cell trait.*

Poirier-Brode, K. Hematological Complications of Pregnancy. In K. R. Niswander (ed.). *Manual of Obstetrics* (3rd ed.). Boston: Little, Brown, 1987. *Quick reference for management of obstetric patients with sickle cell.*

Pritchard, J., MacDonald, P., and Gant, N. Medical and Surgical Illnesses During Pregnancy and the Puerperium. In J. Pritchard, P. MacDonald, and N. Gant, *Williams Obstetrics* (17th ed.). Norwalk, CT: Appleton-Century-Crofts, 1985. Pp. 561–640. *Excellent review of problems and management of sickle cell during pregnancy, including genetic counseling for the disorder.*

15 Chlamydial Infections and Pregnancy

Jose Arevalo

I. The problem

A. Description. Colonization of the pregnant female genital tract with *Chlamydia trachomatis* presents a potentially serious threat to the newborn child as well as conferring on the mother a significant risk of postpartum infection. Numerous reports demonstrate that *C.trachomatis* is a common, sexually transmitted pathogen, and that it may be present without clinical symptoms in many individuals [1,2,3]. Evidence is mounting that implicates this organism in association with prematurity, low birth weight, and perinatal mortality [4,5].

The etiological agent, *C. trachomatis*, is an obligate intracellular parasite resembling a bacterium in that it has cell walls, but differing in its inability to manufacture its own energy. Chlamydia are fastidious organisms that depend on the host cells' metabolic machinery to survive. Thus, they are difficult to isolate and must be cultivated in cell cultures as viruses are [1,2,3].

B. Epidemiology. Carrier rates for chlamydia in women range from 2–37%, with most values between 8–12% [6,7,8]. Both inclusion conjunctivitis (see Chap. 38), which occurs at 1–3 weeks of age, and newborn pneumonia, which presents at 1–4 months of age, have been attributed to perinatally acquired *C.trachomatis* infection. Some 18–50% of infants born through infected cervices will develop clinical chlamydia conjunctivitis [9]. Infants born to women with positive cultures have a 10–20% risk of newborn pneumonia [8]. Thirty to 40% of pneumonias that occur during the first 6 months of life are associated with chlamydia, and 25% of infants with chlamydia will manifest significant complications of dyspnea, tachypnea, and apnea. Schachter has conservatively estimated a potential for 26,000 cases of neonatal pneumonia and 29,000 cases of neonatal conjunctivitis yearly from undiagnosed *C.trachomatis* infections in pregnancy [10].

In a case-control study in Seattle, Martin reported a higher incidence of stillbirth and neonatal death in chlamydia-infected women [5].

Wager, et al. reported the association of chlamydia with intrapartum fever and late postpartum endometritis in patients infected during pregnancy who deliver vaginally [11].

The **risk factors** that place individuals at higher risk of chlamydia infection are shown in Table 15-1.

II. Secondary prevention

A. Early detection

1. Methods

- **a. Description and performance.** See Table 15-2 and Chap. 99.
- **b. Interval and timing of testing.** Testing should be done prenatally, preferably at the first prenatal visit [12]. Follow-up test of cure is controversial, and no firm guidelines have been agreed on. However, because of the potential compliance problems in the chlamydia high-risk populations, strong consideration should be given to a test of cure in the third trimester, preferably around 37 weeks. It is important to note that monoclonal antibody identification may detect dead organisms 3–6 weeks [12] after treatment, and thus test of cure is best accomplished with culture.
- **c. Population** (see Table 15-1). High-risk individuals should be routinely screened for chlamydia.

2. Justification (see Table 15-2).

- **a. Routine risk assessment** and laboratory evaluation of high-risk individuals during pregnancy will identify those women who will benefit from prenatal treatment.

Table 15-1. Chlamydia risk factors

Age younger than 20
Multiple sex partners
History of other sexually transmitted diseases
Single
Use of oral contraceptives
Lower socioeconomic status
Ethnicity*: Black; Latino; White or Asian

*In descending degree of risk.

b. **Risks and side effects.** The risks and side effects of testing are minimal and are based only on the potential for treating false-positives or missing false-negatives.

c. **Costs** (see Table 15-2).

d. **Acceptability.** Acceptability of chlamydia testing is excellent by both the practitioner and patient since testing can be accomplished at the first prenatal pelvic exam and requires minimal extra effort.

B. Early intervention

1. **Methods.** Pregnant women identified as infected with *C.trachomatis* should be treated with erythromycin base 500 mg PO qid for 7 days, or erythromycin ethylsuccinate 800 mg PO qid for 7 days. Alternatively, for patients who are unable to tolerate the recommended regimen, erythromycin base 250 mg (or erythromycin succinate 400 mg) PO qid for 14 days may be used. At the present, there are no proven alternative regimens for patients allergic to erythromycin or who are unable to tolerate erythromycin. Tetracycline, which can be used in the nonpregnant state, is contraindicated during pregnancy. The Centers for Disease Control recommends that sexual partners (within 30 days of last sexual contact) of confirmed positive *C. trachomatis*-infected individuals be examined for the presence of sexually transmitted diseases and treated for chlamydia [13]. (see Chap. 99).

2. **Justification**

a. **Effectiveness.** Schachter, et al. have reported an 85–90% effectiveness utilizing erythromycin, as determined by follow-up cultures and negative routine surveillance follow-up of infants. However, treatment failure may run as high as 9% [14].

Schachter has estimated that a program of routine culturing of high-risk pregnant women would be cost-effective if the prevalence of chlamydia in the population is greater than 12% [14].

b. **Risks and side effects.** Erythromycin in pregnancy is fairly well tolerated, especially when given with meals. In Schachter's study, only 3% of the patients noted side effects significant enough to warrant discontinuation of the medication. The most common side effects are nausea and vomiting, followed by dizziness [14].

c. **Costs.** The usual costs of the medication to the pharmacist varies from $2.03 to $11.90, depending on dosage and duration of treatment [15].

d. **Acceptability.** Once informed of the potential dangers to infants and pregnant women from untreated chlamydial infection, pregnant patients appear to accept treatment at a high rate.

III. Recommendations

A. Early detection. All pregnant females who fall into the high-risk group should be screened for the presence of chlamydia using a culture or the more economical monoclonal antibody test at the first prenatal visit.

B. Early intervention

1. For those patients with positive chlamydia tests, treatment with erythromycin should be instituted early in the pregnancy.
2. Sexual partners (last contact within 30 days) of confirmed chlamydia-infected individuals should be examined to rule out sexually transmitted diseases or to be treated.

Table 15-2. Comparison of chlamydia tests

Test	Type	Costs (range and average)	Sensitivity/ specificity	Comments [12, 16, 17]
Culture	Cell culture	$25–90 ($40)	Unavailable	"Gold Standard" Requires 2–6 days Difficulty in handling/ transfer Not widely available
Microtrak	Fluorescein conjugated monoclonal antibody	$15–60 ($25)	92%/99% (positive predictive value= 91%)	Total processing time 30–40 min Can be done on direct smear Only tested in high-risk populations under optimum conditions
Chlamydi-azyme	ELISA	$10–40 ($20)	82%/98% (positive predictive value= 80%)	Total processing time 4 hr Only tested on high-risk populations under optimum conditions
PAP	Cytological	$10–21 ($14)	Poor	Not recommended for routine screening
Serology	Blood testing		Unknown	Little value in screening Utility only as a research tool

3. Follow-up test of cure (preferably by culture in the third trimester) is strongly advised to assess efficacy of treatment.

4. If follow-up test is positive, repeat treatment with above schedule.

References

1. Schachter, J. Chlamydial infections. *N. Engl. J. Med.* 298(8):428, 1978. *An essentially complete review of the microbiology, clinical manifestations, and treatment of the spectrum of chlamydial diseases, up to 1978 (first of three parts).*
2. Schachter, J. Chlamydial infections. *N. Engl. J. Med.* 298(9):490, 1978. *See reference 1 (second of three parts).*
3. Schachter, J. Chlamydial infections. *N. Engl. J. Med.* 298(10):540, 1978. *See reference 1 (third of three parts).*
4. Harrison, H. R., et al. Cervical chlamydia trachomatic and mycoplasmal infections in pregnancy. *J.A.M.A.* 250(13)1721, 1983. *A prospective study from the University of Arizona identifying risk factors associated with chlamydia, mycoplasma, and ureaplasma infection in pregnancy, and comparing pregnancy and postpartum outcomes.*
5. Martin, D. H., et al. Prematurity and perinatal mortality in pregnancies complicated by maternal *Chlamydia trachomatis* infections. *J.A.M.A* 247(11):1585, 1982. *This prospective study was conducted by the University of Washington and examined the relationship of pregnancy outcome in women with and without positive chlamydial cultures.*
6. Handsfield, H. H., et al. Criteria for selective screening for *Chlamydia trachomatis* infection in women attending family planning clinics. *J.A.M.A.* 255(13):1730, 1986. *This cross-sectional study of women attending two urban family planning clinics examined clinical, behavioral, and demographic characteristics in women requesting contraceptive counseling, and correlated these factors with chlamydial cervical infection.*
7. Khurana, C. M., Deddish, P. A., and delMundo, F. Prevalence of *Chlamydia trachomatis* in the pregnant cervix. *Obstet. Gynecol.* 66(2):241,1985. *This is a study that reviewed*

the prevalence of chlamydial cervical infection in pregnant females seeking care in Fabella Memorial Hospital in Manila, the Philippines.

8. Schachter, J., et al. Prospective study of perinatal transmission of *Chlamydia trachomatis*. *J.A.M.A.* 255(24):3374, 1986. *This is a report of the five-year prospective experience at San Francisco General Hospital following 5531 pregnant women, with 262 chlamydia-positive patients.*
9. Alexander, E. R. and Harrison, H. R. Role of *Chlamydia trachomatis* in perinatal infection. *Rev. Infect. Dis.* 5(4):713, 1983. *A state-of-the-art review of the relationship between maternal cervical infection and prepartum, neonatal, and postpartum complications.*
10. Schachter, J., and Grossman, M. Chlamydial infections. *Annu. Rev. Med.* 32:45, 1981. *Excellent early review of the spectrum of chlamydial infection in infants.*
11. Wager, G. P., et al. Puerperal infectious morbidity: Relationship to route of delivery and to antepartum *Chlamydia trachomatis* infection. *Am. J. Obstet. Gynecol.* 138(7 part 2):1028, 1980. *A study that reviews the relationship of route of delivery and of chlamydia cervical infection to intra- and postpartum fever.*
12. Centers for Disease Control: 1985—STD Treatment Guidelines. *M.M.W.R.* 34(45):75S, 1985. *Most recent recommendations from the CDC on sexually transmitted disease detection, treatment, and follow-up.*
13. Centers for Disease Control: *Chlamydia trachomatis* infections: Policy guidelines for prevention and control. *M.M.W.R.* 34(35):53S, 1985. *A document prepared for the CDC by a distinguished panel of experts, containing recommendations regarding risk assessment, laboratory evaluation, prevention, treatment, and education of chlamydial infections.*
14. Schachter, J., et al. Experience with the routine use of erythromycin for chlamydial infections in pregnancy. *N. Engl. J. Med.* 314(5):276, 1986. *Prospective clinical trial examining the efficacy of erythromycin in the prevention of newborn chlamydial infection.*
15. Oral erythromycins. *Med. Lett. Drugs. Ther.* 27(678):1, 1985. *A review of available oral erythromycin preparations.*
16. Amortegui, A. J. and Meyer, M. P. Enzyme immunoassay for detection of *Chlamydia trachomatis* from the cervix. *Obstet. Gynecol.* 65(4):523, 1985. *A comparison of chlamydiazyme (an E.L.I.S.A. assay) to cell culture for chlamydia detection, with data on sensitivity, specificity, and predictive values.*
17. Quinn, T. C., et al. Screening for *Chlamydia trachomatis* infection in an inner-city population: A comparison of diagnostic methods. *J. Infect. Dis.* 152(2):419, 1985. *A comparison similar to that above of the immunofluorescence slide test to chlamydial cultures, with data on sensitivity, specificity, and predictive values.*

16 Gonorrhea and Pregnancy

Dewey Sandberg

I. The problem

A. Description. Infection of the genital tract with *Neisseria gonorrhoeae* during pregnancy is often asymptomatic and carries with it the potential for acute salpingitis and its sequelae, as well as a number of serious complications of pregnancy [1].

Prior to the twelfth to fourteenth week of pregnancy, when the chorion fuses with the endometrial decidua obliterating the intrauterine cavity, ascending gonococcal infection may cause septic abortion as well as the typical forms of pelvic inflammatory disease. After the sixteenth week, the endocervix is occluded by the chorioamnion, and intraluminal spread is blocked, but chorioamnionitis may occur and cause premature rupture of membranes or preterm labor [2]. Disseminated gonococcal infection,including gonococcal arthritis, also occurs in pregnancy, though there is disagreement in the literature as to whether the pregnant state increases the likelihood of such systemic spread [1].

Maternal gonorrhea exposes the fetus and newborn to risk of intrauterine growth retardation (IUGR), deep tissue infection, arthritis, and, although rare, fetal demise. Direct inoculation of the mucous membranes with infectious material during passage through the birth canal is the most likely cause of infection in the newborn. Ophthalmia neonatorum is the most common form of gonococcal infection in newborns, but the vagina, pharynx, urethra, and rectum may also be colonized. Localized scalp infections, as well as disseminated disease, have been attributed to use of scalp electrodes in the presence of intrapartum gonococcal infection [3,5–7].

B. Epidemiology. The incidence of gonorrhea in the United States increased rapidly between 1960 and 1975 to its present level of about one million cases reported annually, which may represent only half of the cases actually treated [2].

The highest age-specific rates occur in young adults, during peak reproductive years. These rates, ranging from 3–7%, apply equally to pregnant and nonpregnant women. Although as many as 40–60% of young women with gonococcal infections have symptoms [4], pregnant women with gonorrhea are often asymptomatic [1].

There is relatively little quantitative information on maternal, fetal, and neonatal morbidity and mortality. Chorioamnionitis and IUGR may complicate 5% of pregnancies (significantly more than matched controls) of women with gonorrhea detected prior to the intrapartum period. For infections not discovered until the intrapartum period, premature rupture of membranes (PROM), PROM greater than 24 hours, and chorioamnionitis occurred in 63%, 42%, and 26%, respectively, of the cases in one study [1].

As for the newborn, the prominent problem of ophthalmia neonatorum occurs in approximately 28% of infants born to mothers with gonorrhea (see Chap. 38).

High-risk groups include minority women; poor, young, unmarried, urban-dwellers; and those with a history of other sexually transmitted diseases [2].

II. Secondary prevention

A. Early detection

1. Methods [4,5–7]

a. Description. Pregnant women should have an endocervical culture for gonorrhea performed as part of the first prenatal exam, as early in pregnancy as possible. Women at high risk for sexually transmitted disease should have an additional gonorrhea culture performed near the end of the third trimester.

b. Procedure. The endocervical culture is done as an integral part of the vaginal speculum exam. Under direct vision, the exocervix is cleansed of adherent exudate or vaginal secretions, and a sterile cotton-tipped swab is inserted 1–2 cm into the external os and rotated for a few seconds.

The specimen is transferred immediately onto the culture medium—in the clinic if possible. Optimal growth of gonococcus requires high humidity, temperature of 35–37 °C, a 5–10% carbon dioxide atmosphere, and, when collected from the cervix with its complex bacterial flora, a selective culture medium. Therefore, when a nonselective transport medium is used, transport time to the lab should be less than 8 hours and never more than 24 hours. The most commonly used media are Modified Thayer-Martin, which contains antibiotics and is selective for gonococcus, and modifications of Stuart's media, which serve as transport media. A number of culture kits are available for office use and include a crushable carbon dioxide-generating capsule.

c. **Population.** In choosing the patients to screen, the high-risk groups mentioned above must be emphasized, particularly in repeat culturing late in pregnancy, but all pregnant women are to be cultured at the first prenatal exam [4].

2. **Justification**

a. **Test characteristics.** An endocervical culture, with a sensitivity of 80–90%, is the best method available for screening asymptomatic pregnant women. Gram-stained endocervical smears, though having a high specificity, have a sensitivity of 50–70%, making them inadequate for screening. Other rapid diagnostic techniques based on biochemical or immunological detection of gonococcal elements have not yet demonstrated sufficient sensitivity and specificity for use in routine endocervical screening [5–7], particularly in low-prevalence populations.

b. **Cost, risks, and acceptability.** The screening culture is generally accepted by the patient and physician, costs approximately $18–43 (average $32, Sacramento, 1986), and risks are negligible.

B. **Early intervention**

1. **Methods** [8]. For uncomplicated endocervical infection in pregnancy, the same treatment regimen is recommended as for any adult patient: briefly, amoxicillin (3.0 gm) or ampicillin (3.5 gm) PO, or ceftriaxone (250 mg IM) or aqueous procaine penicillin G (4.8 million U IM). Except when ceftriaxone is used, probenecid (1 gm PO) should accompany the antibiotic. Spectinomycin (2.0 gm IM) may be used in patients who are allergic to penicillin (see Chap. 97). In addition, erythromycin base (500 mg) or erythromycin ethylsuccinate (800 mg) PO qid for 7 days should be given (see Chap. 15).

Tetracycline and doxycycline should not be used in pregnancy because of potential adverse effects on the fetus.

Similarly, the recommendations for follow-up cultures, management of treatment failures, simultaneous treatment of chlamydial infection, tracking and treatment of sex partners, prophylactic treatment for known exposure, and serologic testing for syphilis apply to pregnant women as for any adult (see Chap. 97). Note that all women should have a rectal culture performed as part of the posttreatment follow-up exam, regardless of whether rectal infection was sought or found prior to therapy.

2. **Justification**

a. **Effectiveness.** There is little information on the effectiveness of treatment in preventing complications of pregnancy, though one study [9] estimated that about 28% of prenatal patients with untreated gonorrhea developed complications of pregnancy, compared with 5.8% of treated cases and 4% of patients with negative cultures. These, and the figures presented above, argue for early detection and treatment, as well as for repeat cultures late in pregnancy to avoid the serious complications of pregnancy and neonatal health.

b. **Risks.** Although the manufacturers of these medications note that safety for use in pregnancy has not been established, many organizations, including the Centers for Disease Control and the American College of Obstetricians and Gynecologists, recommend their use as outlined above. Assuming that antibiotic allergies are taken into account, the risks of new allergic reactions, gastrointestinal upset, and other mild intolerances of antibiotics are generally accepted as outweighed by the benefits of treatment.

c. **Costs.** The costs of the recommended dosages of antibiotics are included in Table 16-1.

Table 16-1. Costs and dosages of antibiotics used to treat gonorrhea*

Antibiotic	Dosage	Cost
Amoxicillin	3.0 gm PO	$ 7.00
Ampicillin	3.5 gm PO	$ 5.50
Ceftriaxone	250 mg IM	$13.50
Aqueous procaine penicillin G	4.8 million IU IM	$16.00
Spectinomycin	2.0 gm IM	$15.00
Erythromycin base 250 #56	500 mg qid for 7 days	$11.00
EES 400 mg #56	800 mg qid for 7 days	$16.50

*Average costs in Sacramento, California, in 1986.

III. Recommendations

A. Early detection

1. All pregnant women should have an endocervical culture for *Neisseria gonorrhoeae* during the first prenatal visit.
2. A second culture should be done late in the third trimester on all women at high risk.

B. Early intervention

1. Following the same recommendations as for any adult with gonorrhea, amoxicillin or ampicillin PO, IM aqueous procaine penicillin G with probenecid, or ceftriaxone should be given as a one-time dose.
2. Spectinomycin may be used in penicillin-allergic women.
3. A seven-day course of erythromycin should also be given to treat for chlamydial infection that may be assumed to be present in patients being treated for gonorrhea. Tetracycline and doxycycline should not be used in pregnancy.
4. The recommendations for follow-up cultures after treatment, management of treatment failures and sex partners, prophylaxis for known exposure, and testing for syphilis are the same as in nonpregnant patients. All women should have a rectal culture performed during the follow-up exam.

References

1. Edwards, L. E., et al. Gonorrhea in pregnancy. *Am. J. Obstet. Gynecol.* 132(6):637, 1978. *A clinical investigation of the effect of gonococcal infection on outcome of pregnancy.*
2. Hook, E. W., III, and Holmes, K. K. Gonococcal infections. *Ann. Intern. Med.* 102(2):229, 1985. *A broad-scoped review of clinical aspects of gonococcal infection.*
3. Oppenheimer, E. H., and Winn, K. J. Fetal gonorrhea with deep tissue infection occurring in utero. *Pediatrics* 69(1):74, 1982. *A case report and discussion of in utero gonococcal infection and fetal demise.*
4. Gonorrhea and Chlamydial Infections. Chicago: *ACOG Technical Bulletin* No. 89, November 1985. *ACOG recommendations for screening and management of gonorrhea and chlamydial infection, with a section devoted to gonorrhea in pregnancy.*
5. Handsfield, H. H. Gonorrhea and Uncomplicated Gonococcal Infection. In K. K. Holmes, et al. (eds.), *Sexually Transmitted Diseases.* New York: McGraw-Hill, 1984. Pp. 205–220. *Thorough, recent text that includes detailed discussions of all aspects of gonococcal infections.*
6. Brunham, R. C., Holmes, K. K., and Eschenbach, D. Sexually Transmitted Diseases in Pregnancy. In K. K. Holmes, et al. (eds.), *Sexually Transmitted Diseases.* New York: McGraw-Hill, 1984. Pp. 782–816. *See reference 5.*
7. Mardh, P. A. Bacteria, Chlamydiae and Mycoplasmas. In K. K. Holmes, et al. (eds.), *Sexually Transmitted Diseases.* New York: McGraw-Hill, 1984. Pp. 829–856. *See reference 5.*
8. 1985 (STD) Sexually transmitted disease treatment guidelines. *M.M.W.R.* 34(4S Suppl):75S, 1985. *CDC guidelines for treatment of sexually transmitted diseases.*
9. Charles, A. G. Asymptomatic gonorrhea in prenatal patients. *Am. J. Obstet. Gynecol.* 108:595, 1970. *An early study supporting routine screening of prenatal patients for asymptomatic gonorrhea.*

17 Syphilis and Pregnancy

James A. McGregor

I. The problem

A. Description. In the pre-chemotherapeutic era, our medical forebears recognized syphilis as the frequently fatal "great pox," which they deemed "beyond cure." Now that antimicrobials are easily available, we have pronounced syphilis "completely preventable"[1]. Yet it persists because of a web of behavioral, economic, and medical circumstances that impede application of knowledge to recognize, prevent, and eradicate syphilis [2, 3]. As in the past, it is unborn and newborn children who are most commonly caught in this complex web that can entangle and leave them prey to destruction by an easily treatable disease. It is now generally only the fetus and newborn who suffer the full brunt of untreated syphilis.

We can examine means to prevent modern-day children from being born with "great pox." Masterful reviews are available and authoritative sources should be consulted for the most current treatment recommendations [4–10].

B. Pathobiology. Syphilis is caused by *Treponema pallidum*, a thin, delicate spirochete that is about 10–13 μm long, about the diameter of an erythrocyte, and has a characteristic "turning thread" motility on dark-field microscopy. The cell wall contains lipopolysaccharide, and cell division occurs only every 30–33 hours. Other treponemal species include *T. carateum*, *T. pertenue*, and a variant of *T. pallidum*. These mediate, respectively, pinta and yaws in the tropics, and bejel, or endemic syphilis, in the Middle East. Because these generally nonvisceral treponematoses are seroantigenically similar to *T. pallidum*, immigrants from endemic areas may have positive serologic tests for syphilis (STSs).

Syphilis can be contracted by sexual intimacy (including kissing), intrauterine exposure, and rarely, transfusion. Although syphilis can be acquired by direct contact during birth, hematogenous infection of the placenta with spread to the fetus is the primary means of vertical transmission. Up to 95% of women with early syphilis during pregnancy transmit infection to the fetus [11].

On the other hand, syphilis is not a highly contagious disease if exposure is limited to direct contact. A person who has a single sexual encounter with another person with infectious syphilis has approximately one chance in ten of acquiring the disease. Given direct contact, however, only a few microorganisms are required to invade intact mucosa or abraded skin. Entry is rapidly gained into lymphatics and the bloodstream with possible spread to all visceral organs, including the placenta. After a median of 3 weeks (3–90 days), a chancre forms at the site of inoculation.

Primary syphilis is usually manifested by a single, painless chancre, which is most often asymptomatic and inapparent in women. Spirochetemia, with possible spread to the placenta, is heaviest and most sustained during secondary syphilis. Any type of rash can be found, with the general exception of vesiculobular lesions, which are much more common in congenital syphilis. Of note are condyloma lata which are raised lesions on moist areas of the body, including the genitalia. Spirochetes are plentiful in condyloma lata. These lesions may be mistaken for condyloma acuminata (genital warts), and direct contact can lead to infection during intercourse, medical care, or parturition. Spirochetemia diminishes with time but may be episodic for several years, allowing untreated women to give birth to congenitally infected children in successive pregnancies.

T. pallidum can infect the trophoblast or placenta at any gestational age. Harter and Benirschke demonstrated that spirochetes can be found within trophoblast and embryonic tissue in the first trimester [12]. Past failure to recognize syphilitic infection before 18 weeks' gestation is now considered to have been due to the inability of the embryonic/fetal immune system to mount a recognizable response, rather than because of resistance to infection.

Table 17-1. Pregnant women and newborns at increased risk for syphilis*

Women
1. Who were possibly inadequately treated for syphilis in the past
2. With inconsistent or no prenatal care
3. With a history of multiple sexual partners, or who are prostitutes
4. Who are substance abusers
5. With preterm labor or intrauterine growth retardation in high-risk geographic area or populations
6. With findings of a large placenta, fetal edema, or hydrops noted antenatally or at birth

Newborns
1. Of women listed above
2. With any findings suggestive of intrauterine infection (e.g., hepatosplenomegaly, rash)
3. With large placenta, edema, hydrops, intrauterine growth retardation
4. In high-risk geographic areas

*These women and babies should have STS testing done near term or on cord blood samples at birth. All women should have STS evaluation at their initial antenatal visit.

Once *T. pallidum* infects the placenta, the organisms gain hematogenous access to all fetal organs, possibly causing acute, subacute, and granulomatous parenchymal inflammation. Overall, untreated early syphilis during pregnancy results in 40% reproductive wastage, either by spontaneous abortion, stillbirth, or perinatal death. An additional 10% are born with stigmata of congenital syphilis. Only one in 5 "self-heals" or escapes infection [11]. The risks and severity of fetal syphilis are heightened if syphilis is acquired during pregnancy. The venerable "Kassowitz's law" holds that risks of fetal syphilis are inversely related to the length of maternal infection prior to pregnancy. These observations correspond to presumed heavier spirochetemia earlier in infections and transplacental IgG antibody passive immunization after infection is well established. Untreated primary or secondary syphilis in early pregnancy results in abortion or stillbirth in about 50% of pregnancies and congenital syphilis in survivors. In contrast, pregnancies of women with latent syphilis suffer only 10% wastage, 10% preterm delivery, and 10% congenital syphilis [11].

Because fetal syphilis is contracted by hematogenous spread, there is no primary stage. Congenital syphilis resembles secondary syphilis but with greater preponderance of potentially lethal visceral infection. Thus, fetal syphilis most closely resembles the considerable morbidity and mortality of syphilis initially infecting immunologically "inexperienced" Europeans in the fifteenth and sixteenth centuries.

C. Epidemiology. The occurrence of congenital syphilis reflects rates of syphilis in women generally and may differ greatly in varying locations. During 1979 and 1980, different states reported 5.9–74.1 cases of congenital syphilis/1000 women with early syphilis [13]. Since 1981, the incidence of syphilis in women has risen steadily, especially among 15- to 24-year olds, who also have the highest birth rate [14]. Mirroring this trend is a 50% increase of congenital syphilis since 1978. In the early 1980s, the number of reported cases approximated 150–160 yearly [14].

D. Risk groups (see Table 17-1). All types of syphilis are found most frequently in large urban centers, and the disease is most common among young, poor, unmarried women. In developing nations, all types of syphilis are much more common than in industrialized countries. In developing countries, syphilis remains a common cause of perinatal morbidity and mortality.

Regardless of geographic location, pregnant women and health care providers must be alert to the occurrence and real risks of congenital syphilis. Two studies done 30 years apart, first in Massachusetts (1951) and then in Texas (1981), revealed very similar findings [1,15]. Both studied approximately 50 women who gave birth to infants with congenital syphilis. Both noted that approximately one-third received no prenatal care, one-third did not complete treatment, and 10% appeared infected subsequent to an initially negative prenatal serology test. In each series, several infected women were not administered serologic tests for syphilis during their antenatal care [1,15].

Certainly inaccessibility, underutilization, and inadequacies of antenatal care all play important roles in the continued occurrence of congenital syphilis. Forthright and effective steps should be taken to ensure that acceptable antenatal care is available, used, and effectively given.

II. Primary prevention (see Chap. 98).

III. Secondary prevention

A. Early detection

1. **Methods.** Secondary prevention of congenital syphilis involves education of all women regarding the necessity of seeking early and sustained antenatal care, and ensuring that serologic tests are performed on all pregnant women and on women and babies at high-risk at or near term and/or at delivery (see Table 17-1).

   a. **Serologic tests for syphilis (STS).** Serologic tests for syphilis are based on development of antibodies responding to both treponemal and nontreponemal antigens.

      (1) **Nontreponemal antibody tests.** Nontreponemal antibodies (reagin), which react with combinations of cardiolipin and other phospholipids using the Venereal Disease Research Laboratory (VDRL) procedure, card test (RPR) Rapid Plasma Reagin, or the Automated Reagin test (ART), are employed as screening tests and as means to document adequacy of treatment.

      (2) **Treponemal antibody tests.** The most useful treponemal antibody test is the fluorescent treponemal antibody absorption test (FTA-ABS) in which serum is absorbed with nonpathogenic treponemal antigen. Another increasingly employed treponemal test is the microhemagglutination assay for *T. pallidum* (MHA-TP). This test appears to be clinically similar to FTA-ABS but is easier to perform.

   b. **Interpretation** (see also sec. **III.A.2.a** below). Presently available nontreponemal tests are clinically similar and are all subject to misinterpretation around endpoints and in their detection of reagin-antibody that is not caused by treponemal infection. If a nontreponemal screening test is positive, then a treponemal-specific test should be performed to confirm the serologic diagnosis. Once positive, treponemal tests remain positive for life.

      In North America, the most common treponemal disease by far is syphilis. In other parts of the world in which other treponemal infections occur, such as pinta, yaws, and bejel, serologic diagnosis of syphilis may be problematic and rests on clinical findings and history. As noted, immigrants from other areas of the world where these diseases are endemic may give positive nontreponemal and treponemal serologic test results for syphilis. Presumptive treatment is commonly given.

   c. **Evaluation.** It must be remembered that serologic tests for syphilis do not become reliably positive until 4–6 weeks after infection, and roughly 50% of patients with primary disease will be initially sero-negative. Therefore, dark-field examinations of possible primary and secondary lesions in both adults and children are important and can lead to immediate diagnosis. Dark-field microscopy of any primary lesion should be performed by experienced personnel. Referral to local experts or sexually-transmitted-disease clinics may be necessary. If lesions are dark-field negative and syphilis is still a possibility, then STS may be repeated in 2–4 weeks. Patients with secondary syphilis have uniformly positive STS. On rare occasions, these individuals may exhibit a "prozone" effect due to very high titers of antibody and may have a falsely negative test. If secondary syphilis is a possibility, the laboratory should be alerted so that they may further dilute the specimen to reach an accurate endpoint.

   d. **Follow-up.** Serologic evidence of syphilis should prompt expedited evaluation including a carefully done history and physical and a history of exposure, signs and symptoms, and possible prior treatment for syphilis so as to appropriately diagnose, stage, and treat the patient. Local health departments may be contacted to obtain records from other states. All named sexual partners and the possibly infected woman's fetus should be promptly treated.

      Because nontreponemal test results fall and may disappear with treatment (1 year in primary and secondary syphilis, 2 years in early latent syphilis), they are commonly used to document adequacy of treatment. Pregnant women treated for syphilis should be followed with monthly VDRL tests or their equivalent until delivery, and then periodically until sero-negative. Even though treponemal tests remain positive for the life of the individual, reinfection may occur and is associated with increased nontreponemal antibody titer. Both children and adults with prolonged untreated syphilis may become "serofast" and demonstrate no fall in titer even though they are adequately treated. In complex situations, expert consultation may be obtained from local health departments or other sources.

Examination of cerebral spinal fluid (CSF) in syphilitic patients remains controversial. Many authorities recommend lumbar puncture if neurosyphilis is a possibility. In a series of pregnant women evaluated for syphilis, Jones and Harris found that fully 11% of pregnant women with syphilis had positive FTA-ABS-specific IgM CSF examinations. These authors suggest that lumbar puncture be performed in any pregnant woman who is FTA-ABS positive [16].

e. **Population/interval.** Pregnant women should be screened with an STS at the first prenatal visit. It is crucial to understand that in at least 10% of congenitally infected newborns, maternal infection appears to occur after STS testing has been performed. Women at high risk for syphilis should be screened near term as well as when first seen during pregnancy. A list of characteristics of women and newborns who should be screened near term and have cord blood STS testing performed is presented in Table 17-1.

f. **Infants.** Satisfactory diagnosis of infants with congenital syphilis may be difficult [6]. Details of the mother's history, physical findings, serology, and previous treatment must be known. In relatively high-risk settings such as large inner city hospitals, cord blood samples may be STS tested routinely. While newborns with congenital syphilis may be asymptomatic, most present with either prematurity, intrauterine growth retardation, hepatosplenomegaly, abdominal distention, edema, or a variety of rashes or mucosal lesions. Immediate placental examination can be helpful, especially if histologic sections are obtained. Skin and mucosal lesions can be immediately examined by dark-field microscopy. Late congenital syphilis is manifest by "scars" caused by earlier infection causing stigmata, which become apparent after the first 2 years of life. Late congenital syphilis is most famously defined as Hutchinson's triad: notched teeth, interstitial keratitis, and eighth nerve deafness.

Serologic tests, which should be performed on newborns with a history of recognized maternal syphilis during pregnancy and on any other infants who may have syphilis, include titered VDRL, FTA-ABS, and IgM-specific FTA-ABS. While none of these tests is conclusive, any newborn with a positive test should have a CSF examination. Although it is true that a positive STS after 4 months of age is considered prima facie evidence of congenital infection, it is more important to see that newborns possibly suffering from congenital syphilis are treated as promptly as possible so that vagaries of follow-up do not interfere with or delay necessary treatment. Differential diagnosis of congenital syphilis includes bacterial and viral sepsis, blood group incompatibility, other causes of fetal hydrops and dermatitis, nephrotic syndrome, as well as many genetic disorders.

2. **Justification.** Because of the generally asymptomatic nature of syphilis in pregnant women and the lack of knowledge among contemporary health care providers about the signs and symptoms of syphilis, appropriate sampling and interpretation of syphilis test serology remains crucial for identification of infected pregnant women and children.

   a. **Test characteristics.** Up to one-fourth of positive nontreponemal tests occur because of errors in laboratory interpretation or the presence of nontreponemal antibody. These latter tests are called biologic false-positives (BFPs). BFP nontreponemal tests are associated with a large number of conditions including "collagen disorders," subclinical lupus erythematosus, other autoimmune disorders, intravenous substance abuse, recent immunization, and various acute or chronic infections, as well as pregnancy itself. Persistance of BFPs after pregnancy or for more than 6 months is ominous, as the test may be an indicator for subsequent development of systemic lupus erythematosus and other disorders of altered immunity. The presence of BFP test during pregnancy is now also recognized as an indicator of the presence of antiphospholipid antibody, also known as lupus anticoagulant, which is associated with its own greatly increased risks of reproductive wastage [17]. Documentation of BFP positivity should be used as an indicator for partial prothrombin time (PTT) screening for lupus anticoagulant. Paradoxically, the

Table 17-2. Treatment of syphilis during pregnancy[a]

Type of disease	Drug[b]	Dose	Duration
Early syphilis (primary, secondary, latent syphilis of less than 1 year's duration). Cerebral spinal fluid examination preferred in latent syphilis.	Benzathine Penicillin G	2.4 million U IM	Once
Syphilis of more than 1 year's duration (latent syphilis of unknown or more than 1 year's duration, cardiovascular or late benign: treat unknown as though of more than 1 year's duration). Cerebral spinal fluid examination preferred prior to treatment.[c]	Benzathine Penicillin G	2.4 million U IM	Weekly for 3 doses
Neurosyphilis[d]			

[a]From Centers for Disease Control recommendations.
[b]Because of pharmacokinetic alterations during pregnancy, these recommendations should be considered as minimal treatment in late pregnancy. We recommend further dosing with penicillin (ampicillin 500 mg qid for 7–14 days) as adjunctive treatment in advanced pregnancy. Since penicillin is the preferred agent for treatment of syphilis in pregnancy, expedited evaluation and desensitization should be performed if there is a convincing history of penicillin allergy.
[c]Lumbar puncture is generally recommended if neurosyphilis is a possibility.
[d]See first source below.
Source: 1985 STD treatment guidelines. *M.M.W.R.* 34(Suppl 4):75s, 1985; L. Mascola, et al. Congenital syphilis. Why is it still occuring? *J.A.M.A.* 252(13):1719, 1984.

presence of this substance is associated with the increased occurrence of thrombotic disease systemically and focally within the placenta.

False-positive FTA-ABS tests may occur in systemic lupus erythematosus, cirrhosis, and in unexplained circumstances, including pregnancy. If there are questions of a possible false-positive FTA-ABS, then another treponemal test such as MHA-TP should be performed at a reference laboratory.

IgM-treponemal (FTA-ABS) antibodies may be useful in defining fetal infection because IgM does not cross the placenta. Even with removal of rheumatoid factor, IgM test results are not entirely specific or sensitive.

b. **Risks.** The risks of serologic testing in pregnancy relate mainly to false-positives noted above.

c. **Costs and acceptability.** Nontreponemal testing in pregnancy is inexpensive and is considered standard of care. As noted, because treponemal-based tests are expensive and somewhat difficult to perform, they are not employed as screening tests but must be considered in the overall cost since they are employed whenever a nontreponemal screening test is positive.

B. Early intervention

1. Methods

a. **Antenatal (fetal) syphilis.** In every instance of maternal syphilis, the goals are treatment of the mother and prevention of congenital syphilis by treating the mother and the fetus as promptly as possible. Primary, secondary, and latent syphilis (less than 1 year in duration) are appropriately treated with a single dose of benzathine penicillin G, 2.4 million U IM [10]. Treatment of uncomplicated latent syphilis of over 1 year's duration consists of this same regimen of benzathine penicillin G repeated at weekly intervals for three doses (Table 17-2) [10].

To effectively treat the fetus, originally low maternal drug levels must first cross the placental barrier and then achieve spirocheticidal levels in each of the fetal organs, including the central nervous system, by crossing the "blood-brain barrier." Penicillin levels that may be curative within the mother may be insufficient within the fetus. Although the matter remains unstudied, it is likely that only very low levels of penicillin can be found at sites of infection, especially the central nervous system, within the fetus. Therefore, it is reasonable to treat syphilitic pregnant women near term with extra or increased doses of penicillin, so as to increase both maternal and fetal drug levels and improve chances for complete spirochetal eradication within the fetus. We suggest supplementary dosing of 500 mg ampicillin, or an equivalent agent, qid PO for 1–2 weeks. Furthermore, if the mother appears unlikely to complete an outpatient regimen, she should be hospitalized so that penicillin treatment may be supervised. Newborns of women treated near term with penicillin or with alternative agents should be expediently evaluated, including CSF examination after birth, and preemptively treated for congenital syphilis.

At this time, there is no satisfactory alternative to penicillin for the treatment of fetal syphilis. Tetracycline and erythromycin are recommended as alternative treatments in penicillin-allergic adults with syphilis. Tetracycline is contraindicated during pregnancy because of possible damage to fetal dentition and bone. Erythromycin base or succinate 500 mg qid PO for 14–30 days appears adequate for maternal treatment for early and latent syphilis, respectively (see Table 17-2). Because erythromycin does not reliably cross the placenta, however, it is inadequate treatment for fetal syphilis.

Evaluation of other antibiotics that cross the placenta and can eradicate fetal syphilitic infection would be of great interest. Unfortunately, clindamycin has not worked well in animal models, and cephaloridine and rifampin have been anecdotally ineffective.

b. **Postnatal (congenital) syphilis.** Penicillin is the agent of choice for treatment of congenital syphilis after birth as well. Penicillin allergy is not a problem in neonatal therapy, as the responsible IgE antibodies do not cross the placenta. Treatment recommendations for symptomatic congenital syphilis have recently changed. All infants with congenital syphilis should have CSF examinations to provide a baseline for follow-up. Regardless of CSF results, all children should now be treated with a regimen effective for neurosyphilis. These include aqueous crystalline penicillin, 50,000 U/kg IV or IM in 2 divided doses for a minimum of 10 days; or aqueous procaine penicillin, 50,000 U/kg IM, also for a minimum of 10 days. Treatment may be completed on an ambulatory basis or during hospitalizaton if follow-up is not assured. Further treatment of asymptomatic infants whose mothers were adequately treated with penicillin during pregnancy is not necessary if follow-up is assured. If not, then these infants should be treated with a single dose of benzathine penicillin, 50,000 U/kg IM [10].

c. **Follow-up.** Subsequent to treatment of fetal or congenital syphilis, nontreponemal STSs should be obtained at birth, at 1 month, and every 3 months for the first 15 months; and then every 6 months until nontreponemal tests are negative or stable at low titer. Nontreponemal tests (VDRL and RPR) will usually become negative by 3–6 months after birth if the newborn has been effectively treated. If this does not occur, then treatment may be reconsidered after CSF examination. Children with congenital neurosyphilis should have a repeat CSF examination at 6 months in any case. Adequate treatment of congenital syphilis may not necessarily protect against subsequent manifestations of late congenital syphilis.

2. **Justification**

a. **Effectiveness.** These regimens appear to be up to 98% effective in treatment of fetal syphilis [18,19]. Anecdotal information suggests that treatment of fetal syphilis fails more frequently when treatment is given late in pregnancy[20]. Fetal treatment may fail more frequently near term for a variety of reasons. First, the fetus may have been infected for a longer period of time and may be more extensively infected. Secondly, benzathine penicillin treatment provides low, but spirocheticidal, levels of penicillin for several weeks. In pregnancy, intravascular and extracellular fluid spaces are increased, and penicillin is excreted more quickly due to increased glomerular filtration. Therefore, penicillin levels may be lower and more short-lived than in nonpregnant individuals.

b. **Risks**

(1) **Allergy.** Wendel and colleagues have addressed the issue of putative penicillin allergy, which is claimed by approximately 7% of pregnant women who have syphilis [21]. This group used skin testing to determine true number (approximately 2%) of patients who have evidence of anti-penicillin IgE antibodies. The presence of anti-penicillin determinant IgE antibodies to the major determinant antigen (penicilloylpolylysine) and two minor determinant antigens (benzylpenicillin G and penicilloic acid) identifies this group. Skin testing should be done with all three penicillin determinants in consultation with a clinical immunologist. If not truly allergic, syphilitic mothers should be given penicillin. Because of the importance of penicillin treatment in pregnancy, Wendel successfully administered an oral penicillin desensitization protocol that allowed the administration of full penicillin antisyphilitic treatment during pregnancy. Barring use of these methods, children of mothers treated with an erythromycin during pregnancy should also be evaluated and preemptively treated promptly after birth.

(2) **Jarish-Herxheimer reaction.** Pregnant women being treated for syphilis appear anecdotally predisposed to Jarish-Herxheimer reaction [5, 20]. This may be because they are generally young and may have early syphilis more frequently than other patients. The occurrence of Jarish-Herxheimer reaction corresponds with the severity of the infection and the number of organisms destroyed. Antispirochetal antibiotics release cell membrane lipids that likely induce subsequent release of lymphokines, which may directly cause the syndrome. Because of the heavy burden of infection in fetal and congenital syphilis, Jarish-Herxheimer reactions are also of concern during treatment of the fetus or newborn. Reactions are marked by hyperpyrexia, chills, myalgia, tachycardia, and possibly hypertension and shock. Older literature describes "placental shock" with fetal demise occurring soon after the treatment of syphilis during pregnancy [22]. Examination of these stillborn fetuses demonstrated that they were frequently heavily infected [21].

Uterine contractions, decreased fetal movement, and findings of fetal distress have been noted in up to 50% of cases of syphilis treated during pregnancy [21]. It is likely prudent to electronically monitor fetuses of women treated for syphilis in the third trimester. Pretreatment ultrasonic observation of polyhydramnios, fetal edema, or abdominal distention might reasonably be an indication for intensive fetal monitoring during the first 24 hours of maternal and fetal treatment of syphilis. The means to prevent or ameliorate this incompletely understood reaction are under study.

c. **Costs and acceptability.** The cost of penicillin treatment is certainly low compared to the burden of untreated congenital syphilis, and failure to treat is obviously unacceptable.

IV. Recommendations

A. Primary prevention.
Follow recommendations for adults in Chap. 98.

B. Secondary prevention

1. Early detection

a. All women should be effectively encouraged and educated to the necessity of seeking early and sustained antenatal care.

b. STS should be performed at the initial prenatal visit and in women and babies at high risk at or near term or at delivery.

d. Pregnant women with serologic evidence of syphilis should have a careful history and physical performed to assess exposure, contacts, signs and symptoms, and possible prior treatment of syphilis to stage the patient.

e. Many authorities recommend lumbar puncture if neurosyphilis is a possibility.

2. Early intervention

a. Appropriate antibiotic treatment of pregnant women with syphilis must be given (see Table 17-2), based on the stage of disease.

b. Possible risks to the fetus of treatment should be monitored.

c. Appropriate serologic follow-up of the mother to ensure adequate treatment is essential.

d. Evaluation of the newborn of a mother with syphilis is difficult and may involve consultation with experts.

References

1. Congenital syphilis among newborns: Texas—1981. *M.M.W.R.* 31(28): 382,1982. *A succinct analysis of a large collection of contemporary congenital syphilis cases.*
2. Mascola, L., et al. Congenital syphilis. Why is it still occurring? *J.A.M.A* 252(13):1719, 1984. *Excellent review and discussion of means to improve care.*
3. Kaufman, R. E., et al. Questionnaire survey of reported early congenital syphilis: Problems in diagnosis, prevention, and treatment. *Sex. Transm. Dis.* 4(4):135, 1977. *Pointed discussion of where improvements can be made.*
4. Murphy, F. K., and Patamasucon, P. Congenital Syphilis. In K. K. Holmes, et al. (eds.), *Sexually Transmitted Diseases.* New York: McGraw-Hill, 1984. Pp. 352–374. *A superb textbook on STDs.*
5. Rathbun, K. C. Congenital syphilis. *Sex. Transm. Dis.* 10(2):93, 1983. *A classic.*
6. Mascola, L., et al. Congenital syphilis revisited. *Am. J. Dis. Child.* 139(6):575, 1985. *Thorough discussion of diagnostic criteria.*
7. Pickering, L. K. Diagnosis and therapy of patients with congenital and primary syphilis. *Pediatr. Infect. Dis.* 4(5):602, 1985. *Excellent discussion of diagnosis and therapy.*
8. Ingall, D. and Musher, D. Syphilis. In J. S. Remington and J. O. Klein (eds.), *Infectious Diseases of the Fetus and Newborn Infant.* (2nd ed.). Philadelphia: Saunders, 1983. Pp. 335–374. *An encyclopedic review.*
9. Wilfert, C., and Gutman, L. Venereal Disease: Syphillis. In R. D. Feigin and J. D. Cherry (eds.), *Textbook of Pediatric Infectious Disease.* Philadephia: Saunders, 1981. Pp. 338–400. *Review aimed at evaluation and treatment of children.*
10. 1985 STD treatment guidelines. *M.M.W.R.* 34(Suppl 4):75s, 1985. *Most current CDC guidelines.*
11. Stokes, J. H., Beerman, H., and Ingraham, N. R. *Modern Clinical Syphilology.* Philadelphia: Saunders, 1947. *The penultimate review of its day.*
12. Harter, C., and Benirschke, K. Fetal syphilis in the first trimester. *Am. J. Obstet. Gynecol.* 124(7):705, 1976. *An ingenious study with an up-to-date discussion of pathogenesis.*
13. Syphilis trends in the United States. *M.M.W.R.* 30(35):441, 1981. *Recent information on trends in men, women, and children.*
14. Syphilis—United States, 1983. *M.M.W.R.* 33(30):433, 1984. *The most recent updates.*
15. Fiumara, N. J. Congenital syphilis in Massachusetts. *N. Engl. J. Med.* 245:634, 1951. *Another classic of modern syphilology.*
16. Jones, J. E., and Harris, R. E. Diagnostic evaluation of syphilis during pregnancy. *Obstet. Gynecol.* 54(5):611, 1979. *Largest recent series of pregnant women and babies with syphilis.*
17. Lockshin, M. D., et al. Antibody to cardiolipin as a predictor of fetal distress or death in pregnant patients with systemic lupus erythematosus. *N. Engl. J. Med.* 313(3):152, 1985. *Study notes association of cardiolipin antibody and poor fetal outcome.*
18. Thompson, S. E. 3d. Treatment of syphilis in pregnancy. *J. Am. Vener. Dis. Assoc.* 3(2 Pt 2):158, 1976. *Summaries and hard-to-get information on treatment in pregnancy.*
19. Jackson, F. R. Jr, et al. Use of aqueous benzathine penicillin G in the treatment of syphilis in pregnant women. *Am. J. Obstet. Gynecol.* 83:1389, 1962. *A highly regarded reference on treatment.*
20. Mascola, L., Pelosi, R., and Alexander, C. E. Inadequate treatment of syphilis in pregnancy. *Am. J. Obstet. Gynecol.* 150(8):945, 1984. *Case studies and analysis.*
21. Wendel, G. D. Jr, et al. Penicillin allergy and desensitization in serious infections during pregnancy. *N. Engl. J. Med.* 312(19):1229, 1985. *Demonstrates that oral penicillin desensitization to penicillin allergy can be successfully employed in pregnancy.*
22. Ingraham, N. R. Jr. Prevention and treatment of prenatal syphilis. *Am. J. Med.* 5:693, 1948. *Extraordinary review of past perspectives.*

Note: As this book went to press, an important new publication was released: Guidelines for the prevention and control of congenital syphilis. *M. M. W. R.* 37(S-1):1, 1988.

18 Genital Herpes Simplex and Pregnancy

Gary K. Stewart

I. The problem

A. Description. The agent responsible for genital herpes simplex belongs to a family of double-stranded DNA viruses called the herpes viruses. They are composed of a nucleoprotein coat, which is covered with a glycoprotein envelope. They produce at least 24 structural polypeptides.

Genital herpes infections are classified as either primary or secondary, indicating whether they are the first or subsequent infections. In general, first infections are worse, involving more extensive areas and having more constitutional symptoms: fever, myalgias, and malaise.

Infection of the newborn is almost always acquired from an infected mother at the time of delivery, with intrauterine and nosocomial infections occurring only occasionally [1]. The virus can have a devastating effect on the newborn, involving almost all organs, including the central nervous system. About 50% of infected babies will die unless treated, with the survivors having severe neurologic sequelae [2].

B. Epidemiology. In 1984, there were 450,570 consultations [3] for this infection alone, with 5000–20,000 infants [4] being delivered from infected mothers. Binkin surveyed a number of obstetric and neonatal experts and determined an approximate risk of neonatal infection of 1–10% if the newborn delivers through an infected birth canal (mode of 5%)[5].

It has been estimated that 1% of all women have genital herpes during pregnancy. A major obstacle to the prevention of neonatal infection is that over 60% of women who give birth to infected infants are asymptomatic. One study doing random cultures on a population of pregnant women had one positive culture/150 women [6]. Another study using cytologic screening techniques estimated the infection rate at 1 in 1000 [7].

For most women, the primary infection has lesions that will last 14 days, whereas recurrent infections are present only 7–10 days.

These numbers are the basis for the standard recommendation that pregnant women with a history of genital herpes simplex virus infection be checked weekly beginning at 34 weeks' gestation and be delivered vaginally **only** if at least one viral culture before delivery is negative. If the virus is present, a cesarean section is performed to prevent neonatal disease [8]. A recent study by Arvin et al. [9] showed that antepartum screening did not predict which patient would be shedding viruses at term, raising some uncertainty about what should be done in terms of prevention.

II. Secondary prevention

A. Early detection

1. Methods

a. History. Ask all pregnant women about herpes risk factors:

(1) A documented or likely past history of primary or recurrent genital herpes.

(2) A sexual partner with genital herpes.

(3) A prior affected baby.

b. Physical exam. Herpes in any stage, anywhere "below the belt," is an indication for cesarean section if the patient is in labor or has ruptured membranes.

c. Virus culture at weekly intervals, beginning at 34 weeks, should be carried out. Cultures have a positivity rate of 60–90%.

The cultures should be taken from the site of usual recurrence and from the vagina and cervix. The specimen should be collected using synthetic swabs (Dacron, rayon)—**not** cotton. The specimen is to be immersed in the transport media and transported to the lab, preferably on ice.

Ninety-seven percent of positive cultures will be evident within 7 days—usually within 1–5 days. Cultures are not declared negative until after 7 days.

d. **Antigen detection techniques and cytopathology** evaluations have varying degrees of effectiveness and might become the standard for screening.

e. **Other procedures** including immunofluorescence, Papanicolaou (Tzanck prep), and crystal violet cytological preparations appear less reliable, with sensitivities of 40% or less [10].

2. **Justification**

a. **Test characteristics**

(1) **Clinical evaluation.** The justification for clinical evaluation of women at term seems clear—if an active lesion is clinically present, a cesarean section would be indicated. Binkin, et al. estimated that among women with symptomatic recurrences in the week before delivery, 54% would be symptomatic at delivery [5].

(2) **Cultures.** Binkin estimated only one-fourth of infected patients would be detected at delivery. Arvin, et al. followed 414 women with a history of recurrent genital herpes infection. None of these women had positive cultures at delivery [9]. Five of the 354 asymptomatic mothers had positive cultures at delivery, despite repeated negative cultures in the month prior to delivery. It seems clear that antepartum maternal cultures do not reliably predict the infants' risk of exposure to herpes viruses at delivery.

b. **Risks.** Cultures themselves are relatively risk-free; however, false-positives subject a large number of women to cesarean section, and false-negatives may lead to complacent vaginal delivery and possible infection of the infant.

c. **Costs.** Cultures obtained weekly prior to delivery would cost approximately $1.8 million for each case averted and would subject a large number of women to the costs of cesarean sections [5].

d. **Acceptability.** Although the pelvic exam is uncomfortable, most women tolerate it without much complaint. The key issue becomes follow-up of results and keeping everyone informed of the results when available.

B. Early intervention

1. **Methods.** If an active lesion is present at term or if a culture has been positive in the 10 days prior to term (and there is no subsequent negative culture), a cesarean section should be carried out.

2. **Justification**

a. **Effectiveness.** If the herpes virus is present in the delivery canal, contact with the neonate is avoided—thus recommendation of a cesarean section.

b. **Risks.** For cesarean section versus vaginal delivery, there is an increase in maternal morbidity (28% versus 7.6%) and mortality (59.3 deaths/100,000 versus 9.7/100,000) [5]. It is assumed that one avoids the higher probability of neonatal morbidity and mortality when cesarean section is performed. Binkin estimated that in screening a cohort of 3.6 million women, the standard screening would avert 11.3 neonatal deaths and 3.7 cases of severe retardation, but that 3.3 women would die from cesarean sections performed because of culture results [5].

c. **Costs.** Using Binkin's estimates [5], the total cost of screening in the United States would be $41 million. The cost of the cesarean sections and subsequent morbidity would be $20 million. These efforts would prevent an estimated 30.6 cases of neonatal herpes annually. The cost for each case prevented would be approximately $1.8 million.

The cost per culture is about $30, and the cost for a cesarean section is around $5000.

d. **Acceptability.** Most patients are very accepting of recommendations that may prevent fetal damage.

III. Recommendations

A. Early detection

1. Ask all pregnant women about herpes risk factors.
2. Examine all pregnant women for signs of herpes infection.
3. If herpes risk exists, review the plan of management with the often anxious mother and her family.
4. Culture any herpetic lesion at once. (Consider that up to 40% of herpes genitalis patients have other sexually transmitted diseases, and examine accordingly.)

5. If herpes risk exists and no lesions are seen, screen the genital tract, including cervix, vagina, and vulva, at approximately 34 **and** 35 weeks' gestation with a culture, since somewhat less than 5% of women may excrete the virus asymptomatically. The test is performed twice to increase sensitivity. Screening is performed at 34 and 35 weeks since 40% of affected babies are preterm and most infected newborns are born of asymptomatic mothers [11,12]. Whether the cultures should be repeated weekly is controversial.
6. Inquire about any prodromal herpetic symptoms with subsequent visual inspection of the genital tract weekly until delivery.
7. **Repeat** viral culture when the cervix ripens near term (38 weeks) or continue culturing weekly after the intitial culture.

B. Early intervention

1. If all evaluations are negative for herpes simplex virus (HSV), vaginal delivery is encouraged.
2. If the clinical evaluation, culture, or cytologic examination reveals recoverable amounts of herpes simplex virus, then the tests should be repeated twice a week until at least one negative evaluation is obtained along with observed healing of lesions. Recurrent genital herpes commonly heals within a week.
3. Provide careful counseling to ensure prompt care if membranes rupture or labor begins.
4. Cesarean section should be expeditiously performed after rupture of membranes or with the onset of labor if lesions remain unhealed and one negative culture (at least 72 hours old) has **not** been obtained.
5. Cesarean section should be performed within 4 hours of ruptured membranes if there is evidence of genital herpetic infection.
6. Amniocentesis or viral culture need not be performed (at time of labor) since in utero infection is rare and positive viral culture is not predictive of newborn disease [6]. If care is delayed and cesarean section is contraindicated or refused, then precautions are taken: (1) avoid skin puncture with scalp electrode placement or sampling; (2) prep vagina with povidone-iodine once; and (3) caution nursing personnel to handle the exposed newborn with gloved hands until bathing the baby with soap and water [13]. Newborn isolation is appropriate for this circumstance [14].
7. The value of acyclovir treatment of maternal genital herpetic lesions during pregnancy remains untested, as does acyclovir or high titer anti-HSV immunoglobulin in the newborn who is exposed to herpes virus at birth. Overuse of acyclovir in unproven circumstances may lead to increased HSV resistance.

References

1. Light, I. J. Postnatal acquisition of herpes simplex by the newborn infant: A review of the literature. *Pediatrics* 63(3):480, 1979. *An excellent review of the subject.*
2. Visintine, A. M., Nahmias, A. J., and Alford, C. A. The Natural History and Epidemiology of Neonatal Herpes Simplex Virus Infection. In A. J. Nahmias, W. R. Dowdle, and R. F. Schinazi (eds.), *The Human Herpes Viruses.* New York: Elsevier, 1981. P. 599. *A good review of the natural history of the infection in the neonate.*
3. Genital herpes infection—United States 1966–1984. *M.M.W.R.* 35(24): 402, 1986. *Epidemiologic data collected by the CDC.*
4. Sever, J. L., Larsen, J. W. Jr, and Grossman, J. H. III. *Handbook of Perinatal Infections.* Boston: Little, Brown, 1979. *Excellent handbook.*
5. Binkin, N. J., Koplan, J. P., and Cates, W. Jr. Preventing neonatal herpes. The value of weekly viral cultures in pregnant women with recurrent genital herpes. *J. A. M. A.* 251:2816, 1984. *Using decision analysis techniques, the authors examined the benefits, risks, and costs of viral culture screening for women with recurrent genital herpes.*
6. Bolognese, R., et al. Herpesvirus hominis type II infections in asymptomatic pregnant women. *Obstet. Gynecol.* 48(5):507, 1976. *A survey of a population of pregnant women to determine the frequency rate of infection.*
7. Ng, A. B., Reagan, J. W., and Yen, S. C. C. Herpes genitalis. *Obstet. Gynecol.* 36(4):645, 1970. *A cytologic study of a population to determine frequency of occurence of neonatal herpes.*
8. Herpes Simplex Virus Infections. Chicago: *ACOG Technical Bulletin* No. 102, March 1987.

A four-page summary of epidemiology, clinical spectrum, diagnosis, treatment, counseling, and bibliography. An excellent, succinct review.

9. Arvin, A. M., et al. Failure of antepartum maternal cultures to predict the infants' risk of exposure to herpes simplex virus at delivery. *N. Engl. J. Med.* 315(13):796, 1986. *A current herpes screening study showing the lack of accuracy of antepartum screening in predicting infectivity at delivery.*
10. Brown, S. T., et al. Sensitivity and specificity of diagnostic tests for genital infection with herpesvirus hominis. *Sex. Transm. Dis.* 6(1):10, 1979. *Good review of tests for detecting the herpes virus.*
11. Nahmias, A. J., et al. Perinatal risk associated with maternal genital herpes simplex virus infection. *Am. J. Obstet. Gynecol.* 110(6):825, 1971. *Excellent review.*
12. Whitley, R. J., et al. The natural history of herpes simplex virus infection of mother and newborn. *Pediatrics* 66(4):489, 1980. *Excellent review of the subject.*
13. Friedrich, E. G., and Masukawa, T. Effect of povidone-iodine on herpes genitalis. *Obstet. Gynecol.* 45(3):337, 1975. *Authors showed this type of cleansing is helpful.*
14. Valenti, W. M., et al. Nosocomial viral infections: II. Guidelines for prevention and control of respiratory viruses, herpesviruses, and hepatitis viruses. *IC: Infect. Control.* 1(3):165, 1980. *Excellent guidelines.*

19 Toxoplasmosis and Pregnancy

James A. McGregor

"Contact with cats and eating rare meat are normal pleasures."
—Anonymous

I. The problem

A. Description. Toxoplasmosis is a cosmopolitan zoonosis that is contracted by at least one-third of humans in most geographic regions [1–3]. Toxoplasmosis is caused by the obligate intracellular coccidian parasite *Toxoplasma gondii. T. gondii* is distributed worldwide by cats and other felines, which are definitive hosts in which toxoplasma completes its complex sexual cycle [2]. Many animals, including humans and most other mammals studied, serve as incomplete hosts in which toxoplasma invades muscle and central nervous system tissues most heavily. Viable tissue cysts are formed after the development of the host immune response. These persist for the life of the individual.

Acute infections are most important in immunocompromised or pregnant hosts. During pregnancy, toxoplasma may be transmitted transplacentally and cause severe infection in the developing embryo or fetus.

1. **Pathogenesis.** Humans are infected with *T. gondii* by: (1) ingesting the cyst stage from inadequately prepared meat or other animal products (including eggs and milk), (2) ingesting the oocyst stage from feline feces-contaminated soil or food, or (3) transplacental or blood product transmission of tachyzoites [3,4]. Cats shed infectious oocysts in their feces for approximately 2 weeks after being infected, primarily by eating infected prey or raw meat [5,6]. Serologic evidence suggests that 30–80% of domestic cats have had toxoplasma infection. Cats rarely shed oocysts after acute infection unless they become immunosuppressed [5]. Toxoplasma tissue cysts can be isolated from muscle of 5–30% of swine, sheep, and cattle [1,4].
2. **Maternal infection.** Primary toxoplasmosis is asymptomatic in 80–90% of immunologically intact adults, including pregnant women [4]. If symptoms are recognized, the most common presentation is lymphadenopathy (most commonly cervical), with or without a heterophil-negative mononucleosis-like illness with fever and malaise [4]. Approximately 15% of unexplained lymphadenopathy is ascribed to toxoplasmosis [4]. Much less commonly, encephalitis, hepatitis, myocarditis, pneumonia, and chorioretinitis may occur [4]. Both acute and recrudescent infections are important in immunocompromised hosts, including acquired immune deficiency syndrome (AIDS) patients.
3. **Intrauterine infection.** Like rubella, toxoplasmosis is transmitted to the fetus across the placenta only when the organism is spread through the bloodstream during primary infection [1,3,7]. Although Garcia reported the occurrence of congenital toxoplasmosis in two successive siblings, prior toxoplasma infection appears to offer nearly complete protection against intrauterine infection [1,8].

   Remington reported a series of 800 women with toxoplasma infection during a prior pregnancy with no congenital infection in a succeeding pregnancy [1].

   When primary maternal toxoplasmosis occurs during pregnancy, fetal infection rates are directly related to gestational age [9]. First trimester infection is associated with approximately 20% transmission. During the second and third trimesters, fetal infections occur roughly 25% and 65% of the time, respectively. Overall, Desmonts found that primary toxoplasmosis occurring during pregnancy is transmitted to the embryo or fetus 39% of the time [9].

   In contrast to intrauterine transmission, the severity of intrauterine infection is inversely linked with gestational age [9]. First trimester infection is severe in 60%, mild in 20%, and subclinical in 20% of occurrences. Second trimester fetal infection appears intermediate in severity with 30% severe, 25% mild, and 45% subclinical involvement [1,9]. Third trimester infection uncommonly leads to severe disease and is associated with mild disease in approximately 8%, and subclinical infection in 92% of infected children at the time of birth [1,9]. Overall, 72% of congenitally infected newborns will be subclinically infected, while 11% will be severely affected at birth. A further 17% will be less obviously infected with generally only chorioretinitis being physically detectable at birth. Such differences likely reflect decreased embryonic or fetal immunologic development early in pregnancy.

Symptomatic newborns commonly demonstrate one or more findings of the triad of "classic" findings, including hydrocephalus, chorioretinitis, and intracranial calcification [10,11]. Other findings characteristic of intrauterine infection commonly include hepatosplenomegaly, jaundice, thrombocytopenia, and temperature instability. Differential diagnosis includes other congenital infection ("TORCH" infections, e.g., rubella, cytomegalovirus, herpes simplex virus, syphilis), congenital anomalies, neoplasia, vascular anomalies, and other causes of mental retardation and cerebral palsy. Less common neonatal findings include rash (including "blueberry muffin" spots), hepatitis and hepatic calcifications, hearing loss, nephrotic syndrome, and bony defects. Stillbirth and neonatal death occur primarily in perinates with first trimester exposure (9%) [1].

Ultimately, neurologic manifestations predominate in about 60% of symptomatic newborns. Findings include mental retardation, cerebral palsy, epilepsy with associated findings of hydrocephalus, intracranial calcification, and microcephaly. Most patients with significant neurologic impairment have intracranial calcification.

It is important to remember that disease may be progressive after birth. In one study, fully 11 of 13 (85%) asymptomatic newborns developed serious sequelae during an average of 8.3 years of follow-up [12]. As in other studies, damage consisted primarily of chorioretinitis (11 in 13), often with serious vision loss. Mental retardation (2 in 13 or 15%) and severe neurologic disability (1 in 13 or 8%) also occur [12]. Koppe followed seven asymptomatically infected and five treated Dutch children for 20 years, and majorities of both groups developed further chorioretinitis and/or vision losses [13]. Toxoplasmosis may recur and cause serious infection with significant immunosuppression at any time during the individual's life.

Thus it appears that symptomatic, damaging infection eventually occurs in most individuals with intrauterine toxoplasma infection.

B. Epidemiology. Worldwide, toxoplasmosis is one of the most common infections in both animals and humans [14]. Primary factors appear to be the presence of free-ranging felines, poor sanitation and hygiene, and preference for undercooked meats [3]. In populations where toxoplasmosis is most common, infection occurs during childhood; such prepubertal infection protects against subsequent primary infection and transplacental spread during pregnancy.

In North America, the prevalence of toxoplasma antibody at the end of the second decade of life ranges from 3–20% in different geographic areas [2,7]. Rate of acquisition between the ages of 15 and 35 is estimated to be from 0.25–1.2% each year of reproductive life [2,15]. Desmonts estimates that roughly 6 of 1000 pregnant women in the United States will acquire toxoplasmosis during pregnancy [15]. Since up to 39% of these women will give birth to congenitally infected newborns, Desmonts estimates an overall incidence rate of up to 23/1000 live births [15]. Prospective serologic studies from various parts of the United States suggest congenital toxoplasmosis is less common than in Europe, with rates of approximately 7 in 750 in Alabama, 1 in 800 in Oregon, and 1 in 1350 in New York City [2]. Because of limitations in surveillance techniques, these estimates may be low. On the other hand, in the Rocky Mountain region, toxoplasmosis appears to be much less common. Overall, it is estimated that from 2–16 cases of primary maternal infection occur per 8500 pregnancies in the United States [14].

II. Primary prevention

A. Methods

1. **At-risk individuals.** Obviously, toxoplasmosis is better prevented than treated. In the absence of an effective vaccine, certain measures can help to diminish the possibility of acquiring infection [16]. These measures do not necessarily need to be applied to the public at large, but should be reasonably observed by: (1) pregnant women, (2) women who may become pregnant, and (3) all immunocompromised individuals whose anti-toxoplasma serologic status is negative or unknown.

2. **Strategies for avoiding inoculation.** Hands should be washed with soap and water after handling raw meat. Only thoroughly cured or cooked meat products should be eaten. Since freezing (−20°C) kills both trophozoites and encysted organisms, meats that have been frozen are preferred. Unpasteurized milk and uncooked eggs should be avoided. Fruits and vegetables should be thoroughly scrubbed prior to consumption.
3. **Avoid contact with infectious oocysts.** Since excreted oocysts require 2–3 days for sporulation, the litter of domestic cats should be disposed of daily by a nonpregnant member of the household. The emptied litter pan may be filled with near-boiling water to disinfect any residue fecal matter. It is generally cats that are allowed to hunt or eat raw meat that can become infectious. Cats kept indoors and fed prepared foods are less likely to become infected. Working in gardens where cats have defecated should be avoided. Gloves should be used for gardening while pregnant.
4. **Be cautious of possibly infected cells or tissues.** Toxoplasma infection has been transmitted by blood transfusions and organ transplantation. It is wise to check donor anti-toxoplasma antibody states prior to use in pregnant women in endemic areas.

B. **Justification.** The effectiveness of such hygienic measures has not been evaluated. Nevertheless, these biologically based recommendations may be the best means to prevent congenital toxoplasmosis. The risks of these measures are negligible. The education and motivation of health care providers and patients, and the inconvenience of these measures, remain significant obstacles.

III. **Secondary prevention**

A. **Early detection**

1. **Methods.** Diagnosis of toxoplasmosis is often problematic. Clinical signs and symptoms are not specific. In the absence of pathologic or microbiologic evidence, the diagnosis generally rests on interpretation of a variety of incompletely evaluated or standardized tests [12]. Misapplication and misapprehension of anti-toxoplasma serologic tests frequently lead to emotional suffering and sometimes to unnecessary treatment or pregnancy termination. Expert consultation should be sought in most instances in which toxoplasmosis during pregnancy is a real possibility.
   a. **The Sabin-Feldman dye test** is the most sensitive and specific test but requires live, possibly infectious, organisms and is not generally available.
   b. **Indirect hemagglutination (IHA)** antibody testing is useful for screening and for population studies but is not helpful in identifying acute infection, as the test is frequently negative early in the course of the illness.
   c. **Indirect fluorescent-antibody (IFA)** testing is most widely used. Detectable levels of IgG occur beginning approximately 2 weeks after infection, and peak within 1 or 2 months. High titers (>512–1024:1) persist for several months and suggest recent infection [1]. Since test supplies and performance vary, acute and convalescent samples are best tested together. Since test results must be known promptly in pregnancy, it is generally desirable to store a frozen portion of the "acute" or original test sera. In case of a high IFA titer (>512:1), a second, or convalescent, titer may be performed along with the frozen sample in order to validate the original titer and to examine for either significant (fourfold) rise or fall of antibody levels.
   d. **IgM anti-toxoplasma** antibody testing is also available. The presence of IgM antibody suggests acute infection, since it usually appears during the initial weeks of infection and peaks and falls within approximately 3 months. Since technical problems can occur, it is recommended that sera with putatively elevated IgM levels be submitted to reference laboratories for confirmation before such serologic evidence of toxoplasmosis in pregnancy is acted on. Two sources of clinical and serologic expertise are Dr. J. Remington, Palo Alto, CA; and Dr. J. Sever, Chief, Infectious Diseases Branch, National Institutes of Health, Bethesda, MD. Test sera should be kept frozen for 1 year to facilitate possible further studies. In any case, only laboratories that submit themselves to periodic quality assurance testing (including detection of toxoplasma antigens) should be used. Since only a portion (about 39% overall) of toxoplasmosis during pregnancy results in intrauterine infection, means of determining actual fetal infections are highly desirable. Use of advanced ultrasound techniques to obtain samples of fetal blood for anti-

toxoplasma IgM testing, toxoplasma culture with intraperitoneal infection, and lactic dehydrogenase (LDH) and serum glutamic oxaloacetic transaminase (SGOT) determinations, are highly desirable if pregnancy termination is considered. Serial ultrasound assessment (every other week) of possible hydrocephaly or intracerebral or hepatic calcifications may also be considered in order to detect at least some fetal infection. Such evaluation requires consultation with experts.

Diagnosis of toxoplasmosis within aborted tissue on stillborns is also problematic since histologic examinations are limited and culture of toxoplasma requires serial passages of intraperitoneally inoculated tissue in mice.

2. **Justification.** Except in France, large-scale attempts at serologic surveillance and treatment of toxoplasma infection during pregnancy have not been rewarding. If serologic surveillance for toxoplasmosis is undertaken, it should be started prior to pregnancy. Serologic tests can be repeated every 1–2 months. If there is evidence of infection prior to pregnancy, then the patient may be reassured that congenital infection is most unlikely.

B. Early intervention

1. **Methods**

   a. **The mother.** Specific treatment should be given to the mother, as well as to other adults, if she is immunocompromised, has active chorioretinitis, or has damage to vital organs [4,14]. Treatment consists of 3–4 weeks of a combination of pyrimethamine, trisulfapyrimadine, and folinic acid. Treatment regimens are listed in Table 19-1. Interestingly, clindamycin (which reliably crosses the placenta) has been given for ocular infection.

   b. **The fetus.** Intrauterine treatment of a possibly infected fetus is controversial. European authorities recommend maternal treatment with spiramycin, a macrolide, which appears effective but does not cross the placenta well. Controlled evaluation of anti-toxoplasma fetal therapy is difficult. Studies with agents that have anti-toxoplasma activity and cross both placental and perinatal blood-brain barriers, such as clindamycin, and which also may treat intracellular forms, would be of interest. Pregnancy termination is performed in selected circumstances.

2. **Justification.** Specific treatment of pregnant women for acute toxoplasmosis is rarely initiated because: (1) the great majority of infections are asymptomatic; (2) the acute infection is over by the time diagnosis is confirmed; and (3) there is no evidence that anti-toxoplasma treatment hastens recovery in immunocompetent hosts or prevents infection in the fetus.

   There is a recent report from France that supports the use of spiramycin and other antimicrobial agents in the pregnant woman with an infected fetus who is not going to abort [17]. Once again, evaluations of newer agents such as clindamycin appear desirable. Desmonts also reported less severe disease at birth in infected perinates whose mothers received antitoxoplasma therapy [1]. Concerns regarding the teratogenic effects of the antifolate effects of pyrimethamine and sulfadiazine given to the mother along with folinic acid remain theoretical.

IV. Recommendations

A. Primary prevention

1. **Risk assessment**

   a. Serologic testing should optimally begin prior to pregnancy.

   b. Highest-risk individuals include:

      (1) Sero-susceptible pregnant or possibly pregnant women.

      (2) Sero-susceptible immunocompromised or potentially immunocompromised hosts.

2. Since most pregnant women have not had toxoplasma status determined before conception, the following strategies for avoiding infections should be offered to all pregnant women:

   a. Avoid ingestion of infective tissue cysts.

      (1) Ensure that meat is thoroughly cooked (at least at 66°C), smoked, or cured in brine. **Never eat raw or poorly cooked meat.**

      (2) Use frozen meat kept at −20°C for at least 24 hours. Home refrigerators may not achieve −20°C.

      (3) Wash hands thoroughly after handling raw meat.

      (4) Wash all fruits and vegetables well.

      (5) Control insects that may travel between feline feces and food.

Table 19-1. Treatment for toxoplasmosis*

Subject	Medication	Dosage	Duration	Comments
Acutely infected mother	Pyrimethamine plus trisulfapyrimadine plus folinic acid	25 mg once daily 2–6 gm/day 10 mg/day	3–4 weeks 3–4 weeks	Monitor twice weekly complete blood count, platelet count
	OR Spiramycin	2–4 gm/day in 4 doses	3–4 weeks	Available on special request from the FDA
Congenitally infected infant	Pyrimethamine plus	2 mg/kg/day for 3 days; then 1 mg/kg/day† (max. 25 mg/day)	4 weeks†	Monitor twice weekly complete blood count, platelet count.
	trisulfapyrimadine daily dose plus folinic acid	100–200 mg/kg/day 5 mg twice a week	3–4 weeks 3–4 weeks	Prednisone (1–2 mg/kg/day) may be added in patients with active chorioretinitis or central nervous system infection
	OR Spiramycin	50–100 mg/kg/day in 2–3 daily doses	3–4 weeks	

*Appropriateness of treatment, specific agents, and duration of therapy must be considered individually.
†Every 2–3 days for infants; treat congenitally infected infants for 1 year.
Source: Drugs for parasitic infections. *Medical Letter* 30:15, 1988.

b. Avoid contact with infectious oocysts.
   (1) Dispose of cat droppings **daily**.
   (2) Disposal of cat litter should be done by someone who is not pregnant.
   (3) The emptied litter box may be further disinfected by cleansing with near-boiling water.
   (4) Avoid digging or handling possible cat dropping-laden soil (i.e., gardens or sand boxes). Wear gloves and wash hands if this if unavoidable.

c. Be alert to the possibilities of infection from tissue or organ donation.

B. Secondary prevention

1. Serologic screening for toxoplasma antibodies in women during pregnancy is not currently recommended but may be selectively performed.
2. If acute toxoplasma infection is a real possibility in pregnancy, expert advice should be sought to help determine which, if any, tests should be ordered and what, if any, treatment should be considered.

References

1. Remington, J. S., and Desmonts, G. Toxoplasmosis. In J. S. Remington, and J. O. Klein (eds.), *Infectious Diseases of the Fetus and Newborn Infant* (2nd ed.). Philadelphia: Saunders, 1983. Pp. 143–263. *An encyclopedic review by the current experts.*
2. Frenkel, J. K. Toxoplasmosis. *Pediatr. Clin. North Am.* 32(4):917, 1985. *An excellent review of biology and pathogenesis.*
3. Swartzberg, J. E., and Remington, J. S. Transmission of toxoplasma. *Am. J. Dis. Child.* 129(7):777, 1975. *Excellent summary of information concerning transmission of toxoplasmosis.*
4. Krick, J. A., and Remington, J. S. Toxoplasmosis in the adult—an overview. *N. Engl. J. Med.* 298(10):550, 1978. *Good review of adult disease before the AIDS era.*
5. Derrick, P. Toxoplasmosis in cats. *Vet. Ref. Lab. Newsl.* 5:2, 1982. *Complete information about disease in cats.*
6. Dubey, J. P. Reshedding of toxoplasma cysts by chronically infected cats. *Nature* 262(5565):213, 1976. *Shows that cats rarely spread cysts after acute infection.*
7. Feldman, H. A. Editorial: Congenital toxoplasmosis, at long last. *N. Engl. J. Med.* 290(20):1138, 1974. *A valedictory address by one of the leading figures in the field.*
8. Garcia, A. G. Congenital toxoplasmosis in two successive siblings. *Arch. Dis. Child.* 43(232):705, 1968. *A very uncommon occurrence.*
9. Desmonts, G., and Couvreur, J. Congenital toxoplasmosis. A prospective study of 378 pregnancies. *N. Engl. J. Med.* 290(20):1110, 1974. *A classic in the field.*
10. Stagno, S. Congenital toxoplasmosis. *Am. J. Dis. Child.* 134(7):635, 1980. *A good review.*
11. Dische, M. R., and Gooch, W. M. 3d. Congenital toxoplasmosis. *Perspect. Pediatr. Pathol.* 6:83, 1981. *The consummate pathological review.*
12. Sever, J. L. TORCH tests and what they mean. *Am. J. Obstet. Gynecol.* 152(5):495, 1985. *The "Rosetta stone" for serologic interpretation.*
13. Koppe, J. G., Loewer-Sieger, D. H., and deRoever-Bonnet, H. Results of a 20-year follow-up of congenital toxoplasmosis. *Lancet* 1(8475):254, 1986. *A unique contribution detailing a progressive disease.*
14. Elliot, D. L., et al. Pet-associated illness. *N. Engl. J. Med.* 313(16):985, 1985. *Very complete review of zoonosis.*
15. Desmonts, G., and Couvreur, J. Toxoplasmosis: Epidemiologic and serologic aspects of perinatal infection. *Prog. Clin. Biol. Res.* 3:115, 1975. *A complete review with information not available elsewhere.*
16. Wilson, C. B. , and Remington, J. S. What can be done to prevent congenital toxoplasmosis? *Am. J. Obstet. Gynecol.* 138(4):357, 1980. *An extraordinary synthesis with practical recommendations.*
17. Daffos, F., et al. Prenatal management of 746 pregnancies at risk for congenital toxoplasmosis. *N. Engl. J. Med.* 318(5):271, 1988. *A large prospective study from France on testing for and treatment of toxoplasmosis in pregnancy accompanied by an excellent editorial in the same issue.*

Selected Readings

Ladiges, W. C., DiGiacomo, R. F., and Yamaguchi, R. A. Prevalence of *Toxoplasma gondii* antibodies and oocysts in pound-source cats. *J. Am. Vet. Med. Assoc.* 180(11):1334, 1982. *Epidemiologic review of toxoplasmosis in cats.*

Toxoplasmosis. *Br. Med. J.* 282(6260):249, 1981. *Eloquent summary. Contains the line, "Children's sand-pits should be covered when not in use, though a case could be made for encouraging infection in children to provide immunity to toxoplasmosis for pregnant women."*

20 Rubella and Pregnancy

T. Warner Hudson

I. The problem

A. Description. The principal risk from rubella infection is damage to the fetus when a nonimmune pregnant woman is infected by wild rubella virus. The classic **congenital rubella syndrome** (CRS) is characterized by intrauterine growth retardation (IUGR), microcephaly, deafness, congenital heart disease, and mental retardation. Congenital rubella actually includes a much broader spectrum of manifestations (Table 20-1). Intrauterine rubella infection may be followed by spontaneous abortion, stillbirth, or live birth of an affected or unaffected infant. The frequency of congenital infection after confirmed maternal rubella with a rash is 80% during the first 12 weeks, 54% at 13–14 weeks, and 25% at the end of the second trimester. Infection rates rise again to very high levels in the last month of pregnancy. Rubella defects occur in almost all infants infected before 11 weeks, 35% of those infected at 12–16 weeks, and are very uncommon after 16 weeks but appear to include IUGR [1,2].

B. Epidemiology. In 1985, there was a provisional total of 604 cases of rubella reported in the United States, and two cases of CRS in 1984. Since the licensure of rubella vaccine in 1969, reported cases of rubella have declined 99%. Although the majority of rubella cases occur in children under 5 years, in 1984, 48% of reported cases with known ages occurred in individuals 15 years of age or older. Although there has been considerable decline in the attack rates in individuals over age 15, serologic studies in the late 1970s and early 1980s showed that 10–20% of women in the childbearing age group lacked protection against rubella [3]. The vast majority of these susceptible women were never vaccinated [4].

Individuals at risk, then, are unimmunized childbearing-age women. Men, women, and children who can transmit disease to these women are also part of the risk group (see sec. **II.A.1.C.**).

II. Primary prevention

A. Risk assessment

1. Methods

a. Description

(1) **History of clinical rubella** is unreliable [5], and although the history of vaccination is probably somewhat more reliable, it is not sufficiently accurate to be recommended by itself in individuals at risk.

(2) **Documented records** of rubella immunization are presumptive evidence of rubella immunity [4].

(3) **Serologic evidence of immunity** is currently recommended for assessment of rubella susceptibility in all prenatal patients as early as possible in pregnancy, as well as in the groups at risk described below.

b. Interpretation of serology. Women receiving prenatal care should be screened at the first neonatal visit for evidence of immunity to rubella. In fact, it would be ideal to screen preconception so that nonimmune women could be immunized prior to conceiving. Until recently, rubella hemagglutination inhibition (HI) antibody titers were used. Those with any detachable antibodies or titers greater than 1:8 or 1:10 are considered protected from developing viremic infection. Recently, a number of additional serologic measures have become available, including enzyme immunoassay (EIA) tests, latex agglutination, fluorescence immunoassay, passive hemagglutination, and hemagglutination-in-gel. These appear to be more sensitive than the earlier HI tests [4].

c. Risk groups. In the contexts of prenatal care and primary prevention, risk is assessed so that if it exists, the individual(s) can be vaccinated. An alter-

Table 20-1. Manifestations of congenital rubella

Growth retardation (low birth weight)	Central nervous system defects
Eye defects	Psychomotor retardation
Cataracts	Microcephaly
Glaucoma	Encephalitis
Retinopathy	Spastic quadriparesis
Microphthalmia	Cerebrospinal fluid pleocytosis
Deafness	Mental retardation
Cardiac defects	Progressive panencephalitis
Patent ductus arteriosus	Hepatomegaly
Ventricular septal defect	Hepatitis
Pulmonary stenosis and coarctation	Thrombocytopenic purpura
Myocardial necrosis	Splenomegaly
Diabetes mellitus	Bone lesions
Thyroid dysfunction	
Growth hormone deficiency	

Source: Modified from S. Krugman and S. L. Katz. Rubella (German measles). In *Infectious Diseases of Children* (7th ed.). St. Louis: Mosby, 1981.

nate approach is to vaccinate everyone regardless of risk or prior vaccination history. This may be most cost-effective but has some real and theoretical risks. Vaccine side effects, which would be at least troublesome, are also unnecessary if an immune individual is vaccinated and pose theoretical risks to the fetus if a woman is accidentally vaccinated while pregnant.

With this in mind, the following individuals and groups are potentially at risk for passing rubella infection to their future or present fetus, and their immune status must be assessed.

(1) **All children** 12 months of age or older without a record of previous rubella immunization or serologic evidence of immunity should be vaccinated (see Chap. 60), unless there are contraindications.

(2) **Adolescent and adult women** of childbearing age who have not been vaccinated or who lack serologic evidence of immunity should be vaccinated as part of preconception, premarital, or general routine health care (see Chap. 92), with precautions to be certain that the woman is not already pregnant or will not become pregnant in the ensuing 3 months. Family planning clinic visits, hospital discharges, and medical visits when a mother brings the children for well-child care may be especially opportune times.

(3) **All pregnant patients** should be checked for serologic evidence of immunity as early as possible in routine prenatal care. This serves two purposes. Those at risk are known and followed closely during the pregnancy and are vaccinated in the immediate postpartum period.

(4) The next groups include nonimmune **males and females** who have regular contact with potentially pregnant and potentially nonimmune women. Mandatory programs usually are more successful than voluntary ones.
   (a) **Health care workers** exposed to pregnant women.
   (b) **High school and university students and staff.**
   (c) **Military and other** concentrations of male and female employees, including day-care centers, companies, government offices, and industrial sites.

2. Justification

a. Test characteristics. The reliability of HI titers can vary since the red blood cells used by the laboratory, the presence of nonspecific hemagglutinins, temperature, pH, and constituents of the buffers can cause erroneous values. This problem was pointed out in a Centers for Disease Control survey involving 318 laboratories throughout the country. Sera with no antibodies were reported as positive by 11–12% of the laboratories, and 32–60% of the laboratories reported titers so far from actual levels that they were considered "outside the acceptable range" [6]. Less information is available on the newer tests. Therefore, until better laboratory techniques are available, the health care provider should ask the laboratory to save all rubella sera for 6 months to 1 year. If this is not possible, half of each serum sample should be kept in the prenatal clinic freezer for 6 months to 1 year. If a question arises later in the pregnancy, the paired sera can be run together by the same laboratory [7].

b. **Risks and side effects** of serologic testing are negligible except when rare false-negatives or false-positives occur. The impact of this can be minimized by keeping part of each serum specimen as noted above.

c. **Costs.** In Sacramento, California, in May 1987, a routine rubella EIA cost $32, latex agglutination cost $16, and HI cost $16.

d. **Acceptability** to patients and health care providers of serologic testing and vaccination of nonimmune individuals or vaccination of at-risk individuals without prior serologic testing is relatively good. Motivating nonpregnant individuals to follow through with serologic testing or vaccination is difficult.

B. Vaccination

1. Methods

a. **Description.** Only one live rubella virus vaccine is currently available in the United States. RA 27/3 is prepared in human diploid cell culture and distributed singly (LRuV) and in combination with the measles vaccine (MR) and with measles and mumps vaccines (MMR).

b. **Performance.** Rubella vaccine is licensed only for subcutaneous administration.

c. **Dose.** The dose is 0.5 ml of reconstituted vaccine.

d. **Timing/population.** The vaccine is administered to those individuals who are at risk by serology or inadequate documentation of prior vaccination (see **sec. II.A.1.C**). It should not be given to pregnant women, and females of childbearing age who receive the vaccine should be counseled not to become pregnant for 3 months after vaccination. Note that the other **principal effort remains vaccination of all infants older than 12 months of age** (see Chap. 60).

2. Justification

a. **Effectiveness.** Approximately 95% of susceptible persons who receive a single dose of rubella vaccine when they are 12 months old or older develop antibody and have long-term, probably lifelong protection against clinical rubella and viremia. The primary vaccine failure rate is 3–5%, and secondary vaccine failure is a rare event, if it occurs at all.

b. **Risks and side effects**

(1) **Side effects of the vaccine** include rash, lymphadenopathy, arthralgias (up to 40%), frank arthritis (<1%), and paresthesias or pain in arms or legs. The extremity symptoms usually begin 7–21 days after vaccination, last for 1–3 days, and are reversible. The vaccine side effects only appear in nonimmune recipients, so revaccination of immune individuals is felt to be free of side effects, except for local pain or infection and inconvenience [4].

(2) **If a pregnant woman inadvertently receives the vaccine, risks to the fetus** of vaccine-associated malformations are felt by the Centers for Disease Control Advisory Committee on Immunization Practices to be "so small as to be negligible" and "should not ordinarily be a reason to consider interruption of pregnancy"[4]. Thus far, RA 27/3 rubella vaccine virus has been isolated from the products of conception of 1 of 32 (3%) of the pregnant and susceptible recipients of the vaccine. Since the observed risks of CRS to date is zero with this vaccine, any risk of malformation is theoretical only, although it could range from 0–3% [8]. If a pregnant woman does receive the vaccine, she should be advised of the theoretical risks to the fetus, since the vaccine virus can cross the placenta and infect the fetus, and such instances should be reported to the Immunization Division of the Centers for Disease Control (404-329-1836).

(3) **Nursing mothers** who are not immune should be given the vaccine in the immediate postpartum period even though the virus is excreted in the breast milk and the infant may develop a mild infection [4]. If RhIG has been given, serology should be tested in 6–8 weeks to ensure that seroconversion has occurred.

c. **Contraindications and precautions**

(1) **Pregnancy.** Because of the theoretical risks noted above, women should

not receive the vaccine if known to be pregnant, should not become pregnant for 3 months following vaccination, and should be advised of the theoretic risks of vaccination.

(2) **Other.** Patients with severe febrile illnesses, anaphylactic neomycin allergy, or impaired immunity should not be given the vaccine. Breastfeeding is not a contraindication to vaccination, and it is likewise safe to vaccinate an infant in the household of a pregnant woman. Although virus can be recovered from the pharynx of vaccinated children, it is **not communicable** [4]. Pregnant women in the household are at greater risk of acquiring rubella if the child is not vaccinated and acquires wild rubella virus.

d. **Cost.** The total cost of rubella vaccine and administration at the University of California, Davis Medical Center in November 1986 was $27.50.

e. **Acceptability.** Vaccination appears to be very acceptable, although certain groups of health care providers appear to be recalcitrant in accepting vaccination once seronegativity has been established.

III. Secondary prevention

A. Early detection

1. Methods

a. **Clinical recognition** of acute rubella is unreliable and subclinical cases are common. In the classic illness, there may be a history of exposure 2–3 weeks prior to the rash. The rash may be absent 50% of the time and lasts from 1–5 days but is usually present for 3 days. The red maculopapular rash appears first on the face and then spreads to the trunk and extremities, sometimes coalescing. Suboccipital, postauricular, and cervical nodes are typical, and there is often low-grade fever, malaise, anorexia, slight conjunctivitis, and cough. A few individuals have transient arthralgias or arthritis. Unfortunately about one-third of people with rubella do not recognize or report clinical disease. The prenatal health care provider must, therefore, educate pregnant women to report any illness resembling rubella so that appropriate studies can be pursued.

b. **Serologic assessment** is the best technique for assessment of risk and diagnosis of acute infection. **All pregnant women should have rubella titers checked as early as possible during pregnancy, if not before.** Part of the serum should be saved by the laboratory for 6 months to 1 year. The following approach applies to HI titers, and health care providers should speak with their laboratory personnel when using the newer tests.

(1) **A pregnant woman known to be immune** (HI titer $\geq 1:8$) prior to or at the time of exposure to rubella can be reassured that there is no apparent risk to the fetus [9].

(2) **A pregnant woman known to be susceptible to rubella** based on the initial prenatal titer (HI titer $< 1:8$) may be exposed to rubella and develop a rash illness compatible with rubella. After exposure, an acute phase titer should be drawn as soon as possible after exposure and a convalescent titer 28 or more days after exposure. If a rash illness is present, an acute titer should be drawn as soon as possible after the rash and a convalescent specimen 10 or more days after onset of the rash. A fourfold or greater titer rise indicates acute infection. In equivocal cases, IgM-specific antibody can be helpful.

(3) **A pregnant woman whose immune status at the time of exposure is unknown** presents a more challenging problem. The recent algorithms described by Mann [9] and endorsed by the American College of Obstetrics and Gynecology [10] are available for three different categories of time from exposure or onset of rash illness: within 1 week after exposure to rash illness; 1–5 weeks after exposure to rash illness or up to 3 weeks after the onset of rash illness in the pregnant patient; and greater than 5 weeks after the onset of rash illness or a single titer from a pregnant woman with no known exposure and no rash illness. Consultation with experts may be advisable in these situations.

(4) **Titer rises in the absence of exposure or clinical illness in the pregnant patient** can be especially confusing. Fifteen percent of the normal adult population has high HI titers (≥ 256), which do not necessarily mean infection. Twofold titer rises are not significant, and titer rises fourfold or greater in an immune ($\geq 1:8$) individual reflect secondary or rein-

fection, which does not cause viremia and therefore presents no risk to the fetus. Fourfold titer rises from susceptible levels ($<1:8$) indicate primary infection and significant risk to the fetus, particularly in the first trimester [9].

2. **Justification**
   a. **Test characteristics**
      (1) **HI antibody** test reliability is variable but can be ensured by choosing a laboratory that measures it routinely and has good quality control. Serum specimens should be kept by the lab for 6 months to 1 year to allow retesting if questions arise later.
      (2) **EIA and latex agglutination** tests appear to be more accurate than HI antibodies.
      (3) **CF antibodies** may be useful when HI antibodies are elevated and stable [10].
      (4) **Rubella-specific IgM antibodies** are measured by a limited number of laboratories. The presence of elevated rubella IgM indicates acute primary infection. However, because of its short half-life—5 days—it may disappear quickly. Its absence, therefore, does not rule out acute infection.
   b. **Risks and side effects** are negligible except as related to false-negatives and false-positives.
   c. **Costs.** The costs for rubella serologies performed at a private laboratory in Sacramento, California, in May 1987 were as follows:
      (1) HI–$16.
      (2) EIA–$32.
      (3) Latex agglutination–$16.
      (4) CF–$32.
      (5) IgM–$37.

B. **Early intervention**
1. **Methods**
   a. **Voluntary termination of pregnancy** is usually considered if there is evidence of a primary infection occurring in the first trimester. This is a highly personal decision that rests with the individual patient and her physician. Risks must be carefully weighed by the patient and her physician.
   b. **Immune serum globulin (ISG) for postexposure prophylaxis is of uncertain value and is not recommended for routine use.** It may be offered to the woman whose fetus is at risk and who would not consider abortion under any circumstances [4].
   c. **Vaccination** after exposure is not recommended in pregnancy.
2. **Justification**
   a. **Success of pregnancy termination in preventing congenital rubella** depends on the true risk to the fetus, a prediction based on epidemiologic likelihood. The probabilities of congenital rubella are approximately 80% in the first trimester, 28% in the fourth month, and are very uncommon after 16 weeks [2]. The physician must counsel any woman at risk regarding these probabilities.
   b. **Risks and side effects of pregnancy termination** include the possibilities of erroneous diagnosis of maternal infection, aborting an unaffected fetus, and aborting an infected but undamaged fetus. There are, of course, risks to the procedure itself, which increase with gestational age [11].
   c. **Costs to the patient of pregnancy termination** during the first trimester at Planned Parenthood of Sacramento in November 1986 were approximately $225.
   d. **Acceptability.** This is a personal, ethical, religious, and highly individual decision that is best left up to the well-informed patient and her physician.

IV. **Recommendations**

A. **Primary prevention**
1. All children should receive rubella vaccination at 12 months of age or older and their parents should keep copies of the immunization records.
2. Risk groups of individuals without physician-documented records of rubella immunization or detectable antibodies should be vaccinated if not pregnant. Serologic screening to select susceptibles prior to vaccination is preferable to universal reimmunization [12]. Risk groups include:
   a. All prepubertal school children. Age 10–11 years is ideal.
   b. All adolescent and adult women of childbearing age. They should not be preg-

nant and should understand that they should not become pregnant for 3 months. Family planning clinics, routine health care visits for children, and hospital discharges provide excellent opportunities to vaccinate susceptibles.

c. All pregnant women. Check serology at earliest prenatal visit and vaccinate all susceptibles postpartum prior to discharge, including those breast-feeding.

d. Health care workers exposed to pregnant women.

e. High school and university students and staff.

f. Military and other concentrations of male and female employees, including day-care centers, companies, government offices, and industrial sites.

B. Secondary prevention

1. Check rubella antibodies on all pregnant women as early as possible in prenatal care or before pregnancy. Save, or be certain the laboratory saves, part of the serum for 6 months to 1 year in case questions arise later.
2. Educate susceptible pregnant women to avoid anyone with a rash illness and to report any exposure to rash illness to their physician at once.
3. Rubella exposure or suspected infection during pregnancy in a patient known to be immune by serologic testing poses no apparent risk to fetus.
4. If rubella exposure or infection is suspected during pregnancy in a known seronegative patient or in a patient whose immune status is unknown, refer to the algorithms in Mann, et al. [9], speak with your laboratory, and possibly consult with perinatal infection experts.
5. Pregnant patients with initially high HI ($\geq$256) titers and no known exposure or illness may need to be carefully assessed.
6. Rising HI titers may need to be evaluated by other serologic means.
7. The decision to voluntarily terminate pregnancy rests with the patient and her physician and can be considered only after adequately informing the pregnant woman of the risks of congenital rubella and of abortion.
8. Routine postexposure prophylaxis with ISG is not recommended but may be offered to those women who would not consider abortion under any circumstances, provided its equivocal protection, if any, is understood.

References

1. Krugman, S., and Katz, S. L. Rubella (German measles). In *Infectious Diseases of Children* (7th ed.). St. Louis: Mosby, 1981. Pp. 315–31. *Good basic textbook coverage of congenital rubella.*
2. Miller, E., Cradock-Watson, J. E., and Pollock, T. M. Consequences of confirmed maternal rubella at successive stages of pregnancy. *Lancet* 2(8302): 781, 1982. *Large prospective study of fetal outcomes resulting from infection at different gestational ages.*
3. Rubella and congenital rubella syndrome—United States, 1984–1985. *M.M.W.R.* 35 (9):129, 1986. *Figures on distribution and incidence rates of rubella cases.*
4. Rubella prevention. Immunization Practices Advisory Committee. *M.M.W.R.* 33(22):301, 1984. *CDC recommendations for rubella prevention.*
5. Lerman, S. J., et al. Accuracy of rubella history. *Ann. Intern. Med.* 74:97, 1971. *History of rubella has 18% false-positive rate.*
6. Taylor, R. N., et al. Centers for Disease Control diagnostic immunology proficiency testing program results for 1977. *J. Clin. Microbiol.* 8(4):388, 1978. *CDC sent samples with known values to 318 labs throughout the United States to check the validity of their measurements.*
7. Sever, J. L. Rubella serology: A need for improvement. *Obstet. Gynecol.* 56(1):127, 1980. *Editorial on the problems with rubella serology and recommendations.*
8. Rubella vaccination during pregnancy—United States, 1971–1983. *M.M.W.R.* 33(26):365, 1984. *Current information on risks to fetus of maternal vaccination.*
9. Mann, J. M., et al. Assessing risks of rubella infection during pregnancy, a standardized approach. *J.A.M.A.* 245(16):1647, 1981. *Excellent algorithmic approaches to assessment of acute rubella in pregnant women.*
10. Rubella. . . A Clinical Update. *ACOG Technical Bulletin* No. 62, November 1981. *Endorsement of approach in reference 9.*
11. Stubblefield, P. G. Current technology for abortion. *Curr. Probl. Obstet. Gynecol.* 2(4):3, 1978. *Good review of entire subject of abortion.*
12. Fulginiti, V. A. Immunizations: Current controversies. *J. Pediatr.* 101(4):487, 1982. *Good review of recent changes and controversies.*

21 Viral Hepatitis and Pregnancy

James A. McGregor

I. The problem. Several types of viral hepatitis may be transmitted to the perinate at or around the time of birth. Of greatest concern are hepatitis A, hepatitis B, and delta agent. In addition, at least two types of non-A, non-B hepatitis may infect the mother and the newborn or fetus [1–3]. Each of these common viral infections has its own distinctive pathogenesis, epidemiology, and clinical manifestations. Other possible viral causes of hepatitis, including cytomegalovirus (CMV) and Epstein-Barr viruses (EBV), may also be transmitted from the mother to her progeny. Except for the viruses that cause non-A, non-B hepatitis, viral hepatitides possess distinctive serologic or virologic markers and can be specifically identified.

Vertical transmission of hepatitis B virus (HBV) from mother to perinate is well described and plays an important role in the spread of this virus [4–6]. Vertical transmission of other hepatitis viruses is less well documented [4]. An infected pregnant woman's sexual contacts, household contacts, and possibly health care providers also may be at risk from these frequently asymptomatic infections [7]. Preventive strategies may appear complex and are frequently revised; the most current applicable recommendations should be reviewed and applied [7].

Viral hepatitis in well-nourished North American or European pregnant women does not appear to greatly affect the course of pregnancy, nor does the pregnancy adversely affect the course and outcome of hepatitis, except if the disease is severe [8,9]. This is not the case in developing areas of the world where hepatitis appears to occur more commonly in pregnant women, as well as being an increasingly recognized cause of maternal and perinatal morbidity and mortality [10].

II. Hepatitis A

A. Description. Hepatitis A virus (HAV) is a common RNA picornavirus that is spread primarily by fecal-oral contamination. The course of hepatitis A during pregnancy is not significantly different from that in the nonpregnant woman. Infection of the newborn may occur at delivery or if the mother is acutely infected and shedding virus in her stool (if the baby is exposed to fecal contamination). Because normal individuals shed HAV only transiently (most heavily in the late incubation and early prodromal phases, and declining rapidly with onset of symptoms), vertical transmission is rare.

B. Epidemiology. Although hepatitis A is endemic worldwide, recurrent epidemics are a feature. The incidence of reported nonspecific hepatitis in the United States approximates 25 cases/100,000 people. Approximately 45% is considered to be HAV infection, 41% is categorized as HBV, and the remainder is unspecified. The actual incidence is much higher, because infections are most often asymptomatic and only a small proportion of cases are reported [2].

C. Primary prevention

1. Methods

a. Pregnant women who should receive immune-globulin (IG) prophylaxis for HAV exposure include: (1) those with close personal contacts (household or sexual exposure within 2 weeks) of individuals with documented HAV infection, (2) mothers of children in diapers who attend day-care facilities in which HAV infections have recently occurred, (3) employees in custodial institutions who have close contact with prisoners or patients during outbreaks of HAV, (4) those exposed to a common source outbreak in the prior 2 weeks, and (5) travelers who will visit or live in areas with poor sanitation [7]. For postexposure prophylaxis, a single dose of 0.02 ml/kg IM is recommended. For prolonged travel (>2 months), 0.06 ml/kg should be given every 6 months. Individuals who may be subjected to multiple prophylactic immune globulin injections should have IgG anti-HA status determined so as to avoid unneeded treatment.

b. **Newborn infants of acutely ill mothers.** Even though the matter is not well studied, a single 0.5-ml dose of immune globulin IM may reasonably be given as promptly as possible after documented exposure (within 2 weeks). Active vaccination against HAV will be available in the next few years and will likely offer more effective and enduring protection than passive vaccination.

2. **Justification.** Passive immunization is approximately 80–90% effective in adults if given early in the incubation period [7]. Even though hepatitis A is only rarely transmitted to the newborn infant if the mother is acutely ill, vertical infection may be theoretically prevented or ameliorated by prompt administration of immune globulin to an exposed newborn. Cost of HAV passive immunization with IG is minimal (adult doses of immune globulin cost approximately $5).

III. Hepatitis B

A. **Description.** Hepatitis B virus (HBV) is the best studied of the viral hepatitides. HBV is a unique DNA virus that primarily infects hepatocytes [11]. The course and outcome of HBV infection is determined in large part by inoculum and host response. Liver cell damage and disease is primarily mediated by host immunocyte attack, damage, and clearance of infected cells. Relatively immunosuppressed or immunologically "inefficient" individuals, such as newborns, are less likely to clear HBV infection and more likely to become chronic carriers of HBV than are normal hosts. Chronic HBV infection may persist for long periods of time, possibly for life [11].

Although approximately 80% of HBV infection is asymptomatic in North America and northern Europe, acute HBV can cause significant illness and may be fatal (approximately 1 in 1000) [10]. Chronic infection is initially asymptomatic but may be ultimately associated with persistent hepatitis, chronic hepatitis, and cirrhosis [11]. Chronically infected individuals are at greatly increased risk for development of hepatocellular carcinoma after several decades of carriage [11]. Chronic HBV carriage contributes significantly to the worldwide perpetuation of this infection. Spread to others, including sexual partners, recipients of donated blood, tissues, and organs, and offspring, occurs frequently [7]. Chronic HBV carriage may even be perpetuated through generations by vertical transmission. Vertical HBV infection contributes greatly to HBV endemicity in many areas of the world (Southeast Asia, China, sub-Saharan Africa, and the Arctic).

Although previously termed "long incubation" or "serum hepatitis," the incubation period of HBV is largely determined by inoculum size and means of inoculation. Mucous membrane exposure-mediated infection is increasingly recognized and is most probably the mechanism of infection of newborns, young children, and sexual partners [7].

Relatively few fetuses become infected in utero, and the majority of newborn infection is considered to be due to exposure to HBV infectious particles in blood or vaginal secretions during birth [12]. Further exposure to HBV occurs in the course of lactation and from ongoing exposure to infected siblings and parents [13,14]. These features of HBV pathogenesis allow for effective use of coordinated, passive, and active vaccination against HBV for the newborn.

B. **Epidemiology.** Within industrialized countries, it is mainly women who have been exposed to HBV from the following sources who are at highest risk (1–20%) of being asymptomatic HBV carriers: (1) treatment with or exposure to blood or blood products; (2) use of contaminated needles during parenteral substance abuse; (3) recurrent contact with an infectious sexual partner or multiple contacts with possibly infected partners; or (4) being born from a possibly infected mother in an area of the world where HBV is endemic and commonly vertically transmitted. These and other groups of women who are at highest risk for HBV infection and continued chronic HBV carriage are listed in Table 21-1.

C. **Primary prevention**

1. **Methods**

a. **Risk assessment.** At a minimum, high-risk women (Table 21-1) should be evaluated for hepatitis B surface antigen carriage (HBsAg) during pregnancy [7]. Universal screening of pregnant women for HBsAg carriage has recently been advocated [7a].

Because newborns of all HBsAg-positive women should presently receive HBV passive and active prophylaxis, serum markers for increased infectivity (presence of HBeAg, HBV DNA polymerase, high titers of HBsAg, or absence

Table 21-1. Women who should receive HBsAg screening antenatally*

1. Women of Asian, Pacific Island, or Eskimo descent, whether immigrant or native born
2. Women born in Haiti or sub-Saharan Africa
3. Women with histories of:
   a. Acute or chronic liver disease
   b. Work or treatment in a hemodialysis unit
   c. Work or residence in an institution for the mentally retarded or in prison
   d. Blood donation being refused
   e. Repeated blood transfusion
   f. Frequent exposure to blood or blood products (medical or dental care providers)
   g. Household or sexual contact with HBV carrier or dialysis patient
   h. Multiple sexual contacts or multiple episodes of sexually transmitted disease
   i. Parenteral substance abuse

*Patients appearing at very high risk for acquisition of HBV infection should be screened when initially seen and again near term.
Source: Recommendations for protection against viral hepatitis. *M.M.W.R.* 34(22):313, 1985.

of anti-HBe and anti-HBc) in maternal serum need not be determined [7]. (Antibody to hepatitis B need not be evaluated.) Oriental and possibly black racial origin is associated with increased risk of vertical transmission and adds to the urgency of antenatal identification of HBsAg carriage in the mother.

b. **Immunization.** At this time, all newborns of HBsAg-positive mothers should be given hepatitis B immune globulin (HBIG) 0.5 ml IM as promptly as possible after birth (Table 21-2). Active vaccination (0.5 ml HBV vaccine) IM should be initiated within the first 3 days of life (Table 21-2). Active vaccination with 0.5 ml HBV vaccine given in the deltoid muscle should be repeated at 1 and 6 months of life (Table 21-2) [7]. Breast-feeding is not contraindicated for immunologically protected newborns, although continued breast-feeding when nipples are cracked should be discouraged since the dose of HBV infectious material is likely increased by serum or blood contamination. Pregnancy is not a contraindication for HBV passive or active vaccination [7]. Women who plan pregnancy and who are at increased risk for HBV exposure should also be offered active HBV vaccination. Individual adults at increased occupational risk, including health care providers or laboratory technicians commonly exposed to infectious blood products, should be vaccinated as early as possible in their careers [7]. Occurrences of HBV infection in patients, spread by HBV-infected medical and dental workers, are documented [18]. Non-HBV immune pregnant women at high occupational risk for HBV infection should either be vaccinated or reassigned to less hazardous positions.

2. **Justification**

a. **Effectiveness.** Even though commercially available immune globulin contains significant amounts of anti-HBsAg, only high titer ($\geq$1,000,000 units) anti-HBsAg (HBIG) has been demonstrated to passively protect newborns exposed to HBV at birth [15]. HBIG appears to be at least 85% effective if given promptly after birth ($\leq$3 days) [7]. HBV vaccine (Heptovax) is immunogenic and well tolerated in newborns [16]. Currently, passive immunization with high titer ($\geq$1,000,000 units anti-HBsAg) HBIG is considered to be effective in preventing HBV acquisition at birth, and active vaccination is directed at prevention of HBV infection primarily from horizontal infection after birth. Recent preliminary data from China suggests that the currently available vaccine (Heptovax) alone can effectively ($>$90%) prevent both vertical and horizontal HBV infection in the first year of life when active vaccination is initiated immediately after birth [17].

b. **Risks.** Although any blood product may contain antibody to human immunodeficiency virus, no immune globulin, HBIG, or HBV vaccine available in the United States has been shown to mediate infection [7]. Use of these products is not a risk for AIDS infection [19].

c. **Costs.** Screening pregnant women for HBsAg and immunizing their at-risk newborn appears to be cost-effective [7a]. HBV vaccine costs pharma-

Table 21-2. Prevention of perinatal viral hepatitis

	Passive immunization	Active immunization	Comments
Hepatitis A virus			
Mother	0.02 ml/kg IG IM once	None available	Confirm diagnosis in index case. Administer IG if exposed by close contact (household or sexual) or by child attending day-care with another child suffering hepatitis
Newborn	0.5 ml IG once	None available	Not proven but reasonable. Administer if newborn exposed to fecal contamination during incubation (2 weeks) or early symptomatic (10 days) phase of maternal HAV infection
Hepatitis B virus			
Mother	0.06 ml/kg HBIG as soon as possible for postexposure. Also vaccinate actively if at continued risk	1 ml HBV vaccine. *Give in deltoid;* 3 doses; 0, 1, and 6 mo	Confirm diagnosis in index case. Active vaccination not contraindicated during pregnancy. Testing for seroconversion (anti-HBsAg) generally unnecessary
Newborn	0.5 ml HBIG IM given once immediately (by 8h) after birth	0.5 ml HBV vaccine IM within 1st week of life at alternative site. Repeat at 1 and 6 mo	Timely administration requires antenatal identification of maternal carriage or infection (HBsAg+). Temporarily discontinue breast-feeding with cracked nipples
Delta agent			
Mother	Prevented by effective HBV prophylaxis or naturally acquired immunity	Prevented by HBV prophylaxis	Effective HBV prophylaxis prevents coinfection or superinfection with delta agent
Newborn	Same	Same	Same
Non-A, Non-B*			
Mother	0.2 ml/kg IG IM once	None available	Serologic markers for putative NANB virus not yet identified. Consider IG administration since antibody likely occurs in IG
Newborn	0.5 ml IG once	Same	Same

Key: Ig=immune globulin; HAV=hepatitis A virus; HBIG=hepatitis B immune globulin; HBsAg=hepatitis B surface antigen; HBV=hepatitis B virus; NANB=non-A, non-B hepatitis.
*No adequate data. See selected readings.

cies about $80 for 3 adult doses, which is considerably less than the cost of a single adult dose of HBIG ($125–150). The total pharmacy cost for newborn HBV vaccine is $48.

IV. **Delta agent hepatitis.** Delta agent hepatitis is caused by a defective RNA virus that is infectious only in the presence of ongoing HBV infection. Delta agent virus "clothes" itself in HBsAg to complete its virion. Delta agent is increasingly recognized as a coinfection or superinfection of HBV, which may account for much of the morbidity previously ascribed to HBV. Prevention of HBV infection by immunization or prior healed natural infection precludes infection with delta agent.

V. **Non-A, Non-B hepatitis.** Non-A, non-B (NANB) hepatitis is the most common cause of transfusion-associated hepatitis and may presumably be transmitted perinatally [20]. NANB hepatitis is clinically similar to hepatitis B but does not demonstrate any currently recognized serologic markers. Presently, at least two distinct agents appear to be associated with NANB hepatitis. Because antibody to agents of NANB hepatitis is likely to be widely distributed, administration of 0.5 ml IM of immune globulin to the newborn of an acutely infected mother has been suggested as possibly effective in the prevention of NANB hepatitis [20].

Although many issues remain to be resolved, much can be done now to prevent the occurrence of viral hepatitis in pregnant women and their progeny. Rapid advances, including release of recombinant vaccines, will offer new opportunities for viral hepatitis prevention in the near future.

VI. **Recommendations.** Recommendations for perinatal and adult preemptive and postexposure hepatitis immunoprophylaxis are outlined in Table 21-2.

References

1. Snydman, D. R. Hepatitis in pregnancy. *N. Engl. J. Med.* 313(22):1398, 1985. *Good current review.*
2. Shaffer, E. A. Liver disease in pregnancy. *Curr. Probl. Obstet. Gynecol.* 7(15):3, 1984. *Thorough review of liver disease in pregnancy.*
3. Shaw, F. E., and Maynard, J. E. Hepatitis B: Still a concern for you and your patients. *Contemp OB/GYN* special issue. *General Medicine Update*, 24, 1986. *An excellent review of hepatitis B, incorporating the latest CDC recommendations.*
4. Tong, M. J., et al. Studies on the maternal-infant transmission of the viruses which cause acute hepatitis. *Gastroenterology* 80(5 part 1):999, 1981. *Vertical transmission studies.*
5. Lee, A. K., Ip, H. M., and Wong, W. C. Mechanisms of maternal-fetal transmission of hepatitis B virus. *J. Infect. Dis.* 138(5):668, 1978. *Study supporting oral route of infection of infants born to infected mothers.*
6. Hieber, J. P., et al. Hepatitis and pregnancy. *J. Pediatr.* 91(4):545, 1977. *Chart review study of the clinical course of hepatitis in pregnancy.*
7. Recommendations for protection against viral hepatitis. *M.M.W.R.* 34(22):313, 1985. *Recent recommendations for practical prevention of viral hepatitis.*

7a. Arevalo, J. A., and Washington, E. Cost effectiveness of prenatal screening and immunization for hepatitis B virus. *J. A. M. A.* 259:365, 1988. *Decision analysis of costs of screening and immunization in the United States.*

8. Khuroo, M. S., et al. Incidence and severity of viral hepatitis in pregnancy. *Am. J. Med.* 70(2):252, 1981. *A prospective study of viral hepatitis in pregnancy.*
9. Borhanmanesh, F., et al. Viral hepatitis during pregnancy. Severity and effect on gestation. *Gastroenterology* 64(2):304, 1973. *Prospective study on the effects of viral hepatitis on the pregnancy and the fetus.*
10. Francis, D. P. Selective primary health care: Strategies for control of disease in the developing world. III. Hepatitis B virus and its related diseases. *Rev. Infect. Dis.* 5(2):322, 1983.
11. Hoofnagle, J. H. Type A and Type B hepatitis. *Lab. Med.* 14(11):705, 1983. *Good review of serology of hepatitis A and B.*
12. Goudeau, A., et al. Lack of anti-HBc IgM in neonates with HBsAg-carrier mothers argues against transplacental transmission of hepatitis B virus infection. *Lancet* 2(8359):1103, 1983. *Study in Senegal demonstrating transmission to infant during delivery by contamination with maternal blood.*
13. Beasley, R. P., et al. Evidence against breast-feeding as a mechanism for vertical transmission of hepatitis B. *Lancet* 2(7938):740, 1975.

14. Beasley, R. P., and Hwang, L. Y. Postnatal infectivity of hepatitis B surface antigen-carrier mothers. *J. Infect. Dis.* 147(2):185, 1983. *Study supporting greater infectivity of HBcAg-positive mothers.*
15. Beasley, R. P., et al. Efficacy of hepatitis B immune globulin for prevention of perinatal transmission of the hepatitis B virus carrier state: Final report of randomized, double-blind, placebo-controlled trial. *Hepatology* 3(2)135, 1983.
16. Barin, F., et al. Immune response in neonates to hepatitis B vaccine. *Lancet* 1(8266):251, 1982. *Early study of effectiveness of hepatitis B vaccine.*
17. Xu, Z-Y., et al. Prevention of perinatal acquisition of hepatitis B virus carriage using vaccine: Preliminary report of a randomized, double-blind placebo-controlled and comparative trial. *Pediatrics* 76(5):713, 1985. *Large study from China of the efficacy of HB vaccine and HBIG.*
18. Hepatitis B among dental patients—Indiana. *M.M.W.R.* 34(5):73, 1985. *Report of a hepatitis outbreak traced to a dentist.*
19. Hepatitis B vaccine: Evidence confirming lack of AIDS transmission. *M.M.W.R.* 33(49):685, 1984. *There is now considerably more data demonstrating that HB vaccine or HBIG does not contain infectious material.*
20. Siegel, J. D. Prevention of hepatitis. *Pediatr. Infect. Dis.* 4(4):434, 1985. *Good review of recommendations.*

Suggested Reading

Seeff, L. B., and Hoofnagle, J. H. Immunoprophylaxis of viral hepatitis. *Gastroenterology* 77(1):161, 1979. *Good prevaccine review of the subject.*

22 Tuberculosis and Pregnancy

James A. McGregor

I. The problem

A. Description. Pregnant women are at risk for developing tuberculosis primarily in two forms: (1) primary infection with pneumonitis, or (2) much more commonly, reactivation or recrudescence of previously controlled primary infection [1]. Fetuses may rarely acquire tuberculosis in utero by means of primarily hematogenous seeding of the placenta with subsequent spread to the fetal liver. Very rarely, fetal infection originates from the maternal endometrium, with mycobacteria growing through the fetal membranes and causing congenital pneumonia secondary to aspiration of contaminated amniotic fluid. Newborns may also acquire tuberculosis by aspiration of infected vaginal material at birth or by exposure to an infectious mother, household member, or hospital attendant after birth [2]. Because of incompletely understood factors, newborns and infants appear especially susceptible to tuberculosis [2]. Maternal tuberculosis rarely leads to congenital tuberculosis, but if an infectious mother remains untreated, she can infect the newborn up to 50% of the time [3,4]. Newborns and infants are prone to progressive dissemination, which is frequently fatal if inadequately treated [2–4].

Clinically apparent reactivation or postprimary disease in adults may be seen at any time in life after resolution of primary infection. The greatest risk of tuberculosis recrudescence is within the first 5 years of primary infection. As many as 5% of newly infected individuals will reactivate and develop tuberculosis in the first year after primary infection. Among previously infected young adults, approximately 1% who have not been previously treated with isoniazid (INH) may be expected to reactivate their tuberculosis each year [5]. Preventive treatment with INH 300 mg PO qd for 1 year reduces the risk of reactivation to negligible levels [1,5].

Pregnancy has been anecdotally thought to predispose to tuberculosis reactivation by some authorities, but there are no controlled studies on this point. Observations made during the preantibiotic era suggest that active tuberculosis does not affect the course of pregnancy unless the infection is severe. Conversely, pregnancy has not been considered to adversely affect the course of tuberculosis [6–9]. Neither tuberculosis nor antituberculous treatment is an indication for pregnancy termination.

B. Epidemiology. In the United States, the decline in morbidity and mortality from tuberculosis began before the availability of effective chemotherapy and likely stemmed initially from improved living conditions and nutrition. The occurrence of tuberculosis complicating pregnancy reflects the frequency of this disease in the entire population: mortality from tuberculosis in the United States declined from 600/100,000 in the midnineteenth century to the present overall rate of approximately 3/100,000/ year [10]. In 1900, approximately 80% of young adults in the United States were tuberculin-sensitive, and this has been reduced to an overall rate of 3% today [10]. More recently, case rates for tuberculosis have fallen as low as 20/100,000 but may be much higher in various subpopulations [11]. These rates have been increased recently by trends in immigration with movement of infected individuals to this country from Mexico, Central America, the Caribbean, Eastern Europe, and Southeast Asia [11].

C. Risk groups. Now, as always, tuberculosis is most common among the malnourished and socioeconomically deprived [1]. Relatively high rates of tuberculosis have always persisted among the economically disadvantaged, inner city minorities, and native Americans [11]. In addition, recent increases in international travel and living may serve to make tuberculosis relatively more common in all segments of society [11]. Importantly, tuberculosis is increasingly seen as a presenting manifestation of acquired immune deficiency syndrome (AIDS).

II. Primary prevention

A. Methods. Primary prevention of tuberculosis centers around (1) proven epidemiologic practices of evaluation and appropriate treatment of all persons exposed to active tuberculosis, and (2) identification and preemptive antimycobacterial treatment of those who may be at risk for developing tuberculosis that may cause subsequent infection of others, including newborns and infants [1,5]. As always, pregnant women should take pains to avoid contact with possibly infectious individuals.

B. Justification. (See Chap. 96.)

III. Secondary prevention

A. Early detection

1. **Methods.** Prevention of tuberculosis in women and babies requires provision of informed medical care, patient cooperation, and medical care systems that can provide proven prevention and treatment regimens.

   a. **Skin testing**

      (1) **Description.** Women obtaining prenatal care or appearing for a delivery without prenatal care should be screened for *Mycobacterium tuberculosis* infection with the intradermal Mantoux test. Women with a prior history of treated or healed tuberculosis need not be tested.

      (2) **Performance.** A 0.1 ml inoculum of freshly mixed and stabilized (Tween 80) purified protein derivative (PPD) containing 5 tuberculin units (TU) should be placed intradermally on the volar aspect of the forearm. The skin test should be examined 48–72 hours later [1,5].

      (3) **Interpretation.** The diameter of test site induration, not erythema, is measured and is considered positive if greater than or equal to 10 mm. Induration of less than 5 mm is a negative test. Induration between 5 and 9 mm may be due to infection with atypical mycobacteria, prior BCG (bacillus Calmette-Guérin) vaccination, or recent tuberculosis exposure and infection [1,5]. A positive Mantoux test may take from 1–3 months to develop after an initial infection. Pregnancy itself does not alter test reactivity [12]. Prior BCG vaccination is not a contraindication to skin testing because: (1) Mantoux tests are commonly negative or less than 10 mm; (2) BCG vaccination is not considered effective when given after age 10; and (3) BCG is most commonly given in regions of the world where tuberculosis is endemic and thus the patients are at highest risk. Only use of Mantoux tests with PPD-S has been standardized and therefore they are recommended for skin testing over other techniques [1].

   b. **Chest x ray.** Women with a positive skin test should receive a standard 14-×17-in. chest roentgenogram with abdominal shielding. Chest x ray can be delayed until the first 20 gestational weeks are completed, unless active tuberculosis is likely [5]. Approximately 20% of patients with active tuberculosis may have a negative skin test, so a chest roentgenogram with abdominal shielding must be performed if pulmonary tuberculosis is clinically suspected [9]. Routine chest x-ray examination of pregnant women is no longer recommended.

   c. **Contacts.** Discovery of active tuberculosis or skin test conversion in a pregnant woman should lead to prompt skin testing and possible clinical examination of household contacts for active tuberculosis [1,5]. Household contacts with active tuberculosis may have been the source of the mother's infection and may also infect the newborn unless adequately treated. Because patients at greatest risk for tuberculosis may not act conscientiously in health matters, community public health resources should be employed to ensure that indicated household screening for tuberculosis is completed.

   d. **Smears and culture.** Definitive diagnosis of pulmonary tuberculosis is made by isolation of *M. tuberculosis.* Pregnant women with possible pulmonary tuberculosis should have at least three adequate sputum samples, induced if necessary, promptly obtained for acid-fast bacilli microscopic examinations and culture.

2. **Justification.** Tuberculosis screening, diagnosis, and treatment regimens for pregnant women are similar to those described for nonpregnant individuals, with a few exceptions [1,5]. The classic clinical triad of cough, fever, and night sweats rarely occurs except in the most florid cases. Today, most patients are unaware of their disease. Indeed, symptoms such as low grade fever, anorexia, and malaise or lassitude may be attributed to pregnancy [9]. Despite some concerns about the validity of tuberculin skin testing during pregnancy, most experts ac-

cept its validity throughout pregnancy [13]. Consequently, pregnant women should be skin-tested as described. The predictive value, risk, cost, and acceptability are described in Chap. 96.

B. **Early intervention**

1. **Methods.** Recommendations for chemoprophylaxis and treatment of tuberculosis are changing and may require individualization. Indeed, authoritative advice may be conflicting. Therefore, recently updated sources, as well as local consultants, should be accessed for the most current information [1,5,14]. Physicians who treat tuberculosis are advised to be familiar with the expertise and resources of their local public health department [14].

a. **Chemoprophylaxis.** The pregnant woman with a positive skin test but a negative chest x ray who would otherwise qualify for isoniazid chemoprophylaxis were she not pregnant may have the preventive therapy delayed until after delivery. The American Thoracic Society has recently reiterated this recommendation [5].

> Although no harmful effects of isoniazid to the fetus have been observed, preventive therapy generally should be delayed until after delivery. There does not appear to be any substantial increase in tuberculous risk for women during pregnancy. The exception is for pregnant women likely to have been recently infected; in that situation, isoniazid preventive therapy should begin when the infection is documented, but after the first trimester.

When INH is used in pregnancy, supplemental pyridoxine is recommended because of concerns of perinatal neurotoxicity [12]. For dose, duration, and monitoring, see Chap. 96.

b. **Treatment** (see Table 22-1).

(1) **Indications** for treatment of tuberculosis in pregnancy are not different from those in the nonpregnant patient (see Chap. 96). For pregnant patients who have more advanced forms of pulmonary tuberculosis, who may be noncompliant, or who are near term, hospitalization so as to expedite diagnosis and therapy is strongly recommended. Because microscopic examination of stained concentrated sputum may be falsely negative, and cultures may require up to 6 weeks to become positive, appropriate treatment of possible tuberculosis should begin after adequate cultures have been obtained [1,5].

(2) **Antituberculosis agents** most commonly used during pregnancy include isoniazid (INH) (in combination with pyridoxine), rifampin, and ethambutol [5,9]. Each of these agents crosses the placenta and may be found in breast milk. Recent reviews do not conclude that any of these agents are teratogenic when used during human pregnancy [5–9]. Adverse effects from the small amounts of antituberculous agents found in breast milk have not been noted, and breast-feeding is not contraindicated [6]. Current recommendations are to initiate treatment of tuberculosis with INH, rifampin, and ethambutol, especially if INH resistance is suspected [5]. If the recovered microorganisms prove to be sensitive to INH, then ethambutol may be discontinued and INH and rifampin continued to complete at least 9 months of therapy [5]. When noncompliance is suspected or documented, directly administered therapy is mandatory.

Pyrazinamide and streptomycin are also first-line drugs for tuberculosis, and their use in four-drug regimens can decrease the length of therapy to 6 months [5]. However, prolonged streptomycin treatment has been implicated as a cause of ototoxicity in exposed progeny, and data on the use of pyrazinamide during pregnancy are limited [15]. Therefore, these potentially useful agents are not recommended for use in pregnancy unless individually indicated on the basis of microbiologic sensitivities or poor response to treatment.

Because isoniazid (300 mg/day) has been inconclusively linked with neonatal seizures [16] and neurologic deficits in the newborn, it should be given in combination with pyridoxine (50–100 mg/day, vitamin B_6) during pregnancy and lactation. Rifampin teratogenicity appears species-specific and has not been demonstrated in humans [6]. Even though teratogenic effects of ethambutol are well established in laboratory animals, use in humans appears safe and is recommended if INH resistance is a possibility [17].

Table 22-1. Treatment of tuberculosis in pregnant and lactating women and children

Commonly used agents	Dosage				Adverse reactions and comments
	Dosage form	Daily dose	Twice weekly	Maximum	
Isoniazid (INH)	Tablets: 100 mg, 300 mg Syrup: 50 mg/5 ml	10–20 mg/kg	20–40 mg/kg	300 mg/day	Give adjunctive pyridoxine 50–100 mg during pregnancy, lactation, or infancy. Mild liver enzyme elevation. Hepatitis especially in those over 35 yr or with prior liver disease. Neuropathy, neonatal seizures. Check monthly. Do liver function tests if over 35 yr at start of therapy and periodically.
Rifampin	Capsules: 150 mg, 300 mg	10–20 mg/kg	10–20 mg/kg	600 mg	Orange discoloration of urine and secretions. Vomiting, hepatitis. Generally avoid during embryogenesis.
Ethambutol	Tablets: 100 mg, 400 mg	15–25 mg/kg	50 mg/kg	2.5 gm	Optic neuritis (reversible). Decreased acuity. Generally not suited for children unable to perform visual screening. Generally avoid during embryogenesis.
Pyrazinamide	Tablets: 500 mg	30 mg/kg	50 mg/kg	2.0 gm	Hepatitis, hyperuricemia. Generally avoid during pregnancy.
Streptomycin	Vials: 1 gm, 4 gm	20–40 mg/kg IM 5 d/wk	25–30 mg/kg	1.0 gm	Ototoxicity, nephrotoxicity. Avoid in pregnancy.

Further obstetric and postpartum concerns include rifampin's immunosuppressive effects and interference with metabolism of warfarin and oral contraceptive agents [18]. Effective contraception for reproductive-age women being treated for tuberculosis is important, and women using rifampin should take care to avoid missing any birth control pills. Women receiving rifampin may consider using supplementary contraceptive techniques, such as barrier methods.

(3) Care of newborns whose mothers are infected with active tuberculosis demands coordinated care of both mother and child [5,14]. Priorities include identification and treatment of congenitally infected infants and prevention of postpartum neonatal infection. Some authorities recommend that newborns of mothers with possibly infectious pulmonary tuberculosis should be promptly isolated until the mother is presumed not infectious on the basis of the following: (1) at least 2 weeks of adequate antituberculosis treatment, and (2) at least two negative induced sputum examined microscopically for acid-fast bacteria [6]. Other authorities consider the risk to be small if the mother is being treated or if the newborn has been placed on INH [4,14]. Newborns of women with inactive tuberculosis or noninfectious nonpulmonary tuberculosis (i.e., extrapulmonary), or women previously begun on treatment and demonstrated to be noninfectious, need not be isolated from their mothers. Pregnant or postpartum women with possibly infectious tuberculosis should be placed in isolation with full respiratory precautions until appropriate treatment is commenced.

If there is increased risk of congenital tuberculosis on the basis of extensive (miliary tuberculosis or tuberculous meningitis) maternal disease with possible bacillemia, then the newborn should be promptly begun on isoniazid 10 mg/kg/day, pending results of 0.1 ml PPD skin-testing, chest roentgenogram, liver function tests, and cerebrospinal fluid and gastric and/or tracheal aspirate smears and cultures [14,19]. If skin tests or microbiologic tests are positive, appropriate doses of at least two mycobactericidal agents should be initiated and continued to at least 9 months. Newborn PPD skin test results may be falsely negative and treatment should be continued if there is clinical, radiographic, or microbiologic evidence of tuberculosis. Skin test negativity at 1 month of age argues against the diagnosis of congenital tuberculosis.

Infants of mothers with less severe tuberculosis require the same studies but do not require presumptive treatment unless there is clinical or laboratory evidence of infection. If skin tests performed at 2 and 4 months of age are positive, then multidrug treatment should be initiated. If skin tests remain negative and the infant remains clinically well, then one of three management plans may be selected on the basis of the individual family's circumstances:

(a) The infant may be started on isoniazid for 1 year with further skin testing every 2 months for 1 year. If the strain of *M. tuberculosis* is INH-sensitive, this regimen appears to be very effective [4,14]. If the infant demonstrates skin test conversion or clinical evidence of disease, then full multiagent therapy is begun.

(b) If compliance is deemed unlikely or cannot be supervised, then the infant may be repeatedly surveyed with chest roentgenograms, skin tests, and gastric cultures for at least 1 year. Again, infants with any evidence of tuberculosis should be fully treated. Both of these regimens require full, reliable, and systematic parental and medical care, cooperation, and follow-up.

(c) If such treatment and surveillance is not possible or likely to occur, then BCG (bacillus Calmette-Guérin) vaccination may be administered. Although the efficacy of BCG vaccination is doubted in individuals over 10 years of age, an excellent case has been made for BCG vaccine efficacy in infants [3,20]. Infant BCG recipients should also be followed for clinical or roentgenographic evidence of tuberculosis, at least through the first year of life. Newborns exposed to possibly infectious health care providers may be similarly followed.

2. Justification

a. Chemoprophylaxis. (Since it is not currently recommended that pregnant women routinely receive antepartum INH prophylaxis, its use is not discussed.) Limited use of INH chemoprophylaxis during pregnancy is based on theoretical risks of INH toxicity in the fetus, potential litigation, and relatively low risks of tuberculosis in a skin test-positive, chest x-ray negative pregnant woman. If primary infections occurred in the prior 1–3 years, then INH and pyridoxine treatment may be initiated during late pregnancy.

b. Treatment. Even though tuberculosis may not adversely affect obstetric outcome, it is mandatory to identify and treat every tuberculous pregnant woman for the following reasons: (1) to prevent progressive maternal lung injury, (2) to prevent dissemination in the mother and possibly the fetus, and (3) to reduce the possibility of infecting the newborn after birth.

IV. Recommendations

A. Primary prevention

1. Apply current public health advice for evaluation and possible treatment of all individuals exposed to tuberculosis.
2. Specifically identify individuals at greatest risk of tuberculosis—close contacts, recent skin test converters—and start antimycobacterial chemoprophylaxis.
3. In households with possible tuberculosis, rigorously evaluate all individuals who may come in contact with infants.

B. Secondary prevention

1. Early detection

a. Use the Mantoux test to screen for prior tuberculosis infection in pregnant women.

b. Rigorously evaluate pregnant women with findings of possible tuberculosis by appropriate tests, including x rays in conjunction with appropriate abdominal shielding.

2. Early intervention

a. Chemoprophylaxis

(1) Unless there is evidence of recent skin test conversion, INH chemoprophylaxis may currently be delayed until immediately after delivery.

(2) INH may be given during pregnancy along with pyridoxine supplementation if there is concern that reactivation may occur.

b. Treatment

(1) With the general exceptions of streptomycin and para-aminosalicylic acid (PAS), full treatment doses of INH and rifampin along with ethambutol are appropriate for treatment of tuberculosis during pregnancy. Avoidance of drug use during embryogenesis is theoretically appealing.

(2) Antimycobacterial drugs may predispose to contraceptive pill failure. Care should be taken not to miss any pills.

References

1. Leff, A., and Geppert, E. F. Public health and preventive aspects of pulmonary tuberculosis: Infectiousness, epidemiology, risk factors, classification, and preventive therapy. *Arch. Intern. Med.* 139(12):1405, 1979. *Excellent review.*
2. Nemir, R. L., and O'Hare, D. Congenital tuberculosis: Review and diagnostic guidelines. *Am. J. Dis. Child.* 139(3):284, 1985. *Authoritative review.*
3. Kendig, E. L., Jr. Prognosis of infants born of tuberculous mothers. *Pediatrics* 26:97, 1960. *Small classic. An insightful review.*
4. Dormer, B. A., et al. Prophylactic isoniazid protection of infants in a tuberculosis hospital. *Lancet* 2:902, 1959. *Another small medical classic. It must be remembered that INH resistance is now endemic, especially in Southeast Asia and Mexico.*
5. American Thoracic Society medical section of the American Lung Association: Treatment of tuberculosis and tuberculosis infection in adults and children. *Am. Rev. Respir. Dis.* 134(2):355, 1986. *Most current recommendations.*
6. Good, J. T., Jr, et al. Tuberculosis in association with pregnancy. *Am. J. Obstet. Gynecol.* 140(5):492, 1981. *Record review of 27 cases of tuberculosis in pregnancy.*
7. Schaefer, G., et al. Pregnancy and pulmonary tuberculosis. *Obstet. Gynecol.* 46(6):706, 1975. *A classic.*
8. Bjerkedal, T., Bahna, S. L., and Lehmann, E. H. Course and outcome of pregnancy in women with pulmonary tuberculosis. *Scand. J. Respir. Dis.* 56(5):245, 1975. *Study of 542 women with tuberculosis during pregnancy.*
9. Wilson, E. A., Thelin, T. J., Dilts, P. V. Jr. Tuberculosis complicated by pregnancy. *Am. J. Obstet. Gynecol.* 115(4):526, 1973. *Another classic. Not likely to be replicated.*
10. *Reported Tuberculosis Data—1969.* Atlanta, GA: Centers for Disease Control, 1971. *A good epidemiologic review.*
11. Tuberculosis statistics: States and cities, 1972–1977. Atlanta, GA: Centers for Disease Control, Tuberculosis Branch. *Another good epidemiologic review. Further epidemiologic information.*
12. Snider, D. Pregnancy and tuberculosis. *Chest* 86(3 Suppl):10s, 1984. *Excellent current review of recommendations and controversies.*

13. Present, P. A., and Comstock, G. W. Tuberculin sensitivity in pregnancy. *Am. Rev. Respir. Dis.* 112(3):413, 1975. *A unique paper.*
14. Jacobs, R. F., and Abernathy, R. S. The treatment of tuberculosis in children. *Pediatr. Infect. Dis.* 4(5):513, 1985. *A perceptive, but somewhat personal, perspective.*
15. Robinson, G. C., and Cambon, K. G. Hearing loss in infants of tuberculous mothers treated with streptomycin during pregnancy. *N. Engl. J. Med.* 271:949, 1964. *Case reports of an uncommon phenomenon.*
16. McKenzie, S. A., MacNab, A. J., and Katz, G. Neonatal pyridoxine responsive convulsions due to isoniazid therapy. *Arch. Dis. Child.* 51(7):567, 1976. *A case report.*
17. Lewit, T., et al. Ethambutol in pregnancy: Observations on embryogenesis. *Chest* 66(1):25, 1974. *Study of the safety of ethambutol in pregnancy.*
18. Skolnick, J. L., et al. Rifampin, oral contraceptives and pregnancy. *J.A.M.A.* 236(12):1382, 1976. *A case report of pregnancy occurring while taking birth control pills and rifampin.*
19. Brown, Z. Tuberculosis and Pregnancy. In J. Sciarra, D. A. Eschenbach, and R. Depp (eds.), *Gynecology and Obstetrics.* Philadelphia: Harper & Row, 1983. Pp. 1–6. *An excellent short review, espousing BCG vaccinations in selected infants.*
20. Eickhoff, T. C. The current status of BCG immunization against tuberculosis. *Annu. Rev. Med.* 28:411, 1977. *A good review of BCG vaccinations.*

23 Preterm Labor and Delivery

Peter Rogge

I. The problem

A. Definition. Preterm labor is the occurrence of regular uterine contractions accompanied by progressive cervical effacement and dilatation prior to 37 completed weeks' gestation. The term **prematurity**, which in the past was applied to growth-retarded as well as preterm infants, has been abandoned (see Chap. 24).

B. Description. Preterm labor and its consequences, preterm delivery with high neonatal morbidity and mortality rates, are clearly the major problems confronting obstetricians worldwide. In the United States, preterm deliveries may account for as much as 75% of perinatal mortality [1]. A British study of a large hospital's experience with preterm births reported that 85% of the early neonatal deaths, exclusive of lethal congenital anomalies, occurred in this group [2]. In addition to mortality, both short- and long-term morbidity result from preterm deliveries. While the introduction in recent years of sophisticated (and costly) neonatal intensive care techniques has reduced this morbidity and mortality substantially, the small preterm infant's risk of a major neurologic or developmental handicap is still about 10% [2].

C. Epidemiology. The incidence of preterm delivery in the United States is approximately 8% and has remained relatively constant over the last 20 years [1].

Although the etiology of preterm labor is unknown, correlates of preterm labor have been described in many reports. However, methodologic difficulties in most of these studies make firm conclusions difficult. Older studies often included small-for-gestational-age infants with appropriately grown preterm babies; other reports have failed to exclude iatrogenic preterm deliveries or have failed to document fetal or maternal pathology [3]. Most have used the last menstrual period as sole criterion of gestational age [4].

D. Risk factors. With the above limitations in mind, the existing reports were critically reviewed and are summarized in Table 23-1, together with the author's assessment of the significance of each risk factor's association with preterm labor.

II. Primary prevention

A. Methods

1. **General measures** that have been recommended include [5]:
   a. **Family planning assistance**
   b. **Screening for and treatment of serious medical and surgical illnesses** (see Chap. 2).
   c. **Counseling regarding alcohol and tobacco abuse.** No safe lower limits for alcohol intake and smoking have been established; at this writing, complete abstinence is the safest recommendation (see Chap. 4).
   d. **Nutritional supplementation for selected populations** (see Chap. 3).
2. **Specific measures** that have been advocated include [5]:
   a. **Intrauterine device (IUD) removal** if a pregnancy occurs with it in place.
   b. **Cerclage** with a documented incompetent cervix. This is most often performed at 12–14 weeks' gestation (after fetal heart tones are heard). Cerclage techniques have recently been critically reviewed [6].
   c. **Surgical repair** of certain congenital uterine malformations. On diagnosis of a uterine anomaly (generally by hysterosalpingography) and reasonable certainty that this condition has caused preterm labor in the past, referral to a gynecologist who is experienced in the surgical repair of these uncommon conditions is recommended.
   d. **Bed rest** in multiple pregnancies, if recommended, should be initiated early in gestation, because up to 70% of perinatal mortality with twin gesta-

Table 23-1. Risk factors for preterm labor and delivery

Risk factor	
Historical factors	
Previous preterm delivery	A
Congenital uterine anomalies (septate/bicornuate uteri)	A
Maternal diethylstilbestrol exposure with cervicovaginal changes	A
Low socioeconomic status	B
Age <20, >40	B
Race (black)	C
Multiple therapeutic abortions	C
Factors during current pregnancy	
Multiple pregnancy	A
Polyhydramnios	A
Antepartum hemorrhage (includes abruption, placenta previa)	A
Incompetent cervix	A
Chorioamnionitis	A
Pyelonephritis (2nd, 3rd trimester)	B
Preterm cervical effacement/dilatation/engagement of presenting part	B
Long, tiring, stressful work	B
Asymptomatic bacteriuria	C
Threatened abortion	C
Smoking	C
Chlamydial cervicitis	C
Alcohol intake >2 drinks/day	C
Maternal anxiety	C
Coitus	C
Large uterine leiomyomata	C
Other medical/surgical complications of pregnancy (appendicitis, cholecystitis, other conditions requiring laparotomy, hypertension, anemia, renal disease, hyperthyroidism)	A–C

Key: A=association with preterm labor and delivery well established; B=association probable, confirmation needed; C=single study suggests association or results conflict, further studies necessary.

tions occurs prior to 30 weeks [7]. **Cerclage and tocolytic agents** used as prophylaxis in uncomplicated twin gestation are not recommended.

e. Weekly intramuscular **progestogen injections** (17-hydroxyprogesterone caproate) administered between 16 and 36 weeks' gestation have been employed in experimental trials [8].

B. Justification

1. General supportive measures

a. **Effectiveness.** While entirely reasonable, these measures have not been studied prospectively in relation to prevention of preterm labor. The results of existing trials of dietary supplementation during pregnancy suggest that only small increases in gestational age may be effected [9].

b. **Risks and side effects.** Implementation of these measures should be without risk.

2. Specific measures

a. IUDs

(1) **Effectiveness.** When a woman becomes pregnant with an IUD in place, the IUD should be removed. If left in place, there is a strong association with spontaneous abortion, and case reports exist of second and third trimester chorioamnionitis and sepsis (one must, of course, rule out an ectopic gestation as well).

(2) **Risks and side effects.** IUD removal is nearly always uncomplicated if properly performed. If reasonable traction fails to dislodge the device, partial perforation should be suspected; excessive force in this setting may produce uterine lacerations and hemorrhage. There is an increased risk of spontaneous abortion at the time of removal (compared to those who did not have an IUD), but overall reproductive outcome is improved (as compared to those in whom the IUD is left inserted).

b. **Cerclage**
   (1) **Effectiveness.** Cerclage is considered to be the treatment of choice for confirmed cervical incompetence based on studies of infant survival before and after cerclage (20–27% before versus 74–82% after) [6]; however, prospective randomized trials comparing cerclage with other treatment modalities do not exist [6]. Moreover, diagnosis of cervical incompetence may be difficult.
   (2) **Risks and side effects.** Complications of cerclage (uncommon with experienced operators) include hemorrhage, chorioamnionitis, iatrogenic rupture of the fetal membranes, and spontaneous abortion or preterm labor. Late complications (if the cerclage is not removed early in labor) are cervical lacerations and uterine rupture.

c. **Metroplasty**
   (1) **Effectiveness.** Metroplasty is performed by skilled surgeons for septate and bicornuate uteri and has resulted in reduced fetal wastage rates [10,11]. For septate uteri with normal external configuration, incision of the septum via the hysteroscope is a safe and effective alternative (one-day hospital stay, vaginal delivery allowable post-procedure) [12].
   (2) **Risks and side effects.** Complications are chiefly those of major abdominal surgery. In addition, these patients generally have Cesarean section deliveries in future pregnancies, with further attendant risks.

d. **Bed rest**
   (1) **Effectiveness.** The issue of bed rest in multiple gestations is still unresolved, with a suggestion in some studies of benefit [7]. Cerclage and tocolytic agents were not helpful in controlled studies [13].
   (2) **Risks and side effects.** Strict bed rest in patients with multiple gestations often imposes significant economic and psychological hardship, as well as possibly increasing the risk of thromboembolic disorders.

e. **Injections of 17-hydroxyprogesterone caproate**
   (1) **Effectiveness.** In one controlled study of women at risk for preterm labor, this was found to be beneficial, although such therapy is at present investigational and not approved by the Federal Drug Administration (FDA).
   (2) **Risks and side effects.** The teratogenic potential of 17-hydroxyprogesterone has not been fully explored since only small numbers of patients have received the drug.

III. Secondary prevention

A. Early detection

1. **Methods of preterm risk assessment**
   a. **Performance.** Use the method of Creasy, et al. [14,15], and Herron, et al. [16].
   b. **Timing.** Obstetric patients are screened at the first prenatal visit for preterm-birth risk factors (Table 23-2), and a risk score is assigned. Rescreening for preterm labor risk is repeated at 22–26 weeks.
   c. **Interpretation.** If the score is above a critical value (Table 23-2), the patient is placed in the high-risk group and intensive educational efforts are begun, directed toward early self-detection of the symptoms of preterm labor.
2. **Justification**
   a. **Test characteristics.** Evaluation of the effectiveness of screening programs for preterm labor is in its infancy. The first report [16] on the effectiveness of the above screening program was recently published, and a collaborative, multi-institutional study is in progress [17]. Analysis of the first report reveals:
      (1) Nine percent of all primigravidas were classified as high risk; these ultimately accounted for 31% of the primigravid preterm births and 39% of the primigravid preterm labors.
      (2) About 14% of the multigravidas were classified as high risk; these contributed 77% of the multigravid preterm births and 80% of the multigravid preterm labors.
      (3) The overall preterm delivery rate in this early assessment and intervention trial was 2.4%, well below the national mean and below that experienced at the study institution during the year prior to the introduction of the program. Although the results represented an encouraging first step, many qualifications should be noted. The scoring

Table 23-2. Determining risk of preterm delivery*

Points	Socioeconomic status	History	Daily habits	Current pregnancy
1	Two children at home Low socio-economic status	One abortion <1 year since last birth	Work outside home	Unusual fatigue
2	<20 years >40 years Single parent	Two abortions	>10 cigarettes/day	<13-kg gain by 32 weeks Albuminuria Hypertension Bacteriuria
3	Very low socioeconomic status <150 cm <45 kg	Three abortions	Heavy work Long, tiring trip	Breech at 32 weeks Weight loss of ≥2 kg Head engaged Febrile illness
4	<18 years	Pyelonephritis		Metrorrhagia after 12 weeks Effacement Dilatation Uterine irritability
5		Uterine anomaly Second-trimester abortion Diethylstilbestrol exposure		Placenta previa Hydramnios
10		Premature delivery Repeated second-trimester abortion		Twins Abdominal surgery

*Score is computed by addition of the number of points given any item: 0–5=low risk; 6–9=medium risk; ≥10=high risk.
Source: R. K. Creasy, B. A. Gummer, and G. C. Liggins. System for predicting spontaneous preterm birth. Reprinted with permission from The American College of Obstetricians and Gynecologists. (*Obstetrics and Gynecology*, Vol. 55, 1980, p. 692).

system's **specificity** was poor (only about one fifth of the high-risk patients developed preterm labor); and its **sensitivity**, especially for primigravidas, was disappointing (44% of total preterm labors came from the low-risk group). Also, individual components of the system were not evaluated separately.

Other studies have provided insight into the effectiveness of this type of screening and intervention.

In large though uncontrolled series of patients in France and Martinique, a preterm risk assessment system similar to Creasy's was employed [18]. In addition, a concerted effort was made to modify specific risk factors—most important, heavy work, long hours on the job, stressful activities, and any activity resulting in painful uterine contractions [18,19]. Impressive reductions in preterm labor occurred following introduction of the system in both countries.

The Creasy system was recently evaluated in a small prospective study [20] of indigent black patients in Philadelphia, and no significant reduction in the preterm delivery rate could be demonstrated. While the bulk of the literature to date suggests that the Creasy system is helpful, improved (and simplified) risk-screening systems need to be developed and tested in well-controlled prospective studies. Additionally, the cornerstone of the French system—reduction of physical exertion and stress in high-risk women (via work leaves or modifications, household help) [18,19]—needs to be tested for efficacy and cost-effectiveness in the United States.

b. **Risks and side effects.** No significant risks should result from the risk screening.

c. **Costs.** The scoring system in Table 23-2 reportedly requires 2–3 minutes for trained staff to perform at each of the initial and the 22–26 weeks' screen [15]. Considerable additional staff and patient time (i.e., cost) would be required for weekly prenatal visits.

B. Early intervention

1. **Methods.** High-risk patients are seen weekly and are taught to report early symptoms promptly: regular uterine contractions, backache, lower abdominal pressure (different from usual), cramping, or a change in vaginal discharge (spotting, increased mucus). Physicians and staff are trained to respond quickly to these symptoms, and if abnormal contraction activity is suspected, baseline pelvic examination is performed and external fetal monitoring is initiated to assess uterine activity. When early preterm labor is diagnosed and when contraindications to labor suppression are absent, treatment with intravenous ritodrine hydrochloride is promptly started. If preterm labor is successfully suppressed, patients are placed on oral ritodrine hydrochloride and after appropriate observation are discharged, continuing the oral medication until 37–38 completed weeks' gestation.

   Recently, a small series of patients at risk for preterm labor were monitored daily at home for contractions with a newly developed ambulatory tocodynometry system [21]. Patients who subsequently developed preterm labor had increased contraction frequency for 8 weeks prior to labor and experienced further abrupt increases within the 24 hours preceding labor. If confirmed in larger studies, this system might increase the accuracy of risk assessment as well as facilitate early diagnosis of preterm labor.

2. **Justification**

   a. **Effectiveness.** Educating high-risk patients about early symptoms of preterm labor is reasonable, though this strategy has not been evaluated separately in preterm-birth prevention trials. One would expect low **specificity**, as the majority of women report one or more of these symptoms during pregnancy.

   Assuming preterm labor is diagnosed early (intact membranes, cervix dilated <3–4 cm) and no contraindications exist, suppression of labor with intravenous ritodrine hydrochloride currently is the treatment of choice in the United States. Most reports, including a recent large, prospective, randomized, double-blind study [22,23], have demonstrated statistically significant decreases in neonatal mortality and morbidity up to 34 weeks' gestation from such therapy.

   Recently, intravenous magnesium sulfate has been advocated as an acceptable alternative to ritodrine. Side effects of therapy appear minimal, although its efficacy when compared to betamimetic agents has been questioned, and prospective comparison trials with ritodrine are continuing [24]. Preliminary results are encouraging.

   Many clinicians substitute terbutaline for ritodrine as an oral tocolytic; terbutaline's longer half-life allows for more convenient dosage schedules.

   b. **Risks and side effects.** Risks of labor suppression with ritodrine hydrochloride are summarized in Table 23-3.

   c. **Costs.** Total hospital costs for the first day of evaluation and suppression of preterm labor are about \$750–1000, with subsequent daily hospital costs, assuming successful therapy, being somewhat less. A total hospital stay is typically 2–4 days. The cost to the patient of oral ritodrine hydrochloride is about \$14 daily; this cost accrues until 37–38 weeks' gestation. If preterm labor is not or cannot be suppressed and a very small infant is delivered, costs rise astronomically since neonatal intensive care is required. It has been reported that the cost per normal surviving infant in a group of babies weighing less than 1000 gm is \$88,058.25 [25]. Thus, in utero care of preterm infants via suppression of labor, while expensive, is probably cost-effective because of the extraordinary costs of prolonged intensive care of delivered infants. A recent study reported cost savings of \$11,240 per birth when tocolysis was attempted between 26 and 33 weeks' gestation; after 33 weeks, no substantial difference in costs was found [26].

Table 23-3. Adverse effects of ritodrine

Usual effects
Maternal tachycardia (19–40 beats/min increase above baseline)
Increased pulse pressure
Mild increase in fetal heart rate (0–9 beats/min)
Moderate transient elevations of blood glucose and plasma insulin
Moderate transient hypokalemia
Frequent effects
Palpitations (30%)
Tremor (20–25%)
Anxiety (5–10%)
Uncommon effects
Chest pain or tightness, arrythmias
Pulmonary edema

Source: P. T. Rogge and K. R. Niswander. Preterm Labor. In H. J. Osofsky (ed.), *Advances in Clinical Obstetrics and Gynecology.* ©1982, the Williams & Wilkins Co., Baltimore.

IV. Recommendations

A. Primary prevention

1. Perform the **general measures** prior to pregnancy: family planning assistance, screening for and treatment of medical and surgical illnesses, counseling and dissuasion of alcohol and tobacco abuse, and nutritional counseling as required (see Chaps. 3 and 4).
2. **Remove an IUD,** should a pregnancy happen while it is in utero.
3. With a firm diagnosis of incompetent cervix, perform a **cerclage** at 12–14 weeks' gestation. If the diagnosis is uncertain, follow the patient closely with weekly cervical examinations. Patients should be warned to report immediately any contractions, increased pressure, or urinary urgency. If significant cervical changes develop, cerclage should promptly be performed.
4. **Metroplasty** by an experienced surgeon is indicated prior to intended pregnancy for patients with bicornuate or septate uteri if a prior, otherwise unexplained, fetal loss or preterm labor has occurred.
5. Increased **rest** and avoidance of strenuous exertion—both at work and at home—are recommended for patients at risk for preterm labor. Patients at high risk (e.g., with twin pregnancies) should be encouraged to take bed rest as much as possible.

B. Early detection

1. At the initial prenatal visit, all patients are screened for risk factors (see Table 23-2). This risk screening should be repeated at 22–26 weeks' gestation.
2. All patients, especially those at high risk based on this assessment, are instructed about early symptoms of preterm labor and the importance of reporting these promptly if they occur.
3. Scheduling of office visits should be individualized based on risk; patients at high risk should probably be seen every 1–2 weeks between 20 and 36 weeks' gestation. During the visit, a gentle cervical examination may be performed. Patients with significant effacement/dilation or engagement of the presenting part are at increased risk, and closer surveillance is warranted.

C. Early intervention. If preterm labor is diagnosed early in its course and contraindications do not exist, hospitalization and suppression of labor with ritodrine hydrochloride or magnesium sulfate is warranted.

References

1. Rogge, P. T., and Niswander, K. R. Preterm Labor. In H. J. Osofsky (ed.), *Advances in Clinical Obstetrics and Gynecology.* Baltimore: Williams & Wilkins, 1982. Pp. 63–74. *Current concepts of etiology, diagnosis, and treatment of preterm labor.*
2. Lipshitz, J., and Schneider, J. M. Inhibition of Labor. In J. J. Sciarra (ed.), *Gynecology and Obstetrics.* Vol. 3. Philadelphia: Harper & Row, 1980. Chap. 87. *Review of preterm labor, emphasizing treatment; 192 references.*

3. Creasy, R. K., and Herron, M. A. Prevention of preterm birth. *Semin. Perinatol.* 5(3):295, 1981. *Review of epidemiology and prevention of preterm birth.*
4. Berkowitz, G. S., and Berkowitz, R. L. Predicting correlates of prematurity. *Contemp. Obstet. Gynecol.* 20:182, 1982. *Epidemiology of preterm delivery.*
5. Johnson, J. W. C. Options in preventing preterm labor. *Contemp. Obstet. Gynecol.* 20:201, 1982. *Review of prevention strategies.*
6. Cousins, L. Cervical incompetence, 1980: A time for reappraisal. *Clin. Obstet. Gynecol.* 23(2):467, 1980. *Review of cervical incompetence: diagnosis, etiology, and treatment.*
7. Hawrylyshyn, P. A., et al. Twin pregnancies—a continuing perinatal challenge. *Obstet. Gynecol.* 59(4):463, 1982. *Five-year retrospective review of management of 177 twin pregnancies at a large Canadian hospital.*
8. Johnson, J. W., et al. Efficacy of 17-alpha hydroxyprogesterone caproate in the prevention of premature labor. *N. Engl. J. Med.* 293(14):675, 1975. *Prospective study of progestin injections for prevention of preterm labor.*
9. Kristel, A. R., and Rush, D. Maternal nutrition and duration of gestation: A review. *Clin. Obstet. Gynecol.* 27(3):553, 1984. *Review of studies on nutrition and preterm labor.*
10. Musich, J. R., and Behrman, S. J. Obstetric outcome before and after metroplasty in women with uterine anomalies. *Obstet. Gynecol.* 52(1):63, 1978. *Results of metroplasty for various uterine anomalies.*
11. Heinonen, P. K., Saarikoski, S., and Pystynen, P. Reproductive performance of women with uterine anomalies: An evaluation of 182 cases. *Obstet. Gynecol. Surv.* 37(10):627, 1982. *Editorial comment on large study of women with uterine anomalies.*
12. Israel, R., and March, C. M. Hysteroscopic incision of the septate uterus. *Am. J. Obstet. Gynecol.* 149(1):66, 1984. *An alternative to metroplasty for the septate uterus: report of 15 cases.*
13. O'Connoor, M. E., et al. The merits of special antenatal care for twin pregnancies. *Obstet. Gynecol. Surv.* 37(10):14, 1982. *Editorial comment and recommendations for treatment of multiple gestations.*
14. Creasy, R. K., Gummer, B. A., and Liggins, G. C. System for predicting spontaneous preterm birth. *Obstet. Gynecol.* 55(6):692, 1980. *Prospective study of a risk-scoring system for prediction of preterm labor.*
15. Creasy, R. K., and Chez, R. A. How to detect premature labor early. *Contemp. Obstet. Gynecol.* 19:203, 1982. *Discussion of specifics of Creasy's preterm-birth prevention program.*
16. Herron, M. A., Katz, M., and Creasy, R. K. Evaluation of a preterm birth prevention program: Preliminary report. *Obstet. Gynecol.* 59(4): 452, 1982. *Prospective study of a preterm-delivery prevention protocol.*
17. Gonik, B., and Creasy, R. K. Preterm labor—its diagnosis and management. *Am. J. Obstet. Gynecol.* 154(1):3, 1986. *Review article on preterm labor.*
18. Papiernik, E. Proposals for a programmed prevention policy of preterm birth. *Clin. Obstet. Gynecol.* 27(3):614, 1984. *The French experience with preterm birth prevention.*
19. Cole, C. H. Prevention of prematurity: Can we do it in America? *Pediatrics* 76(2): 310, 1985. *Editorial comment on the French preterm birth prevention program.*
20. Main, D. M., et al. Can preterm deliveries be prevented? *Am. J. Obstet. Gynecol.* 151(7):892, 1985. *Prospective randomized study of the Creasy system.*
21. Katz, M., Newman, R. B., and Gill, P. J. Assessment of uterine activity in ambulatory patients at high risk of preterm labor and delivery. *Am. J. Obstet. Gynecol.* 154(1):44, 1986. *Study of ambulatory tocodynamometry in patients at risk for preterm labor.*
22. Merkatz, I. R., Peter, J. B., and Barden, T. P. Ritodrine hydrochloride: A betamimetic agent for use in preterm labor. II. Evidence of efficacy. *Obstet. Gynecol.* 56(1):7, 1980. *See reference 23.*
23. Barden, T. P., Peter, J. B., and Merkatz, I. R. Ritodrine hydrochloride: A betamimetic agent for use in preterm labor. I. Pharmacology, clinical history, administration, side effects, and safety. *Obstet. Gynecol.* 56(1):1, 1980. *Prospective randomized double-blind studies confirming the efficacy and safety of ritodrine hydrochloride for suppression of preterm labor.*
24. Beall, M. H., et al. A comparison of ritodrine, terbutaline, and magnesium sulfate for the suppression of preterm labor. *Am. J. Obstet. Gynecol.* 153(8):854, 1985. *Prospective randomized study of drugs commonly used for preterm labor suppression.*
25. Pomerance, J. J., et al. Cost of living for infants weighing 1000 grams or less at birth. *Pediatrics* 61(6):908, 1978. *Analysis of neonatal costs associated with preterm births.*
26. Korenbrot, C. C., Aalto, L. H., and Laros, R. K. Jr. The cost-effectiveness of stopping preterm labor with beta-adrenergic treatment. *N. Engl. J. Med.* 310(11):691, 1984. *Study of cost-effectiveness of labor suppression between 20 and 37 weeks' gestation.*

24 Intrauterine Growth Retardation

Mary Meyers

I. The problem

A. Definition. Intrauterine growth retardation (IUGR) is most commonly defined as a birth weight at or below the tenth percentile for a given gestational age [1]. Additionally, the diagnosis is made if tissue wasting or fetal malnutrition is evident on physical examination of the neonate, but in this situation the diagnosis is usually referred to as small for gestational age (SGA).

B. Description. Before 1960, a newborn weighing less than 2500 gm was classified as premature, regardless of gestational age. IUGR was first recognized in 1961, and investigators have now established norms for weight, length, and head circumference at various weeks of gestation [2]. By using prenatal and neonatal assessments [3] of gestational age, the low birth weight infant may be classified as preterm, growth retarded, or both.

Because mortality rates are much more sensitive to weight than to gestational age, IUGR increases the risk of perinatal mortality four- to eightfold [4]. During the neonatal period, there is an increased risk of asphyxia, meconium aspiration, hypoglycemia, hypothermia, hyperglycemia, polycythemia, and necrotizing enterocolitis. Long-term morbidity may include decreased height and weight, as well as neurologic and intellectual deficiencies [19].

Studies of growth-retarded infants reveal two basic patterns [6] (Table 24-1). The first, which occurs about 40% of the time, is designated "symmetric" IUGR because all of the body organs tend to be proportionally reduced in size. This reduction in growth potential begins before the third trimester, sometimes as early as conception. The fetus continues to grow throughout the pregnancy, although weight always remains below the tenth percentile.

In contrast, in "asymmetric" IUGR, which occurs in about 60% of cases, some body organs, such as the liver, are affected more than others, such as the brain. Growth in the fetus is usually normal until the third trimester, when slowing and even total arrest of growth is observed.

During the first 20 weeks of gestation, there is a rapid rate of cell division, but the weight gain of the fetus is small. In the second half of pregnancy, fetal growth occurs more by cell hyperplasia than by cell division, and the fetus gains 95% of its weight [7]. It is during this time that the fetus grows much faster than the placenta and is sensitive to even small decreases in placental function. In the first half of pregnancy, all organs are decreased by insults that affect cell division, whereas in the second half of pregnancy, some tissues are more sensitive to insults than others and react with a relative lack of hypertrophy.

C. Epidemiology. The incidence of low birth weight infants in the United States is about 6%, and approximately one third of these infants are affected with IUGR [8]. In countries where the incidence of low birth weight is greater than 10%, the prematurity rate is steady at 5–7%, and the remainder of the low birth weight infants have IUGR. In some developing countries, one third or more of all newborns are affected.

IUGR is associated with a variety of factors (Table 24-2); however, one third to one half of cases will have no known etiology. According to a recent study, the factors most strongly correlating with IUGR are severe preeclampsia, past history of IUGR, multiple pregnancy, and chronic renal disease [9]. Other factors recently noted to be important include smoking (which doubles the risk of delivering an infant weighing <2500 gm), advanced maternal age, lack of prenatal care, and nonwhite ethnicity.

II. Primary prevention.

The best time to intervene to prevent IUGR is before a planned pregnancy is actually conceived. Patients should be encouraged to obtain preconception counseling for optimal pregnancy outcome.

Table 24-1. Types of intrauterine growth retardation (IUGR)

Symmetric or early
Insult is early and prolonged
Decreased cell number
Decreased cell size
Weight, height, and head circumference all below the 10th percentile
Decreased potential for growth after birth
Less birth asphyxia than with asymmetric IUGR
Asymmetric or late
Insult mediated through the placenta
Decreased cell size
Brain relatively spared; markedly decreased size of liver, spleen, and thymus
Catch-up growth is possible
Weight affected more severely than height and head circumference
High incidence of birth asphyxia

Table 24-2. Etiologic factors in intrauterine growth retardation (IUGR)

Factors more closely associated with symmetric IUGR	
Fetal factors	Chromosomal abnormalities
	Congenital malformations
	Intrauterine infections (syphilis, cytomegalovirus, rubella, toxoplasmosis)
Fetal exposures	Smoking
	Alcohol
	Malnutrition
	Drugs (especially narcotics, antiepileptic drugs, chemotherapeutic agents)
	Radiation (10–25 rads) to pelvis in early gestation
	High altitude
	Erythroblastosis fetalis
Factors more closely associated with asymmetric IUGR	
Maternal disease	May affect the placenta and its function
	Preeclampsia, chronic hypertension
	Renal disease, cardiovascular disease
	Metabolic disease
	Sickle cell anemia
	Diabetes
Placental dysfunction	Placental infarction, abruption, or previa
	Multiple gestation
	Ectopic pregnancy
	Prolonged gestation
	Previous IUGR infant
	First trimester bleeding

A. Methods [10]

1. **Proper nutrition.** Patients should be advised regarding proper nutrition before and during pregnancy and should be given nutritional supplements if necessary. Patients should be encouraged to achieve a normal weight before attempting pregnancy, especially if they are underweight, and advised to gain at least 20 lb during pregnancy (see Chap. 3).
2. **Smoking.** Cigarette smoking lowers fetal weight in a dose-related fashion, and the infants of heavy smokers weigh an average of 280 gm less than those of nonsmokers. Patients should be strongly encouraged to quit smoking before pregnancy, or at least to lower their consumption as much as possible (see Chap. 4).
3. **Alcohol consumption.** IUGR, as well as the fetal alcohol syndrome, are known consequences of maternal alcohol abuse. One study suggests that IUGR is 2.7 times as common in infants of heavy drinkers. Since the tolerable dose of alcohol in pregnancy is not known, patients should be cautioned that the safest

course is to avoid alcohol while pregnant or at risk for becoming pregnant (see Chap. 4).

4. **Rubella.** Patients should be screened for immunity to rubella before attempting pregnancy. If vaccination is required, pregnancy should be delayed for 3 months. However, accidental vaccination done during early pregnancy has not caused harmful effects (see Chap. 20).
5. **Other infectious diseases.** Routine screening for prevention and detection of cytomegalovirus (CMV) and toxoplasmosis is not indicated at this time. Patients should be advised to avoid cat litter and raw meat during pregnancy. Syphilis screening is done at the first prenatal visit, and necessary treatment is started as soon as possible.
6. **Congenital anomalies.** If there is a family history of congenital anomalies, preconception and prenatal genetic counseling should be offered and appropriate screening done. If not done preconception, it should be offered at the first prenatal visit. All patients who will be 35 when they deliver should be offered genetic counseling and amniocentesis at 16 weeks to detect Down's syndrome and other chromosomal abnormalities. Some health care providers now routinely offer maternal serum alpha-fetoprotein screening to expectant mothers between 15 and 20 weeks.
7. **Chronic maternal disease.** Patients with chronic disease (e.g., hypertension, renal disease, diabetes) who wish to become pregnant should be advised of the risks of pregnancy to the mother and the fetus and should be followed with special attention (see Chap. 2).

B. Justification

1. **Effectiveness.** These methods are consistent with good prenatal care. They should be effective in preventing some cases of IUGR, but this has not been proved.
2. **Risks.** Rubella vaccination is associated with occasional arthralgias in adults. Amniocentesis is associated with a 1–2% risk to the fetus. Drug and smoking withdrawal may have negative physiologic and social side effects in the short term.
3. **Costs.** These methods do not add to the costs of routine prenatal care, except for the cost of an office visit for prepregnancy counseling. This visit varies between $50–100, depending on the laboratory work necessary.
4. **Acceptability.** Most of the information and screening is acceptable to the patient and to the physician. Behavioral changes, however, may be difficult to initiate.

III. Secondary prevention

A. Early detection

1. **Detect high-risk patients.**
   a. **Method.** At the first prenatal visit, patients should be screened for the high-risk factors discussed earlier. A study by Galbraith, et al. [9] found five factors associated with a greater than five times higher risk of IUGR: prior IUGR, severe hypertension, nephritis, severe preeclampsia, and multiple pregnancy. In their study of 3000 patients, two thirds of the IUGR infants came from the population with risk factors, and one third came from the population with none. Another paper presented a risk-scoring system using eight variables, and the two most strongly weighted variables were no increase in fundal height and smoking. Patients known to be at high risk for IUGR should be followed particularly closely.
   b. **Justification.** There are no prospective studies showing that identifying high-risk patients leads to a decreased incidence of IUGR. Early identification of patients at risk will lead to earlier identification of patients with IUGR, which can improve perinatal outcome.
2. **Establish gestational age.** Accurate estimation of gestational age is a goal in all pregnancies. Poor fetal growth is difficult to detect in the absence of known gestational age. Patients should be seen as early as possible in the pregnancy for the most accurate dating. Methods for accurately dating the gestational age include last menstrual period (LMP), pregnancy tests, physical exam, fetal heart tones, and ultrasound (see Chaps. 25 and 26).
3. **Follow fundal growth.**
   a. **Method.** Fundal height measurements, made from the symphysis pubis "over the curve" to the top of the uterine fundus, correlate well with fetal age, with the fetal age equaling the fundal height in centimeters. Fundal growth should

proceed at approximately 1 cm/week. IUGR may be suspected by one fundal height value greater than 2 cm below the expected value, or three consecutive static or declining values.

b. **Justification.** The measurement of the fundal height at each visit is part of good prenatal care. This currently is the single best way of diagnosing IUGR. Unfortunately, this method detects only 50–75% of IUGR.

4. **Ultrasound.** Ultrasound is the most accurate method for diagnosing IUGR at this time and is used when IUGR is suspected clinically. In the absence of accurate dating of the pregnancy, the diagnosis of IUGR can be difficult or impossible. The fetus may already be affected at the time of the first ultrasound, and the current measurement cannot be compared to the known gestational age.

a. **Crown-rump length**

(1) **Method.** This measurement is made in the first trimester.

(2) **Justification.** The crown-rump length is accurate to plus or minus 5 days between 7–14 weeks and should not be affected by IUGR except in the earliest forms.

b. **Biparietal diameter (BPD)**

(1) **Method.** The BPD is the mainstay for determining gestational age and is most accurate under 20 weeks. As the gestation advances, the BPD may be affected more and more by IUGR, especially symmetric IUGR. In the absence of accurate early dating of the pregnancy, the first BPD is used to date the pregnancy, and repeat scans are done every 2–4 weeks to confirm the expected growth of the BPD [5].

(2) **Justification.** A BPD at 20 weeks or earlier predicts the date of delivery to within 12 days in 95% of cases, which is better than even the LMP.

c. **Femur length**

(1) **Method.** The femur may be identified as early as 10 weeks' gestation.

(2) **Justification.** The femur length is another method of determining the gestational age and is accurate to plus or minus 9.5 days between 12 and 23 weeks. The femur length does not appear to be more accurate than the BPD for assessment of gestational age in IUGR.

d. **Abdominal circumference**

(1) **Method.** The abdominal circumference should be less than the BPD until approximately 36 weeks. Asymmetric IUGR, with relative head sparing, leads to a significant change in the BPD-abdominal circumference ratio and can be used to diagnose IUGR [11].

(2) **Justification.** When the gestational age is known, the abdominal circumference can identify 96% of IUGR [11].

e. **Amniotic fluid volume**

(1) **Method.** An association between oligohydramnios and IUGR is well accepted, and the absence of a pocket of amniotic fluid 1 cm or more in broadest diameter is well correlated with IUGR [12].

(2) **Justification.** Eighty-three percent of fetuses with IUGR were detected with decreased amniotic fluid volume [12].

f. **Other methods.** Placental grading, total intrauterine volume, and estimated fetal weight are less accurate in diagnosing IUGR.

5. **Hormonal assays.** Maternal estriol and human placental lactogen measurements have been popular in the past but do not have sufficient accuracy to diagnose IUGR [11].

B. **Early intervention.** When IUGR is diagnosed, the fetal condition must be assessed to determine if the fetus will be more healthy in the uterus or in the nursery, even if this means premature delivery.

1. **Optimize the in utero environment.**

a. **Aggressive treatment of maternal disease**

(1) **Method.** Maternal diseases that may contribute to IUGR should be aggressively treated in an effort to improve the fetal environment. Diabetes, hypertension, anemia, and renal disease should be brought under optimal control.

(2) **Justification.** Although there are no studies supporting this, it is consistent with good prenatal care.

b. **Bed rest**

(1) **Method.** The uterine blood flow is maximal in the lateral, recumbent position. Therefore, it is reasonable to assume that bed rest may increase fetal growth in IUGR.

(2) **Justification.** There are no studies showing that bed rest improves fetal growth once IUGR has been identified.

c. **Adequate maternal nutrition**

(1) **Method.** The mother must consume adequate nutritious food to support normal weight gain in pregnancy.

(2) **Justification.** There is no evidence that extra nutrition above normal requirements is useful once IUGR has been identified.

2. **Evaluate the fetus.**

a. **Ultrasonography**

(1) **Method.** When the diagnosis of IUGR is considered, the fetus is followed with sonograms every 2–4 weeks. Close attention is paid to the BPD, abdominal circumference, femur length, and amount of amniotic fluid. Continued lack of growth may be a cause for early intervention.

(2) **Justification.** Sonography is currently the best tool for following a fetus with IUGR. A study of 260 cases of IUGR found that 96.8% of IUGR could be detected using the BPD-abdominal circumference ratio.

b. **Antepartum fetal monitoring** [13]. When IUGR is suspected, fetal monitoring is begun to assess the fetus. If there are indications that the fetus is compromised, delivery is recommended.

(1) **Nonstress test (NST)**

(a) **Method.** The nonstress test, performed on a weekly or twice-weekly basis, is the least expensive and time-consuming method of fetal monitoring. Spontaneous decelerations, as well as nonreactivity and decreased variability, should be searched for. A nonreactive NST should be followed by a contraction stress test.

(b) **Justification.** In a review of 3000 cases, the patients with nonreactive NST had a significant increase in cesarean sections, fetal distress, and perinatal deaths. Also, a study of 250 patients with IUGR showed that nonreactive tracings were significantly associated with cesarean sections, fetal distress, a high perinatal mortality, and fetal anomalies.

(2) **Contraction stress test (CST)**

(a) **Method.** The contraction stress test stresses the feto/placental unit and identifies the fetus with diminished or absent placental reserves. It is done in the case of a nonreactive NST and may also be done weekly as a primary test. A negative CST is more reassuring than a reactive NST as the time of labor approaches, since the NST does not assure fetal well-being with contractions.

(b) **Justification.** In a study of 85 fetuses with IUGR, 35% had a nonreactive NST, and 40% had a positive CST. Adverse fetal outcome was predicted by a nonreactive NST and a positive CST in 92% of cases [14].

(3) **Biophysical profile**

(a) **Method.** The biophysical profile looks at fetal movement, tone and breathing, qualitative amniotic fluid volume, and the nonstress test; it may be done weekly or twice weekly.

(b) **Justification.** In a study of 1184 high-risk patients who were evaluated with the biophysical profile, the perinatal mortality rate was 5/1000, which was markedly lower than the historical control population [15].

3. **Time the delivery appropriately.**

a. **Reassuring fetal monitoring**

(1) **Method.** The current recommendation is that the growth-retarded fetus should be delivered at 37–38 weeks, unless fetal growth stops [16]. Amniocentesis will probably be necessary to confirm fetal lung maturity before elective delivery. The lecithin-sphingomyelin (L/S) ratio has classically been used to demonstrate pulmonary maturity when it is greater than or equal to 2. Recent studies indicate that in IUGR, the presence of phosphatidyl glycerol (PG) [17] or a mature foam stability index ($\geq$0.47) [18] indicates lung maturity even in the absence of a mature L/S.

(2) **Justification.** There are no controlled studies to indicate that early delivery is beneficial in the absence of fetal distress. It is very important to prevent the unanticipated delivery of a premature infant who is at risk for respiratory distress and other problems.

b. **Fetal distress**

(1) **Method.** If the fetus exhibits mild signs of fetal distress, such as a nonreactive negative CST, the fetus should be evaluated for delivery with an amniocentesis and attempts should be made to improve the intrauterine environment. In the case of a nonreactive positive CST or a low score on the biophysical profile, immediate delivery should be undertaken, as the fetus is most certainly in danger.

(2) **Justification.** As mentioned above, the NST/CST and the biophysical profile are currently the best methods of predicting fetal distress and intrauterine death.

4. **Manage the delivery properly.**

a. **Method.** Although fetuses with IUGR have a decreased tolerance for hypoxia and labor stress, the majority can tolerate labor and vaginal delivery without fetal distress. The fetus should be carefully monitored with an internal scalp electrode and liberal use of fetal scalp blood pH samples if feasible. Emergency cesarean section should be quickly available. An experienced person should be available to resuscitate and care for the newborn.

b. **Justification.** Close attention during labor is consistent with good prenatal care and is very important in this high-risk situation.

IV. Recommendations

A. Primary prevention at preconception visit

1. The patient should not be underweight before conception, and proper nutrition should be stressed.
2. The patient should stop smoking before conception.
3. All alcohol consumption should be discouraged before conception.
4. Any type of drug use should be discouraged.
5. Patients should be immune to rubella before attempting pregnancy.
6. With a family history of congenital anomalies, genetic counseling should be offered, ideally before conception.
7. Patients with chronic maternal disease should be counseled regarding the risks of pregnancy to themselves and to the fetus.

B. Secondary prevention

1. **Early detection**

a. The gestational age must be accurately known. This may be established by a variety of methods early in pregnancy, or an ultrasound may be done between 16 and 20 weeks' gestation. If an early ultrasound is not available, several ultrasounds may be needed after 20 weeks to rule out symmetrical IUGR and to show good fetal growth.

b. Fundal height must be followed closely to ensure that there is agreement with the gestational age. If there is no agreement, ultrasound is done to look for signs of IUGR.

c. Ultrasound is used to follow suspected IUGR. Many measurements are made during a complete exam, but an increased head-to-abdomen ratio and decreased fluid correlate best with IUGR. The ultrasound exam should be repeated every 2–4 weeks to assess fetal growth.

2. **Early intervention**

a. Fetal monitoring with the NST/CST or biophysical profile should be done once or twice a week when IUGR is suspected.

b. Treatment of IUGR should be attempted with close attention to maternal disease, bed rest, and proper maternal nutrition.

c. In the absence of fetal distress and continued fetal growth, the fetus should be delivered at 37–38 weeks, after assurance of fetal maturity.

d. Fetal distress is an indication for delivery regardless of fetal age.

e. Delivery should be carefully monitored, and an experienced physician should be present to care for the infant.

References

1. Lin, C. C. Intrauterine growth retardation. *Obstet. Gynecol. Annu.* 14:127, 1985. *Long, complete review of IUGR by an expert in the field.*
2. Usher, R., and McLean, F. Intrauterine growth of live born Caucasian infants at sea level: Standards obtained from 7 measurements in infants born between 25 and 44 weeks'

gestation. *J. Pediatr.* 74:901, 1969. *Commonly used standard for neonatal weight by gestational age.*

3. Dubowitz, L. M., Dubowitz, V., and Goldberg, C. Clinical assessment of gestational age in the newborn infant. *J. Pediatr.* 77:1, 1970. *Standard for assessing gestational age of neonate by physical examination.*
4. Seeds, J. W. Impaired fetal growth: Definition and clinical diagnosis. *Obstet. Gynecol.* 64(3):303, 1984. *Recent, practical review of IUGR.*
5. Sholl, J. S., et al. Intrauterine growth retardation risk detection for fetuses of unknown gestational age. *Am. J. Obstet. Gynecol.* 144(6):709, 1982. *Demonstrates need for repeated ultrasound to determine IUGR if the gestational age is unknown.*
6. Villar, J., and Belizan, J. M. The timing factor in the pathophysiology of the intrauterine growth retardation syndrome. *Obstet. Gynecol. Surv.* 37(8):499, 1982. *Good review of types of IUGR.*
7. Vorherr, H. Factors influencing fetal growth. *Am. J. Obstet. Gynecol.* 142(5):577, 1982. *Excellent discussion of why certain factors affect fetal growth.*
8. Villar, J., and Belizan, J. M. The relative contribution of prematurity and fetal growth retardation to low birth weight in developing and developed societies. *Am. J. Obstet. Gynecol.* 143(7):793, 1982. *Discussion of why IUGR is a very serious problem in developing countries.*
9. Galbraith, R. S., et al. The clinical prediction of intrauterine growth retardation. *Am. J. Obstet. Gynecol.* 133(3):281, 1979. *Over 8000 deliveries reviewed looking for clinical predictors for IUGR.*
10. Villar, J., and Belizan, J. M. The evaluation of the methods used in the diagnosis of intrauterine growth retardation. *Obstet. Gynecol. Surv.* 41(4):187, 1986. *Statistical evaluation of 86 reports of methods used in diagnosis of IUGR.*
11. Seeds, J. W. Impaired fetal growth: Ultrasonic evaluation and clinical management. *Obstet. Gynecol.* 64(4):577, 1984. *Review of diagnosis and management of IUGR.*
12. Manning, F. A., Hill, L. M., and Platt, L. D. Qualitative amniotic fluid volume determination by ultrasound: Antepartum detection of intrauterine growth retardation. *Am. J. Obstet. Gynecol.* 139(3):254, 1981. *Discussed oligohydramnios and IUGR.*
13. Thacker, S. B., and Berkelman, R. L. Assessing the diagnostic accuracy and efficacy of selected antepartum fetal surveillance techniques. *Obstet. Gynecol. Surv.* 41(3):121, 1986. *Large, recent review of fetal monitoring techniques.*
14. Lin, C. C., et al. Oxytocin challenge test and intrauterine growth retardation. *Am. J. Obstet. Gynecol.* 140(3):282, 1981. *Oxytose challenge test predicts fetal outcome in IUGR.*
15. Manning, F. A., et al. Fetal biophysical profile scoring: A prospective study in 1,184 high-risk patients. *Am. J. Obstet. Gynecol.* 140(3):289, 1981. *Large review of use of fetal geophysical profile.*
16. Simpson, G. F., and Creasy, R. K. Obstetric management of the growth retarded baby. *Clin. Obstet. Gynecol.* 11(2):481, 1984. *Good, recent review of management of IUGR.*
17. Gross, T. L., et al. Amniotic fluid phosphatidylglycerol: A potentially useful predictor of intrauterine growth retardation. *Am. J. Obstet. Gynecol.* 140(3):277, 1981. *Phosphatidylglycerol predicts lung maturity in IUGR.*
18. Sher, G., Statland, B. E., and Knutzen, V. K. Identifying the small-for-gestational-age fetus on the basis of enhanced surfactant production. *Obstet. Gynecol.* 61(1):13, 1983. *Foam stability index also predicts lung maturity in IUGR.*
19. Allen, M. C. Developmental outcome and follow-up of the small for gestational age infant. *Semin. Perinatol.* 8(2):123, 1984. *Review of effects of IUGR.*

25 Postterm Delivery

Trent MacKay

I. The problem

A. Definition. A postterm delivery is a delivery occurring after 42 completed weeks, or 294 days, from the first day of the last menstrual period.

B. Description. Except in the rare case of known causes such as anencephaly or placental sulfatase deficiency, the cause of postterm pregnancy and resultant postterm delivery is unknown. Until the mechanism of normal human birth is understood, the etiology of postterm delivery will remain a mystery.

The risk of perinatal morbidity and mortality are increased with postterm delivery. There are two areas of concern. First, the incidence of macrosomia is increased, leading to an elevated risk of prolonged labor and traumatic delivery. Second, as the placenta has a finite lifespan, placental insufficiency may develop and lead to fetal hypoxia and malnutrition. Under these circumstances, the fetus will be at increased risk of stillbirth or intrapartum asphyxia or demise. Some of these compromised infants will develop the postmaturity syndrome, with an increased risk of neonatal morbidity and mortality. The incidence of meconium-stained amniotic fluid, with the attendant risk of meconium aspiration, is markedly increased in postterm pregnancy. The incidence of cesarean section for fetal distress and failure to progress is increased two- to threefold in postterm pregnancies.

C. Epidemiology. Up to 14% of all pregnancies continue beyond 42 weeks and approximately 4% continue beyond 43 weeks. The risk of perinatal mortality is lowest between 39 and 41 weeks. By 43 weeks, the perinatal mortality rate is doubled and by 44 weeks it is more than tripled in comparison with the rate at 39–41 weeks. Perinatal morbidity and the need for admission to a neonatal intensive care unit are significantly increased for infants born after 42 weeks.

There are no well-defined risk groups for postterm delivery. There is no evidence that maternal age or parity are contributing factors. All pregnancies are at risk for postterm delivery, although women who have had a previous postterm delivery are at increased risk.

II. Secondary prevention

A. Early detection

1. **Methods.** The single most important factor in the prevention of postterm delivery is accurate dating of the pregnancy. Dating of the pregnancy should occur as early as possible in gestation and should include as many separate pieces of information as can be obtained. If a discrepancy exists among the several clinical methods used to estimate gestational age, a more objective measurement (i.e., ultrasound) should be obtained.

   a. **Last menstrual period (LMP).** The date of the first day of the last menstrual period combined with information on the woman's average cycle length is the single most important indicator of gestational age. However, in women with irregular menses, women using fertility drugs, or women recently discontinuing oral contraceptives, the date of the LMP may be a poor indicator of gestational age. Early identification of pregnancy is tied to more accurate identification of LMP. The liberal use of available pregnancy tests can assist in this effort.

   b. **Physical examination.** Evaluations of uterine size between 6 and 14 weeks and of fundal height between 18 and 28 weeks are useful determinants of gestational age. However, obesity or uterine pathology such as fibroids may make accurate determination of size difficult.

   c. **Fetal movement.** The onset of fetal movement normally occurs at approximately 20 weeks' gestation in primigravidas, and at 18 weeks in multigravid patients. This information is particularly useful if the woman has been advised in advance to look for the onset of fetal movement.

d. **Fetal heart tones.** The fetal heart can normally first be auscultated at approximately 20 weeks with a DeLee stethoscope. Unfortunately, detection of fetal heart tones requires weekly visits.

e. **Ultrasound.** If a discrepancy exists in the above measurements, the patient should undergo ultrasound examination between 16 and 28 weeks. Measurement of the fetal biparietal diameter and femur length during this period of gestation predicts gestational age with a 95% confidence interval of 1.5–2.0 weeks.

2. **Justification**

a. **Effectiveness.** Identification of gestational age is the single most important method of preventing postterm delivery. Information on the LMP, uterine size, presence of fetal heart tones, and appearance of fetal movement is routinely gathered in the course of prenatal care. A reliable LMP, in combination with the other three landmarks, is at least as reliable an indicator of gestational age as early ultrasound.

b. **Risks.** Collection of information from history and physical examination is without risk. The risk of ultrasound examination is unknown, although there is currently no evidence of risk to the fetus or mother. Routine ultrasound examination is not indicated, but ultrasound is justifiable for ascertaining gestational age if clinical information appears unreliable.

c. **Costs.** As an integral part of prenatal care, historical information and physical examination impart no additional cost. Ultrasound examination for gestational age costs $100–200.

d. **Acceptability.** Because the gathering of historic and physical exam information is routinely included in prenatal care, acceptability is not an issue. The use of ultrasound is well accepted by the medical community and generally well accepted by patients.

B. **Early intervention.** In a patient judged to be at 42 weeks or beyond, efforts are directed at detection of placental insufficiency and delivering those fetuses at risk.

1. **Assessment of methods for detecting placental insufficiency.** A variety of approaches have been used for antepartum testing to detect placental insufficiency.

a. **Hormonal methods.** Assays of estriol and human placental lactogen have been used to monitor postterm pregnancy. However, because of the necessity for frequent testing and high false-negative rates, these tests have fallen into disfavor.

b. **Nonstress test and contraction stress test (NST/CST).** The most widely used methods for antepartum surveillance of postterm pregnancies are the NST and the CST. The NST consists of observing two or more accelerations of the fetal heart rate of at least 15 beats/minute lasting at least 15 seconds during a 20–40 minute period of observation. A nonreactive NST requires a follow-up CST. Because of high false-negative rates with weekly tests, nonstress testing should be done twice a week.

The CST consists of producing uterine contractions with either oxytocin or nipple stimulation at a frequency of 3 contractions/10 minutes. A positive (abnormal) test consists of late decelerations occurring with more than 50% of the contractions. Contraction stress testing should be done on a weekly basis.

c. **Ultrasound.** The presence of fetal jeopardy may be assessed by ultrasound measurement of amniotic fluid volume or by a biophysical profile consisting of amniotic fluid volume, fetal movement, muscle tone, and fetal breathing movements. While standards for normal amniotic fluid volume have yet to be established, a normal biophysical profile done twice weekly appears to correlate well with a fetus at low risk.

2. **Delivery.** The timing of delivery in postterm pregnancy is controversial. Routine induction of labor at 42 completed weeks has been recommended for women with well-documented dates. However, while routine induction at 42 weeks may decrease perinatal mortality, it may also markedly increase the cesarean section rate because of the likelihood of many failed inductions. In the future, the availability of prostaglandin gel for cervical ripening may reduce the number of failed inductions.

While routine induction has been recommended by some experts, others have recommended induction in women with well-documented dates only if the cervix is favorable (Bishop score of ≥5) or if there is evidence of fetal jeopardy using one of the above methods of assessment. This approach generally results in a lower rate of cesarean section. Many management schemes call for induction at 43 or 44 weeks, regardless of the status of the cervix, if the woman has well-documented dates. If evidence of fetal jeopardy develops or if an obstetric complication such as preeclampsia develops, delivery is mandatory.

III. Recommendations

A. Early detection. It is important to establish gestational age as early as possible during pregnancy and to use as many parameters for measurement as are available, including last menstrual period, physical exam, fetal heart tones, and ultrasound.

B. Assessment of placental insufficiency. Detection of fetal jeopardy can be accomplished by the use of one or more of the methods of antepartum assessment, including the nonstress test, the contraction stress test, and ultrasound measurement of amniotic fluid volume, or a biophysical profile.

C. Early intervention. In women with well-documented dates, induction of labor should be considered at 42 weeks if the cervix is favorable. If the cervix is unfavorable for induction, the use of antepartum assessment to rule out fetal jeopardy allows temporizing until the cervix is favorable or evidence of fetal jeopardy develops.

Suggested Readings

Depp, R. Management of Prolonged Pregnancy. In J. T. Queenan (ed.), *Management of High Risk Pregnancy.* (2d ed.). Oradell, NJ: Medical Economics Books, 1985. Pp.561–581. *A comprehensive review of the evolution of management of postterm pregnancy.*

Granados, J. L. Survey of the management of postterm pregnancy. *Obstet. Gynecol.* 63(5):651, 1984. *An interesting survey of management in 72 academic institutions.*

Harris, B. A. Jr, et al. The unfavorable cervix in prolonged pregnancy. *Obstet. Gynecol.* 62(2):171, 1983. *An interesting study demonstrating the difficulties with management by routine induction.*

Jimenez, J. M., Tyson, J. E., and Reisch, J. S. Clinical measures of gestational age in normal pregnancies. *Obstet. Gynecol.* 61(4):438, 1983. *A good review of clinical measurement of gestational age.*

Johnson, J. M., et al. Biophysical profile scoring in the management of the postterm pregnancy: An analysis of 307 patients. *Am. J. Obstet. Gynecol.* 154(2):269, 1986. *A good, recent study of the biophysical profile.*

Lagrew, D. C., and Freeman, R. K. Management of postdate pregnancy. *Am. J. Obstet. Gynecol.* 154(1):8, 1986. *An up-to-date review of management.*

O'Brien, G. D., and Queenan, J. T. Growth of the ultrasound femur length during normal pregnancy. Part I. *Am. J. Obstet. Gynecol.* 141(7):833, 1981. *A good review of the use of femur length for gestational age determination.*

Phelan, J. P., et al. The role of ultrasound assessment of amniotic fluid volume in management of the post-pregnancy. *Am. J. Obstet. Gynecol.* 151(3):304, 1985. *Pertinent study of the utility of amniotic fluid volume measurement.*

Resnik, R. Post-term Pregnancy. In R. K. Creasy and R. Resnik (eds.), *Maternal-Fetal Medicine, Principles and Practice.* Philadelphia: Saunders, 1984. Pp.443–448. *An excellent short review of the subject.*

Sachs, B. P., and Friedman, E. A. Results of an epidemiologic study of postdate pregnancy. *J. Reprod. Med.* 31(3):162, 1986. *An up-to-date epidemiologic study.*

26 Prenatal and Intrapartum Asphyxia

Klea D. Bertakis

I. The problem

A. Definition. Fetal asphyxia is defined by hypoxia, acidosis, and an elevated carbon dioxide tension in the blood and tissues. Because there are no uniformly accepted laboratory criteria for fetal asphyxia, the identification of metabolic acidosis based on an umbilical cord artery buffer base of less than 36.1 mEq/liter has been used [1].

B. Description. Factors that interfere at any point along the path of providing normal oxygenated blood flow (with normal acid-base balance) to the fetal brain can contribute to the problem of prenatal and intrapartum asphyxia [2]. Such factors may interfere with:

1. **Providing normal blood flow to the uterus,** for example:
   - **a.** Chronic and acute hypertension.
   - **b.** Hypotension, from regional anesthesia or from the supine position.
2. **Oxygen transfer from the uterus to the fetus.** This can be affected by placental and cord problems such as:
   - **a.** Uterine hyperstimulation with oxytocin.
   - **b.** Placental separation.
   - **c.** Umbilical cord compression.
3. **Fetal circulation,** for example:
   - **a.** Paracervical block with severe bradycardia or cardiac arrest.
   - **b.** Severe cardiac anomalies.

C. Epidemiology. The reported incidence of fetal asphyxia varies. One study reviewing 600 high-risk monitored obstetric patients for evidence of fetal asphyxia at delivery found the overall incidence to be 20%. This is eight times the occurrence in a normal obstetric population [1]. Another study found that asphyxia occurred antepartum in 51% of cases, intrapartum in 40%, and postpartum in 9% [3]. The developmental outcome for these asphyxiated babies presents a major concern. Whereas intrauterine hypoxia and asphyxia remains an unchallenged cause of perinatal death, it is uncertain what sublethal degrees of hypoxia result in brain damage of surviving infants [4,5].

D. Perinatal risk factors for fetal asphyxia. See Table 26-1 [6,7].

II. Primary prevention

A. Methods

1. A meticulous prenatal history, physical examination, and laboratory work-up.
2. Screening and treatment of maternal diseases such as severe hypertension, preeclampsia, renal disease, and diabetes.
3. Adequate maternal nutrition and caloric intake.
4. Abstinence from smoking, alcohol, and drug abuse.
5. Childbirth preparation classes designed to provide prenatal preventive health education and understanding of labor and delivery.

B. Justification

1. **Prenatal history, physical examination, and laboratory work-up**
   - **a. Effectiveness.** A thorough, initial obstetric evaluation will serve to identify most of those women who are at high risk for complications.
   - **b. Risks/side effects** are negligible.
2. **Screening and treatment of maternal diseases**
   - **a. Effectiveness.** Maternal diseases such as hypertension, preeclampsia, renal disease, and diabetes are associated with a significantly higher incidence of neonatal asphyxia [6].
   - **b. Risks/side effects.** Complications are mainly those of the specific medications involved in treatment.

Table 26-1. Perinatal risk factors for fetal asphyxia

Preterm delivery
Postterm delivery
Intrauterine growth retardation (IUGR)
Maternal diabetes
Toxemia of pregnancy
Maternal smoking
Breech presentation at delivery
Compression of prolapsed cord
Premature rupture of membranes
Abruptio placentae
Placenta previa
Tetanic contractions of the uterus
Cord around the neck or body
Short cord
Paracervical block
Regional anesthesia
Narcosis from maternal drugs
Pressure on brain in difficult labors
Operative procedures
Rh isoimmunization

3. **Adequate maternal nutrition and caloric intake**
   a. **Effectiveness.** Poor maternal nutrition with inadequate intake remains a significant cause of intrauterine growth retardation (IUGR). Fetal asphyxia has been found in approximately 50% of newborn infants with IUGR [8].
   b. **Risks/side effects.** There are no risks or side effects.
4. **Abstinence from smoking, alcohol, and drug abuse**
   a. **Effectiveness.** Smoking, alcohol consumption, and drug abuse can cause IUGR. Provider efforts to encourage pregnant women to reduce or discontinue intake of alcohol have been effective and will probably prove to be similarly effective with tobacco [9]. Drug withdrawal and rehabilitation programs can also be effective.
   b. **Risks/side effects.** Symptoms of withdrawal, especially in heavy abusers, are possible side effects.
5. **Childbirth preparation classes**
   a. **Effectiveness.** Most childbirth preparation classes in the United States today use the Lamaze or modified Lamaze method. While it is probably not possible to have childbirth completely without pain, such "psychoprophylaxis" is felt to be associated with the use of less anesthesia. Most of all, however, patients with knowledge about pregnancy, labor, and the tools to assist with labor can avoid or limit risk-taking behavior.
   b. **Risks/side effects.** A risk is incorrect information resulting in unrealistic expectations. Guilt and anxiety can occur when the individual knows about but takes a risk.

III. Secondary prevention

A. Early detection

1. **Methods**
   a. **Serial assessment of fetal growth**
      (1) **Description.** The fundal height is measured by placing a measuring tape at the pubis symphysis and measuring from there to the top of the fundus.
      (2) **Interpretation.** The expected rate of growth is 1 cm/week of gestation.
      (3) **Interval/timing.** The fundal height is measured at each prenatal visit, being most useful from 16–32 weeks' gestation.
      (4) **Population.** All women followed prenatally are routinely screened for fundal height.
   b. **Ultrasound**
      (1) **Description.** Real-time β-scanning produces images at high rates so that the display appears to change continuously with variation in transducer orientation or with motion of the structures imaged.

(2) **Interpretation.** For assessment of gestational age, crown-rump measurements are used optimally from 10–13 weeks. The biparietal diameter is used later in the pregnancy and is most accurate from 16–26 weeks.

(3) **Interval/timing.** Determination of the presence or absence of fetal life is done from 9 weeks' gestation until term. Gestational dating using the crown-rump measurement is most accurately done at 10–13 weeks. The biparietal diameter (BPD) measurement done between 16 and 26 weeks yields an accurate estimate of gestational age ±10 days. At 27–28 weeks' gestation, this variation increases to ±14 days and further increases to ±21 days for fetuses at term [10].

(4) **Population.** Indications for obstetric ultrasound scans, according to the Society of Obstetrical and Gynecological Ultrasonographers, include evaluation of the following: fetal viability, gestational dates, placental location, IUGR, multiple gestation, congenital anomalies, breech presentation, postterm pregnancy, amniotic fluid quantity, molar pregnancy or pelvic mass, and finally, as an adjunct to special procedures such as amniocentesis and intrauterine transfusion [10].

c. Fetal movement monitoring

(1) **Description.** Fetal movement is an indicator of fetal well-being. In primigravidas, fetal movement is ordinarily first detected at 19 ±2 weeks' gestation, whereas in multigravidas motion may be detected 2 weeks sooner. After 26 weeks' gestation, the mother is asked to keep a daily diary of her baby's movements. Patients are instructed to lie in a left lateral recumbent position in a quiet room and to concentrate on fetal movement. This is done at least 1 convenient hour each day. Any perceived movements are recorded on a chart and returned at the next clinical visit for interpretation.

(2) **Interpretation.** Fetal inactivity has been clinically defined as three or fewer perceived fetal movements per hour for 2 consecutive days [11].

(3) **Interval/timing.** Recordings of fetal movement are usually done after 26 weeks' gestation, when fetal viability and maternal perception are more certain [12].

(4) **Population.** Antepartum complications that have been shown to benefit from fetal activity monitoring include any high-risk pregnancy, decreased fetal activity, bloody amniocentesis in the third trimester, and abdominal surgery or trauma [11].

d. Detection of fetal heart tones

(1) **Description.** Fetal heart tones (FHTs) are first detectable with a fetoscope at 20 weeks' gestation, depending on the position of the fetus and thickness of the maternal abdominal wall. Heart tones may be heard with a Doppler instrument by 10–12 weeks.

(2) **Interpretation.** Aside from the occasional detection of a significant bradycardia (<100 beats/minute), tachycardia (>160 beats/minute), profound cardiac arrhythmia, or inability to find fetal heart tones at all, intermittent auscultation of fetal heart rate in the antepartum period is too sporadic to be an accurate measure of fetal well-being. Its use, then, is primarily to identify life or death.

(3) **Interval/timing.** Typically, fetal heart tones are first auscultated with a Doppler instrument at 12 weeks and then monthly until 20 weeks. From 20 weeks through the end of gestation, FHTs are auscultated with a fetoscope at regular prenatal visits.

(4) **Population.** Auscultation of fetal heart tones is a part of the routine prenatal visit during the second and third trimesters of pregnancy.

e. Nonstress fetal heart rate testing

(1) **Description.** The patient is placed in a recumbent semi-Fowler's position. After the fetal heart monitor is attached, fetal activity is noted by the patient and recorded electronically to permanently mark the fetal heart tracing whenever fetal movement is felt. Once a technically satisfactory fetal heart rate baseline is established and the patient can demonstrate that she can use the fetal movement indicator, the nonstress test (NST) is started and conducted for 20 minutes. If adequate fetal movements are noted in the first 20 minutes (defined as at least two fetal movements), the recording is terminated and interpreted. If inadequate fetal movement has occurred, stimulation is used, either physically with

manipulation of the fetus, or chemically by giving fruit juice to raise blood sugar levels [13].

(2) **Interpretation.** Generally accepted criteria for a **reactive** pattern include two accelerations (with an amplitude exceeding 15 beats/minute from the baseline and whose duration is 15 seconds or more) associated with fetal movement, in 20 minutes of observation. The **nonreactive** test is characterized by the lack of qualifying criteria for a reactive pattern over a 40-minute observation time period. If the patient demonstrates a nonreactive pattern for a total of 40 minutes, another NST is performed within 24 hours. If the nonreactive pattern persists, a contraction stress test is carried out.

(3) **Interval/timing.** The timing of initial testing depends largely on the ability to successfully intervene on behalf of the fetus, whether by treatment or by delivery. Most patients undergo antepartum testing in the last 6–8 weeks of gestation.

(4) **Population.** Pregnancies at risk for uteroplacental insufficiency are typical candidates for NST. Patients with maternal risk factors such as postdatism, uncertain dates, diabetes, hypertensive disorders, and suspected IUGR are usually elevated. There are virtually no contraindications for the NST [13].

f. Contraction stress fetal heart rate testing

(1) **Description.** Performance of the contraction stress test (CST) is based on the theory that by stressing the fetus with uterine contractions while externally monitoring the fetal heart rate, we can identify the fetus at risk for uteroplacental insufficiency. The test may be performed with the classic approach, inducing contractions with oxytocin, or may employ nipple stimulation to produce uterine contractions. These uterine contractions temporarily stop intervillous blood flow so that those fetuses that have little reserve will exhibit fetal heart rate change in response to fetal acid-base changes.

The patient is placed in a recumbent semi-Fowler's position and fetal heart rate and uterine contractions are recorded externally for a baseline period of 10–30 minutes. If uterine contractions are taking place at a frequency greater than or equal to three contractions/10 minutes, with a duration of 40 seconds or more, contraction stimulation is not necessary. If the baseline uterine activity is inadequate, a warm moist towel is placed on both breasts for several minutes. The patient is then instructed to massage the nipple of one breast for 10 minutes. If this is still inadequate, both breast nipples are stimulated for another 10 minutes. Once uterine contractions have begun, the nipples are stimulated periodically to maintain the contraction response. If nipple stimulation is not successful in establishing uterine contractions, oxytocin is begun at 0.5 mU/minute and titrated up every 15–20 minutes until three contractions occur every 10 minutes [14].

(2) **Interpretation.** A **negative** result is defined as no late decelerations while the patient is experiencing three contractions/10 minutes. If late decelerations occur with each of the contractions, the test is read as **positive**. A positive contraction test is categorized as reactive if one or more accelerations occur during the entire test, and nonreactive if there are no accelerations. If late decelerations are associated with some, but not all, contractions present, and the uterine criteria have been met, the test is read as **suspicious** and should be repeated within 24 hours [14].

(3) **Interval/timing.** Antepartum testing utilizing the CST is generally begun after 33 weeks' gestation and repeated at weekly intervals until delivery. Many centers begin testing earlier in gestation if warranted by the clinical condition of either the mother or fetus. However, testing prior to 26 weeks' gestation is not justified, as intervention is unrealistic. It is also appropriate to test more frequently than weekly when there is a deterioration of maternal diabetic, hypertensive, cardiac, or asthmatic control, when there is vaginal bleeding, or premature rupture of membranes, or when the fluid from amniocentesis is stained with blood or meconium.

(4) **Population.** Patients who are candidates for testing include those with diabetes, hypertension, previous stillbirth, or discordant twins [14]. In

addition, those patients who have either positive or suspicious NSTs are candidates for CSTs.

g. Fetal heart rate (FHR) monitoring during labor

(1) Description. Continuous FHR monitoring is based on the principle that the fetus is intermittently stressed by uterine contractions that temporarily reduce the flow of oxygenated blood through the intervillous space. When this leads to early hypoxia, abnormalities of the FHR (decelerations during contractions) are seen. In later stages, FHR decelerations become prolonged, extending into the periods between contractions, and the fetal pH falls. In the external method of detecting fetal heart sounds, most centers use phonocardiography, in which fetal heart sounds are detected by a microphone strapped to the maternal abdomen. Heart sounds must be of sufficient intensity to trigger the cardiotachometer, which may be hindered by maternal obesity, fetal movement, or extraneous sounds. The recording may disappear altogether at the peak of a uterine contraction, when it is of most use. In the intrauterine method, direct fetal electrocardiography is employed using a unipolar electrode that is attached directly to the fetus and picks up the fetal electrocardiogram (ECG). A separate electrode lying free in the vagina of the mother picks up her ECG, and this can then be filtered off to avoid interference. Although this is the most reliable method for monitoring continuous FHR during labor, it has the disadvantage of requiring ruptured membranes for its use [15].

(2) Interpretation. The following specific fetal heart rate patterns may be caused by or are associated with hypoxia: late deceleration, prolonged deceleration, reduced beat-to-beat variability, sinusoidal pattern, and baseline shifts. Late decelerations in labor represent an acute reduction in fetal oxygen tension secondary to uteroplacental insufficiency or decreased uterine blood flow. Continuous prolonged hypoxia results in prolonged bradycardia rather than the transient late deceleration. The term "prolonged deceleration" has been defined as a deceleration of the FHR of greater than 30 beats/minute, persisting for more than 2½ minutes [16]. Prolonged decelerations may be caused by prolonged cord compression or prolapse, caine drug anesthesia effect, uterine hypertonus, vagal stimulation of the fetus, narcotic overdose, or maternal seizure. The instantaneous fetal heart rate is influenced by the autonomic nervous system, cerebral centers, and cardiovascular reflexes. Any alteration in these areas may affect fetal rate variability. Major causes of decreased variability include drugs affecting the central nervous system and autonomic function, prematurity, fetal hypoxia, fetal sleep cycle, congenital anomalies, fetal tachycardia, magnesium sulfate, and beta blockers. A sinusoidal pattern has a sine-wave pattern above and below the baseline with a decrease in short-term variability. It apparently represents a loss of central nervous system control of FHR and occurs most commonly in infants with severe fetal anemia (usually from Rh sensitization), high-output heart failure, and hypoxia [16]. Baseline shifts outside the normal range of 120–160 beats/minute may represent fetal compromise, particularly when associated with a decrease in beat-to-beat variability. Electronic fetal monitoring is a screening tool used in early detection of the hypoxic fetus. FHR patterns monitored can only be interpreted as suggestive of fetal distress, and good fetal outcome depends on subsequent appropriate intervention.

(3) Interval/timing. Advocates of electronic fetal monitoring believe that it should be used routinely and is of potential benefit in all labors of pregnancy. Critics have cited its interference with maternal mobility during labor and maintain that it offers no advantage to auscultation in low-risk or even high-risk patients.

(4) Population. It has been argued that continuous electronic fetal monitoring is only appropriate for high-risk mothers. However, fetal distress during labor may develop in patients previously considered to be low-risk. Nonetheless, it is reasonable to monitor the fetus externally when the patient is admitted and if the initial FHR pattern is normal, to allow the patient freedom of movement until membranes rupture, she returns to bed, or she detects unusual uterine activity. In pregnancies characterized by low estimated fetal weight, prematurity, IUGR, medical complications, meconium staining, intrapartum obstetric complication, use of oxytocin in labor, or abnormal auscultatory findings, it is judicious to employ continuous electronic fetal monitoring during labor.

h. **Fetal blood sampling**

(1) **Description.** Blood is usually collected from the fetal scalp, but in cases of breech presentation it may also be obtained from the buttocks. A cone is introduced into the vagina and through the cervix until it is directly against the fetus. A small area of fetal skin is visualized and cleaned with a swab. The skin is first sprayed with ethyl chloride in order to create a reflex hyperemia and then spread with a thin film of silicone gel or liquid paraffin. A small incision is made into the skin and the blood is collected into a glass capillary tube containing dried heparin.

(2) **Interpretation.** The lower limit of normal fetal pH is usually defined as being two standard deviations below the normal mean. This is generally accepted to be a pH of 7.20 with a "preacidosis" borderline range of 7.20–7.24 [15].

(3) **Interval/timing.** For fetal pH less than 7.20, immediate delivery is required as indicated by such factors as cervical dilatation and ability to perform cesarean section. If the pH value is in the borderline range, scalp blood sampling is repeated every 10 minutes until a definite trend is documented. If pH is in the normal range, fetal blood sampling is repeated every 20–30 minutes as long as the worrisome tracing persists [17].

(4) **Population.** Specific FHR deceleration patterns have been definitely associated with disturbances in fetal acid-base balance. This is particularly true for late deceleration and severe variable deceleration patterns. Fetal blood sampling for pH may also be justified for FHR baseline disturbances and moderate variable deceleration.

2. **Justification**

a. **Serial assessment of fetal growth**

(1) **Test characteristics.** Since studies have found fetal asphyxia with moderate or severe metabolic acidosis in 50% of intrauterine growth-retarded infants, it seems reasonable that any decrease in previously normal growth should raise concern [8].

(2) **Risks/side effects.** Risks are only those related to inaccurate measurement.

(3) **Costs.** Cost is negligible by itself, but worrisome growth generates further costs.

(4) **Acceptability.** Serial assessment of fetal growth is acceptable to both patients and physicians.

b. **Ultrasound**

(1) **Test characteristics.** Ultrasound done at the appropriate time is highly indicative of fetal life and predictive of length of gestation. The prevalence of IUGR in fetuses with biparietal diameters (BPDs) falling consistently below the twenty-fifth percentile is 50%. Therefore, the predictive value positive of BPD in the diagnosis of IUGR is 50% [18].

(2) **Risks/side effects.** The available data are insufficient to adequately assess the safety of diagnostic ultrasound. The American Institute of Ultrasound in Medicine (AIUM) Biological Effects Committee has reviewed reports of the effects of ultrasound in animal experiments. Their conclusion is that there are no significant biologic effects in mammalian tissues exposed to intensities below 100 mW/sq cm. Ultrasound is used appropriately where benefit is expected and the minimum exposure is used to attain that benefit [10].

(3) **Costs.** At the University of California, Davis Medical Center in 1985, real-time diagnostic ultrasonography cost the patient $160.

(4) **Acceptability.** Ultrasound is acceptable to both patients and physicians.

c. **Fetal movement monitoring**

(1) **Test characteristics.** Lack of vigorous fetal activity occurs in 4–5% of all pregnancies and happens twice as often in high-risk as contrasted to uncomplicated pregnancies. Approximately half of these inactive fetuses are distressed or stillborn at delivery. There is a positive relation between fetal movement and the results of NST or CST. A normal fetal movement pattern is associated with a 97% likelihood of either a reac-

tive NST or a negative CST. An inactive fetal movement pattern is less predictive but not significantly different from abnormal antepartum fetal heart rate testing in predicting a compromised fetus. Like other surveillance techniques, fetal movement monitoring is limited in predicting acute fetal distress from umbilical cord accidents or acute placental complications [11].

(2) **Risks/side effects.** Maternal anxiety and false-positives are the risks.

(3) **Costs.** Cost is negligible by itself. Positive findings generate the test costs.

(4) **Acceptability.** Monitoring of fetal movement is acceptable to both patients and physicians. Patient compliance is improved when the patient appreciates the nature of the antepartum complication and understands the charting instructions.

d. Detection of fetal heart tones

(1) **Test characteristics.** The presence of fetal heart tones during episodic prenatal visits after the twelfth week of gestation is an indication of fetal life. For a more precise evaluation of antepartum fetal well-being, it is necessary to perform the NST or CST.

(2) **Risks/side effects.** Risks are only those related to false-positives.

(3) **Costs.** There are one-time costs involved in the purchase of a fetoscope and Doptone.

(4) **Acceptability.** The procedure is acceptable to both patients and physicians.

e. Nonstress fetal heart rate testing

(1) **Test characteristics.** A reactive nonstress pattern is associated with fetal death within 1 week of testing in less than 1% of patients.

(2) **Risks/side effects.** There are no risks or side effects.

(3) **Costs.** At the University of California, Davis Medical Center in 1985, nonstress testing cost the patient $84.

(4) **Acceptability.** NST is acceptable to both patients and physicians.

f. Contraction stress fetal heart rate testing

(1) **Test characteristics.** A weekly negative contraction test is associated with low risk for fetal death. This is defined as approximately 0.4/1000 (corrected) compared to 3.2/1000 (corrected) for patients followed by nonstress testing for primary surveillance. Reactive positive contraction tests are associated with a good fetal outcome if the mature fetus is delivered without delay. About 50% of reactive positive CSTs are false-positive, with no significant decelerations occurring during labor [14].

(2) **Risks/side effects.** Although oxytocin contraction stress testing has not been linked to a significantly increased incidence of premature labor, it is contraindicated in patients at high risk for the following: premature labor secondary to premature rupture of membranes, incompetent cervix, multiple gestation, known uterine abnormalities or classical cesarean section scar, third-trimester bleeding, or history of previous premature labor [14].

(3) **Costs.** At the University of California, Davis Medical Center in 1985, contraction stress testing cost the patient $91.

(4) **Acceptability.** CSTs are acceptable to both patients and physicians.

g. Fetal heart rate (FHR) monitoring during labor

(1) **Test characteristics.** Continuous electronic surveillance provides reliable, predictive information about the fetal condition in both the antepartum and intrapartum periods. Investigators have demonstrated a correlation between FHR patterns, fetal pH in utero, and Apgar scores at birth. A normal FHR pattern correctly predicts high 1-minute Apgar scores with 93% accuracy and high 5-minute Apgar scores with an even more impressive 99%. Unfortunately, abnormal patterns are significantly **less** predictive [19].

(2) **Risks/side effects.** Intrauterine monitoring does not seem to significantly increase the risk of maternal or fetal infection (e.g., scalp infections and abscesses). The risk of external fetal monitoring also appears to be minimal.

(3) **Costs.** At the University of California, Davis Medical Center in 1985, electronic fetal monitoring cost the patient $65.

(4) **Acceptability.** In the past decade, there have been many changes in attitudes toward childbirth. These include a growing interest in more family-oriented childbirth with fewer interventional obstetric practices, and concerns regarding the rising cost of health care. Nevertheless, pregnant women who are aware of both the risks and benefits of intrapartum fetal monitoring and have discussed its appropriate use are less liable to have negative feelings about FHR monitoring.

h. **Fetal blood sampling**

(1) **Test characteristics.** There is a good correlation between fetal capillary pH and the infant's clinical condition at birth as measured by the 1-minute Apgar score. In one study, however, 18% of the fetal acid-base status reports were not predictive of the clinical state at birth: 7.6% of the fetuses were acidotic (pH <7.20) but born in vigorous condition, while 10.4% had a pH >7.20 before delivery but were born in a depressed condition [20].

(2) **Risks/side effects.** Small numbers of fetal complications (0.85% in the above study), including postnatal bleeding and infection, have been noted [20].

(3) **Cost.** At the University of California, Davis Medical Center in 1985, a fetal blood pH determination cost the patient $84 (each repeated test is $49).

(4) **Acceptability.** Fetal blood sampling is acceptable to both patients and physicians, although patients exhibit anxiety about the fetal scalp procedure.

B. Early intervention

1. **Methods.** When clinical fetal distress appears in labor, there should be an immediate search for the possible cause of hypoxemia. Since oxytocin may hyperstimulate uterine tone, thus compromising blood flow and oxygen delivery, it should be discontinued. Maternal hypotension from regional anesthesia or the supine position can also reduce uterine blood flow and oxygen delivery to the fetus and is sometimes relieved by changing the patient to a lateral recumbent position and vigorously infusing fluids. Oxygen may be administered to the mother via face mask in the hope of increasing the saturation of fetal hemoglobin. This is usually only of transient benefit since the concomitant acidemia is not corrected. A thorough vaginal examination should be performed to rule out cord prolapse. If subsequent FHR monitoring is normal, it may be assumed that the fetus has recovered from a temporary asphyxial stress, but it is wise to ascertain the condition of the fetus more accurately by means of fetal blood gas analysis. If hypoxemia persists, the fetus should be delivered as promptly as possible, usually by cesarean section [16].

2. **Justification**

a. **Effectiveness.** Before 1965, cesarean-section birth rates were constant at a level of between 2 and 5%. Since then, there has been approximately a threefold increase in the number of cesarean sections done in the United States, mainly for failure to progress in labor and breech presentation. Fifteen percent of the overall increase has been due to surgical intervention for fetal distress. The incidence of severe asphyxia in monitored patients has been found to be significantly lower than in unmonitored patients [21].

b. **Risks/side effects.** Cesarean section is not without complications. Maternal mortality rates of between 20 and 70 cases for every 100,000 patients have been reported. Overall maternal morbidity has been reported to be between 10.4 and 36.4%.

c. **Costs.** At the University of California, Davis Medical Center in 1985, a cesarean birth cost the patient from $3500–$6500, depending on the length of hospital stay.

d. **Acceptability.** Most patients who have an understanding of the possible benefits of cesarean delivery find it an acceptable procedure.

IV. Recommendations [22]

A. Primary prevention

1. Perform a thorough screening prenatal history, physical examination, and laboratory work-up during the first prenatal visit.
2. Treat and/or refer mothers with the following conditions: insulin-requiring diabetes, severe chronic or pregnancy-induced hypertension, sickle cell disease and related disorders, recurrent pregnancy losses, Rh sensitization, and other severe

medical disorders such as chronic renal failure, lupus erythematosus, valvular heart disease, and severe asthma.

3. Advise pregnant patients to maintain adequate nutrition and to abstain from smoking, alcohol consumption, and all drugs except those that are medically approved.
4. Encourage participation in childbirth education and preparation classes.

B. Early detection

1. Regularly assess fetal growth after the sixteenth week of gestation by measuring fundal height. If there is a discrepancy between fundal height and gestational dates, order an ultrasound.
2. An obstetric ultrasound scan is indicated for the evaluation of the following: fetal viability, gestational dates, placental location, IUGR, multiple gestation, congenital anomalies, breech presentation, postterm pregnancy, amniotic fluid quantity, molar pregnancy, and pelvic mass.
3. Caution patients to report any decrease or loss of fetal activity. Monitor fetal movement in such patients and in high-risk pregnancies. Patients sustaining abdominal trauma or surgery in pregnancy or having a bloody third trimester amniocentesis will also benefit from fetal activity monitoring.
4. Regularly auscultate fetal heart tones with a Doppler instrument at 12 weeks and with a fetoscope after 20 weeks' gestation. Inability to auscultate fetal heart tones necessitates expeditious ultrasound examination. Detection of significant bradycardia or tachycardia warrants further evaluation with contraction stress testing.
5. Perform either nonstress or contraction stress fetal heart rate testing on patients with maternal risk factors such as postdatism, uncertain dates, diabetes, hypertensive disorders, or suspected IUGR. If the nonstress test is persistently nonreactive, a contraction stress test is a requisite for further fetal assessment.
6. Continuous FHR monitoring during labor is a reliable predictor of fetal well-being when the tracing is normal. It also serves to forewarn of the possibility of asphyxia when the tracing is abnormal. It is not possible to determine the significance of an abnormal FHR pattern with certainty without a knowledge of fetal pH.
7. Specific FHR deceleration patterns definitely associated with fetal acid-base disturbances include late deceleration and severe variable deceleration patterns. These require additional evaluation by sampling fetal blood for pH.

C. Intervention/treatment

1. Fetal distress in labor demands an immediate search for the possible cause of hypoxemia. Oxytocin, if being used, should be discontinued. Maternal hypotension can sometimes be relieved by a change to a lateral recumbent position and by increasing fluids. Oxygen administered to the mother may also be of transient value. A vaginal examination should be performed to check for cord prolapse.
2. In the absence of any correctable abnormality, persistent hypoxemia requires immediate delivery.

References

1. Low, J. A., et al. The incidence of fetal asphyxia in six hundred high-risk monitored pregnancies. *Am. J. Obstet. Gynecol.* 121(4):456, 1975. *Review of the incidence of fetal asphyxia in obstetric patients with specific high-risk indices.*
2. Adamsons, K., and Myers, R. E. Perinatal asphyxia, causes, detection, and neurologic sequelae. *Pediatr. Clin. North Am.* 20:465, 1973. *Good review of perinatal asphyxia.*
3. Brown, J. K., et al. Neurological aspects of perinatal asphyxia. *Dev. Med. Child. Neurol.* 16(5):567, 1974. *Description of neurological sequelae of fetal asphyxia.*
4. Lilienfeld, A. M., and Parkhurst, E. A study of the association of factors of pregnancy and parturition with the development of cerebral palsy. A preliminary report. *Am. J. Hyg.* 53:262, 1951. *Classic article relating various childbirth conditions to the development of cerebral palsy.*
5. Volpe, J. J. Perinatal hypoxic-ischemic brain injury. *Pediatr. Clin. North Am.* 23(3):383, 1976. *Discusses the pathophysiology of hypoxic-ischemic insults to the brain, and clinical features in the neonatal period.*

6. MacDonald, H. M., et al. Neonatal asphyxia. I. Relationship of obstetric and neonatal complications to neonatal mortality in 38,405 consecutive deliveries. *J. Pediatr.* 96(5):898, 1980. *Multivariate analysis of high-risk factors associated with increased risk of asphyxia.*
7. Hegyi, T., and Hiatt, I. M. Premature rupture of membranes and perinatal asphyxia. *Lancet* 2:913, 1980. *Describes an increased incidence of asphyxia with premature rupture of membranes and amnionitis.*
8. Low, J. A., Boston, R. W., and Pancham, S. R. Fetal asphyxia during the intrapartum period in intrauterine growth-retarded infants. *Am. J. Obstet. Gynecol.* 113:351, 1972. *Demonstrates the association of IUGR with fetal asphyxia.*
9. Rosett, H. L., Weiner, L., and Edelin, K. C. Treatment experience with pregnant problem drinkers. *J.A.M.A.* 249(15):2029, 1983. *Successful integration of therapy for heavy drinking with routine prenatal care.*
10. Nelson, L. H., and Kremkau, F. Real-time diagnostic ultrasound in obstetrics. *Am. Fam. Physician* 25:149, 1982. *Excellent review of the uses of obstetric ultrasound.*
11. Rayburn, W. F. Antepartum fetal assessment. Monitoring fetal activity. *Clin. Perinatol.* 9(2):231, 1982. *Review of fetal movement monitoring.*
12. Sadovsky, E., et al. Correlation between electromagnetic recording and maternal assessment of fetal movement. *Lancet* 1:1141, 1973. *Describes the reliability of maternal perception of fetal movement.*
13. Lavery, J. P. Nonstress fetal heart rate testing. *Clin. Obstet. Gynecol.* 25(4):689, 1982. *Complete discussion of nonstress testing.*
14. Freeman, R. K. Contraction stress testing for primary fetal surveillance in patients at high risk for uteroplacental insufficiency. *Clin. Perinatol.* 9(2):265, 1982. *Describes the test and offers guidelines for its clinical use.*
15. Beard, R. W. The detection of fetal asphyxia in labor. *Pediatrics* 53:157, 1974. *Excellent review of fetal monitoring in labor.*
16. Gimovsky, M. L., and Caritis, S. N. Diagnosis and management of hypoxic fetal heart rate patterns. *Clin. Perinatol.* 9(2):313, 1982. *Summary of fetal heart rate patterns associated with hypoxia.*
17. Collea, J. V. Fetal Monitoring During Labor and Delivery. In A. M. Daze and J. W. Scanlon (eds.) *Code Pink: A Practical System for Neonatal/Perinatal Resuscitation.* Baltimore: University Park, 1981. *A comprehensive look at perinatal asphyxia and its management.*
18. Sabbagha, R. E., Tamura, R. K., and Socol, M. L. The use of ultrasound in obstetrics. *Clin. Obstet. Gynecol.* 25(4):735, 1982. *Describes the use of ultrasound in determining fetal maturity, placental grading, multiple pregnancy, and congenital anomalies.*
19. Schifrin, B. S., and Dame, L. Fetal heart rate patterns: Prediction of Apgar score. *J.A.M.A.* 219:1322, 1972. *Looks at the predictive value of normal and abnormal fetal heart rate patterns.*
20. Bowe, E. T., et al. Reliability of fetal blood sampling: Maternal-fetal relationships. *Am. J. Obstet. Gynecol.* 107:279, 1970. *A large study looking at the correlation between fetal capillary pH and Apgar scores.*
21. Mueller-Heubach, E., et al. Effects of electronic fetal heart rate monitoring on perinatal outcome and obstetric practices. *Am. J. Obstet. Gynecol.* 137(7):758, 1980. *A large study showing that monitored patients had a lowered incidence of severe birth asphyxia than unmonitored patients.*
22. Bertakis, K. D. Fetal asphyxia: Prevention, detection, and intervention. *Am. Fam. Physician* 30(3):203, 1984. *A brief review.*

Infant, Child, and Adolescent Care

Health Promotion

27 Problems of Parenting

Christel Cranston

I. The problems

A. Definition. The term *parenting* as used here refers to the parents' contribution to the parent/child interaction.

B. Description. This interaction is the most critical component of the environment within which nurturance, stimulation, and discipline are provided and within which the child develops and matures. The nature of the parent/child relationship consistently has been found to be the most important variable influencing the psychosocial outcome of the child. The most important characteristics of the interaction in promoting optimal child development are (1) parental acceptance and warmth; (2) parental sensitivity to the signals of the child resulting in appropriate responses to child cues; and (3) the "goodness of fit" between the child's and the parent's temperaments.

1. **Spectrum of parenting problems.** Parenting problems include a wide range of difficulties. At one end of the spectrum are the common problems and frustrations every parent experiences in day-to-day child-rearing, despite adequate parenting skills and healthy parent/child relationships. Examples include coping with age-appropriate behaviors, such as infant crying, two-year-old negativism, the "tall tales" of a four-year-old, and the messiness of a school-age child, or coping with the behavior of temperamentally "difficult" children. In these normal but stressful circumstances, competent, caring parents may become concerned that something is wrong with their child or themselves and may seek advice or support.

   At the other end of the spectrum is dysfunctional parenting: interactions providing insufficient affection, responsiveness to the child's emotional needs, or stimulation, characterized by an inability of the parent or caretaker to meet the individual psychologic or biologic needs of the child. Flagrant evidence of deviant caretaking is common enough (child abuse, neglect, failure to thrive) but is only the "tip of the iceberg." Social and environmental deprivation is considered by many to be responsible for the majority of borderline and mildly retarded children, childhood conduct disorders, and intergenerational cycles of parenting disorders.

2. **Theoretic model of parent/child relationships.** A "transactional" model of the parent/child relationship has been described in which the child and his or her caretaker continually interact, each influencing and changing the other over time. The model emphasizes the malleable character of the parents, infant, and the environment; the child's influence in changing and shaping his or her environment; and a natural "self-righting tendency" toward normalcy. Use of this model helps one understand the dynamics of parenting disorders and also to plan effective intervention.

   Some variables affecting the parent/child relationship are found in Table 27-1.

C. Epidemiology. It is important to note that risk factors do not automatically lead to parenting problems and parenting disorders do not necessarily lead to abnormal development of the child.

1. **Parental risk factors** for the development of parenting problems include unsatisfactory experiences of the parent as a young child, being teenage parents, difficult pregnancies, family stresses (e.g., marital conflict, divorce), certain personality characteristics (e.g., impulsivity, immaturity, self-centeredness), and psychiatric problems of the parents (especially paternal sociopathy or maternal depression).
2. **Risk factors in children** include prematurity, separation from parents in the newborn period, congenital abnormalities or medical problems, developmental dis-

Table 27-1. Some variables influencing the parent/child relationship

Parent	Child	Environment
Parents' age, developmental status, personality characteristics, cultural background, and mental health	Psychosocial development stage	Socioeconomic status of the family
Parents' physical health, including any history of difficult pregnancies	Behavioral characteristics such as social responsiveness	Social support network for the family
Parents' own experiences of being parented as an infant and young child	Temperament characteristics	Family stability
Parents' opportunity for early contact with infant	Cognitive language and motor development	Birth order of the child
Parents' knowledge of child development and child-rearing procedures	Physical health	Community characteristics
	Physical appearance	
	Sex	

abilities, certain temperament characteristics, and being viewed by the parents as "different" for any reason.

3. **Environmental risk factors** include such social stresses as poverty and a lack of support systems (i.e., social isolation).

II. Specific health promotion: Promotion of positive parenting

A. Early assessment

1. Methods of risk assessment

a. **Parental risk factors** (see sec. **I.C.**) should be assessed prenatally when possible and reevaluated on an ongoing basis. An essential part of assessment includes a sensitive inquiry into the family's social circumstances (finances, employment, friends, community involvement), family interactions (marital relationships, interaction with children and extended family, composition of the family at home), and losses and changes in the parents' lives (moves, death of a family member). Experiences of the parents as children, child care arrangements, and the age and maturity of the parents should be ascertained, as well as the appropriateness of the parents' expectations of their child. Several authors have published lists of suggested areas of inquiry and "at risk" responses [1–3].

b. **Child risk factors** (see sec. **I.C.**) during the newborn period are assessed by careful physical examination and by assessing the baby's behavior in the presence of the parents. Any physical handicap in an infant is a major influence on the parent/infant relationship. Behaviorally, newborns vary in their alertness to their environment, their capacity and style of interactive behavior, their ability to cope with disturbing stimuli and control their motor responses, and their cuddliness and soothability. Premature infants may provide parents with few and confusing social clues. An assessment of the infant's behavioral style in the presence of the parents, coupled with discussions with the parents about their infant's behavior and responsiveness, has been found useful in promoting appropriate parenting practices [4].

In the older infant and child, physical health and developmental progress should be assessed. Developmental screening using a tool such as the Denver Developmental Screening Test (DDST) [5], the Denver Prescreening Developmental Questionnaire [6], and the Early Language Milestone Scale (ELM) [7] will identify many at-risk children. An evaluation of child temperament may be done informally by questioning the parents, especially if the infant seems to be "difficult." An Infant Temperament Questionnaire [8] is available to identify temperamental characteristics. Behavioral observations of the child should include the child's response to stress, including adaptive responses (strengths) as well as responses indicating inadequate adaptation.

c. **Environmental risk factors.** Consideration of the environmental variables should include assessment of parental finances, employment, social support system, and community factors.

d. **Evaluation of the parent/child interaction** includes observation of reciprocal behaviors between parents and infants, especially the parents' attention, sensitivity, and responsiveness to infant cues.

As the child grows older, parent behaviors that indicate an awareness of and responsiveness to the child's feelings and needs, and the amount and quality of the interaction between parent and child should be noted at each visit. Assessments include observations of the parent's handling of the child and response to cues, nurturant and loving behavior, and reciprocal behaviors between parent and child. The way the parent talks to the child and responds to exploratory behavior or to efforts to (or refusal to) do things for himself or herself may also be indicators of sensitivity to the child's needs and the appropriateness of parenting skills. Various rating scales and recommendations for assessment of parent/infant interaction are available that are useful in routine well-child care [1, 9, 10].

2. **Justification**

a. **Test characteristics.** Available methods of assessing parenting and parent/child interaction are not optimal, and their predictive accuracy assessment may be uncertain. Developmental screening assessment using the DDST and ELM scales, both of which have high levels of reliability and validity, identifies children at risk of developmental disability. Since (1) such disability is a frequent outcome of environmental deprivation, (2) developmentally handicapped children place special stresses on the parents, and (3) it has been found that developmental delays are often missed unless specifically screened for, routine developmental screening of all children is essential. Evidence of the value of assessing newborn behavior [4] and infant temperament [8] is available.

b. **Risks.** Labeling the parents or child as "at risk" may result in reduced expectations, leading to a self-fulfilling prophecy of poor parenting and developmental delay.

B. **Early intervention**

1. **Methods.** A variety of activities are felt to promote better parenting or to prevent parenting problems.

a. **Establishing a positive relationship between the health care provider and parent.** The ability of the health care provider to empathize with the parents and to acknowledge their skills and strengths as well as their problems can be important to successfully promoting healthy parenting.

b. **Prenatal education.** Prenatal education should include parenting topics presented in the form of individual discussions with a health care provider, as well as classes or printed materials.

c. **Perinatal attachment.** Support of the family should include (1) the presence of a supportive companion for the mother during labor, (2) early contact between the parents and their newborn baby, and (3) a newborn and postpartum ward environment providing warmth and support.

d. **Anticipatory guidance and counseling.** Anticipatory guidance regarding child behavior and parenting has traditionally been a major focus of well-child care in the medical setting. Emphasis should be on supporting parent strengths (e.g., by commenting on appropriate parent behavior), pointing out the child's strengths, eliciting parent opinions and attitudes, and developing a problem-solving approach with the parents rather than simply recommending parenting methods [9]. Individual family issues (e.g., foster care, adoption, nontraditional family structure, divorce) may require particular attention.

Anticipatory guidance lists are only as useful as the pertinence of the topics suggested, and this will vary according to patient and family characteristics. At any given developmental stage, guidance given to parents should be geared to assist them to understand and facilitate the child's mastery of current developmental tasks (Table 27-2). Numerous useful books for parents are available, and the primary care provider should be knowledgeable about the most helpful and be able to recommend appropriate reading.

(1) **First year.** Anticipatory guidance should follow a continuum begun antenatally, as mentioned above under prenatal education. Topics for the first year might include learning to understand the infant's cues and the need to establish a basic sense of trust. Other issues would be needs of parents and siblings, crying, sleep, behavior expectations, discipline, stimulation, separation anxiety, and exploration.

(2) **One to three years.** For the child aged 1 to 3, pertinent areas of anticipatory guidance include exploration, independence testing, the child's need for validation of his or her new skills ("you did it!"), sleep, toilet training, and feeding. The importance of early reading to children should be discussed. Information about day-care may be needed.

Parents of toddlers frequently ask about discipline. Toddlers characteristically are enormously curious and seem to have unbounded energy. They lack both a sense of the consequences of their behavior and "inner controls" to guide their behavior, and they are often "negativistic," disinclined to do what is asked of them. Providing discipline, therefore, may be quite exhausting and frustrating; at best it relies on ample use of distractions (rather than confrontations), manipulating the environment (keeping valuable or fragile items out of reach and safety proofing the home thoroughly), making rules clear and consistent, and keeping the number of rules to a minimum. Anticipatory counseling should be based on consideration of the temperaments of parent and child and individual needs.

(3) **Three to five years.** For the 3–5-year-old child, subjects commonly discussed include sibling rivalry, discipline, rules, parental consistency, positive reinforcement of desired behavior (including validation of new skills), imaginative play, tall tales, and fears. Counseling on preschool or television [11] may be indicated. School readiness [12] should be discussed, with particular emphasis on the results of the child's developmental screening.

(4) **School-age children.** For the school-age child, anticipatory guidance could include discussions of peer relationships, homework, independence, household responsibilities, neatness, discipline, and the child's need for developing a sense of competence and mastery. Behavior modification techniques are effective in improving parent management of a difficult child and can be taught in a well-child setting.

(5) **Adolescence.** Issues in adolescence include school experiences, peer activities, independence, responsibility, sexuality, and the adolescent's need to develop a sense of identity. Parents may need support in "letting go" as their adolescent develops increasing independence.

e. **Office visits.** Increased frequency of visits, duration of contact, and altered visit content are suggested for families with special needs.

f. **Parenting classes and books** are widely available and popular (see **Bibliography** of books for parents).

g. **Community resources. Prenatal and postpartum home-based intervention programs** for high-risk families are increasingly available. **Early intervention programs** designed to promote the development of high-risk and handicapped young children have been rapidly proliferating in the last decade. Often, in-home programs are available for children from birth to 18 months. Center-based toddler programs provide services for 18-month to 3-year-old children and their families. **Head Start programs** for the preschool age group have similar aims for socially disadvantaged children; **public schools** are mandated to provide (and private schools may provide) services for handicapped children between the ages of 3 and 22 years. These programs often include parent involvement and parent counseling.

h. **Therapy.** Family and parent counseling are traditional interventions for the routine problems of parenting. Group counseling for families with special needs is available in many communities. For seriously dysfunctional families or individuals, psychotherapy may be indicated.

2. **Justification**

a. **Effectiveness**

(1) **The positive doctor/patient relationship** is felt to be central to the success of preventive activities but has not been adequately studied.

(2) **Prenatal parenting preparation** is recommended by most developmen-

tal pediatricians and is desired by many parents, although its effectiveness has not been documented.

(3) **Attachment between parent and infant** has received much attention. Results of several studies indicate that providing opportunities for mother/infant contact soon after birth facilitates the development of bonding, as evidenced by increased eye-to-eye contact and parent responsiveness. It has been pointed out that early contact might facilitate attachment in the high-risk groups, but it should not be considered either essential or sufficient for the development of good parent/child interactions.

Another factor that seems to positively influence the mother/infant interaction is the presence of a supportive companion during labor and delivery. Most studies of parent/infant attachment have involved mother only, with the father/child relationship being studied much less. The benefits to the child of extra contact with the father are being studied with increasing interest, however.

(4) **Promoting positive parenting by anticipatory guidance** is a highly regarded activity that is generally considered effective in improving parents' understanding of parenting skills and of children's developmental progress. The author's personal experience and common sense attest to the value of these activities, and research data is beginning to document their usefulness [13].

(5) **Parenting classes and books.** Their effectiveness has not been evaluated by controlled studies.

(6) **Office visits.** The value of counseling by the primary care physician in prevention and early management of parenting problems is beginning to be studied and its effectiveness documented [14].

(7) **Community resources. Home visits** begun prenatally to enhance parenting preparation have been shown—when the child was 1 year old—to significantly reduce mother/infant interaction problems and nonparticipation of fathers, when compared to home visits initiated postpartum or not at all [15]. Studies of **Infant Stimulation** and **Head Start programs** indicate that their effectiveness depends on the involvement of the parent in the program. Improved social skills and educational outcome were shown in several programs having parent involvement [16].

(8) **Counseling and psychotherapy.** While dysfunctional parenting puts the child at high risk of psychiatric disorder and cognitive delays, interventions that result in improved caretaking practices can reverse the effects of earlier deprivation, minimizing or preventing long-term cognitive, social, or behavioral sequelae [17].

b. **Risks/side effects.** Risks of activities to promote better parenting are largely unstudied but they may exist. Guilt or inappropriate expectations may inadvertently be provoked by well-meaning counseling. For example, enthusiasm about bonding may lead some parents to believe that a critical bonding period exists and, if missed, leaves the chances of successful parenting blighted. Anticipatory guidance may increase parental anxiety without improving the parent/child interaction.

c. **Cost and acceptability.** The time that should be devoted to these activities, and therefore the cost, may be substantial, and the cost is not specifically covered by most third-party payment plans. Many parents desire guidance about parenting from their health care providers (at reasonable cost), but, unfortunately, some high-risk families are quite resistent to it when offered.

III. Recommendations

A. Early assessment

1. Assessment of risk factors in parent.
2. Assessment of risk factors in child as determined by physical examination, neonatal behavioral assessment, developmental screening, evaluation of temperament style.
3. Assessment of risk factors in the home environment.
4. Assessment of parent/child interaction.

B. Early intervention

1. Establishment of positive parent/physician relationship.
2. Prenatal education.
3. Perinatal facilitation of parent/infant attachment.
4. Anticipatory guidance and counseling.

Table 27-2. Schema for anticipatory guidance and parental counseling

Age	Psychosocial stage (Erickson)	Psychocognitive stage (Piaget)	Stage of ego development and object relations (A. Freud, M. Mahler, S. Freud)	Language development	Gross motor development	Fine motor development	Age-appropriate difficult behavior
0–18 mo	Basic trust vs. basic mistrust	Sensori-motor: exploration and manipulation of objects	**0–9 mo:** symbiotic **9–18 mo:** beginning of separation and individuation	**Birth–6 mo:** visual attention; gestural social interaction **3 mo:** coos reciprocally **6 mo:** imitates sounds **9 mo:** da-da-da, non-specific **12 mo:** follows 1-step command; first word **18 mo:** 6–10 words; jargon	**3 mo:** head up when prone **4 mo:** no head lag **6 mo:** strong tonic neck reflex gone **9 mo:** pulls up to stand **9–14 mo:** walks	**3 mo:** hands open **4 mo:** reaches, grasps **6 mo:** transfers hand to hand **9 mo:** pincer-grasp	**Early:** Crying; sneezing; colic; straining at stool; irregular breathing; temperamental variations **Late:** Fears of separation; exploratory behavior
18 mo –3 yr	Autonomy vs. shame and doubt		Completion of separation and individuation	**2 yr:** 2–3 word phrases **3 yr:** 3–4 word sentences	**18 mo:** walks upstairs holding on **2 yr:** runs, throws ball **3 yr:** pedals tricycle	**18 mo:** makes tower[a], 2 cubes **2 yr:** tower, 4 cubes **3 yr:** tower, 8 cubes	Negativism: stubbornness, tantrums Messy eating Toileting problems Sleeping problems "Poor appetite" Little self-control Trouble sharing toys
3–5 yr	Initiative vs. guilt	Preoperational: symbolic activity; make-believe play; magical thinking	Oedipal	**4 yr:** 4–5 word sentences; speech understandable **5 yr:** counts to 10; asks why	**4 yr:** hops, stands on 1 foot 5 seconds **5 yr:** skips, catches bounced ball	**4 yr:** copies +, DAP[b] (draws 4 parts) **5 yr:** copies □, DAP (draws 8 parts)	Tall tales; stealing; sex play; nightmares; fears of imaginary creatures and injury; pretend playmates; guilt about divorce, illness; sassiness; bathroom talk

5–12 yr	Industry vs. inferiority	Concrete operations: logical thinking bound to concrete real world, develops "rules"	Latency	Sentence length in words approximates chronological age **6 yr:** sounds out written words **9 yr:** automatic reading	**8 yr:** rides 2-wheeler **8–12 yr:** learning soccer, baseball, etc.	**6 yr:** prints alphabet **9 yr:** writes short stories **12 yr:** writes neat reports	Clannishness Scapegoating of younger or weaker children Resistance to performing chores Messiness Preoccupation with rules of game and fairness Fear of failure
12–18 yr	Identity vs. role confusion	Formal operation: abstract thinking	Genital	Language reflects abstract thinking and questioning of values and ideals Reads for comprehension, organizes information	Motor coordination reaches peak	May be skilled at notetaking, typewriter, musical instrument	Increased clannishness, idealism and hero worship Challenge of parental authority Falling in love Overconcern with physical appearance and sexuality Rule testing and pranks

[a]Using 1-in. cube
[b]Draw a person.

Table 27-2 (continued)

Age	Appropriate parenting tasks: Safety	Discipline	Development	Physician tasks
0–18 mo	**Prenatal:** carseat, crib **0–4 mo:** auto safety, prevention of falls; water heater temp.; crib safety **4–6 mo:** remove or lock up drugs, poisons, dangerous objects Secure or remove electric cords Turn pot handles in Safety-proof electric outlets Use stair barriers Fence pool Have ipecac on hand	**0–4 mo:** Response to crying: You can't spoil a young infant **4–9 mo:** Remove dangerous and valuable items; use distraction **9–18 mo:** Child understands NO but forgets rules	**Prenatal:** Physical preparation Decision regarding nursing Emotional readiness Support system **Infant:** Holding child, eye contact Support other caregiver Provide appropriate environment re temperament Play to foster growth in language, psychosocial, and motor development	**Establish relationship** with parents and child **Evaluate parent needs:** Parent/child relationship Family stress Knowledge of growth and development Accident prevention skills **Evaluate child's health status, temperament, and development** including: Social: parent/child relationship, peer relationship School: achievement and behavior **Provide appropriate parent education re:** Developmental tasks of child Problem-solving Accident prevention, considering: child development status; parent stress and organization; physical environment Discipline Special issues: sleep, feeding, daycare, TV, toilet training, nursery school, divorce, school readiness, peer group activities (e.g., scouts, 4H, sports), school success (importance of talking with teachers, homework), promotion
18 mo –3 yr	Auto safety Review home safety Provide safe environment while promoting development of sense competence and mastery	Consistency, firmness when limits tested "Time out" Minimal attention for negative behavior Positive attention for desired behavior	Support development of sense of mastery by encouraging self-help skills Provide stimulating emotional and physical environment Provide opportunity for peer play (parallel)	
3–5 yr	Auto safety Review home safety Water safety and swimming lessons	Child able to remember rules most of the time (inner control) Avoid long lectures and arguments about rules "Positive reinforcement" "Natural consequences"	Assist child to sort out reality/fantasy while enjoying sharing fantasies Provide support for supervised peer play (interactive) Provide stimulating environment and activities: sand, water, paint, crayons, trucks, dolls, puppets, books, visits	

5–12 yr	Auto safety Sports and recreation safety Drug, alcohol, and tobacco education Sex education	Positive reinforcement of desired behaviors Active listening Consistency	Appreciation of child's need for success and parental ability to create situation in which child can succeed Balance supportive home with encouragement of peer friendships Support school program and homework Promote increasing independence and responsibility	of independence and responsibility, drug education, "letting go" of older adolescent
12–18 yr	Auto safety Driver's education Drug, alcohol, and tobacco education Sex education Sports and recreation safety	Positive reinforcement of desired behaviors Active listening Consistency Increasing self-responsibility of child	Appreciation of clannishness, idealism, challenging behavior, etc., as normal means of clarifying identity Parental support balanced with encouragement of peer friendships, school and community activities, and increased independence and responsibility	

5. Enhanced office visits for guidance and counseling for high-risk families.
6. Parenting classes and books.
7. For high-risk situations, infant early intervention programs, Head Start programs, and public and private school programs.
8. Parenting counseling, family counseling, and psychotherapy, if indicated.

References

1. Children and Family Assessment: The Family Inventory. In H. J. Grossman, et al. (eds.), *The Physician and Mental Health of the Child* Vol. 1. Chicago: American Medical Association, 1979. *Concise outline with good lists of sample screening questions and "at risk" responses.*
2. Assessing Parental Capabilities. In H. J. Grossman, et al. (eds.), *The Physician and Mental Health of the Child* Vol. 1. Chicago: American Medical Association, 1979. *Concise overview with developmental format and practical suggestions.*
3. Sasserath, V. J., and Hoekelman, R. H., (eds.). *Minimizing High Risk Parenting.* Skillman, NJ: Johnson and Johnson Child Development Publications, 1982. *Concise and readable little book full of practical information.*
4. Widmayer, S. M., and Field, T. M. Effects of Brazelton demonstrations for mother on the development of preterm infants. *Pediatrics* 67(5):711, 1981. *Teaching mothers the amazing skills of their newborns seems to facilitate parent/child interaction, which in turn may contribute positively to infant development.*
5. Camp, B. W., et al. Preschool developmental testing in prediction of school problems. Studies of 55 children in Denver. *Clin. Pediatr.* 16(3):257, 1977. *Follow-up of children given the DDST as preschoolers.*
6. Frankenburg, W. K., et al. The Denver Prescreening Developmental Questionnaire (PDQ). *Pediatrics* 57(5):744, 1976. *Description of the PDQ.*
7. Coplan, J., et al. Validation of an early language milestone scale in a high risk population. *Pediatrics* 70(5):677, 1982. *Description of ELM Scale.*
8. Little, D. Parent acceptance of routine use of the Carey and McDevitt Infant Temperament Questionnaire. *Pediatrics* 71(1):104, 1983. *Brief article discussing practical use of temperament assessment in anticipatory guidance.*
9. Telzrow, R. W. Anticipatory guidance in pediatric practice. *J. Cont. Educ. Pediatr.* 1978. Pp. 14–27. *Excellent review of process and content of anticipatory guidance.*
10. Casey, P. H., and Bradley, R. H. The impact of the home environment on children's development: Clinical relevance for the pediatrician. *J. Dev. Behav. Pediatr.* 3(3):146, 1982. *Review of the impact of home environment on children and their development and available instruments for screening home environment.*
11. Strasburger, V. C. Television and adolescents. *Pediatr. Ann.* 14(12):818, 1985. *A variety of helpful articles are available in this issue.*
12. Oberklaid, F., and Levine, M. D. Precursors of school failure. *Pediatr. Res.* 2(1):5, 1980. *Excellent, brief review of epidemiology, and early assessment and intervention.*
13. Casey, P. H., and Whitt, J. K. Effect of the pediatrician on the mother/infant relationship. *Pediatrics* 65(4):815, 1980. *Anticipatory guidance provided by the pediatrician during routine well-baby visits was effective in positively influencing the mother/infant relationship and infant development.*
14. Cullen, K. J. A six-year controlled trial of prevention of children's behavior disorders. *J. Pediatr.* 88(4, part 1):662, 1976. *Study of the effect of preventive counseling during infancy and preschool on the behavior of six-year-olds.*
15. Larson, C. P. Efficacy of prenatal and postpartum home visits on child health and development. *Pediatrics* 66(2):191, 1980. *Study supporting the efficacy of home visits started prenatally.*
16. Provence, S. On the efficacy of early intervention programs. *J. Dev. Behav. Pediatr.* 6(6):363, 1985. *Comprehensive, brief overview of information available about effects of preschool educational programs for disadvantaged children.*
17. Fraiberg, S., Adelsen, E., and Shapiro, V. Ghosts in the nursery. A psychoanalytic approach to the problems of impaired infant-mother relationships. *J. Am. Acad. Child. Psychiatry* 14(3):387, 1975. *Description of therapeutic approaches with case examples.*

Suggested Readings

Allmond, B. W., et al. *The Family Is the Patient: An Approach to Behavioral Pediatrics for the Clinician.* St. Louis: Mosby, 1979. *Excellent introduction to "family focused pediatrics" and family therapy; written for pediatricians.*

Bennett, F. Rationale for Early Identification and Treatment. In W. K. Frankenburg, et al. (eds.), *Pediatric Developmental Diagnosis.* New York: Thieme-Stratton, 1981. Pp. 7–13. *Excellent short summary chapter on early identification and treatment of developmental disorders. The well-organized, concise text is very useful for primary care practitioners.*

Dixon, S., et al. (eds.). *Encounters with Children: Pediatric Behavior and Development.* Chicago: Year Book, 1986. *Written for the primary care practitioner; guide for integrating developmental and behavioral assessment into the routine office visit.*

Levine, M. D., et al. (eds.). *Developmental-Behavioral Pediatrics.* Philadelphia: Saunders, 1983. *See especially Chapters 4, 5, 13A, B, C, D, 23, and 53. These concise, practical chapters summarize important issues in developmental-behavioral pediatrics. Excellent text for primary care practitioner.*

Bibliography of Books for Parents

Caplan, F. (ed.). *The First 12 Months of Life.* New York: Grosset & Dunlap, 1973. *Month-by-month review of behavior and development with much information and advice.*

Caplan, F. (ed.). *The Second 12 Months of Life.* New York: Grosset & Dunlap, 1977. *Similar to book above for parents of the one-year-old.*

Dreikurs, R., and Grey, L. *A Parent's Guide to Child Discipline.* New York: Hawthorn Books, 1970. *Useful approach to discipline; this book is shorter and more readable than some of Dreikurs' others.*

Elkind, D. *The Hurried Child: Growing Up Too Fast Too Soon.* Reading, MA: Addison-Wesley, 1981. *Excellent discussion of stresses and pressures to achieve.*

Fraiberg, S. H. *The Magic Years. Understanding and Handling the Problems of Early Childhood.* New York: Charles Scribner, 1984. *Classic, beautifully written description of the development of children up to age 6 with practical advice for parents.*

Ginott, H. G. *Between Parent and Teenager.* New York: Macmillan, 1969. *Useful parenting suggestions.*

Gordon, T. *PET: Parent Effectiveness Training.* New York: New American Library, 1975. *Excellent practical discussion of basic principles of communication and resolution of conflict between parent and child.*

Patterson, G. *Living with Children.* Champaign, Ill: Research Press, 1976. *Every parent's easy introduction to behavior management.*

Satir, V. M. *Peoplemaking.* Palo Alto, CA: Science & Behavior Books, 1972. *Excellent, readable book without technical terminology or jargon; discusses the child in the family.*

Spock, B. M. *Baby and Child Care.* New York: Simon & Schuster, 1977. *Classic reference book for parents—comprehensive and sensible.*

28 Accidental Death and Injuries

Albert Chang

I. The problem

A. Definition. Accidents are unintentional events that result in injury or death. Deaths from homicide and suicide are intentional and are excluded from this definition.

B. Description. Although accidents are unexpected and felt by many to be due to chance, they are not totally random events. In large part they are predictable and preventable. There are human biologic, environmental, life-style, and health system factors involved, as well as preevent, event, and postevent phases of injury. Each of these components can potentially be modified by providers to decrease risk.

C. Epidemiology. Accidents are the leading cause of mortality in children or youth from 1 to 19 years old. They are responsible for more years of life lost before age 65 than any other cause of death. Although accidents hold fourth place as the cause of death of infants under one year, it should be noted that infants still have the highest mortality due to accidents in the pediatric age group. In 1983, the three leading causes of mortality due to accidents for the following three pediatric age groups were: (1) for infants under one year: motor vehicle (190 deaths), ingestion of food or object (189 deaths), and mechanical suffocation (174 deaths); (2) for children 1–4 years: motor vehicle (1,043 deaths), drowning (655 deaths), and fires and burns (638 deaths); and (3) for children 5–14 years: motor vehicle (2,241 deaths), drowning (711 deaths), and fires and burns (422 deaths).

In addition to the high mortality, accidents can also cause permanent impairment, disabling injuries, bed-disability days, and considerable loss of time from school. In a given year, one out of every five children or youths, 0–19 years, will have an injury serious enough to require medical treatment. In 1980, about 6.7 million children under 6 (35.2% of this age population) and 15.7 million children in the 6–16 age range (40.4% of this age population) suffered injuries requiring medical attention or involving at least one day of restricted activity. Time lost from school because of injuries amounted to 50.7 days per 100 boys and 29.0 days per 100 girls [1]. (National Center for Health Statistics, 1981.)

Information from the 1981–1982 National Health Interview Survey provides us with some information on risk factors in children 16 years and under: more injuries occur in boys, more injuries occur in white children than black children, and slightly more occur in children from higher income families and in children living in rural areas. Interestingly, the incidence rate between younger children (under 6 years) and older children (6–16 years) is about the same (35.2 versus 38.7 injuries per 100 persons per year), but the causes of injury are different.

In the 50 years since 1930, there has been a steady downward trend in the mortality from accidents in children. In 1930 the mortality per 100,000 for young children (1–4 years) was 61.2, and for older children (5–14 years) it was 36.1. In comparison, in 1983 the mortality was 21.8 (a 64% reduction since 1930) and 12.7 (a 65% reduction), respectively [2]. Continuing efforts in the prevention and in early management of accidents will undoubtedly continue the reduction of accidental deaths and injuries in children and adolescents.

II. General health promotion

A. Methods. One of the areas of greatest potential benefit in health promotion is the prevention of accidental injuries and deaths in children and adolescents. The American Academy of Pediatrics (AAP) [2] has stated that "anticipatory guidance for injury prevention should be an integral part of the medical care provided for all infants and children." While some clinicians are doing an effective job, the vast majority could do much more, since it appears that little time and effort is currently spent in anticipatory guidance [3].

Table 28-1. Early childhood safety counseling schedule

Preventive health visit	Minimal safety counseling		
Age	Introduce	Reinforce	Materials
Prenatal/newborn	Infant car seat Smoke detector Crib safety		
2–4 weeks	Falls	Infant car seat	
2 months	Burns—hot liquids	Infant car seat Falls	Questionnaire 1 Safety sheet 0–6 months
4 months	Choking	Infant car seat Falls Burns—hot liquids	Safety sheet 0–6 months
6 months	Poison Burns—hot surface	Falls Burns—hot liquids	Safety sheet 7–12 months Ipecac syrup Poison center sticker
9 months	Water safety Toddler car seat	Poison Falls Burns	Safety sheet 1–2 years
1 year		Poison Falls Burns	Safety sheet 1–2 years
15 months	Specific to need—optional		Questionnaire 2
18 months		Poison Falls Burns	Safety sheet 1–2 years
2 years	Falls—play equipment, tricycles Auto—pedestrian	Auto—restraints Poison Burns	Questionnaire 3 Safety sheet 2–4 years
3 years		Auto—restraints, pedestrian Falls Burns	Safety sheet 2–4 years
4 years		Auto—restraints, pedestrian Falls—play equipment Burns	Specific to need

Source: American Academy of Pediatrics. Committee on Accident and Poison Prevention. *The Injury Prevention Program.* Evanston, IL: 1983. With permission.

Enhancing the effectiveness of a provider as counselor is well described in a recent review [4], and some important principles the provider-counselor can use in focusing his or her efforts also have emerged. It is likely that the provider can succeed in getting patients to do those things that once done, provide long-lasting protection, e.g., install a smoke alarm, turn down the hot water temperature to below 130°F, or purchase a child-restraint device. It is far more difficult to get them to comply with accident prevention advice that requires ongoing implementation, e.g., using a child restraint device correctly. If we expect compliance with advice in this latter category, we need to remind patients on an ongoing age-appropriate basis, as suggested by the American Academy of Pediatrics [1] (Table 28-1), to monitor success, and at times to legislate compliance. Ideally, this should take place in collaboration with other interested individuals from either public or private agencies such as health departments, departments of motor vehicles, the American Automobile Association, the American Red Cross, the National Safety Council, hospitals, schools, and the media.

B. Justification. Advising parents to install smoke alarms is effective [5], so we can suppose that, in the absence of proof, anticipatory guidance directed at other similar one-time accident prevention behaviors may be similarly successful. Much less effectiveness has been demonstrated in areas requiring ongoing compliance with the preventive behavior, but some small successes have been achieved [6]. Community-wide prevention programs can be successful as evidenced by the pediatricians in Tennessee who were largely responsible for the enactment of mandatory safety seat and safety belt legislation for children in that state. Other health professionals also have an important role. Home visits by health professionals reduce the accident rate for children 12 and 18 months old, if initiated prenatally [7]. Thus, a substantial involvement by the clinician in accident prevention activities is both justified and desirable.

Vehicle-Related Accidents

I. The problem

A. Description. Motor-vehicle-related accidents involving children and adolescents as passengers or pedestrians represent the leading cause of accidental death in the age group 1–19 years. It should be noted that although significant reduction in mortality has taken place in other types of accidental deaths, motor-vehicle-related deaths have not decreased substantially over the last 50 years; in fact, such deaths have increased since 1960 for adolescents [2]. Even when all causes of death in this age group are considered, motor vehicle accidents account for almost 30% of the mortality.

B. Epidemiology. In the age group between 1 and 10 years, mortality is evenly divided between passengers and pedestrians; at the older age, passenger casualties predominate. Passenger mortality is higher in infancy and late adolescence: in the former case, infants, top-heavy because of their higher center of gravity, are missiles hurled against solid interior components of the motor vehicle; in the latter case, adolescents begin to drive and are at higher risk for traffic accidents. There is an increase in passenger mortality during the warmer months when more children and adolescents are traveling. Young drivers 16–24 years old constitute 17% of the U.S. population, but were involved in accidents producing 48% of the fatalities [8].

Pedestrian deaths constitute roughly half of the motor-vehicle-related deaths from 1–10 years, and 10–15% of all deaths from 13–19 years. Children under 15 represent 50% of all pedestrian deaths. The highest risk group is the 1- to 8-year-old children; they are ambulatory but their limitations in both perceptual and physical abilities make them more vulnerable. Most pedestrian injuries occur near the child's home and during daylight hours. It used to be thought that the fault was always with the pedestrian victim, but more recent studies indicate driver negligence.

Bicycle accidents were the most common cause of head injury in hospitalized children in one review [9]. The cyclist is at fault in about 50% of the cases. Twenty percent of injuries occur in accidents with autos, 14% of which are fatal [10].

Over 30% of motorcycle fatalities occur in persons under 20 years of age, and deaths increased about 50% in states in which laws requiring helmet use were repealed. Motorcyclists have a sevenfold greater risk of death per mile driven than automobile drivers, with the highest incidence of injuries in males 15–24 years old. Approximately three-fourths of motorcycle accidents involve collisions with a motor vehicle; in most cases the other driver is at fault, often not having seen the motorcycle [11].

A recent serious concern has been the increased use of all terrain vehicles (ATVs), injuries from which showed a dramatic increase—from 8,600 injuries in 1982 to 85,900 in 1985. These numbers represent injuries that were treated in hospital emergency rooms; in 1985 there were 200 fatalities. Since almost half of the injured persons were children under 16 years of age, ATVs should not be driven by children under 16.

II. General health promotion

A. Methods. Primary care providers should focus their activities in clinical practice, the community, media, hospitals, legislation, and medical education in at least the following areas.

1. **Child restraint devices (CRDs).** The most opportune time for initiating the child passenger message is just before or just after the birth of a baby. Instructions

and demonstrations of car seat use can be conveniently incorporated into prenatal classes, a prenatal pediatric visit, or during the first educational session with the new mother. Emphasis should be on face-to-face counseling and demonstration. Visual aids such as posters, movies, and videotapes also are helpful. At present, the AAP is involved in a nationwide campaign to promote the concept of "The First Ride—A Safe Ride." Since compliance increases briefly but diminishes rapidly after counseling, continued reinforcement at each visit to enhance compliance is important. AAP's Injury Prevention Program (TIPP) kit includes materials that can be used to enhance patient and provider compliance in this and other accident prevention areas (see **Suggested Readings**).

Currently there are basically three groups of restraint devices available for purchase: (1) for infant only, (2) for infant and toddler/preschooler (also called a "convertible"), and (3) for toddler/preschooler and school-age child (also includes the newer booster seats). The choice is essentially between a sequence of seats and a convertible model. The former begins with the use of an infant safety seat, progressing to a toddler/preschooler convertible seat, then a booster seat, and eventually to a regular lap belt when the child is 4 years old or 40 lb. Disadvantages include the greater cost and trouble of buying a second seat. A more reasonable option may be to use a convertible seat only. Over 25 dynamically tested CRD models are now available at most juvenile retail and discount stores. A recent Consumers Union evaluation of these seats found that the Century 200 convertible model offered the best value.

It should be noted that some of the older convertible seats and toddler/preschooler seats as well as some newer booster seats require a top anchoring strap for effective use. Many clinicians have reported that many families do not securely install this anchoring strap. It is important to remind families who may have such seats to correctly install this strap before they use the seat. The safest location for the car seat is in the rear, not the front seat; it also should be noted that, except for infants, a safety belt is better than no restraint at all.

2. **Lap and shoulder belts.** Lap belts are strongly recommended beginning when the child is 4 or weighs 40 lb. Shoulder restraints should be added when the child is tall enough (usually 55 in.) that the shoulder harness does not cut across his or her face or neck. For provider counseling in this area to be effective, reminders at each visit are important.
3. **Pedestrian safety.** Pedestrian safety should also be emphasized beginning at the age of 2. The most important measures are adequate adult protection and education. Parents, relatives, friends, and teachers should acquaint young children with the traffic environment and emphasize hazards. Children should not play in the street or driveway. An excellent set of brochures has been developed by the Automobile Club of America, and the AAP TIPP sheets (see **Suggested Readings**) can also be used.
4. **Cyclist safety.** Approved helmets should be worn by all bicycle and motorcycle riders. Approved motorcycle helmets bear the Snell, DOT, or ANSI labels. Bicycle helmets have been tested recently and will bear safety labels in the future. The National Safety Council also recommends the following for motorcycle riders; above-the-ankle boots, heavy gloves, face guards, and bright heavy clothing, and windshields and decreased engine size [11].
5. **ATVs.** ATV riders should also wear helmets. Equally important are the following recommendations: riders should receive training from certified instructors, riders should never carry passengers, riders should not ride on paved roads, and riders should not speed.
6. **Alcohol and drug use.** Because of the tremendous risk to adolescents of drinking and using alcohol, this problem must be approached by working at all levels of preventive intervention (see Chap. 32).

B. Justification

1. Child restraint devices

a. Effectiveness. Great potential exists for significantly reducing child passenger deaths and injuries with the regular use of restraint devices. Restrained children are 50–70% less likely to be injured or killed in an automobile accident than unrestrained children [12, 13]. By 1986, all 50 states and the District of Columbia had enacted legislation requiring some use of restraint devices (either safety seats or safety belts) in the preschool-age population. Initial evaluation of these laws indicates a reduction in deaths. Although the impact of pediatricians counseling in this area has been small, education and counseling remain acceptable and practical strategies for promoting child passenger safety.

b. **Risks.** Known risks have mostly been due to incorrect seat use, such as a seat that requires tethering not being tethered. Some skin burns from hot metal seat parts have been reported.

c. **Costs.** CRDs cost from $26 to $78 but average around $50. In some localities, voluntary agencies have established car seat loaner programs at only a nominal charge.

d. **Acceptability.** Public acceptance of these devices has been suboptimal and only a minority of physicians and hospitals routinely provide information on child restraint devices. Despite this, legislation in Tennessee increased CRD use from 9.1% in 1977 to 32% in 1981 [13].

2. **Lap and shoulder belts**

a. **Effectiveness.** In the U.S., safety belt use can decrease fatalities and injuries by 50% and 65%, respectively [13].

b. **Risks and side effects.** Intraabdominal injuries may occur in 0.5% of belted crash victims, but these are much less common and serious than those seen in unbelted occupants. Rarely, spinal fractures may occur. Although some people feel that seat belts may increase risk by preventing a person from being thrown free of a vehicle in a crash, the risk of death or injury from ejection is five times greater for the ejected than the restrained person.

c. **Costs.** Since belts are standard equipment on all new cars sold in the United States, cost does not constitute a significant barrier to their use.

d. **Acceptability.** Voluntary seat belt use in the United States remains low, around 20%. Compulsory safety belt legislation in other countries increases use to 50–80% [13]. By January 1986 about 12 states had enacted mandatory safety belt use in older children and adults. The value of physician-initiated patient education efforts in this area is uncertain.

3. **Pedestrian safety.** Some evaluation with encouraging results has been done on pedestrian safety education with children. Additional success in decreasing injuries has been accomplished through measures such as use of crossing guards, use of light-reflecting clothing (at night), or a physical separation between pedestrians and motor vehicle traffic.

4. **Cyclist safety.** Nonhelmeted motorcyclists are five times more likely to sustain severe or critical injury than helmeted riders [13]. Although there is less data on bicycle helmets, because the components and mechanism of injury are similar, it is anticipated that benefits are similar [9]. Risks of helmet use are low if approved helmets are correctly used. The principal barrier to helmet use is acceptance by riders, although this can be dramatically increased by legislating use. The effectiveness of physician advocacy of helmet use may be limited in the office setting.

5. **ATVs.** It is too early in the course of this epidemic to determine the effectiveness of the measures described.

6. **Alcohol and drug use.** In 1981 almost half of the fatal single-vehicle accidents among drivers 16–24 years old involved alcohol. Young drivers in motor vehicle accidents involving alcohol are 49% more likely to be killed than those with zero or unknown alcohol involvement [8]. This is another problem that must be approached at all levels of preventive intervention. The reader should note the additional discussion on this topic in Chap. 32.

Drowning

I. **The problem**

A. **Description.** Drowning is the second leading cause of accidental death in the age range 1–19 years. For children under 10, drowning occurs most often when bathing or playing unattended near water. Private swimming pools present the greatest hazard for this group, while salt water, bathtubs, fish ponds, and hot tubs are involved in smaller numbers of drownings. For teenagers, drowning usually occurs when they swim in an "unorganized" facility, i.e., places not officially designated as swimming areas [14], and includes a significant number of diving injuries.

B. **Epidemiology.** Not surprisingly, drowning occurs more frequently during the warmer months, May through August, when children and adolescents are more involved in swimming and other water-related activities [14]. Boys are at much higher risk than girls, presumably because boys take more risks. Teenage boys are at increased risk of drowning when drinking and are at risk for spinal cord injuries when diving, surfing, or waterskiing.

II. **General health promotion**

A. **Methods.** Providers should point out the importance of adequate **adult supervision** of swimming activities. In localities where private or public pools are popular, recommendations on adequate **fencing and enclosure** should be made [15]. Unfortunately, pools in apartment and condominium complexes often lack adequate fencing. For families who are receptive, the clinician should suggest **water safety instruction** for children 3 years or older, but no young child, particularly a preschooler, can be considered "water-safe" [15]. The AAP currently recommends that swimming lessons for infants under age 3 be on a one-to-one basis with a parent or responsible adult. Parents who own swimming pools should be encouraged to know lifesaving and **cardiopulmonary resuscitation techniques.**

The clinician can help others who work in this area of prevention. Schools, health departments, parks and recreation centers, the Red Cross, the National Safety Council, and other agencies play a significant role in public education and in the creation of safety legislation, and they can be aided by clinician input.

B. **Justification.** The single most effective method of prevention is adequate adult supervision. The clinician is most effective when reminding parents that babies and preschoolers should never be left unattended or with preschool-age siblings in or near water. Adequate fencing is effective in reducing swimming pool drownings [16], although the clinician's effectiveness in encouraging implementation is uncertain. On the other hand, well-organized public education programs can substantially reduce drownings in swimming pools [17]. Parents' knowledge of cardiopulmonary resuscitation techniques can significantly increase the survival of drowning victims when such measures are instituted early. The effectiveness of providers in averting alcohol and diving-related drownings and injuries in teenagers is uncertain, but their efforts are more likely to be of value when integrated into community-wide prevention activities.

Fires, Burns, and Scalds

I. **The problem**

A. **Description.** Fires and burns are the third leading cause of accidental death in children and adolescents and actually lead drowning as a cause of accidental deaths in infant boys and girls and in young girls aged 1–9 years. Three-fourths of all fire-related deaths result from house fires, nearly one-half of which are started by cigarettes and many of which involve alcohol [18]. The mechanism of death in house fires is most often smoke inhalation and not burns. Although most burn deaths result from fire, the most frequent cause of burns is contact with hot liquids (scalds). Some of the most severe burn injuries in children are due to hot tap water. Such burns occur most frequently in the kitchen and are most often related to food preparation activities.

B. **Epidemiology.** Deaths and injuries from fires and burns occur more often during the colder months, November through April, presumably because more indoor heating units, e.g. radiators, wood stoves, and fireplaces, are being used and children are indoors more. Young children under 3 are at highest risk of burn injuries, most of which occur during food preparation and consumption activities. Serious tap water burns are most common in infants and young children, and their occurrence in certain patterns may be due to child abuse.

II. **General health promotion**

A. **Methods.** The clinician should **inform families** of the situations that increase the possibility of burns or uncontrolled fires: unsupervised infants or children near hot liquids, particularly hot foods, cookware, stoves, and tap water; open flame; radiators and space heaters; matches; and cigarette smoking. A safe place for an infant while the adult caretaker is cooking, eating, or cleaning up is in a playpen.

The family should be encouraged to install **smoke detectors**, either of the photoelectric type (PSD) or ionization type (ISD), both of which are now readily available for home purchase and easy to install and maintain. At least one should be installed between the sleeping area and the area most used by the family during waking hours (the kitchen and the living room). The family should carefully follow instructions on placement and maintenance of these warning devices. The family should be encouraged to develop and rehearse an **escape plan** should a fire occur: identify possible escape routes, maintain availability of a rope or metal ladder to rooms above ground, assign each family member specific duties during the escape (e.g. call the fire department, care for young children), leave the premises immediately, check for fire behind closed doors, and arrange a specific meeting place after evacuation of the home [19]. Important also is the purchase of small **fire extinguishers** that are appropriate for the type of fire to be contained (i.e., type A, B, and C fires). The family should be instructed to **lower the hot water heater temperature** to below 130°F. They should also be instructed to store combustible materials in safe locations secured by childproof latches, reduce electric cord accessibility to growing infants, and seal electric outlets with protective guards. Should a burn injury occur, the parent should know to place the burned area in cold water immediately.

B. Justification. As in drowning, the most effective method of prevention is **adult supervision**, particularly in the kitchen. Smoke detectors reduce the potential for serious injury or death in 90% of the fires that occur when all occupants are asleep [18]. Physician counseling of parents to install smoke detectors is effective one-third of the time, while uncounseled parents rarely install smoke detectors on their own [5]. Concerns have been raised about radiation hazards of smoke detectors employing ionizing radiation, although the risk is negligible. The cost of smoke detectors ranged from $4–$25 in 1987; home fire extinguishers cost from $15–$35 in 1987.

A preplanned escape route with a specified meeting place away from the fire can maximize the successful evacuation of potential victims and permit immediate accounting of all individuals at risk.

Although the individual health care provider can have some impact on burn prevention through anticipatory guidance, education is not sufficient. Clinician input to modify product and home design through legislation is also important.

Full thickness burns from hot liquids occur in 10 minutes at 120°F, in 30 seconds at 130°F, and in 5 seconds at 140°F [20]. Although many home water heaters are set at over 160°F, and a majority over 140°F, no household need requires tap water temperature greater than 130°F. Laundering and dishwashing work well at these temperatures, and turning the hot water heater setting to 130°F or to the "low" setting, is a one-time activity that may have long-lasting preventive benefits as well as generate savings on energy bills.

Poisonings

I. The problem

A. Description. Ingestions of toxic medicinal and nonmedicinal substances constitute the fourth leading cause of accidental death among children 1 to 4 years of age. Although ingestions of medicinal products regulated by the Poison Prevention Packaging Act of 1970 (e.g., aspirin) have decreased dramatically, ingestions of unregulated products (e.g., acetaminophen) have increased. Aspirin, acetaminophen, antihistamines, and vitamins comprise the bulk of medicinal ingestions, while household products such as cleaners, bleach, rubbing compounds, cosmetics, and pesticides constitute another large group. Plants, gasoline, and lead poisoning are also part of the problem (see Chap. 47).

B. Epidemiology. Children 1 to 2 years of age are at highest risk for accidental poisoning. As noted above, medications and household products cause the majority of poisonings.

II. General health promotion

A. Methods. All parents should be given a 1-oz bottle of **syrup of ipecac at the six-month visit.** They should also be given the nearest **poison center telephone number,** which should be on a sticker they can attach to the telephone. If an ingestion occurs, they should call the poison center immediately for instructions. They should not follow instructions listed on the toxin container as they may be misleading. They should also wait until the poison center instructs them to give ipecac.

Parents should be instructed to **store all toxic substances up and away** from the reach of preschool children, to **install safety latches** on drawers and doors where these substances are stored, and to **place "Sgt. Ugh" or "Mr. Yuk" stickers** on dangerous substances. Providers should also continue their involvement in efforts to expand the number of substances sold in child-resistant containers to include all those that are commonly involved in childhood poisonings. Lead poisoning prevention is discussed in Chap. 47.

B. Justification. Ipecac is safe and effective. If used as instructed by a poison control center or physician, it also shortens the time to emesis, compared to the delay that occurs when parents have to obtain it from a pharmacy or health care facility if its use becomes necessary. Ipecac is inexpensive and well accepted by health care providers and parents. Stickers with the poison center telephone number and "Mr. Yuk"-type stickers are helpful when used. Protective latches like Kindergards are effective, but physicians' advice may not result in more utilization than in a control group, even when people are given the latches free [21]. Reported poisonings by regulated substances (those now sold in child-resistant containers) have decreased 65% since the regulation was introduced, while poisonings involving unregulated substances have increased [22].

Other Accidents

I. The problem

A. Description. Other common causes of accidental injury and death in children and adolescents mentioned in this section include falls, being struck or cut by an object, inhalation of food or other objects, mechanical suffocation, and sports. Sports injuries are discussed in Chap. 34. Most of these accidents can be termed "home accidents" and most are due to consumer products.

B. Epidemiology. Current research into these types of accidents is beginning to identify children at higher risk: for example, furniture and fixtures affect younger children while sports and recreational equipment affect older children [23]. Falls are the leading cause of injury to toddlers and young children. The majority are associated with stairs and steps, but other household structures and furniture, including porches, beds, tables, chairs, and cribs, are commonly involved. Being struck or cut is the next most common cause of injury and is more common after age 5. Foreign body aspiration usually involves peanuts, popcorn, beads, candy, or other small objects and is most common at 2 and 3 years, while mechanical suffocation is most common among infants.

II. General health promotion

A. Methods. Obviously, the clinician cannot cover the entire gamut of causes in one anticipatory guidance session with the family. Age-appropriate counseling to prevent accidents at home is an ongoing process. This task is greatly facilitated by the availability of several publications written for families, especially the TIPP questionnaires and handouts designed by the American Academy of Pediatrics and the Home Safety Checklist (Fig. 28-1). Important topics include falls; inhalation of objects; toy safety for infants and toddlers; and bicycle, firearm, and sports safety. The text entitled *Child Safety is No Accident: A Parents' Handbook of Emergencies* [24] by Arena and Bachar is excellent. The suggested reading list also lists a number of short safety pamphlets published by the American Academy of Pediatrics safety organizations, or commercial companies. Families should be counseled to use gates on stairways and doors and window guards above the first floor [25].

Frequent or poorly explained "accidents" may indicate family dysfunction or child abuse (see Chap. 41), in which case detailed evaluation and intervention is indicated.

B. Justification. Discussion of this compilation of home accidents is important because of the very high incidence of nonfatal injuries. The efficacy of anticipatory guidance is not known, however, and although probably limited, this could represent a large number of injuries prevented considering the large number of accidents involved. Physicians have been important in identifying dangerous household items and reporting these to the U.S. Consumer Products Safety Commission, which can then intervene to improve the safety of the item or remove it from the market. The effectiveness of window guards in preventing fatal falls and in the area of removing environmental hazards is unquestioned. The use of stair gates probably reduces the incidence of nonfatal injuries in young children.

1. Bicycles
   - ______ See that brakes are working.
   - ______ Make sure chain guards are secure and all screws and bolts are tight.
   - ______ Make sure they have front, rear, pedal, and spoke reflectors and headlights and taillights.
2. Stairs, ramps, and landings
   - ______ Fix poor lighting.
   - ______ Fix loose handrails and broken steps.
   - ______ Tack down loose carpeting and remove objects that people trip over.
3. Home playground equipment
   - ______ Make sure swing sets, gym sets, and other playground equipment are installed on soft surfaces and at least 6 ft from obstructions such as fences or walls.
   - ______ They should be anchored firmly in the ground, and any exposed bolts or screws should be covered with plastic caps or taped over.
4. Bathtubs
   - ______ Place nonskid bath mats or adhesive strips on the bottom of tubs and showers.
   - ______ Make sure that all bathroom rugs and mats have slip-proof backings.
5. Ladders
   - ______ Install slip-resistant rubber or plastic to the feet and steps.
   - ______ Make sure rungs are sturdy and not cracked, and braces are secure.
6. Electrical cords and outlets
   - ______ Make sure only one appliance is plugged into each socket.
   - ______ Install plastic plug-in safety caps or rotary cap outlets in unused wall sockets.
   - ______ Have frayed cords, exposed wires, and loose plugs repaired.
   - ______ Make certain that all fuses are of the correct amperage.
7. Furniture
   - ______ Move all upholstered furniture well away from stoves, space heaters, floor and wall furnaces, and anything else that could set the upholstery on fire.
   - ______ Also make sure that furniture is not placed where people will trip or stumble over it.
8. Glass doors and panels
   - ______ Make sure doors and panels have safety glazing. For visibility, stick decals or colored tape on them at both adults' and children's eye levels.
9. Liquid fuels
   - ______ Store all flammable liquids in properly labeled, tightly capped, non-glass safety containers, away from heat and flame.
10. Fire safety
    - ______ Install a smoke detector in your home so your family will have an early warning and an excellent chance for escape if a fire starts.
    - ______ Develop and practice a fire escape plan.

Fig. 28-1. Home safety search checklist. (From United States Consumer Product Safety Commission.)

Recommendations

The following health promotion activities should be incorporated into appropriate prenatal, postpartum, infant, child, and adolescent care on an ongoing basis.

I. Motor-vehicle-related

A. All providers caring for children should develop a child passenger safety program, including: brochures; counseling; demonstrations; audiovisual materials or CRD models on display, or both.

B. Infants should use an approved safety seat on the first ride home from the hospital and a child restraint device on every ride thereafter until reaching 4 years or 40 lb. The CRD must be installed properly in the car and be age or size appropriate for the infant or child. The provider should remind the parents at each subsequent visit to continue using the CRD.

C. Parents must set an example by using a safety belt themselves whenever they are in an automobile.

D. When a child reaches 40 lb or 4 years, he or she should always use a lap belt in the car. A shoulder harness should be added when sufficient height is attained, and when the harness does not cut across the face or neck.

E. Emphasize pedestrian safety; emphasize adult supervision during play in driveways or streets.

F. Encourage approved headgear for all bicycle and motorcycle riders, in conjunction with other safe operation anticipatory guidance.

G. Include anticipatory guidance to prevent adolescents from driving while using drugs or alcohol. This should be reinforced in the office setting and pursued with other ongoing preventive efforts in the family, community, schools, media, and legislation (see Chap. 32).

H. Participate in local organized community activities that promote child passenger safety: local child passenger safety committees, health departments, chapters of the National Safety Council, the state Automobile Club, the Red Cross, schools, voluntary organizations, private corporations, and law enforcement agencies.

II. Drowning (guidelines for parents)

A. Never leave babies and toddlers unattended in the water, no matter the depth of the water.

B. All children 3 years old or older should learn water safety and should be taught to swim. Swimming lessons for infants, when desired by parents, should be on a one-to-one basis with a parent or trained instructor.

C. No infant or young child can be considered water-safe.

D. Never allow children to play alone near an unfenced or unguarded pool or other natural pool of water (e.g., lakes, rivers, ocean).

E. Never allow a child or adolescent to swim alone.

F. Never allow a child to become exhausted in the water or be exposed to dangerous conditions (e.g., strong waves at the seashore).

G. Advise children not to hyperventilate before swimming.

H. Always place a fence around all sides of a pool and securely lock the entrance.

I. Always make sure that there is adult supervision at both private or public pools.

J. Advise children to never dive into water without first knowing the depth and likelihood of unseen objects.

K. The ingestion of alcoholic beverages before or during water- or swimming-related activities should be discouraged.

III. Fires, burns, and scalds (guidelines for parents)

A. Never allow infants and children near an open fire, radiators, or space heaters without supervision.

B. Never allow children near hot liquids or materials that could be inadvertently spilled or touched. Be especially cautious in the kitchen and during food preparation and mealtimes.

C. Place smoke detectors (at least one) in important areas of the house.

D. Place fire extinguishers in locations in which fire could occur.

E. Set water heater at below 130°F.

F. Develop and practice (at least once a year) a fire escape plan for the family.

G. Never allow children to play with matches.

H. Place combustible materials away from flames and store them securely in well-ventilated areas.

I. Assist parents to quit smoking and seek help for problem drinking.

J. Prevent access to electric cords by crawling infants and young children. Seal all electric outlets with guards.

K. If a burn injury occurs, place the burned area in cold water immediately.

IV. Poisonings

A. Give all parents of infants a 1-oz bottle of syrup of ipecac at the six-month visit, with instructions to call the poison control center or emergency room immediately in case of an ingestion.

B. Give parents the nearest poison control center or emergency room telephone number, preferably on stickers that should be placed on their telephone.

C. Advise parents to store toxic substances, labeled with Mr. Yuk-type stickers, up and away from the reach of children or behind Kindergard-type latched doors or drawers.

V. Other accidents

A. Recommend each family conduct a safety check (see Fig. 28-1) each year.

B. Recommend or provide printed literature on home accidents (e.g., toy safety, bicycle safety, firearm safety).

C. Based on a home hazard assessment, which may be aided by a questionnaire such as TIPP, recommend changes to improve home safety.

D. Advise use of gates on stairs and steps and window guards, as well as safety catches, on windows above the first floor.

E. Participate in workshops on home injury prevention for parents, teachers, youth organizations, day-care centers, nursery schools, and schools.

References

1. Jack, S. S. *Current Estimates from the Health Interview Survey: United States, 1980.* Washington, DC: Government Printing Office, 1981. *Provides data on persons injured and disability days due to injuries; obtained by periodic national health surveys.*
2. *Better Health for Our Children. Vol. 3. A Statistical Profile.* Washington, DC: Department of Health and Social Services, 1981. *A rich compilation of health data on children, collated from publications from the National Center for Health Statistics.*
3. Reisinger, K. S., and Bires, J. A. Anticipatory guidance in pediatric practice. *Pediatrics* 66(6):889, 1980. *A small but informative report on educational activities for parents provided by the pediatrician.*
4. Lovejoy, F. H., Jr., and Chafee-Bahamon, C. The physician's role in accident prevention. *Pediat. Rev.* 4(1):53, 1982. *Excellent discussion of suggested activities for physicians in the area of accident prevention.*
5. Miller, R. E., et al. Pediatric counseling and subsequent use of smoke detectors. *Am. J. Public Health* 72(4):392, 1982. *Describes a successful example of home safety promotion in the office and clinic setting.*
6. Reisinger, K. S., et al. Effect of pediatricians' counseling on infant restraint use. *Pediatrics* 67(2):201, 1981. *A well-planned program of child passenger safety. There was an increase in safe practice during 6 months of the health supervision schedule.*
7. Larson, C. P. Efficacy of prenatal and postpartum home visits on child health and development. *Pediatrics* 66(2):191, 1980. *A decrease in reported accidents during the first year of life occurred in families receiving home visits by trained educators.*
8. Alcohol-related highway fatalities among young drivers—United States. *M.M.W.R.* 31(48):642, 1982. *Young drivers have the highest mortality risk in motor-vehicle-related accidents, and alcohol consumption is a major factor in this increased risk.*
9. Ivan, L. P., Choo, S. H., and Ventureyra, E. C. Head injuries in childhood: A 2-year survey. *Can. Med. Assoc. J.* 128(3):281, 1983. *Reports on 880 children hospitalized with head injuries. The single most common cause of injuries was bicycle accidents. Wearing of helmets is recommended.*
10. Guichon, D. M., and Myles, S. T. Bicycle injuries: One-year sample in Calgary. *J. Trauma* 15(6):504, 1975. *Reports on 107 patients hospitalized for bicycle-associated injuries. Craniocerebral trauma was involved in 67%, and 20% involved a bicycle-automobile collision. Children under 16 years were at highest risk.*
11. Doolittle, R. P., Brown, R. T., and Boshell, A. Adolescents and motorcycle safety: The case for health advocacy. *Pediatrics* 64(6):963, 1979. *An appeal to medical practitioners to emphasize the possible risks of unsafe use of motorcycles.*
12. Scherz, R. G. Fatal motor vehicle accidents of child passengers from birth through four years in Washington state. *Pediatrics* 68(4):572, 1981. *Documents the significant reduction in mortality risks (90%) in children using safety restraints.*

13. State action to prevent motor vehicle deaths and injury among children and adolescents. *M.M.W.R.* 31(35):488, 1982. *A progress report on child-passenger-related activities at the state level.*
14. Accidental drownings by cause and site. *Stat. Bull. Metropol. Insur Co.* 58(6):9, 1977. *An extensive description of drowning mortality collated from periodicals nationwide.*
15. Swimming instructions for infants. *Pediatrics* 65(4):847, 1980. *This statement recognizes the increasing popularity of water instruction for infants but warns of its possible "false sense of security" effect. Recommends adult supervision, installation of fencing, and use of flotation equipment.*
16. Pearn, J. H., et al. Drowning and near-drowning involving children: A five-year total population study from the city and county of Honolulu. *Am. J. Public Health* 69(5):450, 1979. *Excellent study of pediatric submersion injuries in a community, and possible benefits of fencing regulations.*
17. Lawson, J. S., and Oliver, T. I. Domestic swimming pool drowning in children: Positive results of a practical prevention program. *Aust. Paediatr. J.* 14(4):275, 1978. *An interdepartmental committee in New South Wales addressed drowning prevention by a public education campaign and promoting legal requirements for adequate fencing.*
18. Mierley, M. C., and Baker, S. P. Fatal house fires in an urban population. *J.A.M.A.* 249(11):1466, 1983. *More than half of the deaths resulted from cigarette-ignited fires. Residents of poorer neighborhoods were at higher risk.*
19. Reisinger, K. S. Preventing Deaths Due to Fire. In A. B. Bergman (ed.), *Preventing Childhood Injuries.* Report of the Twelfth Ross Roundtable on Critical Approaches to Common Pediatric Problems. Columbus, OH: Ross Laboratories, 1982. Pp. 44–49. *Provides practical measures to early detect home fires and plans for rapid evacuation. Prevention of fire hazards in the home is also emphasized.*
20. Katcher, M. L. Scald burns from tap water. *J.A.M.A.* 246(11):1219, 1981. *Describes 33 hospitalized patients admitted over a 10-year period in a Wisconsin community. Patients in the extremes of age (under 5 years and over 70 years) were at highest risk for mortality. Suggests setting of hot water temperature between 120–125* °F.
21. Derschewitz, R. A. Will mothers use free household safety devices? *Am. J. Dis. Child.* 133(1):61, 1979. *Describes educational activities at a prepaid health plan. Limited success when measured by safety practices at home.*
22. Unintentional poisoning among young children—United States. *M.M.W.R.* 32(9):117, 1983. *Although childproof packaging of medicines has significantly reduced poisoning deaths in young children, preventable poisoning deaths continue to occur in this age group.*
23. Rivara, F. P. Epidemiology of Childhood Injuries. In A. B. Berman (ed.), *Preventing Childhood Injuries.* Report of the Twelfth Ross Roundtable on Critical Approaches to Common Pediatric Problems. Columbus, OH: Ross Laboratories, 1982. Pp. 13–18. *Summary of epidemiological aspects of pediatric injuries in the United States.*
24. Arena, J. M., and Bachar, M. *Child Safety Is No Accident: A Parents' Handbook of Emergencies.* Durham, NC: Duke University Press, 1978. *An excellent, complete, concise, and very readable guide for parents. Part 2 emphasizes developmental stages and relationship to hazards and avoidance.*
25. Spiegel, C. N., and Lindaman, F. C. Children can't fly: A program to prevent childhood morbidity and mortality from window falls. *Am. J. Public Health* 67(12):1143, 1977. *Describes effective intervention in preventing falls from high-rises. One of the few truly "successful" injury prevention projects.*

Suggested Readings

Accident Facts. Chicago: National Safety Council, 1986. *The most complete and current single compilation of accident information in the United States. Published annually.*

American Academy of Pediatrics. Committee on Accident and Poison Prevention. *The Injury Prevention Program.* Evanston, IL: 1983. *Provides a general statement of the importance of injury prevention in the pediatrician's office, and age-specific questionnaires and counseling sheets.*

American Automobile Association. *Preschool Children in Traffic: A Practical Approach to Reducing Pedestrian Accidents Among Children Ages 3 to 6.* Falls Church, VA: American Automobile Association, 1976. *Very comprehensive guidelines for traffic safety for the young pedestrian. Excellent illustrations. Available on request.*

Arena, J. M., and Bachar, M. *Child Safety Is No Accident: A Parents' Handbook of Emergencies.* Durham, NC: Duke University Press, 1978. *An excellent, complete, concise, and very readable guide for parents. Part 2 emphasizes developmental stages and relationship to hazards and avoidance.*

Bergman, A. (ed.). *Preventing Childhood Injuries.* Report of the Twelfth Ross Roundtable on Critical Approaches to Common Pediatric Problems. Columbus, OH: Ross Laboratories, 1982. *An excellent up-to-date compilation of current research and activities on childhood accident prevention.*

Feldman, K. W. Prevention of childhood accidents: Recent progress. *Pediatr. Rev.* 2(3):75, 1980. *Concise review of most common injuries seen by pediatricians. Includes a good schedule of child-safety counseling topics by developmental age.*

Smith, G. S. Measuring the gap for unintentional injuries: The Carter Center Health Policy Project. *Public Health Rep.* 100(6):565, 1985. *Discusses the potential for preventing injuries through the application of broad-based mixed strategies: motor-vehicle-related fatalities and injuries (75% reduction), home injury deaths (50% reduction), and alcohol-related fatal and serious injuries (25% reduction).*

29 Infant Nutrition

Kathryn Dewey

Breast-Feeding

I. The problem

A. Description. The Committee on Nutrition of the American Academy of Pediatrics [1] recommends that breast-feeding be strongly encouraged. However, the incidence of breast-feeding among American women is lower than desirable, especially among low-income and minority groups.

B. Epidemiology. Although the incidence of breast-feeding in the United States has increased dramatically in the past 15 years—from 25% (at hospital discharge) in 1971 to 61% in 1983 [2]—we are still far from the U.S. Public Health Service (PHS) goal of 75% by 1990. Similarly, although the duration of breast-feeding has increased, with the percent of infants breast-fed at 5–6 months rising from 6% in 1971 to 27% in 1983, the PHS goal is 35% by 1990. The incidence of breast-feeding is lower than average among blacks (32%), Hispanics (54%), mothers with grade school (41%) or high school (54%) education, low-income mothers (44%), and teenagers (43%).

II. Health promotion

A. Methods

1. **Breast-feeding.** Ideally, women should be encouraged to breast-feed for 6 months or more. This encouragement begins with education in schools and through mass media, continues through prenatal instruction, and includes support by maternity wards in promoting breast-feeding. Maternity wards can support breast-feeding by (1) avoiding excessive sedation or anesthesia during labor and delivery so that suckling by the infant is not impaired; (2) avoiding separation of the mother and infant for long periods of time; (3) allowing for breast-feeding "on demand" by providing alternatives to a rigid 3–4 hour schedule, e.g., rooming-in; (4) avoiding routine use of formula, water, bottles, pacifiers, and nipple shields for breast-fed infants so that they can learn to suck from the breast without other potentially confusing stimuli; and (5) maintaining a positive and supportive attitude towards breast-feeding on the part of all staff.

   Breast-feeding for even a couple of weeks benefits the mother and her infant. Health care personnel should provide instructions in proper breast-feeding techniques [3], anticipate potential problems, and give information regarding proper nutrition (Table 29-1) and drug avoidance. In particular, mothers should be aware that infants cry for reasons other than hunger and that normally their breasts will feel less full after the initial period of engorgement, even though the milk supply is adequate. Switching the infant to bottle-feeding without attempting to maintain lactation should be discouraged.

   If a woman cannot breast-feed for medical reasons or if she chooses not to breast-feed, she should not be made to feel guilty or inadequate, as this may increase tensions and be detrimental to her and her infant. However, mothers who choose not to breast-feed should be aware that it is difficult to reinitiate lactation later on if the infant shows an adverse reaction to infant formula.

2. **Recommendations regarding supplementary vitamins and minerals** for breast-fed infants are as follows:

   a. A single dose of vitamin K, 0.5–1 mg IM or 1–2 mg PO, to all newborns [4] (see Chap. 37).

Table 29-1. Dietary allowances for lactating women*

Nutrient	Recommended additional dietary allowances
Energy	+500 kcal
Protein	+20 gm
Calcium	+400 mg
Phosphorus	+400 mg
Magnesium	+150 mg
Iron	+30–60 mg
Zinc	+10 mg
Iodine	+50 μg
Vitamin A	+400.0 μg RE
Vitamin D	+5.0 μg
Vitamin E	+3.0 mg TE
Vitamin C	+40.0 mg
Thiamin	+0.5 mg
Riboflavin	+0.5 mg
Niacin	+5.0 mg NE
Vitamin B_6	+0.5 mg
Folacin	+100.0 μg
Vitamin B_{12}	+1.0 μg

*Above intakes recommended for nonlactating women.

Key: RE=retinol equivalents; TE=tocopherol equivalents; NE=niacin equivalents.

Source: Reproduced by permission from Worthington-Roberts, Bonnie S.: Lactation and Human Milk: Nutritional Considerations. In Worthington-Roberts, Bonnie S., Vermeersch, Joyce, and Williams, Sue Rodwell: *Nutrition in Pregnancy and Lactation,* St. Louis, 1985, Times Mirror/Mosby College Publishing; modified from Food and Nutrition Board, National Research Council, National Academy of Sciences: Recommended Dietary Allowances (9th ed.). Washington, D.C., 1980, U.S. Government Printing office.

Table 29-2. Recommended supplemental fluoride dosage schedule according to fluoride concentrations in drinking water

Age (years)	Fluoride dosage (mg*/day) for drinking water with fluoride concentrations (ppm) of		
	<0.3	0.3–0.7	>0.7
Birth–2	0.25	0	0
2–3	0.50	0.25	0
3–13	1.00	0.50	0

*2.2 mg sodium fluoride contains 1 mg fluoride.

Source: F. J. Margolis. Flouride supplements for children. *Am. J. Dis. Child.* 134:865, 1980. Copyright 1980, American Medical Association.

b. Fluoride, in unfluoridated areas, according to the fluoride content of the local water supply [5, 6] (Table 29-2) (see Chap. 45).

c. Vitamin D (400 IU daily) [4, 7], if the mother has a low dietary intake of vitamin D and is exposed to little sunlight. Although rare, rickets has been reported in a few unsupplemented breast-fed infants under these circumstances.

d. Supplemental iron is generally not necessary until after the infant reaches 6 months and can then be provided from solid foods (see section in this chapter on formula and solids).

e. Other vitamin and mineral supplements are unnecessary unless the mother's diet lacks fruits and vegetables and other foods rich in vitamins A, C, and B_6. Mothers whose diets are low in iron and calcium may benefit from a balanced mineral supplement, but maternal mineral intake is generally unrelated to mineral levels in breast milk [8].

B. Justification

1. Benefits

a. Breast-feeding. Abundant evidence demonstrates the advantages of breast-feeding [8]. Although commercial infant formulas are manufactured to approximate human milk as closely as possible, a number of important differences remain.

(1) The types of proteins found in human milk differ from those in infant formulas. Formulas contain beta-lactoglobulin (not found in human milk), which is one of the proteins considered to be responsible for allergic reactions to cow's-milk-based formulas. Allergic reactions to human milk are rare. Formulas are also low in the protective substances secretory IgA, lactoferrin, and lysozyme, all of which contribute to the antimicrobial effect of human milk. A greater proportion of the nitrogen content of human milk is made up of nonprotein nitrogen (25%). The nutritional significance of this difference is not yet known, but it is possible that an imbalance in protein concentrations could be detrimental during the rapid growth of early infancy [2, 9].

(2) The lipid, carbohydrate, and mineral content of human milk also differs from that of formulas. Formulas have less cholesterol than human milk, which may affect proper cholesterol metabolism in young infants [2]. Lipids in human milk are generally more easily digested than those in formulas. The carbohydrates in both human milk and infant formulas are primarily lactose. In some formulas, however, sucrose is substituted for lactose, giving a sweeter taste to the formula and perhaps leading to consumption of a greater volume. In general, the levels of minerals are higher in formulas, with the result that the contribution of formulas to the renal solute load may be higher than optimal for young infants [9]. Although the iron content of human milk is low relative to fortified infant formulas, a much higher percentage of iron is absorbed. The incidence of anemia in exclusively breast-fed infants before 6 months of age is very low [10].

(3) Human milk has antimicrobial factors [2, 3, 9]. It contains: (1) antibodies effective against both viral and bacterial infections; (2) lactoferrin, an iron-binding protein that has a bacteriostatic effect by binding available iron, which promotes resistance to *Escherichia coli* and *Candida albicans* in particular; (3) lysozyme, a milk protein with bactericidal activity; (4) lymphocytes, neutrophils, and macrophages (in colostrum primarily), which have been shown to be active as viable cells in vitro; and, (5) the *Lactobacillus bifidus* factor, a growth factor promoting the colonization of *L. bifidus* in the infant's intestine, which aids in the infant's resistance to enteric pathogenic bacteria. Even under optimal sanitary conditions, breast-feeding has been associated with lower rates of morbidity than bottle feeding [11].

(4) Human milk is thought to protect against allergies by preventing early exposure of the gastrointestinal tract to foreign food antigens [2].

b. Supplementary vitamins and minerals

(1) Vitamin K. See Chap. 37.

(2) Fluoride. See Chap. 45.

(3) Vitamin D. Vitamin D supplementation can prevent rickets when maternal intake and exposure of the infant to the sun are inadequate.

(4) Routine iron supplementation of breast-fed infants is not recommended because of the risk of saturating the lactoferrin in human milk and thus obliterating its bacteriostatic effect.

2. Risks

a. Breast-feeding

(1) Hemorrhagic disease of the newborn is more likely in breast-fed neonates. It is rare today, but before vitamin K prophylaxis was routine, it was commonly seen in breast-fed infants, while it was uncommon in formula-fed infants.

(2) Environmental contaminants such as polychlorinated biphenyls (PCBs) may be present in breast milk. If high levels of toxic substances are found in a sample of a mother's milk, breast-feeding may be contraindicated [3]. Moderate to heavy smoking (more than 20 cigarettes/day) can result in relatively high nicotine levels in breast milk and may diminish milk production. Moderate maternal alcohol and caffeine intake are not known to be harmful to the breast-fed infant, although both substances do pass into breast milk [3].

(3) Although the physical and psychological strains of breast-feeding are easily tolerated by most women, the need to be constantly available to the infant can be overwhelming for some mothers. Such mothers can be shown how to express their milk so that others may feed the infant. Alternatively, a combination of breast-feeding and formula-feeding may be appropriate for some women and is better than no breast-feeding at all.

(4) Occasionally, a highly motivated woman may insist on breast-feeding exclusively even when her infant is not thriving. In such cases, counseling, including a physical examination of the breasts and observation of the infant sucking, is necessary to uncover the root of the problem.

b. Supplementary vitamins and minerals

(a) Vitamin D toxicity is seen with amounts in excess of 1800 IU given daily for periods of greater than one month.

(b) Fluoride can also be toxic in large amounts.

3. Costs. In 1977, breast-feeding, including the added value of the lactating woman's diet, cost about 50–60% of the price of commercially prepared formula [13]. This is still generally true.

4. Acceptability. Breast-feeding is widely accepted among well-educated women in the United States, but it is not as popular among women with less education and among black and Hispanic women. Some women find it embarrassing to breast-feed, especially in public in a culture in which exposure of the breasts is not commonly accepted.

III. Recommendations. Breast-feeding can be encouraged and supported through the following.

A. Information about breast-feeding should be part of nutrition and sex education classes in the schools for both boys and girls and should also be presented in public communications media.

B. Prenatal instruction should include information to encourage breast-feeding, practical advice on techniques, and information on the kinds of problems that may be encountered [2, 14]. Organizations such as the La Leche League may, in some areas, provide advice and support for breast-feeding mothers.

C. Attitudes and practices in maternity wards should be geared toward promoting successful breast-feeding.

D. Health care providers should encourage women to breast-feed during the first 6 months. They should provide instructions in proper breast-feeding techniques, be aware of the usual problems encountered during breast-feeding and be prepared to offer advice and encouragement in solving these problems, and give information on proper nutrition and drug avoidance during lactation.

E. Supplementary vitamins and minerals should be given to the breast-fed infant as specified in sec. **II.A.**

F. Postpartum follow-up of breast-feeding mothers should take place within 5–7 days of discharge from the hospital.

Formula and Solids

I. The problem

A. Description. Commercially prepared infant formulas are the most appropriate alternative for the first 6 months if breast-feeding is discontinued or never initiated. However, early introduction to cow's milk (prior to 6 months) and solid foods (prior to 4 months) is commonplace in the United States.

B. Epidemiology. Although there has been a decrease in the proportion of infants fed cow's milk in the early months, approximately 20% of infants in 1980 received cow's milk or evaporated milk by 5–6 months [1]. If low-income mothers choose not to breast-feed, they may be unable to afford prepared formulas and may use cow's milk instead, despite its inadequacy for infant feeding in the early months. Some parents give their infants skim or low-fat milk under the mistaken impression that it will be healthier for them, even though skim milk is inadequate for normal growth and has an excessive solute concentration [15].

Solid foods are not recommended until 4–6 months of age, yet the majority of infants in the United States receive solid foods before 4 months [16]. The early introduction of solids is most likely due to social pressures to conform to the norm and to the widespread myth that solid foods will help the infant sleep through the night.

II. Health promotion

A. Methods

1. If breast-feeding is discontinued or never initiated, commercially prepared infant formulas are the most appropriate alternative for at least the first 6 months. After that age, the Committee on Nutrition of the American Academy of Pediatrics [17] states that whole cow's milk (vitamin D-fortified) may be introduced if the infant is consuming at least one-third of his or her total calories from supplementary foods containing adequate iron and vitamin C. Otherwise, infant formula is more appropriate for the first 12 months. Evaporated milk formulas are not recommended because of the excessive lead concentrations.
2. Milks with reduced fat content are not recommended during infancy.
3. Supplementation of bottle-fed infants should include the following.
   a. **Fluoride**, according to the fluoride content of the local water supply (see Table 29-2 and Chap. 45).
   b. **Iron**, through the use of iron-fortified formulas for the first 4–6 months. After that, additional iron may be provided by iron-fortified cereal. Ten tablespoons of dry cereal (1 mg Fe/tablespoon) should provide sufficient iron while other foods rich in iron (such as meats) are introduced into the diet.
   c. A good source of **vitamin C** is essential for infants fed whole cow's milk.
4. Solid foods should not be introduced until 4–6 months of age [16]. At this age, appropriate foods include iron-fortified infant cereal, fruits, and vegetables. At 6–8 months, meat, egg yolks, and other foods may be introduced. Egg whites should be delayed until the infant is 10 months because of potential allergic reactions. In families with a history of allergies, foods such as cow's milk, wheat, and chocolate should be withheld until after the child is 9–12 months.

B. Justification

1. Benefits

a. Infant formulas are the most appropriate alternative to breast milk because they are specifically designed to approximate the nutritional composition of human milk.

For example, commercial formula presents a smaller solute load to the immature kidney than does whole cow's milk. In addition, heat-treatment of whole cow's milk protein, on which most formulas are based, renders them less allergenic and less likely to cause gastrointestinal blood loss [9]. Recent information indicates that after 6 months of age, there is no significant difference in gastrointestinal blood loss between infants fed whole cow's milk and those fed heat-treated formula [17]. Therefore, whole cow's milk after that age may not be harmful if iron and vitamin C intakes are adequate. Neither low-fat nor skim milk is recommended during infancy because of their high protein and mineral content and low caloric density. Infants fed low-fat or skim milk do not increase their volume intake sufficiently to meet energy requirements [15].

b. A delay in the introduction of solid foods until 4–6 months is beneficial for the following reasons.

(1) At this time, solid foods can begin to provide the growing infant with needed nutrients, including calories, protein, iron, and vitamin C. Another reason for delay is that the extrusion reflex makes it difficult for the infant to successfully swallow semisolid foods prior to 4–6 months [16]. By 4–6 months the infant has adequate neuromuscular head control for eating semisolid foods, can indicate desire for food, and can signal when he or she has had enough.

(2) In early infancy, the gastrointestinal tract may be more permeable to large allergenic macromolecules. Although the relationship between the introduction of solids and allergies is not certain, there is sufficient concern to justify delaying solids, especially in infants with a family history of allergies.

(3) Solid foods given too early may also interfere with iron absorption. There is a possibility that solids reduce the bioavailability of iron from human milk, thus increasing the risk of anemia [9].

(4) Although the relationship between early introduction of solids and subsequent risk of obesity is controversial [18, 19], foods of high caloric density may contribute to excess adiposity.

2. Risks

a. Errors in production of infant formulas may cause problems such as inadequate or unsafe electrolyte levels.

b. Some parents may delay introduction of solid foods until long past 6 months, thereby increasing the risk of inadequate intakes of certain nutrients such as iron.

3. Costs. Commercial infant formulas are more expensive than cow's milk, with the ready-to-feed types being most costly [13]. Delaying solid foods until 4–6 months is less costly than early introduction of foods.

4. Acceptability. Commercial infant formulas are well accepted, even though parents do not always fully understand the rationale for their use. Delaying the introduction of solids until 4–6 months is sometimes a problem because of social and family pressures.

III. Recommendation. Appropriate infant feeding practices can be encouraged through the following:

A. Care providers should be aware that parents often receive conflicting advice from grandparents, peers, the media, and other health care providers regarding feeding cow's milk and solid foods. It is useful to point out that recommendations regarding infant feeding have changed since the parents themselves were infants.

B. The context in which infant feeding occurs should be noted: who feeds the infant and when, what are other family members eating, and so forth. Cultural pressures to feed infants certain foods should be investigated.

References

Breast-feeding

1. American Academy of Pediatrics, Nutrition Committee of the Canadian Paediatric Society and the Committee on Nutrition of the American Academy of Pediatrics. Breastfeeding. *Pediatrics* 62(4):591, 1978. *Review of the advantages of breast-feeding and the means to promote it.*
2. *Report of Surgeon General's Workshop on Breastfeeding and Human Lactation, Rochester, NY,* June 11–12, 1984. Presented by U.S. Department of Health and Human Services, Public Health Service, Health Resources and Services Administration, Bureau of Health Care Delivery and Assistance, Division of Maternal and Child Health, in cooperation with the University of Rochester Medical Center. D.H.H.S. Publ. No. HRS-D-MC84-2. Rockville, MD: The Maternal and Child Health Division, 1984. *Proceedings of a workshop on the value of promoting breast-feeding.*
3. Lauwers, J., and Woessner, C. *Counseling the Nursing Mother. A Reference Handbook for Health Care Providers and Lay Counselors.* Wayne, NJ: Avery Publishing Group, 1983. *Comprehensive guide for counseling nursing mothers.*
4. American Academy of Pediatrics, Committee on Nutrition. Vitamin and mineral supplementation needs in normal children in the United States. *Pediatrics* 66(6):1015, 1980. *AAP statement.*
5. Schusterman, S. More on fluoride in breast milk. *Pediatr. Alert* 5:99, 1980.
6. Schusterman, S. Fluoride supplements for children. *Pediatr. Alert* 5:83, 1980. *Leading periodontist's interpretation of the literature [5,6].*
7. Markestad, T. Serum concentrations of vitamin D metabolites in exclusively breast-fed infants at 70 degrees north. *Acta Paediatr. Scand.* 73(1):29, 1984. *Recent investigation of vitamin D issue.*
8. American Academy of Pediatrics, Committee on Nutrition. Nutrition and lactation. *Pediatrics* 68(3):435, 1981. *AAP statement.*
9. Brostrom, K. Human Milk and Infant Formulas: Nutritional and Immunological Characteristics. In R. M. Suskind (ed.), *Textbook of Pediatric Nutrition.* New York: Raven, 1981. Pp. 41–64. *This chapter reviews the nutritional and immunological differences between human milk and infant formulas. This textbook has numerous chapters relating to infant nutrition, all written by authorities in each of the subfields discussed.*

10. Siimes, M. A., Salmenperä, L., and Perheentupa, J. Exclusive breast-feeding for 9 months: Risk of iron deficiency. *J. Pediatr.* 104(2):196, 1984. *Investigation of iron status of breast-fed infants.*
11. Cunningham, A. S. Morbidity in breast-fed and artificially fed infants. *J. Pediatr.* 90(5):726, 1977. *Often-cited article demonstrating reduced frequency of illness in breast-fed infants in a United States community.*
12. American Academy of Pediatrics, Committee on Nutrition. *Pediatric Nutrition Handbook* (2nd ed.). Elk Grove Village, Il: The American Academy of Pediatrics, 1985. *Comprehensive AAP text.*
13. Lamm, E., Delaney, J., and Dwyer, J. T. Economy in the feeding of infants. *Pediatr. Clin. North Am.* (24)1:71, 1977. *Review of costs of different foods for infants.*
14. Lawrence, R. A. *Breast-feeding, A Guide for the Medical Profession* (2nd ed.). St. Louis: Mosby, 1985. *Very good guide to the physiology and anatomy of lactation, biochemistry of human milk, and the management of nursing mothers and infants.*

Formulas and Solids

15. Pipes, P. L. *Nutrition in Infancy and Childhood* (3rd ed.). St. Louis: Times-Mirror/Mosby, 1985. *Good general text.*
16. American Academy of Pediatrics, Committee on Nutrition. On the feeding of supplemental foods to infants. *Pediatrics* 65(6):1178, 1980. *Reviews rationale for delaying the introduction of solid foods until 4–6 months of age.*
17. American Academy of Pediatrics, Committee on Nutrition. The use of whole cow's milk in infancy. *Pediatrics* 72(2):253, 1983. *Recommendations regarding the use of cow's milk.*
18. American Academy of Pediatrics, Committee on Nutrition. Nutritional aspects of obesity in infancy and childhood. *Pediatrics* 68(6):880, 1981. *AAP statement.*
19. Mallick, M. J. Health hazards of obesity and weight control in children: A review of the literature. *Am. J. Public Health* 73(1):78, 1983. *Excellent review of this issue.*

30 Nutrition for Children and Adolescents

Kris Koski

I. The problem

A. Definition. Malnutrition can be defined as a deficiency or an excess of calories or of a single, specific nutrient. Poor nutritional status manifests itself as abnormal anthropometry, an altered biochemical index, or an overt clinical sign [1].

B. Description. Poor nutritional status in American children most commonly occurs from inappropriate food choices.

C. Epidemiology. National nutrition surveillance studies describe **all** children and adolescents living in the United States at risk for developing any of these nutrition problems: calorie excess (obesity); calorie deficits (growth retardation); and a dietary lack of vitamins A, C, and riboflavin and the minerals calcium or iron, or both. Most children and adolescents consume adequate amounts of protein unless dieting [2, 3, 4].

1. **Risk groups.** Individuals at highest risk include members of low-income families, preschool children, vegetarian children, and adolescents, especially those pregnant or on weight reduction diets.

II. Recommendations

A. General health promotion

1. To promote optimal nutrient intake, it is recommended that the clinician follow the modified basic four guidelines (Table 30-1). Consumption of the designated number of servings in each of the food groups guards against malnutrition, because this intake approximates the Recommended Dietary Allowances for each nutrient [5]. Similar guidelines and charts have been developed for the vegetarian child [6].
2. The American Academy of Pediatrics states that there is no evidence that routine vitamin and mineral supplementation is necessary for the properly nourished child [7].
3. The physician should promote routine exercise (1 hour/day) for all patients.

B. Specific health promotion

1. **Screening** for nutritional problems should form part of a routine physical examination.
2. Plot height, weight, and skinfold thickness, and compare with norms for evidence of underweight, overweight, or high body fat.
3. Do 24-hour recall of all foods eaten and compare number of designated servings with the recommendations given in Table 30-1. Obtain biochemical confirmation of possible nutrient or calorie deficiency or excess.
4. Interview the patient and family to determine if there are abnormal eating behaviors (e.g., anorexia nervosa, bulimia, fasting, excessive dieting).

C. Early intervention

1. If the child is at risk for specific nutritional deficiency or excess, modify dietary intake accordingly. Consult with a dietitian for more extensive evaluation and modifications.
2. Begin to promote routine exercise in the early stages of weight gain or increased body fat, long before the weight problem becomes serious and while modifications in behavior are more easily instituted.
3. If abnormal eating behaviors (anorexia nervosa, bulimia, fasting, excessive dieting) are identified, immediate medical attention is required.

Obesity

I. The problem

A. Definition. Obesity is defined as the presence of excess body fat. The most widely used definitions are the National Center for Health Statistics' growth standards (weight for height values > 95th percentile [see Chap. 35]), and those based on minimum triceps skinfold thickness (Table 30-2) for obesity.

B. Description. Obesity is a genetic, psychological, and environmental disorder that develops when calorie intake is greater than output, due either to excessive intake or to a decrease in physical activity [8]. Endocrine causes are rare and they are always accompanied by short stature and delay in bone development. Elevated blood pressure (see Chap. 49), hyperinsulinemia hypertriglyceridemia, hypercholesterolemia, and a lowered level of high density lipoproteins can accompany obesity in children and adolescents. The oral glucose tolerance test may or may not be normal. Moderate weight loss, using minimal calorie restriction and increased activity, improves an abnormal metabolic profile [9, 10].

Adjustment problems and emotional illness accompany obesity. Thus, even without any primary medical implication, the psychosocial consequences necessitate the treatment of obesity [11].

C. Epidemiology. Obesity is a major health and social problem affecting 10% of preschool and school-age children, 15% of adolescents, and 30% of adults. Obesity in childhood and adolescence, if untreated, will usually persist into adulthood. The most conservative estimates are that 50–65% of obese children remain obese throughout adulthood. For obese 12-year-olds, the odds against having normal weight as adults are 4 : 1; if weight loss is not accomplished by the end of adolescence, the odds rise to 28 : 1 [12].

II. Health promotion [3, 4, 8]

A. Methods. Since **prevention remains the best treatment for obesity,** the physician should provide guidelines for the appropriate caloric intake (see Table 30-1) and foster in any child the development of a lifelong habit of regular physical exercise. Treatment of the obese child or adolescent falls into two broad categories: exercise management and dietary management. Before treatment can begin, clinician, parent, and patient must agree on the nature of the problem and on the need for change, since changes in attitude precede reductions in weight.

1. **Exercise management.** Decreased activity characterizes obese American children. Weight management programs with an exercise component have had more success than simple medical treatment programs. Moderate exercise (1 hour/day) depresses the appetite and increases the basal metabolic rate; while this produces only minimal weight reduction, weight gain is stopped and significant reductions in body fat are observed.
2. **Dietary management.** Nutritional consultation is important in providing dietary treatment for children and adolescents because of their growth needs.
   a. Energy requirements for a child or adolescent can be estimated by using the height of the reference adolescent for each age and sex and multiplying it by the recommended kcal/cm for that height (Table 30-3). However, the most accurate calorie requirements are calculated from individual food intake and exercise records.
   b. **Weight loss cannot be recommended** for obese children and adolescents who are still growing. A calorie intake that promotes weight maintenance is preferred, since obese children show increased body weight on a developmental basis. It has therefore been suggested that changes in percent overweight (lbs overweight ÷ ideal weight × 100) is a convenient method for calculating weight loss in a still growing child. Thus, a child who maintains his or her weight but grows 1 in. in height during a 2-month period will have a new ideal weight, and he or she may go from being 20% overweight to 17% overweight, even though he or she has not lost an ounce.
   c. Only adolescents who have completed their growth spurt should be given a calorie-restricted diet.
      (1) No diet should go below 1200 calories. This caloric intake ensures adequate intake of all other nutrients and meets the minimum number of servings of the basic four guidelines (see Table 30-1).
      (2) Weight loss should be gradual—no more than 1 lb/week (500 calorie deficit/day; 1 lb=3500 kcal).

Table 30-1. Feeding guidelines for the growing years

Food Group (approximate kcal listed for each food item)	Recommended no. of servings/day	Suggested Serving Size: Toddler (1–2)	Preschool (3–5)	School-age (6–10)	Adolescent (11–18)
Milk or equivalent					
½ cup milk, 4 oz, (40–85)* equals:	4	½–¾ cup	¾ cup	¾–1 cup	1 cup
2 tbsp powdered milk (50–70)*					
1 oz cheese (50–100)					
¼ cup evaporated milk (75)					
½ cup cottage cheese (100)					
1 serving custard, 4 servings from 1 pt milk (205)					
½ cup pudding (200)					
½ cup yogurt (40–85)					
Meat, fish, poultry, or equivalent					
1 oz meat (55–100)* equals:	2 or more	1.5 oz (3 tbsp)	2 oz (4 tbsp)	3–4 oz (6–8 tbsp)	4 oz or more
1 egg (80)					
1 frankfurter (124)					
1 oz cheese (55–100)*					
1 cold cut (55–100)					
2 tbsp peanut butter (172)					
¼ cup tuna fish or cottage cheese (50–100)*					
½ cup dried peas or beans (70)					
Vegetables and fruits to include:	4 or more to include:				
Citrus fruit or equivalent	1 or more	½ cup (4 oz)	½ cup (4 oz)	½–¾ cup (4–6 oz)	½–¾ cup (4–6 oz)
1 citrus fruit serving (40) equals:					
½ cup orange or grapefruit juice					
½ cup grapefruit or cantaloupe					
¾ cup strawberries					
1 medium orange					
½ citrus fruit serving (20–25) equals:					
½ cup tomato juice or tomatoes, broccoli, chard, collards, greens, spinach, raw cabbage, brussels sprouts					
1 medium tomato, 1 wedge honeydew melon					

Yellow or green vegetables, or equivalent:	1 or more	¼ cup	¼ cup	⅓ cup	½ cup
1 serving equals:					
½ cup broccoli, greens, spinach, carrots, squash, pumpkin (40)					
5 apricot halves (40)					
½ medium cantaloupe (80)					
Other fruits and vegetables	2 or more				
Other vegetables, including potatoes (average 25–70/½ cup)		2–3 tbsp	4 tbsp	⅓–½ cup	¾ cup
Other fruits, including apples, bananas, pears, peaches (average 40/½ cup)		½ medium apple	½–1 medium apple	1 medium apple	1 medium apple
Bread and cereals or whole grain or enriched equivalent	4 or more				
1 slice bread (70) equals:		½ slice	1 slice	1–2 slices	2 slices
¾ cup dry cereal		½ cup	¾ cup	1 oz	1 oz
½ cup cooked cereal, rice, spaghetti, or macaroni		1 tbsp	¼–½ cup	½–1 cup	1 or more
1 roll, muffin, or biscuit					
Miscellaneous					
Butter or margarine (45/tsp)		2–3 tsp	2–3 tsp	2–3 tsp	2–3 tsp
Approximate caloric range, kcal		600–1000	850–1250	950–2100	1200–2200
Recommended calories, kcal/kg body weight		100	90	80	50–60

*Depends on fat content.
Source: *Infant Feeding Guide.* Washington State Department of Social and Health Services, Health Services Division, Nutrition Unit, 1972.

Table 30-2. Fifteenth (lean) and eighty-fifth (obese) percentile cutoff values for triceps skinfold thickness in children and adolescents

	Males		Females	
Age (yr)	15th percentile	85th percentile	15th percentile	85th percentile
1	6.0	9.0	—	—
2	7.0	13.0	5.0	12.0
3	7.0	13.0	7.0	12.0
4	6.0	12.0	7.0	12.0
5	6.0	12.0	7.0	12.0
6	6.0	12.0	7.0	13.0
7	6.0	12.0	7.0	14.0
8	6.0	12.0	7.0	12.0
9	6.0	15.0	7.0	14.0
10	6.0	15.0	7.0	15.0
11	7.0	17.0	8.0	18.0
12	7.0	19.0	8.0	20.0
13	7.0	18.0	8.0	20.0
14	6.0	18.0	9.0	20.0
15	6.0	20.0	9.0	22.0
16	5.0	19.0	10.0	23.0
17	5.0	14.0	11.0	23.0

Source: S. Garn. Growth, body composition and development of obese and lean children. In M. Winick (ed.), *Adolescent Nutrition.* New York: Wiley, 1975. P. 27. Reprinted by permission of John Wiley & Sons Inc.

Table 30-3. Recommended energy intakes

	Daily total (kcal)		Daily total (kcal/cm height)	
Age (yr)	Median[a]	Range[b]	Median[a]	Range[b]
Children				
7–10	2400	1650–3300	18.2	14.8–22.1
Males				
11–14	2700	2000–3700	17.2	15.1–20.9
15–18	2800	2100–3900	15.9	13.5–20.8
Females				
11–14	2200	1500–3000	14.0	11.2–17.5
15–18	2100	1200–3000	12.9	7.9–17.3

[a]Median energy intake of children followed in longitudinal growth studies.
[b]10th and 90th percentiles of the children's energy intake.
Source: Food and Nutrition Board, National Academy of Sciences, National Research Council. *Recommended Dietary Allowances* (9th ed.). Washington, D.C., 1980.

B. Justification

1. **Effectiveness.** Clinically significant weight loss is rare, and when it occurs, it is usually short-lived. Some moderate successes have been achieved with a combination of dietary counseling, exercise programs, and behavior modification. Preventing obesity, particularly in children at genetic risk for it, may be the most effective treatment program [13].
2. **Risks.** Calorie restriction to the point of weight loss in children and adolescents, even obese ones, experiencing the growth spurt cannot safely be recommended. Growth and development are stunted due to negative nitrogen balance [14, 15, 16]. Drug therapy for obesity is of little value since the use of most agents is contraindicated in children under 12, and such use has not been proven to be safe or effective in those above this age.
3. **Cost.** Highly variable.

4. **Acceptability.** Highly variable since it depends on the patient's motivation and the appropriateness of the program's goals.

III. Recommendations

A. A weight loss/maintenance program should not begin unless there is a long-term commitment to solving the problem by the physician, patient, and family. Otherwise, there will be another failure that is detrimental to the individual's self-esteem.

B. A thorough physical and psychological evaluation will be necessary to develop a working understanding of the weight problem and to direct intervention toward specific aspects of the problem.

C. Evaluation of food intake cannot be completed reliably during the first few visits. Obese individuals cannot precisely describe what they eat because over the years they have ignored the question. Others may be aware of what they eat but are unable or unwilling to report consumption accurately. The health care provider should not plan a management program until he or she has reliable food intake data and an exercise profile.

D. The initial goal is usually weight maintenance. In some cases an even more basic change from rapid to slow gain is appropriate.

E. The initial focus for the patient should **not** be based on changes in weight but on positive changes in food-related behavior or exercise patterns, or both.

F. Fasting, "crash diets," and the use of pills and laxatives should be discouraged by pointing out their lack of effect in the long term.

G. The patient should be helped to establish realistic goals and to realize that the program is long term. The use of support groups and registered dietitians should be encouraged.

Iron Deficiency

I. The problem [3, 4, 17]

A. **Definition.** Insufficient dietary intake of iron is the most common cause of iron deficiency. Nutritional iron deficiency commonly leads to anemia in children and adolescents, as well as to nonhematologic manifestations, including behavioral changes [18].

B. **Description.** The Recommended Dietary Allowances (RDA) for iron are 15 mg in children 1–3 years, 10 mg in children 3–10 years, 18 mg between the ages 11 and 18. For a further description and diagnostic evaluation, see Chap. 46.

C. **Epidemiology.** Dietary iron intakes are reportedly 50% of the RDA. While prevalence of anemia will generally provide an estimate of the prevalence of iron deficiency, it underestimates the magnitude of the problem. Iron deficiency is most common in young children between the ages of 6 months and 3 years; it increases again in adolescents during the growth spurt, although it can occur at any age [3].

II. Health promotion

A. **Methods.** Health care providers should promote the increased intake of iron. If speedy improvement is desired, supplementation with medicinal iron is required. However, diet modification to increase total iron consumption is necessary to prevent reoccurrence of the condition. Iron-rich foods should be routinely prescribed. Table 30-4 lists the iron content of typical food groups. A simple summation of the iron content of food eaten over a 24-hour period will determine those children and adolescents who are consuming too little iron, and specific iron-rich foods can be recommended.

B. **Justification**

1. **Effectiveness.** The prevalence of anemia among children from lower-income families who have consistently participated in the Special Supplemental Food Program for Women, Infants, and Children (WIC) has declined by 60% since 1975. The changes are related in part to improvements in dietary iron intake during infancy and childhood [19].
2. **Risks.** Acute accidental iron poisoning can occur [20] if iron tablets are brightly colored, sugar-coated, and taste like candy. Long-term use (>1 month) of therapeutic doses of iron can interfere with the absorption of other trace elements and should be recommended only for the treatment of overt iron deficiency anemia. Vitamin pills containing the RDA for iron are recommended for the treatment of iron deficiency.
3. **Costs** are minimal.
4. **Acceptability.** Increasing dietary iron by modifying the diet is more difficult to institute than advising the patient to take an iron supplement.

Table 30-4. Iron content of foods

Food	Iron (mg)	Unit
Milk	0.5	liter
Eggs	1.2	each
Cereal, fortified	3.0–5.0	ounce
Vegetables		
Yellow	0.1–0.3	ounce
Green	0.3–0.4	ounce
Meats		
Beef, lamb, beef liver	0.4–2.0	ounce
Pork liver, bacon	0.6	ounce
Fruits	0.2–0.4	ounce

Source: P. Lankkowsky. Iron deficiency in adolescents. In M. Winick (ed.), *Adolescent Nutrition.* New York: Wiley, 1982. P. 80. Reprinted by permission of John Wiley & Sons Inc.

III. Recommendations

A. Iron deficiency should be prevented by promoting routine supplementation or increased dietary intake, or both, to the level of the RDA. Enrollment of eligible patients (pregnant and lactating women, infants, and children ages 1 to 5) in the local WIC program should be encouraged.

B. The composition of the diet is often unfavorable for iron absorption. Elimination of dietary factors that impede iron absorption (e.g., tannic acid in tea, antacids, phytates, phosphates) and incorporation of foods that increase bioavailability of iron (e.g., meat protein, vitamin C) is necessary.

C. The consumption of iron-rich foods (whole grains, fortified cereals, meats, eggs, legumes) should be encouraged. Milk is not a good source of iron.

1. Heme iron is absorbed more readily than non-heme iron, so meat and egg consumption should be preferentially promoted.
2. Simultaneous consumption of meat protein and 25–75 mg of ascorbic acid with non-heme or elemental iron should be encouraged, since that combination increases the percentage of iron absorbed.

Hypercholesterolemia

I. The problem

A. Description. Elevated blood cholesterol has been associated, since the Framingham Study, with increased morbidity and mortality in adults. The view that the treatment of hypercholesterolemia in children and adolescents will reduce adult morbidity is necessarily based on extrapolation from the controlled clinical trials in middle-aged, high-risk hypercholesterolemic adult males. Long-term intervention trials have not been done in children.

B. Epidemiology. Surveys conducted in the past 10 years have documented higher plasma lipid concentrations in children in the United States than in children of other populations in which adult atherosclerotic disease is less frequent. About 5% of 5–18-year-old American children have total plasma cholesterol levels greater than 200–220 mg/dl [21].

1. **Risk groups.** The National Institutes of Health Consensus Conference made the following recommendations [22]:
   a. Children and adolescents at high risk should be identified primarily by family histories (hypercholesterolemia or coronary heart disease in a parent before the age of 50–60, or both) [23]. Routine screening before children enter puberty is recommended in all other cases [24].
   b. Those with blood cholesterol levels between the 75th and 90th percentile (170–185 mg/dl) should be counseled regarding diet and other risk factors and followed up at 1-year intervals.

c. Those with levels above the 90th percentile (>185 mg/dl) require special dietary instruction and close supervision by a dietitian.
d. A child with blood cholesterol above the 95th percentile (200 mg/dl) on two occasions may have one of the hereditary hypercholesterolemias. Strict dietary intervention is indicated and will be sufficient for many children. Nonresponders will require drugs.

II. Health promotion

A. Methods. The American Heart Association recommended that healthy children older than 2 years should have a fat intake of about 30% of total calories, with 10% or less from saturated fat, 10% from monounsaturated fat, and less than 10% from polyunsaturated fat. The daily cholesterol intake recommended for this age group is 100 mg of cholesterol per 1000 calories, not to exceed 300 mg/day. Carbohydrate intake, derived primarily from complex sources, should be 55% of total calories [21].

These recommendations are not endorsed by the American Academy of Pediatrics, which says that they are predicated on too little data. They recommend that the current dietary trends toward a decreased consumption of saturated fats, cholesterol, and salt, and an increased intake of polyunsaturated fats, should be followed with moderation in the general population of children, with the more strict guidelines being followed in children having abnormal lipid profiles.

Guidelines and menu plans for children and adolescents requiring a fat controlled "prudent" diet have been developed [25, 26].

B. Justification

1. **Effectiveness.** There is no controlled study demonstrating that reducing dietary cholesterol during childhood will decrease the incidence of coronary heart disease in adults. However, a recent study showed that hypercholesterolemia at age 12 is predictive of adult hypercholesterolemia in the majority of individuals [9].
2. **Risks.** Cholesterol-lowering regimens in children over 2 years old appear to be safe. Low-fat, low-cholesterol diets, particularly the use of skim milk, in children less than 2 is not recommended. There is some concern about the need for fatty acids in the myelinization of the central nervous system, the induction of certain enzyme systems, and preservation of skin integrity. Furthermore, introduction of skim milk should be avoided because of its high renal solute and sodium loads. Cholesterol-lowering drugs do not affect growth and development; however, the regular use of resins (cholestyramine and cholestipol) interferes with absorption of fat-soluble vitamins, so multivitamins with minerals are recommended.
3. **Costs.** There are as yet no long-term studies assessing costs and benefits of mass screening, although some studies are ongoing [27].
4. **Acceptability.** Early dietary intervention is justified because permanent dietary modification is more likely to occur during childhood and adolescence.

III. Recommendations

A. Regular exercise and maintenance of desired body weight should be promoted.

B. Diets should be planned with the basic four guidelines in mind (see Table 30-1), with the following additional dietary specifications:

1. Use of snack foods high in fat (e.g., pizza, salami, bologna-type meats) and sugar should be decreased. Fresh fruits and vegetables, fruit juices, and whole grain crackers, popcorn, or pretzels should be substituted.
2. Alternatives to whole milk should be used, keeping in mind that children and adolescents may need 4 servings/day of dairy foods for calcium.
   a. Whole milk should be diluted with reconstituted skim milk from powder.
   b. Low-fat cheeses (not cheddar), sherbet, or ice milk should be used.
3. Alternatives to fatty meats should be used. The strategy is to emphasize more consumption of poultry, fish, and legumes (pinto beans, dried peas), all of which are lower in fat.
   a. The consumption of deep-fried fast-foods should be drastically reduced, since hydrogenated beef tallow is most commonly used in frying.
   b. One-half low-fat meat and one-half poultry should be the goal.
   c. Foods should be broiled or baked, with drippings discarded.
   d. The use of polyunsaturated soft margarines, which are lower in saturated fat, should be recommended.

Table 30-5. Calcium content of foods (mg per serving)

100+ mg	150+ mg	200+ mg	250+ mg
10 Brazil nuts	1 cup ice cream	1 cup beet greens	1 cup almonds
1 medium stalk broccoli	1 cup oysters	1 oz cheddar cheese	1 oz cheese (Swiss or Parmesan)
1 cup instant Farina	1 cup cooked rhubarb	1 cup cottage cheese	1 cup cooked collards
3 oz canned herring	3 oz canned salmon with bones		1 cup cooked dandelion greens
1 cup cooked kale	1 cup cooked spinach		4 oz self-rising flour
1 tbsp blackstrap molasses	3 oz soybean curd (tofu)		1 cup milk
3 tbsp light (regular) molasses			3 oz sardines
1 cup cooked navy beans			1 cup cooked turnip greens
1 cup cooked soybeans			1 cup yogurt
3½ oz soybean curd (tofu)			
3½ oz sunflower seeds			
5 tbsp maple syrup			
2 corn tortillas (lime)			

Source: American Academy of Pediatrics, Committee on Nutrition. *Pediatric Nutrition Handbook* (2nd ed.). Evanston, IL: American Academy of Pediatrics, 1985.

Dietary Calcium Deficiency

I. The problem [28–30]

A. Definition. A surprising number of American children and adolescents do not consume sufficient daily calcium.

B. Description. The current RDA for calcium is 800 mg/day for children ages 1–10, increasing to 1200 mg/day for individuals 11–18 who are not pregnant or lactating.

Since peak skeletal mass is attained during the first 3 decades of life, calcium intake during childhood and adolescence has a significant impact on achievement of peak bone density and prevention of osteoporosis in later years. Adequate calcium intake is crucial during periods of rapid skeletal growth, such as infancy, childhood, and adolescence, when the body absorbs it most efficiently. Forty-five percent of the total adult skeleton develops during adolescence.

C. Epidemiology. A recent 3-year study of school nutrition programs reported that less than one-half of students consumed 100% of the RDA for calcium and 30% consumed less than two-thirds. Unfortunately, this suboptimal intake continues throughout adult life.

II. General health promotion

A. Methods. Two methods—increased dietary intake or calcium supplementation—can be used to meet the 800–1200 mg RDA.

1. **Food sources.** Milk and milk products are the richest sources of calcium in the American diet, but other foods can be used to entirely meet the dietary requirement (Table 30-5). If individuals are variably intolerant of milk because of intestinal lactase deficiency, Lact-aid (a product that is added to the milk) can be recommended.
2. **Calcium supplements.** Bone meal and dolomite should not be recommended because of reported contamination by toxic metals such as arsenic, mercury, lead,

Table 30-6. Available calcium supplements

Name	Form	Calcium (%)	Tablet size (mg)	Elemental calcium (per tablet [mg])	Vitamin D (per tablet [IU])
Alka 2*	Calcium carbonate	40	500	200	0
Biocal 250*	Calcium carbonate	40	625	250	0
Biocal 500	Calcium carbonate	40	1250	500	0
Caltrate 600	Calcium carbonate	40	1500	600	0
Caltrate 600+D	Calcium carbonate	40	1500	600	125
Centrum	Calcium phosphate, dibasic	29		162	400
Lilly	Calcium gluconate	9	486	44	0
Lilly	Calcium gluconate	9	324	29	33
Lilly	Calcium lactate	13	648	84	0
One-A-Day Plus Iron	Calcium carbonate	40		300	400
Os-Cal 250	Calcium carbonate	40	625	250	125
Os-Cal 500	Calcium carbonate	40	1250	500	0
Tums*	Calcium carbonate	40	500	200	0

*Chewable form.
Source: M. Fanelli, Promoting women's health. *Dietetics Curr.* 12(4):19, 1985.

and cadmium. Table 30-6 lists the currently available calcium supplements. The supplements should be taken between meals unless gastric hyperacidity occurs, in which case supplements can be taken with a meal. If more than one tablet is taken, they should be ingested at different times throughout the day.

B. Justification

1. **Effectiveness.** The presence of lactose or hydrolyzed lactose (Lact-aid) facilitates the absorption of calcium.
2. **Risks.** Excessive intakes of calcium can lead to kidney stones in susceptible individuals.
3. **Costs.** The costs are variable.
4. **Acceptability** is quite variable.

III. Recommendations

A. Exercise should be promoted. Increasing calcium intake by foods or supplements alone will not increase bone mass. Physical activity is a necessary component.

B. Excessive consumption of foods that interfere with calcium absorption or promote urinary calcium loss, such as the following, should be prevented:

1. Phytates: bran and some vegetables.
2. Fiber: cereal fibers.
3. Protein: high-protein diets consisting primarily of purified proteins.
4. Caffeine: coffee, tea, cola.
5. Foods with phosphate-containing additives: carbonated beverages, processed meats, refrigerated bakery goods.

C. Long-term use of drugs that interfere with calcium absorption, such as tetracycline, antacids, laxatives, cortisone, and thyroid medication, should be prevented.

Sugar and Dental Caries

I. The problem [31–35]

A. Definition. Dental caries is a pathological process of localized destruction of tooth tissues by microorganisms (see Chap. 45).

B. **Description.** Evidence points to sugar in snacks as the major factor in the etiology of caries. Existing data show that children and adolescents who consume sugar-filled foods between meals have more decayed, missing, and filled teeth than children who eat those same sweets with meals. Snacking has become a significant part of the eating habits of Americans, with the USDA Food Consumption Survey indicating that 59% of the respondents consumed snacks daily.

Sucrose (table sugar) and fructose (invert sugar) both promote caries. Some alcohol derivatives of sugar, like sorbitol and xylitol, are less readily metabolized by oral bacteria and therefore are not considered to contribute substantially to caries activity [32].

C. **Epidemiology.** The incidence of caries in the United States is greater than 60%. By age 17, American children have an average of over 11 decayed, missing, or filled tooth surfaces.

D. **Risk groups.** Since dental caries is nearly universal, all children would benefit from diet modification. The following groups, however, may be considered to be at especially high risk for dental caries [33].

1. Infants and children put to sleep with baby bottles filled with any substance that contains fermentable carbohydrate. With sleep, saliva protection falls off and food is not cleared from the mouth.
2. Children taking drugs that decrease saliva flow, such as antidepressants, diuretics, narcotic analgesics, antihypertensives, and anticholinergics.
3. Children receiving frequent medication in the form of syrups, particularly at bedtime.
4. Individuals who, in spite of their strict restriction of sucrose, consume more retentive or sticky foods, such as dried fruits, nut butters, honey, molasses, and health-food fudges [34].

II. Health promotion

A. **Method.** Practical dietary advice for caries prevention can take several forms. First, children should receive fluoride according to guidelines set down in Chap. 45. Second, realizing that eliminating sugar from the diet is impractical, the aim of the diet modification is to reduce the frequency and duration of exposure of the teeth to fermentable carbohydrate, particularly sucrose and fructose.

B. **Justification**

1. **Effectiveness.** Diets completely lacking in sucrose produce few if any caries. One longitudinal study in which the sugar substitute xylitol was used reported a 56% reduction in decayed, missing, and filled surfaces after 1 year, and 60% after 2 years. Other studies in which other saccharide alcohols (sorbitol, maltitol) were used have been less conclusive.
2. **Risks.** There are no known risks.
3. **Cost.** There are no significant costs.
4. **Acceptability.** The message that sugar causes cavities is easy to convey to the public.

III. Recommendations

A. Avoid as much as practicable all foods, beverages, and confections to which sugar has been added in such quantities that there is an overly sweet taste.

B. Avoid foods with high concentrations of natural sugars, such as honey, molasses, and dried fruits.

C. If sweets are to be eaten, they should be eaten at mealtime.

D. Restrict between-meal eating of any baked goods, confections, and beverages sweetened with sugar. If snacks are to be eaten between meals, items of low cariogenicity are preferred.

1. Foods with low caries potential include vegetables; milk; cheese; meat; nuts; legumes; and candy, gum, or beverages sweetened with saccharin, sorbitol, xylitol, or aspartame.
2. Foods with intermediate caries potential include starches and popcorn.
3. Foods with high caries potential include fruits, particularly dried fruits; beverages and baked goods sweetened with sucrose, glucose, fructose, or corn syrup; and potato chips, french fries, and corn chips.
4. Chewing gum and candy have the highest caries potential.

E. Fibrous carbohydrates, such as raw fruits and vegetables that require vigorous chewing, are most desirable, because they increase salivary flow and therefore the oral clearance of retained food. The buffer capacity of saliva can also help neutralize the plaque acidity.

References

1. Zerfas, A. J., Shorr, I. J., and Neumann, C. G. Office assessment of nutritional status. *Pediatr. Clin. North Am.* 24(1):253, 1977. *Excellent overview of the anthropometric, biochemical, clinical, and dietary determinants for the pediatric population.*
2. American Academy of Pediatrics, Committee on Nutrition. *Pediatric Nutrition Handbook* (2nd ed.). Evanston, IL: American Academy of Pediatrics, 1985. *AAP sourcebook.*
3. Pipes, P. L. *Nutrition in Infancy and Childhood* (3rd ed.). St. Louis: Times Mirror/Mosby College Publications, 1985. *Comprehensive textbook on all aspects of normal and abnormal childhood nutrition.*
4. Mahan, L. K., and Rees, J. M. *Nutrition in Adolescence.* St. Louis: Times Mirror/Mosby College Publications, 1984. *Comprehensive textbook on all aspects of normal and abnormal adolescent nutrition.*
5. King, J. C., et al. Evaluation and modification of the basic four food guide. *J. Nutr. Educ.* 10(1):27, 1978. *Nutritional justification for basic four food guide is presented, as are practical serving guidelines for nutritionally adequate diets if no meat, milk, or legumes are consumed.*
6. Vyhmeister, I. B., Register, U. D., and Sonnenberg, L. M. Safe vegetarian diets for children. *Pediatr. Clin. North Am.* 24(1):203, 1977. *Practical guidelines for nutritionally adequate vegetarian diets.*
7. American Academy of Pediatrics, Committee on Nutrition. Vitamin and mineral supplement needs in normal children in the United States. *Pediatrics* 66(6):1015, 1980. *AAP policy statement.*
8. Wells, K., and Copeland, B. Childhood and adolescent obesity: Progress in behavioral assessment and treatment. *Prog. Behav. Modif.* 19:145, 1985. *A review.*
9. Freedman, D. S., et al. Relationship of changes in obesity to serum lipid and lipoprotein changes in childhood and adolescence. *J.A.M.A.* 254(4):515, 1985. *Study showing that an increase in childhood obesity is accompanied by an increasingly atherogenic lipoprotein profile.*
10. Kahle, E. B., et al. Moderate diet control in children: The effects on metabolic indicators that predict obesity-related degenerative diseases. *Am. J. Clin. Nutr.* 35(5):950, 1982. *Presents practical approach for normalizing metabolism in obese male children.*
11. American Academy of Pediatrics, Committee on Nutrition. Nutritional aspect of obesity in infancy and childhood. *Pediatrics* 68(6):880, 1981. *AAP policy statement.*
12. American Academy of Pediatrics, Committee on Nutrition. *Pediatric Nutrition Handbook.* Evanston, IL: American Academy of Pediatrics, 1979. *Reference text covering all aspects of clinical nutrition.*
13. Stunkard, A. J., et al. An adoption study of human obesity. *N. Engl. J. Med.* 314(4):193, 1986.
14. Mallick, M. J. Health hazards of obesity and weight control in children: A review of the literature. *Am. J. Public Health* 73(1):78, 1983. *Discusses risk factors associated with significant weight loss in children.*
15. Pugliese, M. T., et al. Fear of obesity: A cause of short stature and delayed puberty. *N. Engl. J. Med.* 309(9):518, 1983. *A study showing that self-imposed calorie restrictions by children and adolescents may cause decreased stature and delay puberty.*
16. Dietz, W. H., Jr., and Hartung, R. Changes in height velocity of obese preadolescents during weight reduction. *Am. J. Dis. Child.* 139(7):705, 1985. *Presents data that indicate that mildly restrictive diets may be associated with a linear reduction in growth velocity.*
17. Reeves, J. D., et al. Iron deficiency in health and disease. *Adv. Pediatr.* 30:281, 1983. *Review article that discusses prevalence, etiology, diagnosis, and treatment of iron deficiency in sick and healthy children.*
18. Scrimshaw, N. S. Functional consequences of iron deficiency in human populations. *J. Nutr. Sci. Vitaminol.* (30)1:47, 1984. *Review of evidence that iron deficiency impairs resistance to infections, cognitive performance, physical capacity, and work output.*
19. Centers for Disease Control. Declining anemia prevalence among children enrolled in public nutrition and health programs—selected states, 1975–1985. *M.M.W.R.* (35)36:565, 1986. *Documents reduction in prevalence of anemia by WIC participants.*
20. Henretig, F. M., and Temple, A. R. Acute iron poisoning in children. *Clin. Lab. Med.* 4(3):575, 1984. *Describes the pathophysiology, clinical manifestations, management, and treatment of acute iron poisoning in children.*
21. Weidman, W., et al. AHA Committee Report. Diet in the healthy child: Task Force Com-

mittee of the Nutrition Committee and Cardiovascular Disease in the Young, Council of the American Heart Association. *Circulation* 67(6):1411a, 1983. *Position paper on diet and cardiovascular disease in the young by American Heart Association Task Force.*
22. Glueck, C. J. Pediatric primary prevention of atherosclerosis. *N. Engl. J. Med.* 314(3):175, 1986. *Excellent short summary article on guidelines for pediatric prevention programs.*
23. Newman, W. P., 3d., et al. Relation of serum lipoprotein levels and systolic blood pressure to early atherosclerosis. The Bogalusa Heart Study. *N. Engl. J. Med.* 314(3):138, 1986. *A study showing that elevated blood pressure and low density lipoprotein cholesterol in children was associated with fatty streaks at autopsy.*
24. Watkins, L. O., and Strong, W. B. The child: When to begin preventive cardiology. *Curr. Probl. Pediatr.* 14(6):1, 1984. *Monograph discussing the feasibility of primary prevention of coronary artery disease in the pediatric population.*
25. American Academy of Pediatrics, Committee on Nutrition. Toward a prudent diet for children. *Pediatrics* 71(1):78, 1983. *Position paper on diet and cardiovascular disease in children and adolescents by the American Academy of Pediatrics Committee on Nutrition.*
26. Dwyer, J. Diets for children and adolescents that meet the dietary goals. *Am. J. Dis. Child.* 134(11):1073, 1980. *Guidelines and menus for a modified fat intake in children.*
27. Orchard, T. J., et al. Cholesterol screening in childhood: Does it predict adult hypercholesterolemia? The Beaver County experience. *J. Pediatr.* 103(5):687, 1983. *Results suggest that screening for hypercholesterolemia at age 12 is fairly predictive of adult values.*
28. Fanelli, M. Promoting women's health. *Dietetics Curr.* 12(4):19, 1985. *List of available calcium supplements.*
29. Amschler, D. Calcium intake: A lifelong proposition. *J. Sch. Health* 55:360, 1985. *Discusses need to include significant amounts of calcium in the diet during the first 30 years.*
30. Spencer, H., et al. Calcium requirements in humans: Report of original data and a review. *Clin. Orthop.* 184:270, 1984. *Evidence that an intake of 1000–1200 mg/day is preferred, as it increases calcium balance.*
31. Newbrun, E. Sugar and dental caries: A review of human studies. *Science* 217:418, 1982. *Excellent review.*
32. Shannon, I. L., Edmonds, E. J., and Madsen, K. O. Honey: Sugar content and cariogenicity. *A.S.D.C. J. Dent. Child.* 46(1):29, 1979. *Discusses relative cariogenicity of sweeteners.*
33. Laven, G. T. Preventive nutrition guidelines for children. *Ala. J. Med. Sci.* 19(4):382, 1982. *Presents practical suggestions for diet intervention for children with hypertension, atherosclerosis, obesity, and dental caries.*
34. Tiegen, V. E., Sintes, J. L., and Dwyer, J. T. A model for evaluating cariogenicity applied to vegetarian diets. *A.S.D.C. J. Dent. Child.* 48(4):278, 1981. *Classification system for cariogenic potential of vegetarian diets.*
35. Watson, M. L. The relationship between dietary factors and dental caries. *J. Sch. Health* 52(1):39, 1982. *Practical dietary advice for parents for caries prevention.*

31 Adolescent Pregnancy

Robert A. Hatcher and
James Trussell

One out of ten women aged 15–19 in the United States becomes pregnant each year. There is an overwhelming consensus that teenage pregnancy is a serious problem. Approaches to this problem include encouraging **delay in the onset of sexual intercourse; sex education,** with attention to the consequences of early sexual intercourse, teenage pregnancy, and contraception; and promoting the consistent use of effective **contraceptives** by sexually active adolescents to prevent unintended pregnancies [1, 2].

I. The problem

A. Definition. Adolescent pregnancy is any pregnancy in a woman under 20 years of age leading to a spontaneous miscarriage, termination of pregnancy, or birth of an infant.

B. Consequences of teenage pregnancy

1. **Health consequences for the mother.** Adolescents who become pregnant are less likely to receive adequate prenatal care, to eat well during pregnancy, or to have support systems that stress the importance of avoiding alcohol, smoking, or dieting during pregnancy. Rates of caesarean section are slightly higher for young teenagers than for adults. Teenagers experience slightly higher abortion complication rates than older women, even when complications are controlled for gestational age. But the major reason for the increase in the rate of such complications is that teenagers terminate pregnancies later than do older women.
2. **Health consequences for the child.** The negative consequences for the child born to a teenage mother include the following: delivery at a low birth weight; high fetal, perinatal, neonatal, postneonatal, and infant mortality; and slower rates of subsequent cognitive development [1].
3. **Socioeconomic consequences for the mother.** Women who are young at the time they give birth to their first child experience more closely spaced subsequent births, have more unwanted and out-of-wedlock children, face greater marital instability, are more poorly educated, and have fewer assets and lower incomes later in life [1].

   Measures of academic progress, educational plans, and scholastic aptitude were available to Card and Wise [3] from a longitudinal study of high school students. For each teenager who subsequently became a mother before age 18, Card and Wise found a control teenager who did not bear a child before 18 but who otherwise was as similar as possible in socioeconomic status, academic achievement, aptitude, and educational expectations. This matched sample was used to study differences between groups for selected outcome variables. By age 29, only half of the women in the youngest childbearing group (under age 18) had received high school diplomas, whereas nearly all those who postponed childbearing until after age 20 received high school diplomas. Similar results hold for college degrees: Only 2% of those who bore a child before age 18 obtained a degree by age 29, compared with 22% of those who did not have a child by age 24 [3].

C. Epidemiology

1. **Age and trends over time.** In 1981, 1.4% of 14-year-old girls in the United States became pregnant. This proportion rose steadily with age to 15% of women aged 19. The fraction of pregnancies ending in a birth also rose with age, from 39% among those aged 14, to 60% among those aged 19. Birthrates among 15- to 19-year-old women declined steadily from 1971 to 1978, then remained rather constant through 1982. In contrast, abortion rates rose steadily from 1973 (the year abortion was legalized) to 1979, and then remained rather constant through 1981. The increase in abortion rates initially more than outweighed the decrease in birthrates, however, so that pregnancy rates rose steadily from 1973 to 1980. Since 1980 they have fallen slightly [4].

2. **Marital status and race.** In 1981, four of five pregnancies among teenagers were conceived out of wedlock. Of these, over half (53%) were terminated by abortion, one-third (34%) resulted in an out-of-wedlock birth, and the remainder (12%) resulted in a marital birth because the woman married before the delivery. Approximately 18% of 18- to 19-year-old women are pregnant at marriage compared with one-third of brides under 18. Overall, 8% of 15- to 19-year-old women were enumerated as married in the 1980 census; the proportion rose from 1% of those age 15 to 20% of those age 19. Of the one in five pregnancies conceived in marriage, the vast majority (87%) were carried to term. Thus, although married teenagers are three times more likely to conceive (1 in 4) than are unmarried teenagers (1 in 12), there are relatively so few married that they contribute only a minority of the total pregnancies each year [4].

   Teenage pregnancy rates among blacks are nearly twice as high as those among whites (163.2 per 1000 black women aged 15–19 in 1981 versus 83.4 per 1000 white women). Furthermore, whites are more likely to abort a pregnancy than are blacks, so that the differential in birthrates is even larger: 96.9 births per 1000 black women aged 15–19 versus 44.7 per 1000 white women [4].

3. **Intentional versus unintentional pregnancy.** Intentional pregnancies comprise only 23% of all conceptions among women aged 15–19, 76% of conceptions among married women, and only 9% of conceptions among unmarried women [4]. Hence, each year 1 of every 14 women becomes unintentionally pregnant—for two primary reasons. First, in 1982 only 1 of every 2 women aged 15–19 was still a virgin, and 4 of 10 had experienced intercourse within the previous 3 months. Among never-married women, the corresponding figures are approximately 4 in 10 and 1 in 3, respectively. Second, teenagers are poor users of contraception. Among those surveyed in 1982, only 1 of every 2 reported use of a contraceptive at first intercourse; of these, 47% used the condom, 27% relied on withdrawal, and only 17% used oral contraceptives [5]. Among premaritally sexually active women in a 1979 survey, 27%, 39%, and 34% reported that they never, sometimes, and always used a contraceptive, respectively [6]. Why do so many teenage girls fail to use contraceptives? In a 1976 survey, among unmarried women who did not use a method at the time they last had intercourse, even though they did not want to get pregnant, half thought that they could not conceive. Of the remainder, 80% stated that they had not expected to have intercourse [7].

II. General health promotion: Preventing teen pregnancy

A. Sex education. It is beyond the scope of this chapter to describe the numerous innovative sex education programs that have been developed in the United States. Programs designed to teach young people and their parents how to communicate about their sexuality, and to provide specific information about reproductive physiology, contraceptives, and pregnancy are extremely important. Boys and girls, as well as young men and young women, must also be taught how to make effective decisions about sex. One of the best evaluated sex education programs in the country has demonstrated that a comprehensive approach to sexual information and decision-making delays slightly the onset of sexual intercourse, leads to increased utilization of contraceptives by sexually active teenagers, and decreases the rate of teenage pregnancies [8].

B. Contraception. Each of the fertility control options that may be open to teenagers is discussed below in the order in which they appear in Tables 31-1 and 31-2.

1. **Abstinence.** Abstinence has tremendous advantages for teenagers. Abstinence protects a couple from pregnancy, infections, cervical dysplasia, and infertility later in life. In most cultures, abstinence is considered the right or moral or good thing to do. However, abstinence may be very difficult for some young couples to adhere to, and pregnancies may occur when a couple practicing abstinence decides to start having intercourse.
2. **Withdrawal or coitus interruptus.** Withdrawal is always available, and it is inexpensive, does not require a visit to a clinician, encourages male involvement, and does not have medical complications. However, withdrawal requires a level of discipline that some couples find extremely difficult to achieve. At a point when intercourse is very pleasurable, the penis must be withdrawn from the vagina. Because this timing is so difficult and pre-ejaculate secretions may contain sperm, effectiveness is poor.
3. **Alternatives to sexual intercourse.** Intimate sex without intercourse is one of the contraceptive options often chosen by teenagers. Noncoital forms of sexual intimacy ("outercourse") exist in many cultures, encompassing a continuum of

activities from holding hands, hugging, kissing, and dancing, to mutual masturbation, petting, and oral genital sex [2, 9].

Alternate forms of sexual pleasure are always available and require no medical intervention, produce fewer medical complications, do not cost money, can be purchased anonymously, and definitely involve the male as well as the female in the decision-making process. Some people argue that alternatives to sexual intercourse are the ideal contraceptive for teenagers, preventing most infections and unwanted pregnancies while permitting young people to explore their sexual feelings.

4. **Condom** [9]. Highly effective if used consistently and correctly, condoms are the most effective means of preventing sexually transmitted infections. Fear of herpes, chlamydia, condyloma accuminata, gonorrhea, and acquired immune deficiency syndrome (AIDS) is causing dramatic increase in the use of condoms.

   Certain infectious agents have been found in semen, and these agents may be deposited in a woman's vagina at the time of intercourse. Viruses found in semen are the AIDS virus, group B hepatitis, and cytomegalovirus. The bacteria found in semen are gonorrhea, *Chlamydia trachomatis*, mycoplasma, ureaplasma, and group B streptococcus. The protozoan agent *Trichomonas vaginalis* is also transmitted in semen.

   Condoms are inexpensive, available without a visit to a physician, safe, and have a protective effect against cervical dysplasia. While not all couples are willing to use condoms, those who do tend to use them more consistently and correctly than couples choosing to use diaphragms, sponges, foam, or suppositories. By prolonging the plateau phase of the sexual response cycle for men, condoms can make intercourse more pleasurable for the man and the woman. On the other hand, condoms interrupt spontaneity, cannot be controlled by the woman as readily as some methods, are considered messy by some couples, and are aesthetically unpleasing to some couples. Most condom failures are due to incorrect or inconsistent use.

5. **Aerosol foam.** Foam has the twin advantages of being available without a prescription and of having no medical complications. Spermicidal foams may also have some protective effects against sexually transmitted infections. However, foam is bulky to carry about, it is messy, it tends to be used inconsistently, it interrupts sexual spontaneity, and it may cause vaginal irritation.

6. **The sponge** [9]. Many of the advantages of the Today contraceptive sponge for teenagers relate to its convenience. It is available without prescription and anonymously; it is small, easy to carry, nonobtrusive if carried in a pocketbook, and fairly inexpensive. It is soft and nonthreatening. Its insertion may be separated by hours from sexual intercourse, and one sponge can protect a woman from several acts of sexual intercourse over a 24-hour period. It is safe and may have some protective effects against sexually transmitted infections.

   The sponge failure rate is about the same as that of the diaphragm among nulliparous women. The failure rate is much higher among multiparous women. At times, women have difficulty removing the sponge, and occasionally, the sponge causes vaginal irritation. The relationship of the sponge to the toxic shock syndrome is not completely clear. For couples having daily intercourse, it may be expensive. Disposal of the sponge may be an inconvenience for some couples.

7. **Diaphragm with spermicide** [9]. While young teenagers tend not to use the diaphragm, some university-age women find the diaphragm an attractive option. Its major advantages are that it is nonhormonal and quite safe. It appears to have a protective effect against upper genital tract infections (pelvic inflammatory disease [PID]) and cervical dysplasia. Its use familiarizes the woman (and sometimes her partner) with her reproductive anatomy. Diaphragms might be more consistently used by young couples if they realized that the diaphragm can be inserted as long as 6–8 hours prior to intercourse.

   Some women have great difficulty learning to insert and remove their diaphragm. The initial cost of the medical visit for diaphragm fitting, cost of the diaphragm itself, and the recurrent cost of tubes of spermicide may be fairly high. For some young women with vaginismus, diaphragm fitting should be delayed a week or so and the patient taught how to manually dilate the opening of her vagina. The diaphragm may be forgotten on trips or if a woman has intercourse in a place other than her own home. It is the careless and inconsistent use of the diaphragm that contributes to its high failure rate. The first-year failure rate for women under the age of 22 is 33%. The one medical complica-

Table 31-1. Relative advantages of fertility control options

Advantage	Contraceptive method							
	Abstinence	Withdrawal	Alternatives to sexual intercourse	Condom	Aerosol foam	Foaming tablets	Sponge	Diaphragm with spermicide
Effective	***		***	**	*	*	*	*
Easy to use	*	*	**	**	*	**	**	
Inexpensive	***	***	***	***	*	***	*	*
Does not require trained personnel	***	***	***	***	***	***	***	
Follow-up not required	***	***	***	***	***	***	**	*
May be separated from act of intercourse	***		***		*		**	*
Safe	***	***	***	***	***	***	***	**
Prevents sexually transmitted diseases	***	*	***	***	*	*	*	**
Prevents cervical dysplasia	***	*	***	***	*	*	*	**
Teaches reproductive anatomy		*	**	*	*	*	**	**
Encourages male involvement	***	***	***	***				
Prevents postcoital discharge	***	**	***	***			**	
Decreases menstrual cramps, pain								
Noncontraceptive benefits				**	*	*	*	*

Advantage	Contraceptive method								
	Cervical cup with spermicide	Fertility awareness methods	Combination birth control pills	Postcoital pills	Hormone injections	IUD	Tubal sterilization	Vasectomy	Abortion
Effective	*		***	*	***	**	***	***	***
Easy to use			*	*	**	***	***	***	
Inexpensive	*	*	*	*	*	**	*	**	
Does not require trained personnel				*	*				
Follow-up not required	*	*		*	*		**	*	
May be separated from act of intercourse	**	*	***		***	***	***	***	***
Safe	*	***	*	**	**	*	**	***	**
Prevents sexually transmitted diseases			**		**		*	*	
Prevents cervical dysplasia	*								
Teaches reproductive anatomy	***	***	*		*	**	*	*	*
Encourages male involvement		*						***	*
Prevents postcoital discharge									
Decreases menstrual cramps, pain			***		***				
Noncontraceptive benefits	*	*	***		**				

Key: ***=very advantageous; **=moderately advantageous; *=slightly advantageous.
Source: Substantial portions of this table were derived or taken directly from 1984 and 1985 editions of R. Hatcher, et al. *Contraceptive Technology 1986–1987*.

Table 31-2. Relative disadvantages of fertility control options

Disadvantage	Contraceptive method							
	Abstinence	Withdrawal	Alternatives to sexual intercourse	Condom	Aerosol foam	Foaming tablets	Sponge	Diaphragm with spermicide
Difficult to use	**	**	**	*	**	*	*	***
High cost per year					*		**	**
Interrupts sexual spontaneity	***	***	*	***	**	**	*	**
Vaginal manipulation required					*	*	**	**
Awkward to carry				*	***	*	*	**
Male involvement required	***	***	***	**	*	*		
Side effects or complications		*		*	*	*	*	*
Removal may be difficult							*	*
Disposal may be difficult				*	*		**	
Vaginal irritation				*	**	**	*	**
Vaginal discharge					**	**	*	**
Vaginal odor							*	*
Vaginal abrasion							*	*
Breakthrough bleeding or spotting								
Pelvic infection								

Disadvantage	Contraceptive method								
	Cervical cup with spermicide	Fertility awareness methods	Combination birth control pills	Postcoital pills	Hormone injections	IUD	Tubal sterilization	Vasectomy	Abortion
Difficult to use	***	***	*	*	*	*	*	*	***
High cost per year	**	*	**	*	*	*	*	*	***
Interrupts sexual spontaneity	*	***							
Vaginal manipulation required	***	**				*			
Awkward to carry	*		*						
Male involvement required		***						***	
Side effects or complications	*		**	*	*	**	*	*	**
Removal may be difficult	**				***	**			
Disposal may be difficult									
Vaginal irritation	**					*			
Vaginal discharge	*					**			*
Vaginal odor	**					*			
Vaginal abrasion	**								
Breakthrough bleeding or spotting			**	*	**	**			*
Pelvic infection						**			*

Key: ***=very disadvantageous; **=moderately disadvantageous; *=slightly disadvantageous.
Source: Substantial portions of this table were derived or taken directly from 1984 and 1985 editions of R. Hatcher, et al. *Contraceptive Technology 1986–1987*.

tion of the diaphragm is that a woman is more likely to develop urethritis or cystitis, which may be caused by the pressure of the rim of the diaphragm against the urethra.

8. **Fertility-awareness methods** [9]. No method teaches a young woman more about her reproductive anatomy and physiology than the various fertility awareness techniques. Moreover, these approaches are readily accepted by all religious and cultural groups. Fertility awareness methods include the rhythm method (or "calendar" method), the basal body temperature (BBT) method, the mucous method (or Billings method), and the symptothermal method. Each approach helps a woman determine when during the menstrual cycle she is most likely to be ovulating and hence capable of becoming pregnant. Fertility awareness methods are free of medical complications, may involve the male partner, and may be used when a couple is trying to become pregnant as well as when trying to avoid pregnancy. However, these approaches tend to be very difficult for women having irregular menses. The extensive periods of abstinence may be difficult to adhere to. The failure rate is typically high.
9. **Combined birth control pills** [9]. Birth control pills are the most widely available and the most effective reversible approaches to contraception for teenagers. Taking the Pill is separated from the act of intercourse, which is a major advantage. The noncontraceptive advantages of the Pill, such as decreased menstrual cramps, decreased menstrual blood loss, more regular menses, lowered risk of hospitalization for PID, prevention of fibrocystic breast disease and functional ovarian cysts, and the prevention or even treatment of acne, may be important considerations for the sexually active teenager or university student who is trying to choose between myriad contraceptive options. Since the Pill and condoms stand out as the best contraceptive options for young women (with the exception of abstinence), the instructions for the use of these two contraceptives are included in this chapter (Figs. 31-1, 31-2).

   The Pill may also have disadvantages as a contraceptive for young sexually active women. Since the Pill requires a prescription in many cultures throughout the world, teenagers fear that they may lose their anonymity by using this approach to birth control. The cost of the Pill ($9.95–$19.95 per cycle) may also deter some individuals from using this method, as may fear of complications or side effects such as nausea, spotting, breakthrough bleeding, scanty menses, headaches, and breast tenderness. If problems or questions arise regarding birth control pills, the support systems the young teenagers might utilize may be quite limited.
10. **Postcoital pills** [9]. If safe and effective postcoital contraceptives were readily available for teenagers who have unprotected intercourse, they would become popular methods of birth control. Recent studies have indicated that Ovral, which contains 50 μg of ethinylestradiol and 0.5 mg of dl-norgestrel, is an effective postcoital contraceptive. Two Ovral tablets are taken within 72 hours of coitus, and 2 more are taken 12 hours later. Yuzpe, in two multicenter trials in Canada, tested this approach on a total of 1300 women [10, 11]. The failure rate in the first trial was 0.16% and in the second was 1.6%.

    While postcoital pills are safe, easy to use, inexpensive, and fairly effective, they have some disadvantages too. Many clinicians are unfamiliar with their use; they can produce nausea, vomiting, or breakthrough bleeding; and they tend to raise some of the same moral and ethical questions as do abortions. Given the unpredictable pattern of sexual intercourse for many young teenagers and for some university-age students, however, postcoital contraception, if widely available, could prevent many unwanted pregnancies.
11. **Hormone injections and implants.** The subcutaneous Norplant implant, which releases very low levels of levo-norgestrel over a 5- to 7-year period, is more likely to gain Food and Drug Administration approval than Depo-Provera. The effectiveness of the Norplant implant, its acceptability to women in a number of cultures throughout the world, and the safety and reversibility of this approach suggest that it may play a major role in fertility control programs serving teenagers throughout the world in the near future. However, the need for physician involvement may present an obstacle to adolescent use.
12. **Intrauterine devices (IUD).** Although IUDs—which may be left in place for a number of years—are effective, easy to use once inserted, inexpensive, require no effort at the time of intercourse, and are usually safe, they are not an appropriate contraceptive for teenagers who may have a number of different sexual part-

1. The combination pill is made up of two hormones—estrogen and progestin. It works by stopping ovulation (release of an egg). If there is no egg to unite with a sperm, pregnancy cannot occur. The pill is very effective if you follow these directions carefully and faithfully.
2. Choose a backup method of birth control (such as condoms or foam) to use along with your first pack of pills. The pill may not fully protect you from pregnancy during the first month. Keep the backup method handy at all times. Learn to use it well in case you:
   a. Run out of pills.
   b. Forget pills.
   c. Experience pill danger signals.
3. There are several ways to start taking your pills; there is no single "right" way. You should start your pills in the way your physician suggests. You may be told to:
   a. Start your first pack on the day you begin bleeding during your period.
   b. Start your first pack on the first Sunday after your period begins.
   c. Start your first pack on the fifth day after you start your period.
   d. Start your pills today if there is absolutely no chance that you could be pregnant. Check with your physician to see how long to use a backup method.
4. Be sure to read the package insert for the pills you are using. The Food and Drug Administration (FDA) now requires that all drugstores give each pill user a copy of an extensive pamphlet to read. The pamphlet is produced by your pill manufacturer and approved by the FDA. It gives you excellent and detailed information about the pill's benefits and risks. Read the whole pamphlet carefully.
5. Take one pill a day until you finish the pack. Then:
   a. If you are using a 21-day pack, stop taking the pills for one week and then start your new pack.
   b. If you are using a 28-day pack, begin a new pack immediately.
6. Try to associate taking your pill with something else that you do at the same time every day, such as going to bed, eating a meal, or brushing your teeth. This may make it easier to remember. The pill works best if you take one about the same time every day; this keeps a steady level of hormones in your system.
7. If you have bleeding between periods, try to take your pill at the same time every day. If you have spotting (light bleeding between periods) for two or more cycles, call your doctor. You may need a different pill.
8. Check your pack of birth control pills each morning to make sure you took your pill the day before.
9. If you miss one pill, take the forgotten one (yesterday's pill) as soon as you remember it and take today's pill at the regular time. You probably will not get pregnant. To be certain, use your backup method until your next period.

Fig. 31-1. Instructions for combination pill users

ners before beginning their childbearing. Pelvic inflammatory disease is the most important serious complication that may occur in IUD users.

13. **Tubal ligation and vasectomy.** Clearly, sterilization is not an appropriate contraceptive option for most teenagers.
14. **Abortion.** Abortion is a more attractive option for some teenagers than carrying a pregnancy to term, and approximately 45% of all pregnancies in United States teenagers ages 15–19 result in pregnancy termination procedures. However, the use of contraceptives or abstinence to prevent unwanted pregnancies has clear advantages over abortion to terminate them.

III. Recommendations

A. Comprehensive sex education designed to outline the serious implications to teenagers of early pregnancy and the methods of avoiding teenage pregnancy if a person is sexually active should be instituted for children age 10 and above [8].

B. Abstinence and alternatives to sexual intercourse should be encouraged in teenagers.

1. The condom is a rubber or membrane sheath that is placed on the erect penis before intercourse to keep sperm from getting into the vagina.
2. The most important rule is to use condoms every single time you have intercourse. When condom-using couples have an unplanned pregnancy, it is almost always because they did not use condoms correctly each time they had intercourse.
3. Use of spermicidal condoms is recommended. These condoms have spermicide suspended in a lubricant. The two brands of spermicidal condoms currently available are Prime Spermicidal and Ramses Extra. Spermicidal condoms are not recommended if either partner has an allergy to the spermicide or if the couple prefers not to use prelubricated condoms.
4. Roll the rim of the condom all the way to the base of the penis before the penis is put in the vagina. If the condom does not already have a nipple tip (reservoir), leave about one-half inch of empty space (not filled with air) at the tip of the condom to catch the sperm.
5. Do not use Vaseline or other petroleum jelly with your condom because it may deteriorate the rubber. If you want to use lubrication on the outside of the condom to help the penis enter the vagina, K-Y Jelly, contraceptive foam, and saliva may be used. One of these should certainly be used if the woman does not feel sufficiently lubricated, since the condom could tear when the penis first enters the vagina.
6. Condoms are more effective if used along with another method of birth control, such as a spermicide, the sponge, or a diaphragm.
7. After intercourse, hold onto the rim of the condom as you remove the penis from the vagina. Be careful not to spill any semen near the woman's vagina. The penis should be withdrawn soon after ejaculation because the condom may slip off into the vagina if the man loses his erection, allowing sperm to escape and a possible pregnancy to occur. This possibility is one of the reasons why condoms that contain spermicide are recommended; if any sperm spill out of the condom, they may already be immobilized by the spermicide.
8. Check the condom before you throw it away. A quick look will tell you if it is torn or not. If the condom tears or comes off in the vagina, insert contraceptive foam or jelly immediately. Although the insertion of foam or jelly does not assure that pregnancy has been prevented, it may help kill some sperm and it is certainly better than doing nothing.
9. After you have used a condom once, throw it away. This is especially important if you are using condoms to protect against sexually transmitted diseases. You may be able to buy condoms cheaply or obtain them free at clinics.
10. Store condoms in a cool, dry place. Do not keep condoms in a wallet or other hot place for a long time because heat (even body heat) can cause rubber to deteriorate. If condoms are kept relatively dry and away from heat, they will probably last 5 years.

Fig. 31-2. Instructions for condom users.

C. Contraceptives should be readily available to those teenagers who are sexually active and do not want to become pregnant. Birth control pills and condoms together would be an ideal approach to prevention of both pregnancy and sexually transmissible infections.

D. Abortion should be available as an option to those teenagers who fail to use contraceptives or who have contraceptive failures and are faced with an unwanted pregnancy.

References

1. Trussell, J. Adolescent Pregnancy. In R. A. Hatcher, et al. (eds.), *Contraceptive Technology 1986–1987.* New York: Irvington Publishers, 1986. *A well-referenced chapter by James Trussell on causes, consequences, and recommendations for the prevention of adolescent pregnancy, in a practical manual on methods of contraception.*

2. Withington, A. M., Grimes, D. A., and Hatcher, R. A. *Teenage Sexual Health.* New York: Irvington Publishers, 1983. *Textbook outlining the magnitude, consequences, and methods of prevention of teenage pregnancy. Emphasis is on counseling techniques designed to improve compliance in teenagers.*
3. Card, J. J., and Wise, L. L. Teenage mothers and teenage fathers: The impact of early childbearing on the parents' personal and professional lives. *Fam. Plann. Perspect.* 10(4):199, 1978. *Case control study of the consequences of teenage pregnancy.*
4. Jones, L., et al. *Teenage Pregnancy in Developed Countries.* New Haven: Yale University Press, 1986.
5. Pratt, W., et al. Understanding U.S. fertility: Findings from the National Survey of Family Growth, Cycle III. *Popul. Bull.* 39(5):1, 1984. *Summary of results from the 1982 National Survey of Family Growth.*
6. Zelnik, M., and Kantner, J. F. Sexual activity, contraceptive use and pregnancy among metropolitan area teenagers: 1971–1979. *Fam. Plann. Perspect.* 12(5):230, 1980. *Results from three surveys of teenagers.*
7. Zelnik, M., Kantner, J., and Ford, K. *Sex and Pregnancy in Adolescence.* Beverly Hills: Sage Publications, 1981. *Results from several surveys of teenagers on sexual behavior, childbearing, contraceptive practice, and marriage.*
8. Zabin, L. S., et al. Evaluation of a pregnancy prevention program for urban teenagers. *Fam. Plann. Perspect.* 16(4):181, 1984. *An early analysis of what may well be the most sophisticated teenage sex education developed thus far in the United States, indicating that sex education delays the onset of sexual intercourse and increases male involvement in the use of contraceptives in school systems in which sex education programs have been implemented.*
9. Hatcher, R., et al. *Contraceptive Technology 1986–1987.* New York: Irvington Publishers, 1986. *Practical manual on methods of contraception.*
10. Yuzpe, A. A., Smith, R. P., and Rademaker, A. W. A multicenter clinical investigation employing ethinyl estradiol combined with dl-norgestrel as a postcoital contraceptive agent. *Fertil. Steril.* (37)4:508, 1982. *Comprehensive article on the postcoital method of contraception used by most American and Canadian clinicians.*
11. Yuzpe, A. A., and Lancee, W. J. Ethinylestradiol and dl-norgestrel as postcoital contraceptive. *Fertil. Steril.* 28(9):932, 1977. *Initial report of what has come to be called the "Yuzpe approach" to postcoital contraception.*

32 Adolescent Substance Abuse

Richard L. Jones and
Robert B. Shearin

I. The problem

A. Definition. Substance use is or becomes abuse when it endangers the immediate or long-term health of the individual.

B. Description. Human use of herbs, potions, spirits, and chemicals to alter mood and relieve feelings of fatigue, sadness, and stress has been recorded throughout human history [1, 2]. In the United States, adolescent drug and alcohol use and abuse have become significant health problems since the 1950s [2, 3, 4].

Initial experimentation with mood-altering drugs often occurs prior to teenage years and usually involves the "gateway drugs": marijuana, alcohol, and cocaine (plus tobacco), or, to a lesser extent, inhalants such as solvents, aerosol sprays, degreasers, and gasoline [5–10]. Factors predisposing to early experimentation are described below.

The movement from experimentation to dependency is insidious but often recognizable by dysfunctional behavior(s) [5–10] (Table 32-1). Abusive use may be manifested by physical illness, especially if there is a predisposing history of seizures; latent mental illness; learning disabilities; attentional deficit disorders (ADDs); asthma; and cardiac, hepatic, or gastrointestinal disease [11]. The dysfunctional adolescent with chronic fatigue, cough, gastritis, peptic ulcer disease, hepatitis, pancreatitis, or recurrent accidents or injuries may be manifesting signs of alcohol and substance abuse (Tables 32-2 and 32-3).

C. Epidemiology [12]. Among adolescents, accidents (through automobiles, falls, fires, drownings), homicides, and suicides are the three leading causes of death. Alcohol or drug intoxication, or both, are important factors in a majority of these deaths [13]. Adolescents failing in school and involved in crime and vandalism are often abusive drug users. Unquestionably, the use of mind-altering drugs by adolescents may result in a pattern of prolonged use or abuse; an increased incidence of acute or chronic disease(s), or both; delayed or arrested psychosocial maturation; and decreased productivity as a member of society [5–10].

Males use more alcohol, drugs, and other illicit substances than females, but females exceed males in cigarette use [14]. Three-fourths of male and two-thirds of female high school seniors used alcohol during the previous month. More worrisome is that 51% of the males and 39% of the females admit having more than five drinks in a row during the previous two weeks [15]. In 1977, the proportion of high school seniors who smoked a half-pack or more daily was about 20%, although this figure has been declining slightly since that time. Marijuana use at any time by high school seniors seems to have leveled off at around 30% and 40% for females and males, respectively; less than 10% are daily marijuana users. Phencyclidine and cocaine have achieved more recent widespread use, and use rates of the latter are rising [16].

D. Risk factors. While rates of substance abuse by teenagers have increased dramatically from the 1950s and the substances selected for abuse have changed over time, the type of young people most at risk seems relatively constant. Major factors that increase risk of substance abuse among adolescents include the following [9,10,15,17–19]:

1. **Age** [1,5–7,9,10,17–19,20]. Early (pre- and early adolescent) adoption of abusive habits tends to predict later use, and urban males are at highest risk for early experimentation.
2. **Male sex** [4,6,9,10,15,17,19]. Males abuse more substances (except cigarettes) at younger ages than females.
3. **Family history** [5–10,19]. Alcoholism on either side of the family and family problems—including divorce, abuse, inconsistent or impulsive parenting—

Table 32-1. Behavioral parameters seen in substance and alcohol abusers

- A worsening in school performance
- School truancy
- Symptoms of acute or chronic depression, or both
- Unexplained or recurrent accidents or fights
- Repeated overt intoxications
- Preoccupation with social activities where alcohol or drugs, or both, might be present
- Decrease in communication with other family members
- Drug-using peer group
- Changes in dress and personal habits of hygiene
- Runaway behavior
- Court involvement regarding charges such as drunken or disorderly conduct or driving while intoxicated

Source: R. L. Jones. Identification and management of the toxic adolescent. *Semin. Adolesc. Med.* 1:239, 1985.

Table 32-2. Physical examination for target organ damage—signs and symptoms of alcohol and substance abuse by adolescents

- Central nervous system
  - Behavioral
  - Neurologic
    - Decreased short-term memory
    - Mixed dominance
    - Decreased fine motor movements
    - Symptoms compatible with attentional deficit disorder
- Gastrointestinal
  - Dyspepsia, epigastric or abdominal pain, melena, weight loss, poor oral hygiene
  - Epigastric rebound tenderness, liver enlargement
- Skin
  - Multiple bruises, evidence of old injury(s), gynecomastia, poor hygiene, tracks (rare among adolescents), poor nail hygiene
- Repiratory
  - Foul-smelling or cigarette breath, stained teeth, chronic cough, bronchitis (recurrent)
- Cardiac
  - Tachycardia, evidence of deconditioning
- Musculoskeletal
  - Evidence of multiple trauma; poor muscle tone, size, and strength; evidence of deconditioning
- Genitourinary
  - Testicular bogginess or atrophy, evidence of sexually transmitted diseases (condylomata, herpes, cervical dysplasia)
- Eyes
  - Injected conjunctiva
- Nose
  - Chronic nasal discharge, recurrent nosebleeds, nasal mucosal irritation or hemorrhage
- Auditory
  - Decreased auditory acuity (conductive)

Source: R. L. Jones. Identification and management of the toxic adolescent. *Semin. Adolesc. Med.* 1:239, 1985.

Table 32-3. Laboratory clues to alcohol and substance abuse (screening tests)

Test	Comments
Complete blood count	Look for macrocytosis and anemia
Liver function tests	Elevations in SGOT (ALT), SGPT (AST) or GGT enzymes may suggest chemical hepatitis. (If enzyme elevation is present, other causes of hepatitis must be ruled out.)
Blood alcohol level	
Urine alcohol level[a]	
Urine screens for drugs[a, b]	
Nicotine metabolites	If present when the patient is denying cigarette or chewing tobacco use, presence of nicotine may indicate a falacious history.
THC	Indicates marijuana use in recent past (7–10 days)
Stimulants	If present may indicate more extensive drug experimentation/abuse than has been admitted.
Cross-addictive drugs (sedatives, tranquilizers, methylqualone)	If present probably indicates serious, multiple drug use
Narcotics	Not usually tested for in most adolescents; if present, extensive drug abuse/addiction has probably occured
Tests for amylase, occult blood in the stool, and sexually transmitted diseases may be indicated; chest x-ray may be indicated.	

Key: SGOT=serum glutamic-oxaloacetic transaminase; ALT=alanine aminotransferase; SGPT=serum glutamic-pyruvic transaminase; AST=aspartate aminotransferase; GGT=gamma glutamyl transpeptidase.

[a]All urines should be collected with direct visual or auditory, or both, confirmations, especially when the patient has not been cooperative or is a sophisticated drug user.

[b]When patient contamination of a urine sample submitted for drug testing is suspected, do a complete urinalysis. A pH greater than 7.0 or the presence of microscopic contamination (e.g., red blood cells, mucus) may render the spectrophotometric test for THC (e.g., EMIT) falsely negative. Repeat the test.

Source: R. L. Jones. Identification and management of the toxic adolescent. *Semin. Adolesc. Med.* 1:239, 1985.

increase the risk of substance abuse. A family history of teetotalism decreases risk. Poor relationships with parents and perceived parental drug use increase risk.

4. **Availability** [5–10,19] of alcohol and drugs increases risk.
5. **Peer modeling** [7–10]. Adolescents tend to adopt the behavior of their peer groups; preference for a drug-using peer group increases risk. Lack of social conformity, sensation-seeking, and perceived peer drug use increase risk.
6. **Psychopathology, attention deficit disorder, and/or learning disabilities** [7,9] increase risk. Depression, isolation, and low self-esteem increase risk.
7. **Poverty, education, religiosity, and ethnicity** [10,17,19,20] influence risk. Low grade point average and lack of religiosity increase risk.

II. General health promotion

A. Methods. Delaying early drug experimentation may offer the best approach to the prevention of abusive drug use by adolescents. Techniques that can be used include the following:

1. **Anticipatory guidance.** The American Academy of Pediatrics Committee on Drugs concluded that:

> The [health care provider's] best recourse, at present, is to become active in efforts at prevention. Before they reach the age of greatest risk, **school-age children** should be well informed about the physiological and psychological effects of marijuana, alcohol, [tobacco], and other psychoactive agents. The physician's role is to provide such information. . . [C]aveats must be accurate and not overstated if the child is to continue to look to the practitioner as a source of truthful information [21].

Note that these efforts begin with the elementary school child, since efforts started later are less likely to succeed. The parents' substance abuse behaviors and attitudes should also be considered (see Chaps. 66 and 67). Strategies for discouraging teenage smoking [22,23] are given below [19].

- **a.** Only casually mention the long-range health effects of smoking.
- **b.** Review the immediate physiological effects of tobacco use. (This is done to remind the adolescent of the short-term health consequences of smoking.)
- **c.** Suggest alternatives to smoking as ways of establishing an independent, mature, sophisticated social image.
- **d.** Discuss in detail short-term negative cosmetic effects of smoking, including those on teeth, breath, and skin.
- **e.** Mention the secondary health effects on nonsmokers from passive smoking as well as the increasing exclusion of smokers from selected public gathering places.
- **f.** Provide the older child and young adolescent with strategies for dealing with peer pressure to smoke.
- **g.** Provide in the physician's office information regarding the effects of smoking.

2. Multilevel efforts. Successful preventive strategies focus on individual children and adolescents, their small groups (families and peers), schools, and communities. Programs should incorporate the following [17,18,23,24].

- **a.** Efforts to foster personal and social growth combined with drug education to enhance the individual's skills to resist substance experimentation and abuse.
- **b.** Coordination of the resources of the government and the community.
- **c.** Utilization of the expertise of several disciplines (education, religion, law, and medicine).
- **d.** Incorporation of a variety of approaches.
- **e.** Monitoring results to achieve accountability [9,20,25].

Health care providers should play an active role in such efforts, which again are more likely to succeed if focused on elementary and junior high school children.

B. Justification

1. Effectiveness. The likelihood that anticipatory guidance can, by itself, avert substance abuse is remote. Nonetheless, it may be additive with other activities at home, school, church, and in the community.

Multilevel efforts that teach students the skills to resist social pressures have been effective in lowering the rates of smoking, alcohol, and drug use by junior high school students [18,23,24].

2. Risks. An authoritarian approach, inaccurate information, or efforts begun too late may actually enhance the likelihood of experimentation [18].

3. Costs and acceptability are difficult to estimate and vary widely depending on the approach taken.

III. Specific health promotion

A. Early assessment

1. Methods. Early detection methods do not appear to have evolved to the point that a specific test or tests exist that should be administered to all adolescents of a certain age or at certain intervals, and on which we can predictably rely in assessing the need to intervene. However, it does appear that providers who care for adolescents should be sensitive to the risk factors and behavioral parameters (see Table 32-1), as well as signs and symptoms of substance abuse (see Table 32-2). In that way, when they appear, more specific assessments can be made, including use of questionnaires, additional history, physical examination, and/or lab evaluation [26, 27, 28].

The presence of one or more major risk factors should increase the physician's concern about an adolescent's possible progression toward substance abuse. The use of specific questionnaires like the Michigan Alcoholic Screening Test

(MAST) [9,29] (Fig. 32-1), Adolescent Failure Syndrome Test [10] (Fig. 32-2), or the CAGE Questionnaire [30] (Fig. 32-3), given in a nonconfrontive, confidential manner, may help to assess the likelihood and seriousness of a problem.

The most reasonable screen for smoking at this time is simply to ask the teenager if he or she smokes.

Staging the severity of the adolescent's progression from experimentation to addiction (stages I–IV) [6,10] can help determine the kind of intervention needed.

2. **Justification.** With the exception of risk factors [9,19] and the MAST test, predictive accuracy of the early assessment devices described is not clearly defined for use with adolescents. The risks, costs, and acceptability are also not yet well known.

B. Early intervention

1. **Methods.** Primary medical care of children and adolescents can provide a confidential setting in which prevention through education and early intervention can occur [9,10,17,18,24,25,31]. Some intervention strategies that can take place in a primary care setting are given in Table 32-4. Allaying parental fears regarding drugs through education and reassurance, assessing the degree of drug use, and counseling the adolescent with the intent to inform, not reform, can and should be done in a primary care setting. Counseling done before or after office hours offers the best circumstances under which to further evaluate the scope of the adolescent's drug involvement and determine if referral is needed [7,9,10,25]. A medical-counseling evaluation procedure is given in Fig. 32-4.

   Evaluation and treatment of adolescents with serious substance abuse problems is complex and will often necessitate both working on drug withdrawal and educating, as well as psychotherapy. Often, multiple drugs are involved. For many patients, recognition and referral by those in primary care may be the appropriate action.

2. **Justification.** The effectiveness, risks, costs, and acceptability of the above interventions are difficult to assess but do represent current opinions of experts.

IV. Recommendations

A. General health promotion

1. Children and adolescents' education with respect to alcohol/drug/tobacco abuse can and should be effectively done in the primary care setting.
2. Children and adolescents should be strongly encouraged through education to abstain from or postpone tobacco (cigarettes or chewing tobacco), drug, and alcohol experimentation.
3. Physician involvement in community-based drug, alcohol, and tobacco education programs is important.
4. Health care providers should support efforts aimed at limiting drug and alcohol availability that have been shown to help prevent **early** experimentation (i.e., increasing the drinking age to 21, restricting drug paraphernalia).

B. Specific health promotion

1. Providers should be sensitive to the possibility of substance abuse in all adolescents and should use specific historical, physical, and laboratory data to help determine the extent of substance abuse (see Tables 32-1 to 32-3 and Figs. 32-1 to 32-3).
2. Smoking and less serious cases of substance/alcohol abuse (stages I, II) [8,9,10] should be treated by the primary care provider within the limits of his or her training (see Table 32-4).
3. Referral of serious substance/alcohol-abusing teenagers (stages III, IV) [8,9,10] usually requires collaboration between the primary care physician and treatment specialists.

Circle the response "Yes" or "No" depending on whether the statement says something true or not true about you. Please answer all questions. The test can be scored to let you know where you lie on a scale from a social drinker to addictive drinker.

	Question			
1.	Do you feel you are a normal drinker?	yes	**no**	2
2.	Have you ever awakened the morning after some drinking the night before and found that you could not remember a part of the evening?	**yes**	no	2
3.	Do your friends or family ever worry or complain about your drinking?	**yes**	no	1
4.	Can you stop drinking without a struggle after 1 or 2 drinks?	yes	**no**	2
5.	Do you ever feel bad about your drinking?	**yes**	no	1
6.	Do friends and relatives think you are a normal drinker?	yes	**no**	2
7.	Do you ever try to limit your drinking to certain times of the day or to certain places?	**yes**	no	0
8.	Are you always able to stop drinking when you want to?	yes	**no**	2
9.	Have you ever attended a meeting of Alcoholics Anonymous (AA)?	**yes**	no	5
10.	Have you gotten into fights when drinking?	**yes**	no	1
11.	Has your drinking every created problems with you and your friends or family?	**yes**	no	2
12.	Have your friends or any family member ever gone to anyone for help about your drinking?	**yes**	no	2
13.	Have you ever lost friends or a spouse because of your drinking?	**yes**	no	2
14.	Have you ever gotten into trouble at work or school because of your drinking?	**yes**	no	2
15.	Have you ever lost a job because of your drinking?	**yes**	no	2
16.	Have you ever neglected your obligations, your family, or your school work for two or more days in a row because you were drinking?	**yes**	no	2
17.	Do you ever drink before noon?	**yes**	no	2
18.	Have you ever been told you have liver trouble?	**yes**	no	1
19.	Have you ever had delirium tremens (DTs), severe shaking, heard voices, or seen things that were not there after heavy drinking?	**yes**	no	5
20.	Have you ever gone to anyone for help about your drinking?	**yes**	no	5
21.	Have you ever been in a hospital because of your drinking?	**yes**	no	5
22.	Have you ever been a patient in a psychiatric hospital, or in a psychiatric ward of a general hospital, where drinking was part of the problem?	**yes**	no	2
23.	Have you ever been seen at a psychiatric or mental health clinic, or gone to a doctor, social worker, or clergyman for help with an emotional problem in which drinking played a part?	**yes**	no	2
24.	Have you ever been arrested, even for a few hours, because of drunk behavior?	**yes**	no	2
25.	Have you ever been arrested for drunk driving or driving after drunk?	**yes**	no	2

Your score is ____________ :

Score	
0–3	Probably not alcoholic
5–10	80% of alcoholism
10 or above	Definitely alcoholic

Fig. 32-1. Michigan Alcoholism Screening Test (MAST) Questionnaire about drinking habits. (From M. L. Selzer. Michigan Alcoholism Screening Test The quest for a new diagnostic instrument. *Am. J. Psychiatry* 127:1653, 1971. Copyright 1971, the American Psychiatric Association. Reprinted by permission.)

	Does Not Apply	Possibly Applies	Definitely Applies
1. A change in the family's communication with adolescent. Refusal to take part in discussions concerning unacceptable behavior. Previous closeness may dissipate, and disciplinary talk interrupted either by "he tunes me out" or angry outbursts.	0	1	2
2. Refusal of the adolescent to recognize the impact on the family of unacceptable behavior, e.g., arguments, intoxicated events, or delinquent acts.	0	2	4
3. Concern expressed by others, e.g., siblings, classmates, teachers, other family members, or authority figures, concerning personality changes, suspected drug usage, or traveling with the "wrong crowd."	0	2	4
4. Expressed concern for oneself, e.g., "I'm worried I might get involved with drugs or alcohol," or "My life is meaningless, and I want to die."	0	2	4
5. Involvement in hard rock music, preoccupation with rock stars, attendance at rock concerts.	0	1	2
6. "Rebellious" dress style, e.g., rock-beer commercial T-shirts, army jackets, worn jeans, long hair.	0	1	2
7. Poor choice of friends, choosing to be with kids known or suspected of being delinquent and/or involved with drugs and alcohol.	0	2	4
8. Mysterious comings and goings, frequent telephone calls and visits by unfamiliar youth.	0	2	4
9. Change in social group, grade school friends left behind for a more "down and out group."	0	2	4
10. Incidents of untrustworthiness, particularly incorrect explanations of absence from school or lies about location of parties or parental chaperoning.	0	2	4
11. Unexcused absences from school or missed classes.	0	1	2
12. Minor or major delinquent involvement, especially where participants were intoxicated or drugs were involved.	0	2	4
13. Any violence or threat of violence toward parents or siblings.	0	2	4
14. Any violent episode away from home, including injury to self or others.	0	1	2
15. Minor or major automobile accidents.	0	1	2
16. Vocal disrespect for parents, teachers, or other authorities.	0	1	2

Fig. 32-2. Adolescent Failure Syndrome Test. (Copyright by David G. Logan, M.D., and Ronald E. Harrison, 2217 Packard Road, Suite 13, Ann Arbor, MI 48104. Used with permission.)

17. Unhealthy relationships. This includes a variety of unfortunate social styles, e.g., isolation from any close friends, choice of older, perhaps delinquent friends, or choice of a single friend to the exclusion of all others. No healthy involvement or interest in the opposite sex.	0	1	2
18. Premature adult behaviors, e.g., seductive dress or behavior, pseudo-sophisticated "existential" concerns, unreasonable questioning or rejection of family values, especially regarding "recreational" drug usage.	0	1	2
19. Early sexual involvement, e.g., concerns of pregnancy or discovery of birth control materials.	0	2	4
20. Mood swings, such as depression, irritability, or unexplained euphoria and talkativeness.	0	2	4
21. Sleep disturbances, particularly staying awake for long periods at night, or going to bed immediately after supper or on returning home.	0	2	4
22. A drop in grade averages, perhaps accompanied by a stated loss of interest in academic pursuits.	0	1	2
23. Money problems: missing money from purses or coin collections at home or babysitting jobs or homes of grandparents, or holds a steady job but does not show money in savings.	0	2	4
24. Annoyance or tantrums occur when questioned, e.g., about possible drug involvement.	0	2	4
25. Cigarette smoking.	0	2	4
26. Discovery of marijuana, pills, or alcohol. Missing bottles of liquor or diluted liquor in the family supply.	0	2	4
27. Discovery of a diary recounting drug experiences or involvement with the drug scene or finding notes stating usage or drug exchange.	0	2	4
28. Episodes of intoxication, either marijuana or alcohol.	0	2	4

Parents should score their children on each item: 0 for not at all; the intermediate column for possible or single occurrence; and the "definitely applies" column where it applies without question or there has been more than one instance. The entire score on all items should then be added. A total of 8 should be viewed as suggestive, that is, worthy of gathering further information; a score of 12 or more is probable for harmful involvement with drugs worthy of further data gathering and an evaluation by a knowledgeable person. A score of 16 or more should be viewed as nearly diagnostic; a full evaluation should be carried out, and serious consideration should be given to seeking treatment.

Fig. 32-2 (continued)

Have you ever felt you ought to **C**ut down on your drinking?
Have people **A**nnoyed you by criticizing your drinking?
Have you ever felt bad or **G**uilty about your drinking?
Have you ever had a drink first thing in the morning to steady your nerves or get rid of a hangover (**E**ye-opener)?

Fig. 32-3. CAGE Questionnaire for alcoholism. (From J. A. Ewing. Detecting alcoholism: The CAGE Questionnaire. *J.A.M.A.* 252(14):1905, 1985. Copyright 1985, American Medical Association.)

1. Appropriately done by clinicians who are:
   a. familiar with the patient/family.
   b. familiar with the risk factors and behavioral toxicities common to adolescent/young adult drug abusers (Stage 2–Stage 4).
   c. have some interest and/or experience in counseling-assessment.
2. Evaluation process should involve 1–5 visits, including a physical examination and appropriate laboratory evaluation, **which should be done during the initial visit.**
3. The visits after the initial interview/physical examination/mental status assessment may number 2–4, depending upon the clinician's ongoing assessment. The clinician should, however, estimate for the family the **total number of expected visits** at that time.
4. Patients should be seen for 30–60 minutes for each visit. Counseling-assessment is best done **before or at the end of office hours** (noontime or prior to the afternoon hours is appropriate as well).
5. The limits of confidentiality should be defined **during the first visit.** Although a complex issue, continued confidentiality with the patient should be judged by the dictum, "If the patient is going to hurt himself/herself, someone else, or run away, then the clinician must bargain/plead to convince the patient how–to whom–what–when the information will be shared with the family."
6. Additional counseling-assessment sessions are used to:
   a. obtain the patient's/family's confidence so that more extensive and reliable history can be obtained;
   b. explore relevant family issues (i.e., divorce, parenting, emotional issues, potential/existing parental alcohol and/or substance abuse);
   c. obtain additional history through the use of questionnaires like the Michigan Alcoholism Screening Test (see Fig. 32-1) and the Adolescent Failure Syndrome Test (see Fig. 32-2).
   d. provide the patient and family with drug-alcohol education;
   e. encourage and educate parent(s) to use appropriate community support groups (e.g., Alcoholics Anonymous, Alanon, Tough Love) and to more closely monitor the patient's behavior (e.g., phone calls, friends, curfew) and search for drugs/drug paraphernalia (in the patient's room, car);
   f. provide ongoing urine monitoring for drug(s)—if appropriate and requested by the parent(s) and/or the patient;
   g. reach agreement with the patient about what information needs to be shared **(in the clinician's judgement)** at the summary session.

Fig. 32-4. Medical-counseling evaluation. (From R. L. Jones. Alcohol and substance abuse: Guidelines for clinicians, office procedures. *State Art. Rev.* 1:3, 1986.)

7. The summary visit should be spent reviewing with the patient and parent(s) simultaneously pertinent risk factors, behavioral parameters, physical examination, and laboratory results, including urine results.
8. Recommendations: The interpretive report should provide the patient and family several treatment options that may or may not continue to involve the clinician:
   a. If the problem(s) prompting evaluation do not seem alcohol- and drug-related, appropriate referral to other counseling, therapy, or school resources is indicated. Experimental drug use should warrant guidance with regard to risk factors and dysfunctional behaviors.
   b. If alcohol and drug use is occurring but only as a covariable in the adolescent's life, referral as above should occur along with the option to provide further management and, one would hope, abstinence from the alcohol/drug use through random urine screening or referral to an ambulatory drug treatment program;
   c. If the adolescent's alcohol/drug use is abusive and the clinician believes it is a **primary cause** of the dysfunctional behavior and physical abnormalities, either a comprehensive ambulatory or in-patient substance abuse program should be recommended;
   d. If the patient's evaluation suggests a primary psychiatric etiology, referral to a psychiatrist or therapist may be warranted. If the patient has concomitant alcohol/drug experimentation and has any risk factors, referral should be to a psychiatrist, who can continue to monitor for the development of abusive alcohol/drug use. Offering to screen the patient's urine for drugs as he or she continues to work with the parents and therapist may be valuable.
9. If the clinician and family decide to attempt an outpatient treatment program, the clinician may suggest the family require a "contract" to be agreed to by the patient.

Fig. 32-4 (continued)

Table 32-4. Intervention strategies in a primary care setting [5, 8, 9, 10, 20, 25]

1. Consider substance abuse in any child over 10 years old with symptoms or signs suggestive of such abuse.
2. Encourage patient and parental discussion (both separately and together) of drug-related issues.
3. Provide factual, up-to-date information through literature and verbal discussions. Encourage questioning.
4. Inform patients of the possible medical and social consequences of their drug use. Do not try to reform them.
5. Stress confidentiality in discussions with adolescents (**unless** their drug use is destructive, in which case mutual agreement to share the scope of the problem with parents must be **insisted** on).
6. Show a willingness to discuss the social implications of drug use and abuse.

References

1. Wilford, B. B. (ed.). *Drug Abuse, A Guide for the Primary Care Physician.* Chicago: American Medical Association, 1981. *This extensive review should be in the primary physician's library.*
2. O'Brien, R., and Cohen, S. *The Encyclopedia of Drug Abuse.* New York: Facts on File, 1984. *An excellent extensive compendium covering the history of drug abuse; contains an excellent drug compendium chart, appendixes, and bibliography.*
3. *A Drug Retrospective: 1962 to 1980.* Rockville, MD: National Institute on Drug Abuse, 1980. *A historical perspective.*
4. Johnston, L. D., O'Malley, P. M., and Bachman, J. G. *National Trend in Drug Use and Related Factors Among American High School Students and Young Adults, 1975–1986.* DHHS Pub. No. (ADM) 87-1535. Rockville, MD: National Institute on Drug Abuse, 1987. *Johnston's surveys are the most concise, epidemiologic chronology of drug abuse trends of adolescents.*
5. Jones, R. L. *Drug Use and Abuse.* In R. B. Shearin and R. Wientzen (eds.), *Clinical Adolescent Medicine: Morbidity and Mortality.* Boston: Hall Medical Publishers, 1983. Pp. 218–227. *An innovative review of the clinical problems seen in adolescents. Needs updating, however.*
6. Newton, M. *Gone Way Down: Teenage Drug Use is a Disease.* Tampa, FL: American Studies Press, 1981. *A thoughtful guide to understanding the progression toward drug abuse and addiction.*
7. Jones, R. L. Identification and management of the toxic adolescent. *Semin. Adolesc. Med.* 1:239, 1985. *A clinical approach with excellent tables. Tables 32-1, 32-2, and 32-3 added to this chapter with permission of author.*
8. DuPont, R. I. *Getting Tough on Gateway Drugs: A Guide for the Family.* Washington, DC: American Psychiatric Inc., 1984. *Good for parents.*
9. Jones, R. L. Alcohol and substance abuse: Guidelines for clinicians, office procedures. *State Art. Rev.* 1:3, 1986. *Excellent review.*
10. MacDonald, D. I., and Newton, M. *Drugs, Drinking, and Adolescents.* Chicago: Year Book, 1984. *One of the best texts for clinicians and parents.*
11. Eckardt, M. J., et al. Health hazards associated with alcohol consumption. *J. A. M. A.* 246(6): 648, 1981. *Has over 300 references.*
12. DuPont, R. I., Goldstein, A., and O'Donnell, J. (eds.). *Handbook on Drug Abuse.* Rockville, MD: National Institute on Drug Abuse, 1979. *Practical and concise. Aimed at the adolescent population.*
13. DeLuce, J. R. (ed.). *Fourth Special Report to the U.S. Congress on Alcohol and Health from the Secretary of Health and Human Services.* Rockville, MD: National Institute on Alcohol Abuse and Alcoholism, 1981. *An excellent epidemiologic compendium on the impact of alcohol on our society.*
14. Green, D. E. *Teenage Smoking: Immediate and Long-term Patterns.* Washington, DC: Government Printing Office, 1979. *A wealth of material now somewhat outdated.*
15. Johnson, L., Bachman, J. G., and O'Malley, P. *Student Drug Use, Attitudes, and Beliefs: National Trends, 1975–1982.* Rockville, MD: National Institute on Drug Abuse, 1984. *Excellent review.*
16. Gold, M. S. *800-Cocaine.* New York: Bantam Books, 1984. *Excellent review of the cocaine abuse problem.*
17. McAlister, A. L. Tobacco, Alcohol and Drug Abuse: Onset and Prevention. In *Healthy People, The Surgeon General's Report on Health Promotion and Disease Prevention. Background papers, 1979.* Rockville, MD: Department of Health, Education, and Welfare, 1979. Pp. 197–206. *Background paper and a classic government document.*
18. Faigel, H. C. Preventing drug and alcohol abuse. *Pediatr. Rev.* 2(1):19, 1980. *Excellent review article.*
19. Newcomb, M. D., Maddahian, E., and Bentley, P. M. Risk factors for original use among adolescents. Concurrent and longitudinal analyses. *Am. J. Public Health* 76:525, 1986. *Ten risk factors demonstrated to be predictive of increased use of cigarettes, alcohol, marijuana, and hard drugs.*
20. Resnik, H. S. *Drug Abuse Prevention for Low-Income Communities: Manual for Program Planning.* Rockville, MD: National Institute on Drug Abuse, 1980. *A community-oriented approach.*
21. American Academy of Pediatrics. *Statement on Drug Abuse.* Evanston, IL: American Academy of Pediatrics, 1979. *Official AAP recommendations; still current.*

22. Wong-McCarthy, W. J., and Gritz, E. R. Preventing regular teenage cigarette smoking. *Pediatr. Ann.* 11(8):683, 1982. *A concise statement of the problem.*
23. McAlister, A. L., Perry, C., and Maccoby, N. Adolescent smoking: Onset and prevention. *Pediatrics* 63(4):650, 1979. *Excellent review article.*
24. McAlister, A. L., et al. Pilot study of smoking, alcohol, and drug abuse prevention. *Am. J. Public Health* 70(7):719, 1980. *A successful primary prevention project.*
25. Masland, R. P., Jr. Drug and alcohol use: How to deal with it. *Consultant* 20(6):190, 1980. *A practical clinical review.*
26. Stewart, D. C. The use of the clinical laboratory in the diagnosis and treatment of substance abuse. *Pediatr. Ann.* 11(8):669, 1982. *A basic review of lab issues. Newer trends have emerged since this was published.*
27. Tennant, F. S., Jr., Day, C. M., and Ungerleider, J. T. Screening for drug and alcohol abuse in a general medical population. *J.A.M.A.* 242(6):533, 1979. *General approach is still appropriate, but the drugs of abuse have changed since this was published.*
28. Schuckit, M. A. *Drug and Alcohol Abuse: A Clinical Guide to Diagnosis and Treatment.* New York: Plenum Medical Book, 1979. *A concise review.*
29. Gitlow, S.E., and Peyser, H. S. (eds.). *Alcoholism: A Practical Treatment Guide.* New York: Grune & Stratton, 1980. *The best in its field. Excellent practical text for treating adult alcoholics, with applications to adolescents.*
30. Ewing, J. A. Detecting alcoholism: The CAGE Questionnaire. *J.A.M.A.* 252(14):1905, 1985. *This questionnaire is good for use with adolescents as well.*
31. Senay, E. C., et al. (eds.). *The Primary Physician's Guide to Drug and Alcohol Abuse Treatment.* Rockville, MD: National Institute on Drug Abuse, 1982. *Excellent review.*

33 Suicide in Children and Adolescents

Robert McConaughy

I. The problem

A. Definition. Suicide is the taking of one's own life.

B. Description. Suicide is the third leading cause of death in adolescents and is a complicated and painful subject, one that can be viewed from a variety of sociocultural, ethical, psychological, and interactive systems perspectives. For the primary care practitioner, it is a preventable cause of death and is particularly compelling when seen in children and adolescents. It can be conceptually viewed on a continuum beginning with normal thoughts of one's own death, as diagrammed below.

Normal		*Emotionally Disturbed*		*Suicidal Behavior*		*Completed Suicide*
Thoughts of one's own death	→	More preoccupied with thoughts of death	→	Acting on death thoughts but unsuccessful	→	

1. **Normal.** There is a developmental progression of children's views of death, with most children up to 5 or 6 seeing death as reversible and as a separation, while school-age children see it as permanent and personified (the "bogeyman"); adolescents 10 and over recognize death as a biologic process [1]. Understanding the concept of death may help a younger child work through subsequent actual losses [2], while the adolescent's establishment of a separate identity may be related to integration of personal loss experiences and realization of one's own potential mortality.

   Suicidal thoughts in normal populations may also show a developmental trend from more ideation in early childhood (54% of 50 school-age children) [3], decreasing in adolescence (22% of 385 teenagers 11–18) [4], but still above the adult range of 13–14%. This would reflect the use of more realistic coping mechanisms and other maturational factors, and may partially explain why adults (including parents and physicians) seem to be blind to such problems in troubled youths. However, more rigorous studies of populations of school-age children [5] and adolescents [6] show 12% of 101 children 7–11 and 7% of 184 adolescents 14–15 with suicidal ideation, which is closer to adult levels.

2. **Emotionally disturbed.** There may be a temporary reaction to loss such as a **grief reaction** following loss of a parent when it is normal to have thoughts of death and one's own mortality. Similar thoughts could be triggered by a near miss accident, a pet's death, or a friend's death, but the child would be expected to revert back to normal over time. There is some evidence that children and adolescents with chronic illness or a history of early losses (e.g., a parent's death) have more highly determined thoughts about their own death; this may be perceived as disturbed by others, but may be relatively normal for similar children. The nonsuicidal child, even though he or she may have thoughts of giving up ("life isn't worth it" and "I wish I were dead") is able to control these feelings and not act on them.

   More chronic emotional disturbance is usually noticed by the child or adolescent and those around him because of **psychiatric symptoms and syndromes** of depression, conduct disorder, and anxiety associated with decreased school, social, or interpersonal functioning and concomitant low self-esteem. In one study of young people seen in an outpatient psychiatry clinic [7], 45% had no suicidal thoughts, 45% had mild thoughts, and 12% had severe suicidal ideation. Although depression increased with severity of suicidal ideation (a major depressive disorder in 83% of the last group), the history of prior suicidal behaviors was not significantly different between the mild and the severe groups. Thus, other factors may influence active and often impulsive suicidal behaviors.

3. **Suicidal behavior** (sometimes called parasuicidal) is any deliberate self-injurious behavior and includes **suicide attempts** and **suicide gestures** (thoughts or actions without risk of injury). *Behavior* is preferable to *attempt* or *gesture*, both of which have frequently been seen as not serious or manipulative.

   A variety of factors can contribute to a nonlethal outcome, ranging from a simple error or lack of cognitive sophistication to ambivalence about dying or lack of serious intent. Degree of **lethality** (high risk versus low risk) needs to be carefully assessed clinically (see Chap 69). Pfeffer [5] and others have shown that degree of **assaultive behavior** toward others is also important, particularly in school-age children; it is measured along a similar continuum of ideation through nonlethal and lethal actions [5].

4. **Completed suicide.** Serious intent is primary. For males, active and physically damaging acts are most frequent—jumping from windows and running in front of cars for younger children; hanging and gunshot wounds for adolescents (although single motor vehicle accidents are also suspect). For females, less active and less physically damaging acts are most frequent—drug overdoses and wrist-cutting, although more violent means may be on the rise [3].

C. Epidemiology

1. **Rates** [8, 9]

   a. **Completed suicide in school-age children** is rare and constant, with two cases through age 9 in the United States in 1982. The youngest child reporting an attempt was age 3, and there were only rare attempts before age 5. Qualitatively, suicide in young children may be a different phenomenon, due to their relative dependency and level of cognitive and emotional development. One study of 15 suicidal preschoolers ages 2½ to 5 showed that 81% had a history of child abuse or neglect [10].

      Suicide accounts for 3.87% of all deaths **in young adolescents** (10–15 years), with a suicide rate of 1.11/100,000; the rate begins to increase at ages 13–14. Between ages 15–19 **(older adolescents)**, suicide accounts for 10.15% of all deaths at a rate of 8.73/100,000—8 times that of the young adolescent group. The number of older adolescent suicides has increased by more than three times that of 20 years ago, although it plateaued between 1979 and 1982. In the 15–24 age group, it is the third leading cause of death (Fig. 33-1).

   b. **Suicidal behaviors.** Population estimates in younger children are not available. **For adolescents,** there has been **an increase** in the 1970s, with one estimate of 1% of 15- to 19-year-old girls in Edinburgh having attempted suicide [11]. A more recent report indicates 8.6% of 382 American high school students make an attempt [12], indicating a possible further increase.

2. **Sex, race, geography**

   a. **Completed suicides. Boys outnumber girls** 4-5 to 1 in all youth-age categories, with white males being the highest risk group (15.5/100,000). Between 1979 and 1982, male completers increased from 1.1 to 1.7/100,000 [9] in the 10–14 age group.

      Native American Indian youth have two and a half to three and a half times **more suicides** than all other races [13]. This may be associated with alcoholism and the breakdown of traditional cultures. Older teenage and young adult suicides are also **more frequent in nine Rocky Mountain and Western states** (Alaska, Nevada, New Mexico, Wyoming, Arizona, Montana, Colorado, California, and Idaho) than in other parts of the country. This parallels other violent causes of death and possibly reflects the effects of population density and use of firearms [14].

   b. **Suicidal behaviors. More preadolescent boys than girls make attempts,** with both sexes showing a similar spectrum of severity [5]. Thus, suicidal behavior in this group may be similar to populations who complete suicide. However, **older adolescent girls outnumber boys** by 9-10 to 1, with girls' attempts more generally considered to be mild with low lethality. This pattern is much different from populations who complete suicide and makes risk assessment studies in adolescent noncompleters questionable.

      In one study, **black adolescents** and young adults **may have two to three**

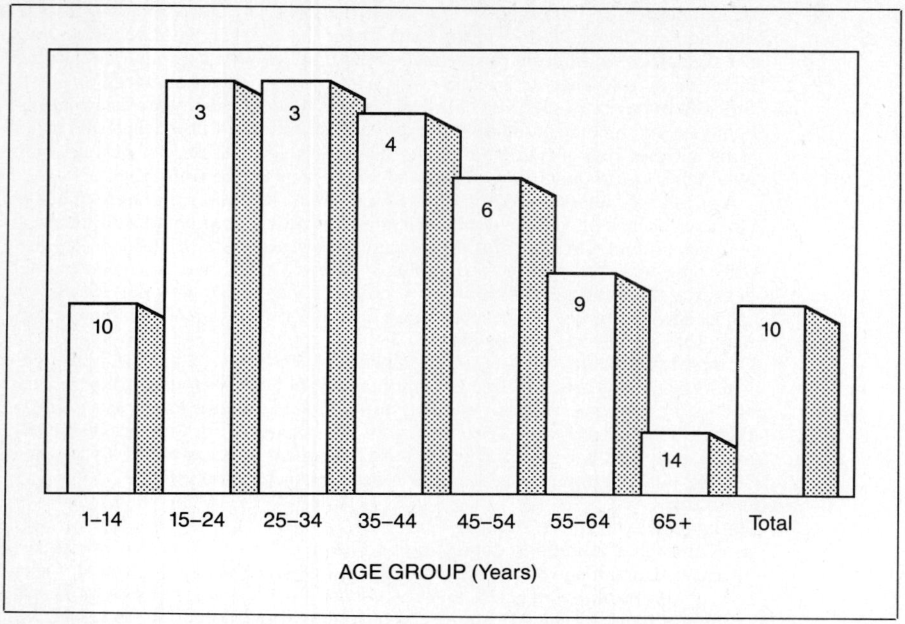

Fig. 33-1. Rank position of suicide among 15 leading causes of death by age group in the United States in 1980. (From Suicide: United States, 1970–1980. *M.M.W.R.* 34(24):353, 1985.)

times as many suicide attempts as whites, possibly related to other violent behaviors and socioeconomic status [15].

3. **Genetic/biological.** Danish adults adopted as children who committed suicide had biological families with an almost five times higher rate of suicide than their adoptive families [16].

   Adult suicides may have decreased brain serotonin, while decreased cerebrospinal fluid serotonin is also associated with suicide attempts and aggression [17]. Receptor studies of H^3-imipramine may show decreased frontal cortex binding in suicidal patients [17].

   These adult research studies, while currently of no clinical value, suggest similar effects in younger patients.

4. **Family/social.** Quarrels or the threat of loss of important relationships frequently precipitates suicidal behaviors. The developmental shifts of these important relationships by age are seen in Table 33-1 from an Israeli study. Clearly, parental relationships are important for all ages, but with an increasing shift from parent and sibling to peers and heterosexual relationships with increasing age.
   a. **Parents/family.** Suicide attempts frequently occur at home and often use parental medication or weapons. Numerous studies link suicide attempts with broken homes (divorce, separation, death of a parent) and parental psychopathology (depression, suicide, aggression, lack of warmth or interest in the child). Maternal depression with suicidal ideation is prominent in the school-age suicidal child [5]. Socioeconomic status may also have a significant influence. Broken homes and other increasing family stresses throughout childhood may differentiate children hospitalized with suicidal behavior from depressed children and other psychiatric controls [19], but may not be associated with completed suicide [20]. Youth who are both depressed and antisocial who have completed suicide have a greater than 50% family history of suicide attempts [21].
   b. **Peer/media.** A known phenomenon in adolescent and young adult psychiatric settings is contagion of suicidal behaviors [22], which has also been seen in

Table 33-1. Primary motive for attempted suicide in 343 adolescents aged 10–18

	Age (number of adolescents)			
Motive	10–13 (11)	14–15 (74)	16–17 (136)	18 (72)
Quarrels in relationships	91%	75%	62%	58%
Type of relationship:				
Parent	55%	42%	38%	25%
Sibling	27%	16%	8%	5%
Peer	9%	14%	3%	1%
Boyfriend, girlfriend, spouse	0	3%	14%	26%

Source: Modified from M. Amir. Suicide among minors in Israel. *Isr. Ann. Psychiatry* 11:219, 1973.

epidemics of suicidal behaviors in high school students [23] and young adult Native American Indian males [24], among others. Such imitative suicidal behaviors show the special relevance of peer relationships and modelling for adolescents, pointing to the value of school-based interventions in vulnerable youth.

Televised movies dealing with suicide have been associated with increased attempted or completed teenage suicides within 2 weeks [25]. During a 6-year period television news stories about suicide were associated with an increased national daily suicide rate in teenagers but not in adults [26].

5. **Populations at risk.** Schrut [27] and more recently Shaffer [28, 21] and Pfeffer [5] describe characteristics of groups at risk for suicide:
   a. **Suicidal-assaultive.** Most frequently, the individual is prone to aggressive or violent outbursts, is impetuous, rebellious, and sensitive to criticism. There is often associated drug or alcohol abuse, runaway behavior, or school problems. They may initially angrily deny suicidal ideation or intent, may not be overtly depressed, and may identify with parental acting out. Motivation may be retaliation for some real or perceived loss of self-esteem.
   b. **Suicidal-depressed.** Less frequently, the anxious or depressed, isolated, withdrawn, but apparently relatively stable child or adolescent may decompensate under the influence of extreme environmental stressors, which frequently includes the loss of a loved or trusted person [29]. This may be the first manifestation of underlying major depressive disorder or undiscovered sexual abuse.
   c. **Psychosis** is rare but often quite violent or lethal, with symptoms of social withdrawal and covert auditory hallucinations. It is sometimes masked by drug use.
   d. **Previous suicidal behaviors.** Motto [30] initially followed hospitalized depressed and suicidal 10- to 19-year-old males for 4–10 years and found the following clinically relevant factors to be mildly but significantly predictive of subsequent suicide: (1) clear communications of intent; (2) fears of "something wrong with me" (going crazy or an unusual disease); (3) active search for help before attempt; (4) hypersomnia; (5) moderate ability to communicate with others (good and poor communicators not at risk); (6) ambivalent or negative attitude toward the interview situation; (7) feelings of helplessness; and (8) apathy, psychomotor retardation [30].
   e. **Communication of intent.** One-third of Motto's at-risk sample who initially communicated clear intent completed suicide. Between 40% [20] and 85% [31] of completed suicides have communicated to someone in their environs. Shafii [31] found (1) a breakdown in communication with parents or friends; (2) contact with a physician for a variety of physical complaints during the previous 4–6 weeks, with emotional state not assessed or taken seriously; and (3) a desperate attempt to contact a friend by phone. Friends are often made to enter a secrecy pact, where they promise not to tell of their suicidal friend's intent, but the friends may also experience guilt over such responsibility for another's life.

Of a teenage psychiatric hospital sample of 48 who had communicated suicidal intent, 83% had talked with parents or spouses, 42% with other relatives or friends, and 15% to professionals (physician, teacher, counselor) [32]. Another study of 101 completed suicides found that 8% were known to pediatricians, whereas 40% had medical visits prior to the actual suicide [33].

II. **General health promotion**: Reducing risks for the whole population

A. **Methods**

1. **Families in need of special services** should be identified. These include those who show poor coping with several losses or accumulated life stresses or both; have parental or family history of suicide, depression, alcohol use (correlating with depression in children); or have poor impulse control. The health care provider should watch for history of poor interaction (or attachment) between child and parent, leading to a withdrawn child, or disordered communication between child and parent, leading to an impulsive child.
2. **Help to families with special needs** should be provided. The health care provider should aim to provide support and guidance for parents in replacing poor coping styles and in handling withdrawn or impulsive children. Directing parents to ancillary services, such as parent groups, courses in child developmental problems or parent-effectiveness, and a range of social services may be useful. Parenting skills should focus on reducing any suicidal or aggressive behaviors in the family, working through issues of loss, and understanding the child's need to develop the following attitudes [34]:
   a. Sufficient positive self-esteem to feel oneself worth protecting.
   b. Capacity to anticipate situations of risk.
   c. Ability to control impulses.
   d. Pleasure in mastering situations of risk.
   e. Sufficient knowledge of oneself and the outside world for survival.
   f. Ability to be self-assertive to protect oneself.
   g. Ability to choose others as friends who will enhance one's protection and not jeopardize one's safety.
3. **Access to dangerous windows and heights** for younger children should be reduced by talking with parents about such safety measures.
4. **The availability of lethal doses of drugs, alcohol, and toxins** at home should be reduced by talking with parents about safety measures and by being careful in prescribing practices.
5. **The availability of firearms** should be reduced through similar discussions with parents regarding safety measures.
6. Health care providers should participate in activities that encourage, reinforce, reward, or mandate **seat belt use and responsible, nonalcoholic driving** by young drivers.
7. Children need to feel loved, valuable, and hopeful of the future. Health care providers should encourage activities by families that promote these feelings.

B. **Justification.** Data on the effectiveness and costs of these measures is sparse. Suicide barriers on bridges have had a positive effect on adult suicidal behaviors, and the elimination of coal gas in Great Britain temporarily reduced the national suicide rate for both adults and teenagers. There is much debate about access to handguns and firearms related to acts of aggression, but the impact on suicides is less clear. Although there are costs in provider time, possible benefits are great even though difficult to measure.

III. **Specific health promotion**

A. **Early assessment** (of at risk individuals)

1. **Methods**
   a. The most important step is for the health care provider to recognize suicide as a potential and serious health problem (even for superficially normal youth) and to take action in its identification and prevention.
   b. **In the community**, as part of talks on child and adolescent health, the physician can emphasize at risk variables. He or she can also be aware of community mental health referral sources, including suicide prevention centers.
   c. **In the school,** the physician can consult with principals, school psychologists, and school nurses regarding suicide as one aspect of a preventive health program for students; **emphasis should be placed on teachers** as adults most likely to first identify such cases **and on students** themselves. Particular attention should be paid to "promising not to tell" in light of competing ethi-

cal questions regarding friendship, confidentiality, and risk of death to the suicidal young person.

d. **In the office**

(1) It is imperative for the physician to have a trusting but separate **relationship** with both parents and child.

(2) Using the model of **anticipatory guidance** (see Chap. 27) **from early childhood,** the continuity of a sharing, working relationship between the physician, patient, and family should be emphasized, with the physician showing an attitude of patience, tolerance, and acceptance.

(3) **In school-age years,** the physician should spend some time with the child alone to get to know him or her and be available to answer any questions or worries concerning health.

(4) At the beginning of **junior and senior high school,** or in conjunction with clinical visits where appropriate, the physician should discuss a variety of health maintenance issues and redefine his or her role for the young adolescent. The young person should be encouraged to think of him or her as not just the giver of shots, associated with pain and illness, but instead as a resource and adviser about health matters and other concerns, including those personal issues of sexuality and thoughts of dying. An individual and confidential relationship apart from parents should be offered, reassuring the youth that discussion of such issues does not automatically mean that he or she will be "locked up" or labeled crazy. A phone number to call if there are crises or emergencies should be given.

(5) In the course of an office visit, the physician should explore the following areas in a directive but open-ended manner: (1) peers, (2) school, (3) age-appropriate stressors (grades, dating), (4) sexual concerns, including pregnancy for teenage girls, and (5) family and other intimate relationships.

Particular attention should be given to signs and symptoms of depression: (1) reactions to recent or past losses, (2) feelings of hopelessness, (3) lowered self-esteem, (4) social withdrawal, (5) poor school performance, (6) crying spells, (7) decreased appetite, (8) apathy, (9) sleep disturbance, (10) irritability or frustration, and (11) impulsivity.

Clues to suicidal ideation may be found in jokes with morbid themes; statements that "everything is boring;" giving away prized possessions; or dreams of black, unknown, peaceful territory, of falling, or of being in an enclosed space (coffin).

Following open-ended questions, **focused questions of intent and lethality,** including access to different methods (pills, guns, automobile, rope) are appropriate when there is a question of suicidal ideation.

(6) A similar interview is warranted when there is either **repetitive or unexplained accidents or trauma,** either in or out of hospitals.

(7) **Any mention of suicide or self-destructive behavior** (by either patient, peers, or parents) **should be pursued by the physician** or other responsible adult. Perhaps the most difficult aspect of such investigation is the patient's or parents' denial by saying "it wasn't important" or "it won't happen again." It may be useful to verbalize the aggressive intent behind the behavior, including the patient's underlying anger at others or self at the time of the event.

(8) The existing data should be assessed in the following manner [35]:

(a) Is there a longstanding history of preceding problems?

(b) Has there been an escalation of previous problems?

(c) Is the stage set for a finale characterized by a chain reaction dissolution of the patient's meaningful relationships?

(9) Once the physician has established that there is a reasonable suicide risk, he or she should consult with psychology or psychiatry colleagues regarding further outpatient evaluation or admission to either a medical or psychiatric hospital, depending on the severity of the problem and available resources. Even in this moment of relative crisis, it is imperative that patient and family be allowed to rebuild hope and reestablish healthy ties among family members.

(10) If an adolescent patient or his or her parents refuse a psychiatric refer-

ral, the physician should **insist** that it take place; the physician should consult with a referral source or local involuntary treatment agency (or child abuse agency for a younger child) if refusal persists. **If the physician is worried about the case, he or she should make every effort possible to make sure that psychiatric referral is completed.**

B. Justification. The accuracy, risks, costs, and acceptability of risk assessment as described above have not been adequately studied. However, the accepted rationale for risk assessment was well stated by the American Academy of Pediatrics in 1980 [36]:

> The pediatrician [and family physician] can provide a significant resource in preventing adolescent suicide by identifying youngsters at high risk and recognizing the behavioral clues in youngsters contemplating suicide. . . . if a pediatrician suspects that a [child or] teenager is contemplating suicide, he should ask the [child or] adolescent directly about suicidal thoughts. Inquiring about suicide does not cause suicide. . . .The pediatrician may wish to make a full evaluation and follow some patients himself. . . . however, most pediatricians who choose to do so should consult with psychiatric colleagues to confirm a "low risk assessment."

C. Early intervention

1. Methods

a. At-risk groups should be identified, especially teenage males with depression, conduct disturbance, and a history of self-destructive or life-threatening behavior. Appropriate hospitals, schools, jails, or juvenile detention facilities should be contacted, **and a direct service intervention program should be established, combined with a health education curriculum** and liaison for teachers, probation officers, and human service workers who have daily contact with adolescents, as described by Reykin [37].

b. Ongoing educational and therapeutic groups should be established for teenagers with suicidal ideation or behaviors, either **in mental health** or suicide prevention center **settings** [38], **or in schools** [39]. Discussion of suicides of peers, community figures, or persons televised or portrayed in the media should be actively encouraged. Also, student or peer group leaders should be involved if concern over contagion or an epidemic develops.

2. Justification. The estimated risk of a recurrent attempt is 1% per year after the initial attempt, with lack of ongoing follow-up possibly creating greater risk for completed suicide. Assessment of the program described in sec. **III.C.1.a.** is in process, with a positive impact reported in selected cases. The method in sec. **III.C.1.b.** has also had a positive impact; it has helped create a social network for identified teenagers with no known repeat attempts or completed suicides two years after termination of involvement with the program. Both approaches seem useful if outcome can be adequately assessed.

IV. Recommendations

A. Primary prevention. Primary care physicians potentially have an important longitudinal role in their communities and schools. They can effectively raise appropriate developmental concerns regarding youth suicide. Awareness of the possibility of suicidal ideation and the importance of helping resolve issues of self-control, loss, and helplessness during adolescence are crucial in preventive contacts with a child and his or her family over time. A specific method of interviewing, physician assessment, and appropriate management and referral is suggested for specific cases. Preventive safety guidelines are also offered.

B. Secondary intervention. Two methods are proposed to help at-risk individuals and at-risk populations of teenagers. Primary care physicians, in conjunction with mental health colleagues and educators, are in a unique position to identify youths with suicidal behaviors at the time of the episode and to channel cases into individual intervention or group treatment settings. An ongoing problem is that of denial or resistance to follow-up of those individuals who may be at greatest risk. Intervening in cases actively in the home and community (see sec. **III.C.1.a.**) and in the school or mental health center (see sec. **III.C.1.a.,b.**) offer viable alternatives to current limited sources of intervention.

References

1. Nagy, M. The Child's Theories Concerning Death. In C. R. Pfeffer (ed.), *The Suicidal Child.* New York: Guilford Press, 1986. *Useful introductory chapter on cognitive changes with development.*
2. Furman, E. *A Child's Parent Dies: Studies in Childhood Bereavement.* New Haven, CT: Yale University Press, 1974. *Readable, sensitive, in-depth exploration of the child's reaction to loss. Recommended.*
3. Lourie, R. S.: Clinical studies of attempted suicide in childhood. *Clin. Proc. Child. Hosp.* 22:163, 1966. *Limited clinical utility.*
4. Kaplan, S. L., Hong, G. K., and Weinbold, C. Epidemiology of depressive symptomatology in adolescents. *J. Am. Acad. Child. Psychiatry* 23(1):91, 1984. *Shows how a checklist depression inventory can screen for depression in a teenage population. Limited clinical utility.*
5. Pfeffer, C. R. (ed.). *The Suicidal Child.* New York: Guilford Press, 1986. *Best overall book for the clinician interested in a balanced, in-depth perspective. Highly recommended.*
6. Rutter, M., et al. Adolescent turmoil: Fact or fiction? *J. Child. Psychol. Psychiatry* 17(1):35, 1976. *Useful population study showing the incidence of depression and other psychopathology. Recommended.*
7. Carlson, G. A., and Cantwell, D. P. Suicidal behavior and depression in children and adolescents. *J. Am. Acad. Child. Psychiatry* 21(4):361, 1982. *Largely technical; limited clinical utility.*
8. Suicide: United States, 1970–1980. *M.M.W.R.* 34(24):353, 1985. *Statistical overview; limited clinical utility.*
9. Frederick, C. H. An Introduction and Overview to Youth Suicide. In M. L. Peck, et al. (eds.), *Youth Suicide.* New York: Springer, 1985. *Useful, descriptive, statistical overview and commentary.*
10. Rosenthal, P. A., and Rosenthal, S. Suicidal behavior by pre-school children. *Am. J. Psychiatry* 141(4):520, 1984. *Useful description of suicidal behavior in this age group.*
11. Hawton, K. *Suicide and Attempted Suicide Among Children and Adolescents.* Vol. 5, *Developmental Clinical Psychology and Psychiatry.* Beverly Hills: Sage Publications, 1986.
12. Harkavy, J. M., and Asnis, G. Suicide attempts in adolescence: Prevalence and implications (letter). *N. Engl. J. Med.* 313(20):1290, 1985. *Limited utility.*
13. Frederick, C. J. Suicide in Young Minority Group Persons. In H. S. Sudak, A. B. Ford, and N. B. Rushford (eds.), *Suicide in the Young.* Boston: Wright-PSG, 1984. Pp. 31–44. *Statistical and descriptive overview. The most comprehensive multiauthored book on suicide in young adolescents and children. Book is recommended.*
14. Seiden, R. H. Death in the west—a regional analysis of the youthful suicide rate. *West. J. Med.* 140(6):969, 1984. *Limited general utility.*
15. Earls, F., and Jameson, A. Suicidal Behavior in American Blacks. In G. L. Klerman (ed.), *Suicide and Depression Among Adolescents and Young Adults.* Washington: American Psychiatric Press, 1986. *Useful chapter in a thought-provoking multiauthored book on suicide in adolescents and young adults. Recommended.*
16. Shulsinger, F., et al. A Family Study of Suicide. In M. Schou, and E. Strömgren (eds.), *Origin, Prevention and Treatment of Affective Disorders.* Orlando, FL: Academic Press, 1979. *Review of Danish adoption findings; limited utility.*
17. Stanley, M. Neurochemical Factors in Suicide Attempts and Completers. Paper presented at the American Association of Child Adolescent Psychiatry Annual Meeting, October 1986.
18. Amir, M. Suicide among minors in Israel. *Isr. Ann. Psychiatry* 11:219, 1973. *Large, descriptive study with limited general utility.*
19. Cohen-Sandler, R., Berman, A. L., and King, R. A. Life stress and symptomatology: Determinants of suicidal behavior in children. *J. Am. Acad. Child Psychiatry* 21(2):178, 1982. *Stimulating but technical paper. Limited utility.*
20. Sanborn, D. E., and Cimbolic, P. Two years of suicide: A study of adolescent suicide in New Hampshire. *Child Psychiatry Hum. Dev.* 3(4):234, 1973. *Brief and limited study of completed suicides.*
21. Shaffer, D. New York Youth Suicide Study. Paper presented at the American Association of Child Adolescent Psychiatry Annual Meeting, October 1986.
22. Walsh, B. W., and Rosen, P. Self-mutilation and contagion: An empirical test. *Am. J. Psychiatry* 142(1):119, 1985. *Useful, brief review; limited general utility.*
23. Robbins, D., and Conroy, R. C. A cluster of adolescent suicide attempts: Is suicide contagious? *J. Adolesc. Health Care* 3(4):253, 1983. *Useful case reports.*

24. Fox, J., Manitowabi, D., and Ward, J. A. An Indian community with a high suicide rate—5 years after. *Can. J. Psychiatry* 29(5):425, 1984. *Brief article; limited utility.*
25. Gould, M. S., and Shaffer, D. The impact of suicide in television movies: Evidence of imitation. *N. Engl. J. Med.* 315(11):690, 1986. *Stimulating study.*
26. Phillips, D. P., and Carstensen, L. L. Clustering of teenage suicides after television news stories about suicide. *N. Engl. J. Med.* 315(11):685, 1986. *Useful companion article to reference 25.*
27. Schrut, A. Suicidal adolescents and children. *J.A.M.A.* 188(13): 1883, 1964. *Useful article. Recommended.*
28. Shaffer, D. Suicide in childhood and early adolescence. *J. Child. Psychol. Psychiatry* 15(4):275, 1974. *Most thorough, published article of completed suicides to date.*
29. Mack, J., and Hickler, H. *Vivienne: The Life and Suicide of an Adolescent Girl.* New York: Mentor Books, 1982. *Excellent in-depth case report. Highly recommended for all audiences.*
30. Motto, J. A. Suicide in Male Adolescents. In H. S. Sudak, A. B. Ford, and N. B. Rushford (eds.), *Suicide in the Young.* Boston: Wright-PSG, 1984. Pp. 227–244. *Longest follow-up study of adolescent male at-risk population. Book is recommended.*
31. Shafii, M., et al. Psychological autopsy of completed suicide in children and adolescents. *Am. J. Psychiatry* 142(9):1061, 1985. *Most recent published report of completed suicides. Also see references 13 and 30. Clinically useful.*
32. Stevenson, E. K., et al. Suicidal communication in adolescents. Study of two matched groups of 60 teenagers. *Dis. Nerv. Syst.* 33(2):112, 1972. *Limited clinical utility.*
33. Hodgman, C. H., and Roberts, F. N. Adolescent suicide and the pediatrician. *J. Pediatr.* 101(1):118, 1982. *Useful population study. Limited clinical utility.*
34. Khantzian, E. J., and Mack, J. E. Self preservation and the care of the self: Ego instincts considered. *Psychoanal. Study Child.* 38:209, 1983. *Excellent psychoanalytic overview. Recommended for mental health and child development professionals.*
35. Teicher, J., and Joseph, D. Suicide and Suicide Attempts. In J. D. Noshpitz (ed.), *Basic Handbook of Child Psychiatry.* Vol. 2: Disturbances in Development. New York: Basic Books, 1979. *Thorough overview. Recommended.*
36. American Academy of Pediatrics, Committee on Adolescence. Teenage suicide. *Pediatrics* 66(1):144, 1980. *Clear position statement; also useful for family physicians.*
37. Reykin, E. Y. Adolescent Suicidal and Self-destructive Behavior. In G. L. Klerman (ed.), *Suicide and Depression Among Adolescents and Young Adults.* Washington: American Psychiatric Press, 1986. *First published description of innovative intervention project. Recommended.*
38. Ross, C. P., and Motto, J. A. Group Counseling for Suicidal Adolescents. In H. S. Sudak, A. B. Ford, and N. B. Rushford (eds.), *Suicide in the Young.* Boston: Wright-PSG, 1984. Pp. 367–392. *Useful overview of another innovative project. Recommended.*
39. Berkovitz, I. H. The Role of Schools in Child, Adolescent and Youth Suicide Prevention. In M. L. Peck, N. L. Farberow, and R. E. Litman (eds.), *Youth Suicide.* New York: Springer, 1985. Pp. 170–190. *Thorough overview of school-based interventions. Recommended.*

34 Sports Safety

Jeff Tanji

I. The problem

A. Description. Although no data exist that document the type and extent of untoward effects of sports in the pediatric age group, intuitively it is obvious that soft tissue and bone injuries are the most common. Less common causes for morbidity include exacerbations of underlying conditions—for example, acute infections (influenza, mononucleosis, hepatitis A and B), respiratory conditions (allergies and asthma), hematologic disorders (iron deficiency anemia, sickle cell anemia), cardiovascular disease (hypertension, valvular disease), and genitourinary disorders (single testicle, kidney anomalies). The adverse effects of sports can thus be categorized into two broad areas: (1) Direct trauma, whether acute or chronic, can result from participation; and (2) The exacerbation of an underlying condition, such as asthma, can result in morbidity as a result of participation.

B. Epidemiology. It has been estimated that between 17 and 25 million children and adolescents participate regularly in an organized sports activity [4, 5]. Furthermore, it is known that about 23% of all injuries reported in school-age children are sports-related [3]. Since many children do not participate in formally organized sports but do participate in loosely organized sports, we believe that these estimates are conservative, reflecting only a portion of those children actually involved in all sports and recreation activities.

Factors that alter risk for injury and illness associated with sports depend on the specific sport. Shaffer [4] has offered a classification of activity that has gained considerable popularity among sports medicine physicians. The outline is concise, with each sport categorized into collision, contact, noncontact, and other (Table 34-1).

There are many other risk factors for morbidity other than the type of sport. Unfortunately, because of controversy and little data a clear evaluation of the risk factors is not possible. These factors include facilities (playing surface, setting), equipment, and growth and maturity of the participant. An example of a current controversy about playing surface is the issue of the relative safety of astroturf and grass. It is assumed that the incidence of football injuries is greater on astroturf than on grass because of the hardness of the surface. However, there is currently no methodologically precise study that analyzes this question.

II. Specific health promotion

A. Early assessment. The purpose of having a screening examination prior to competition in sports is to assess the child's capability of handling the potential trauma, as well as to rule out serious underlying disorders that might be exacerbated in the course of competition.

1. **Methods (the preparticipation examination).** Every child participating in an organized sport or recreational activity should have an initial preparticipation examination by a physician one month prior to competition. The purpose of this lead time is to allow for treatment or rehabilitation, or both, for conditions that **will not disqualify** a child from competition. Children with recognized, ongoing medical problems that do not disqualify them from activity, and children who are undergoing rehabilitation from a previous injury, ought to receive preparticipation examinations at least once a year. Those children with no identified problems who had an initial evaluation without any problems being detected should be examined prior to participation upon entering an educational institution and then on an as-needed basis.

   A physician's examination and clearance prior to a child's participation in organized sports is a legal requirement in 37 states [5]. There are two states, unfortunately, that do not yet require a preparticipation examination, while the

Table 34-1. Classification of sports

Strenuous—contact
Football
Ice hockey
Lacrosse (boys)
Rugby
Wrestling
Strenuous—limited contact
Basketball
Field hockey
Lacrosse (girls)
Soccer
Volleyball
Strenuous—non-contact
Crew (rowing)
Cross-country
Fencing
Gymnastics
Skiing
Swimming
Tennis
Track and field
Water polo
Moderately strenuous
Badminton
Baseball (limited contact)
Curling
Golf
Table tennis
Nonstrenuous
Archery
Bowling
Riflery

Source: T. E. Shaffer. The health examination for participation in sports. *Pediatr. Ann.* 7(10):27, 1978.

remaining 11 conditionally require such an examination. Although many experts [1, 6, 7] have called for nationally standardized preparticipation examination for a child by a physician, there is yet no standard format. We include our history and physical format (Fig. 34-1), which is thorough, as an example. There are, however, several nationally published formats for such examinations [8, 9], and the following set of guidelines are based on them.

a. History. The history should emphasize the following points:

(1) History of not being allowed to participate in competition.
(2) Episodes of loss of consciousness.
(3) Sudden death in a relative.
(4) Use of contact lenses, dentures, or prosthetic devices.
(5) History of fractures or dislocations.
(6) History of heat strokes or heat exhaustion [10].
(7) Menstrual history.
(8) Record of previous performance in sports.
(9) Name and telephone number of nearest relative and physician.
(10) Any chronic medical problem, operations, medications, recreational drugs, or allergies.

b. Physical examination. The physical examination should focus on the following, with specific abnormalities kept in mind:

(1) General: height, weight, body habitus (especially for weight-determined sports).
(2) Skin: jaundice, herpetic lesions, impetigo, severe acne.
(3) Visual acuity: severe myopia, amblyopia, single eye.

HISTORY

Name: ____________________ Date of birth: ____________________

Address: ____________________ Telephone: ____________________

____________________ Family M.D. ____________________

In case of emergency, notify: ____________________

Address: ____________________

Telephone: ____________________

Date of last tetanus booster: ____________________

Date of last examination (approx.) by a doctor: ____________________

The following questions are to be answered by either yes or no. Please check the appropriate space.

	Yes	No
Have you been under a doctor's care in the last 12 months?	( )	( )
Have you been in the hospital in the last 12 months?	( )	( )
Have you ever had any type of surgery?	( )	( )
Do you want to talk to a doctor about a health problem or any injury?	( )	( )
Has anyone in your immediate family ever had:		
Diabetes (high sugar in blood)?	( )	( )
Allergies (hay fever or asthma)?	( )	( )
Migraine headaches?	( )	( )
Heart trouble?	( )	( )
High blood pressure?	( )	( )
Has anyone in your family, under age 50, died suddenly?	( )	( )
Have you had or do you now have:		
Brain concussion (head injury)?	( )	( )
Tendency to lose consciousness (faint)?	( )	( )
Skull fracture?	( )	( )
Convulsions or epilepsy?	( )	( )
Neck injury?	( )	( )
Have you had or do you now have:		
Very bad (impaired) vision in one eye?	( )	( )
Temporary loss of vision?	( )	( )
To wear glasses or contact lenses?	( )	( )
Have you had or do you now have:		
Hearing loss?	( )	( )
Perforated eardrum?	( )	( )
Discharge from ear(s) (recurrent infections)?	( )	( )
Sinus infections?	( )	( )
Broken nose?	( )	( )
Dental plate (dentures)?	( )	( )
Orthodontia (teeth straightened)?	( )	( )
Have you had or do you now have:		
Hernia?	( )	( )
Kidney problems?	( )	( )
Loss of function or absence of testicles (boys)?	( )	( )
Menstrual problems (girls)?	( )	( )

Age at onset of menstruation? ____________

Fig. 34-1. Preparticipation evaluation—history and physical.

	Yes	No
Have you had or do you now have:		
Bone fracture?	( )	( )
Joint dislocation?	( )	( )
Foot problems?	( )	( )
To wear a cast?	( )	( )
Have you had or do you now have:		
Back injury or frequent backaches?	( )	( )
Knee injury (sprain) or recurrent pain?	( )	( )
Ankle injury (sprain) or recurrent pain?	( )	( )
Other joint problems, e.g., swelling, pain, decreased range of motion?	( )	( )
Bone infection?	( )	( )
Have you had or do you now have:		
Diabetes (high sugar in blood or urine)?	( )	( )
Tendency to bleed or bruise easily?	( )	( )
Anemia ("tired" blood)?	( )	( )
Weight problem (under- or overweight)?	( )	( )
Have you had or do you now have:		
Asthma (wheezing)?	( )	( )
Hay fever?	( )	( )
Hives or rash?	( )	( )
Bee-sting reactions (allergy)?	( )	( )
Reaction to medicine (allergy)?	( )	( )
Do you:		
Smoke?	( )	( )
Take any medicine regularly?	( )	( )
If YES, name of medication ____________________		
Take medicine for emergency use?	( )	( )
If YES, name of medication ____________________		
Have you had or do you now have:		
Heart trouble or murmur?	( )	( )
High blood pressure?	( )	( )
Persistent cough?	( )	( )
Chest pain with exercise?	( )	( )
Dizziness or faintness with exercise?	( )	( )
Have you had or do you now have:		
Recurrent rash?	( )	( )
Fungus infection?	( )	( )
Athlete's foot?	( )	( )
Recurrent boils (skin infection)?	( )	( )
Do you wish to discuss an emotional problem with the doctor?	( )	( )
Have you ever been told to give up sports because of a health problem?	( )	( )

If you have answered yes to any of the above questions, please explain below.

Please be advised that this is a preparticipation screening physical exam and in no way constitutes a complete physical exam.

Fig. 34-1 (continued)

PHYSICAL

1. Height ________________ Weight ________________

2. B.P. (sitting) ________ / ________

3. Vision: L 20 / ________ : R 20 / ________

	Check if within normal limits
4. Skin	( )
5. Mouth	( )
6. Eyes	( )
7. Ears	( )
8. Neck	( )
9. Lymphatics	( )
10. Respiratory	( )
11. Cardiovascular: Heart	( )
Pulses	( )
12. Abdomen	( )
13. Genitalia	( )
14. Extremities	( )
15. Neurological	( )
Reflexes	( )
16. Orthopedic: Cervical spine/back	( )
Arm/Elbow/Wrist/Hand	( )
Knees	( )
Ankles	( )

PHYSICIAN'S STATEMENT OF HEALTH:

I certify that I have examined ____________________ and have found no gross evidence of any abnormality that will interfere with his or her participation.

____________________, M.D.

Fig. 34-1 (continued)

(4) Funduscopic exam: detached retina, early atherosclerotic changes, diabetic retinopathy.
(5) Lungs: asthma, bronchitis.
(6) Cardiovascular: murmurs, uncontrolled hypertension, cyanosis.
(7) Abdomen: hepatosplenomegaly, masses.
(8) Back: scoliosis, kyphosis, lordosis.
(9) Genitourinary: single testicle, hernia, sexual maturity (Tanner staging [11], Table 34-2).
(10) Musculoskeletal: unstable knee and ankle ligaments, recurrent shoulder dislocation, assessment of elbow stability, painful Osgood-Schlatter disease, assessment of muscular development.
(11) Neurologic: gross coordination or gait abnormalities.

c. Laboratory. We do not recommend routine laboratory testing in the preparticipation examination [6, 12].

2. Justification

a. Assessment characteristics. Between 1 and 3% of standard preparticipation examinations for children in sports will detect an abnormality requiring follow-up. The value in such screening is heightened when one realizes

Table 34-2. Maturity staging guidelines

	Boys		
Stage	Pubic hair	Penis	Testis
1	None	Preadolescent	
2	Slight, long, slight pigmentation	Slight enlargement	Enlarged scrotum, pink slight ruga
3	Darker, starts to curl, small amount	Longer	Larger
4	Coarse, curly, adult type but less quantity	Increase in glans size and breadth of penis	Larger, scrotum darker
5	Adult, spreads to inner thighs	Adult	Adult

	Girls	
Stage	Pubic hair	Breasts
1	Preadolescent (none)	Preadolescent (no germinal button)
2	Sparse, lightly pigmented, straight medial border of labia	Breast and papilla elevated as small mound; areolar diameter increased
3	Darker, beginning to curl, increased	Breast and areola enlarged; no contour separation
4	Coarse, curly, abundant, but less than adult	Areola and papilla form secondary mound
5	Adult female triangle, spreads to medial surface	Mature; nipple projects, areola part of general breast contour

Source: J. M. Tanner. *Growth at Adolescence* (2nd ed.). Oxford: Blackwell, 1962.

that for some children, the preparticipation examination is the only examination by a physician they may have in a large number of years. Unfortunately, there are no data to assess the effectiveness of the preparticipation examination in the prevention of injury and illness in children. When a standardized preparticipation examination is nationally accepted, the methodology for such research will be simplified and the data will be available.

b. **Risks.** The risks of such an examination are the stigma for the child of not being allowed to compete with peers and the possibility of being labeled a nonparticipant.

c. **Costs.** The average cost in 1987 was $7 to $10 per participant per examination.

d. **Acceptability.** Preparticipation examinations are widely accepted.

B. **Early intervention.** The successful realization of the objectives of early intervention after a preparticipation examination largely depend on being able to perform the examination early, before the start of the sports season. For this reason we recommend that preparticipation evaluations be performed one month prior to the start of the first game.

1. **Methods.** The objectives of early intervention fall into a hierarchy of categories, depending on the nature of the findings of the examination.
   a. To diagnose conditions that will disqualify a child from participating in a specific sport (Table 34-3).
   b. To determine if a correctable condition exists that would allow later participation (i.e., ankle sprain) in a specific sport.
   c. To determine if preventative measures could be taken for a diagnosed condition that would allow for participation.
   d. To reclassify a youth for another acceptable sport if disqualification should occur for the initially desired sport.
   e. To assess the general medical status of the child and to recommend treatment for a potentially serious non-sports-related condition.

Table 34-3. Disqualifying conditions for sports participation

Conditions	Collision[a]	Contact[b]	Non-Contact[c]	Other[d]
General				
Acute infections: respiratory, genitourinary, infectious mononucleosis, hepatitis, active rheumatic fever, active tuberculosis	X	X	X	X
Obvious physical immaturity in comparison with other competitors	X	X		
Hemorrhagic disease: hemophilia, purpura, and other serious bleeding tendencies	X	X	X	
Diabetes, inadequately controlled	X	X	X	X
Diabetes, controlled jaundice	X	X	X	X
Eyes				
Absence or loss of function of one eye	X	X		
Respiratory				
Tuberculosis (active or symptomatic)	X	X	X	X
Severe pulmonary insufficiency	X	X	X	X
Cardiovascular				
Mitral stenosis, aortic stenosis, aortic insufficiency, coarctation of aorta, cyanotic heart disease, recent carditis of any etiology	X	X	X	X
Hypertension on organic basis	X	X	X	X
Previous heart surgery for congenital or acquired heart disease	X	X		
Liver				
Enlarged liver	X	X		
Skin				
Boils, impetigo, and herpes simplex gladiatorum	X	X		
Spleen				
Enlarged spleen	X	X		
Hernia				
Inguinal or femoral hernia	X	X	X	
Musculoskeletal				
Symptomatic abnormalities or inflammations	X	X	X	X
Functional inadequacy of the musculoskeletal system, congenital or acquired, incompatible with the contact or skill demands of the sport	X	X	X	
Neurologic				
History or symptoms of previous serious head trauma, or repeated concussions	X			
Controlled convulsive disorder				
Convulsive disorder not moderately well controlled by medication	X			
Previous surgery on head	X	X		
Renal				
Absence of one kidney	X	X		
Renal disease	X	X	X	X
Genitalia				
Absence of one testicle				
Undescended testicle				

[a]Includes football, rugby, hockey, lacrosse.
[b]Includes baseball, soccer, basketball, wrestling.
[c]Includes cross-country, track, tennis, crew, swimming.
[d]Includes bowling, golf, archery, field events.
Source: American Medical Association, 1979.

2. **Justification**
   a. **Effectiveness.** The physician should have more leverage in the sports setting, as compared to the general medical setting, for altering health behavior in children for two reasons. First, most children are motivated to participate in a specific sport and would naturally work toward that goal. Second, the physician often has the authority to qualify or disqualify a child from participating in a specific sport. This leverage can often be effective in insuring compliance with suggested interventions.
   b. **Risks.** Children and adolescents, coaches, and parents can become angry if they do not understand the reason for disqualifying a youth from a particular sport. Open communication cannot be overemphasized when dealing with this very delicate and sometimes volatile issue.
   c. **Cost** depends on the specific intervention.

III. Recommendations

A. Early assessment

1. Every child participating in an organized sports or recreational activity should have an initial preparticipation examination by a physician one month prior to the start of competition.
2. Children with no identified medical conditions should have preparticipation examinations upon entering an educational institution, and thereafter on an as-needed basis.
3. Children with identified medical conditions should have at least annual preparticipation examinations.
4. A nationally standardized format for the preparticipation examination should be available in the next few years. Until that time, at a minimum, the guidelines for the history and physical examination given above (see Fig. 34-1) should be followed.
5. Laboratory testing is not routinely indicated in the standard preparticipation examination.

B. Early intervention

1. It is ultimately the responsibility of the physician to either qualify or disqualify a child from participation in a specific sport based on his or her evaluation. If the physician is overruled by the coach or parent, it is the task of the physician to inform the coach or parent that their decision is at odds with medical judgement.
2. We recommend that the preparticipation examination be used to assess whether a correctable condition exists that would allow later participation in the specific sport.However, if doubt exists, balancing the long-term health of the child with the short-term gain of participation, we recommend the conservative course of nonparticipation.
3. If a child is disqualified from a specific sport, we recommend that the preparticipation examination be used as a vehicle for reclassifying him or her into another acceptable sport.
4. Realizing that the preparticipation examination prior to athletic competition may be the only recent history and physical examination for some children, we recommend its use for the assessment and follow-up of potentially serious non-sports-related conditions. We also realize, however, that the preparticipation examination is a screening exam, and it should not be misconstrued as a complete history and physical.

References

1. Gress, J. R., and Spindler, K. P. Screening school-age athletes. Part 1. *Ration. Drug Ther.* 15(9):56, 62, 69, 1985. *Concise, readable overview for screening guidelines.*
2. Smith, N. J. Medical issues in sports medicine. *Pediatr. Rev.* 2(8):229, 1981. *Good overview of general issues.*
3. Boyce, W. T., et al. Epidemiology of injuries in a large, urban school district. *Pediatrics* 74(3):342, 1984. *A specific epidemiologic study of injuries.*
4. Shaffer, T. E. The health examination for participation in sports. *Pediatr. Ann.* 7(10):27, 1978. *A good review.*
5. Smilkstein, G. Health evaluation of high school athletes. *Physician Sports Med.* 9(8):73, 1981. *Review of each state's standards for the preparticipation examination.*

6. Smith, N. J. (ed.). *Sports Medicine: Health Care for Young Athletes.* Evanston, IL: American Academy of Pediatrics, 1983. *Excellent reference, from a variety of perspectives.*
7. Garrick, J. G., and Smith, N. J. Pre-participation sports assessment. *Pediatrics* 66(5):803, 1980. *A classic article proposing guidelines for the examination.*
8. Puffer, J. C. Sports medicine and the adolescent: The preparticipation evaluation. *Semin. Fam. Med.* 2(3):201, 1981. *A good review.*
9. American Medical Association, Committee on Sports Medicine. *Medical Evaluation of the Athlete: A Guide.* Pamphlet OP 209. Chicago: American Medical Association, 1976. *Proposes a nationally accepted format.*
10. American Academy of Pediatrics, Committee on Sports Medicine. Climatic heat stress and the exercising child. *Pediatrics* 69(6):808, 1982. *Position statement that recommends awareness of heat stress in pediatric athletes.*
11. Tanner, J. M. *Growth at Adolescence* (2nd ed.). Oxford: Blackwell, 1962. Pp. 28–39. *Classic article for categorization of stages of sexual maturity.*
12. Peggs, J. F., Reinhardt, R. W., and O'Brien, J. M. Proteinuria in adolescent sports physical examinations. *J. Fam. Pract.* 22(1):80, 1986. *Argues against routine urinalysis in screening exams.*

II

Disease Prevention

35 Growth Disorders

Michael A. Reinhart

The obvious changes in body size, shape, and appearance during infancy and childhood are influenced by a host of factors, including genetic background, prenatal and postnatal environments, and health status [1]. Children identified as smaller or larger than most others are statistically unusual in the population, not necessarily abnormal or diseased; most of them are, in fact, quite normal. However, some of these children have been adversely affected by one or more of the many factors influencing growth and maturation; those with identifiable and, it is hoped, remediable factors are the target of these screening activities. Generally speaking, nutritional problems are the most important cause of growth problems, with short-term deficiencies affecting weight primarily, and more chronic deficiencies influencing length and head circumference [2].

A further purpose of screening, and one more difficult to evaluate, is to acquire the data to reassure patients and parents that growth is progressing at the expected rate. The value of growth measurements, then, cannot be estimated only by the amount of disease discovered but must include a recognition of the importance of normal measurements to patients and parents.

I. The problem

A. Neonatal period.

Growth must be assessed in conjunction with the gestational age, so both factors are discussed here.

1. Description

a. Immaturity. Significant abnormalities of function occur in essentially every organ system in the very immature child (e.g., born at less than 28 weeks' gestation); different or lesser abnormalities are seen as the duration of gestation increases. Neonatal mortality is up to a hundredfold greater in the neonate born at less than 28 weeks' gestation than in a term infant [3]. Subsequent long-term morbidity is significant, although now occurring far less frequently than in the past.

b. Advanced maturity (postmaturity, postdates). The majority of infants born at a gestational age of more than 42 weeks show evidence of "placental insufficiency" and a resulting decreased rate of growth. Perinatal asphyxia, meconium aspiration, and hypoglycemia occur more commonly in these infants. In the minority of postdate infants who continue to grow, the large size achieved increases the risk of birth injury. Overall, neonatal mortality is increased by approximately 40% compared to a 40-week gestation.

c. Decreased intrauterine growth (small-for-gestational-age, [SGA], intrauterine growth retardation). Poor fetal growth may be caused by factors intrinsic to the fetus, such as chromosomal abnormalities, malformation syndromes, or inborn errors of metabolism. Specific maternal medical problems such as infections with rubella or cytomegalovirus (CMV) during early gestation, severe toxemia or hypertension, or severe chronic illness of almost any type may be responsible for fetal growth deficits. Other maternal factors are even more common, e.g., low socioeconomic status, poor nutrition, extreme maternal age (low or high), high altitude, and substance abuse (alcohol, cigarettes, opiates). Abnormalities of the placenta and cord may also affect growth.

Because organs are affected differently by each condition, the patterns of growth impairment differ as to the ultimate rates of morbidity and mortality. Common neonatal complications include birth asphyxia, meconium aspiration syndrome, hypocalcemia, hyper- or hypoglycemia, and hyperviscosity syndrome. Factors that affect growth in early gestation tend to cause the greatest long-term morbidity.

d. **Increased intrauterine growth** (large-for-gestational-age [LGA]). Associated with large maternal size, large maternal gestational weight gain, maternal diabetes, and a few uncommon conditions, these infants are at increased risk of birth trauma and birth asphyxia due to their large size alone. The underlying condition may carry with it additional morbidity, e.g., maternal diabetes causing hypoglycemia in the infant. Implications of high birth weight for later well-being are uncertain at present.

2. **Epidemiology**

a. **Immaturity** is present overall in approximately 5–10% of newborns, and much higher frequencies are found in populations with such identified risk factors as low socioeconomic status, young maternal age, inadequate prenatal nutrition, inadequate prenatal care, and closely spaced pregnancies.

b. **Advanced maturity** occurs in approximately 10% of newborns depending on the population studied. Risk factors are poorly understood.

c. **Decreased intrauterine growth.** By definition, 10% of newborns should be small for gestational age, but the actual prevalence in a given population varies depending on the rates of underlying conditions noted in sec. **I.A.1.c.**

d. **Increased intrauterine growth** is increasingly common, with prevalence rates varying widely depending on the definition used and the population being studied. Most of the recent increase is composed of normal, large infants. Higher rates are found at sea level, in Caucasians, and in multiparous mothers.

B. **Infancy, childhood, and adolescence.** Measurement **trends** are of far more value than isolated measurements. Every effort should be made to put the most recent measurement into the context of the child's past growth patterns.

1. **Description**

a. **Short length or stature.** Height-for-age less than the fifth percentile is most commonly associated with short parental stature, constitutional delay of growth and adolescence, short birth length, and low socioeconomic status. Organic disease (generally of an obvious nature) is responsible for about one-sixth of cases. Only a small minority of the total population of short children have remediable organic or nonorganic etiologic conditions.

b. **Low weight.** Weight-for-age less than the fifth percentile is found in genetically small children, children with any of a vast array of organic diseases (most commonly gastrointestinal or neurologic), and malnourished children (whether due to extreme poverty, psychosocial family disorders, or ignorance of proper nutrition). Early malnutrition may affect future growth potential, with the most critical effect being on the brain. In severely malnourished children, immunologic competence is decreased. Early recognition of many causative conditions improves prognosis.

Weight loss in childhood, whether chronic or acute, merits prompt investigation, although few data are available on the occurence rates of specific etiologies.

c. **Small head circumference** [4] is an important indicator of both general growth deficiency and specific deficiency of brain growth. Race, parental head size, congenital malformations, metabolic disorders, prenatal infections, toxic substances, postnatal infections, trauma, and malnutrition may all affect head size. A small head circumference is statistically associated with decreased performance of the children on intelligence tests and an increased prevalence of other central nervous system symptoms such as seizures. Some microcephalic children, however, will be normal intellectually and neurologically.

d. **Tall stature.** Identified as a problem almost exclusively in girls, it is generally an accepted (and often valued) trait in boys. The condition is most often due to genetic, parental influences and rarely treated. Children with exogenous obesity generally are tall for age in the prepubescent years. Other causes of tall stature are uncommon and generally have other obvious manifestations. They include chromosomal disorders (Klinefelter's syndrome, XYY syndrome), genetic disorders (homocystinuria, Marfan's syndrome), malformation disorders (Soto's syndrome, Weaver's syndrome), and endocrine excess syndromes (growth hormone, thyroid hormone, sex steroids).

e. **Overweight.** Children with a high weight-for-age and excess body fat most commonly have exogenous obesity. In less than 10% do endocrine disorders cause the obesity, and when they do, short stature is associated with it. While medical consequences of obesity are minimal in childhood, obesity that continues into adulthood may increase the risk of a variety of conditions. Psychologic complications are frequently seen beginning in childhood.

High weight-for-height without increased fat mass and with increased muscle mass is not known to be associated with morbidity.

f. **Large head circumference** can be due to a variety of conditions, including hydrocephalus, subdural fluid collection, megalencephaly, and pseudotumor cerebri, as well as being a normal variant. Each of these conditions has been associated with or caused by a number of specific etiologies. The specific causes vary widely with respect to outcome in the untreated state and with respect to the type and effectiveness of treatment. In general, early identification of treatable conditions improves eventual outcome.

2. **Epidemiology**

a. **Short length or stature.** In the subpopulation of the United States for which data were submitted to the Nutrition Surveillance Unit of the Centers for Disease Control, height-for-age less than the fifth percentile was found in 9–10% of children. The National Health Survey data (1963–1965) identified low socioeconomic status as a major risk factor for short stature. Asian children tend to be somewhat shorter than whites and blacks.

b. **Low weight.** Weight-for-age less than the fifth percentile was found in 6.6% of the sample of American children reported to the Nutrition Surveillance Unit in 1977; weight-for-height was low in 4%. However, failure-to-thrive is reported in up to 10% of outpatients and 2–5% of hospitalized children. As above, lower socioeconomic groups are at higher risk for poor weight gain.

c. **Small head circumference.** The prevalence of this condition depends on the rates of occurrence of the numerous prenatal, intrapartum, and postpartum conditions that affect brain growth. Parental head size affects a child's potential head growth.

d. **Tall stature.** Other than familial or constitutionally tall stature, most causes are rare. Girls are usually identified as having the "problem," although acceptance of tall girls seems to be increasing.

e. **Overweight.** Over 9% of American children have a high weight-for-height ratio. Poverty and parental obesity are major risk factors. Having one obese parent (especially the father) increases the risk, and it is increased even more if both parents are obese. Obesity is more common in females; overweight due to increased muscle mass and without excess fat is more common in active adolescent males.

f. **Large head circumference.** As with small head circumference, the risk of having a large head depends on the rates of occurrence of a number of different conditions. Many of these conditions are found at increased rates in family members.

II. Secondary prevention

A. Early detection

1. **Methods**

a. **Gestational age** (GA)

(1) **Techniques.** Methods of postnatal estimation of GA of use to the clinician in the routine care of newborns are based on the neurologic examination and physical examination of the neonate's external characteristics [5, 6]. Other methods such as electroencephalogram patterns, radiographs of ossifying bones, nerve conduction velocity, sleep patterns, and biochemical techniques are impractical. In 1970, Dubowitz and associates published a system of GA estimation based on the combination of external characteristics and the neurologic examination; that technique soon became the most widely used [7]. However, it is difficult to administer the complete examination to a severely ill neonate and illness may have a greater effect on neurologic criteria. For this reason, numerous systems have since been developed that eliminate some or all of the neurologic criteria and may add additional physical examination characteristics. Each of the systems requires careful performance of the examinations and scoring by the published criteria. Because experience with the techniques has been shown to improve the correlation of the assigned GA to the GA established by prenatal methods, training with an experienced examiner is useful. The methods of Dubowitz and Ballard are considered here. The reader is referred to Dubowitz and Dubowitz [7] and Bal-

lard [8] for descriptions of the methods. Very sick infants will not tolerate portions of the Dubowitz examination at all (e.g. ventral suspension), and some objections to the less stressful manipulations (e.g., heel-to-ear) required by the Ballard have been raised.

In term infants, both of these methods are very successful in assigning GA to within 2 weeks of the "actual" age derived from maternal history. In preterm infants (especially 30 weeks or less), the examinations tend to assign a GA that overestimates the "actual" GA; they also tend to overestimate the GA of small-for-gestational-age infants. Asphyxiated infants, infants with respiratory distress syndrome, and infants of diabetic mothers will tend to have underestimated GA by either the Dubowitz or Ballard methods.

b. Weight

(1) Equipment. Charts based on Lubchenco's work, while not truly representative of a normal population because of altitude effects and other influences, remain widely used and useful standards for the neonate [9]. While other neonatal standards exist (e.g., Usher and McLean's [6]), none is without some methodologic concern, and none is so widely available. The National Center for Health Statistics (NCHS) charts should be used for infants and children [10]. Beam scales are widely available; they are accurate if calibrated every 3 to 4 months and zeroed daily and after moving the scale. A table model is appropriate for infants, and a floor model for children [11].

(2) Technique. Weighing after a large meal should be avoided. Nude weights are most accurate. If a child is weighed in a dry diaper or underclothes, clothing weights should be subtracted from the total. Weighing should be performed until two agree within 10 gm (½ oz) in infants and 100 gm (¼ lb) in children.

(3) Variation and accuracy. The NCHS charts are generally appropriate for all racial groups in the preschool years, but children of Asian ethnicity are assigned inappropriately low percentiles after that age [10]. Since day-to-day weight may fluctuate as much as 200 gm, intrasubject differences are generally substantially greater than inter- or intraobserver variations of measurements made by trained personnel.

(4) Frequency of measurement. In general, weighing at each visit for health care is recommended. However, the frequency of recommended weighings is highly variable, Illingworth having recommended 18 weighings in the first year and the American Academy of Pediatrics only 6. This is an area in which investigation of screening yield is needed.

(5) Adjustments. The chronologic age of a child who was born **prematurely** should be adjusted during the first 24 months of life, i.e., subtracting the number of weeks the child is premature. After that age, in one carefully performed study [1], differences became insignificant.

c. Length and height

(1) Equipment. Lubchenco's charts are adequate standards for the neonate and NCHS charts for infants and children. For special applications, Himes, Roche, and Thissen's charts, which adjust for parental height, may be useful [12]. Height velocity charts will find wider use in the future. For children less than 2–3 years, the measuring table should have a rigid, fixed headboard and a movable footboard, with linear scale(s) measured in millimeters and ⅛ in. gradations. For children over 2–3 years, use a wall-mounted measuring tape with movable headpiece or a stadiometer. Scale-mounted measuring rods are too inaccurate for clinical use.

(2) Technique

(a) Recumbent length. For children less than 2–3 years old two examiners are necessary. The child lies face up with the body straight. The assistant (parent) holds the head against the headboard so that the plane through the auditory canals and the lower margin of the orbits is perpendicular to the table. The measurer holds the child's knees and ankles with one hand and with the other brings the footboard firmly against the infant's heels. This should be repeated until two measurements are within ¼ in. (6 mm), and the latter of the pair should be recorded to the nearest ⅛ in. (3 mm).

(b) **Stature.** If the child is over 2–3 years of age, he or she should stand with bare heels together, back straight, and heels, buttocks, and shoulders touching the vertical measuring surface. The plane through the auditory canals and lower orbital margins should be horizontal. A headpiece should be brought down firmly to the top of the head and the measurements read before the child moves away.

(c) **Variation/accuracy.** Recumbent length is 0.7 to 1.7 cm (¼–⅔ in.) greater than stature. Gentle stretching while supine and standing reduces postural variations. The standard deviation of differences between replicate measurements approximates 0.2 cm (1/12 in.) for one observer and 0.7 cm (¼ in.) for two well-trained observers.

(d) **Frequency.** Measurement at each visit for routine health care is recommended, although no effectiveness studies are available to indicate the yield of the procedure at various ages.

(e) **Adjustments.** The chronologic age of children who were **premature** should be adjusted, as for weight, until they are approximately 3½, after which time differences become insignificant. Adjustment for **parental stature** should be performed before embarking on extensive workups for short stature.

d. **Head circumference**

(1) **Equipment.** Flexible metal or fiberglass tapes less than 1 cm wide are optimal. Paper tapes can be used reliably when small amounts of hair are present and the head is dry. They become unreliable if reused many times, if allowed to get wet, or if used in a child having thick hair that must be compressed. NCHS charts should be used with infants and children and Lubchenco's with neonates.

(2) **Techniques.** The tape is passed around the forehead above the supraorbital ridges, around each side of the head at the same level, and over the most prominent point of the occiput. Hair is compressed by tension on the tape. The measurement is read to the nearest 0.1 cm (1/25 in.).

(3) **Variation/accuracy.** Thick hair causes significant variation. For example, hair 0.5 cm thick will increase the circumference of a 47-cm head by 0.8 cm; in a 1-year-old girl that would mean the difference between the 50th and 75th percentile. Because of variability in tape positioning, variability in tension used to compress hair, and molding and edema in neonates, the variability of head circumference measurements is greater than that of length or stature, but it is adequately reliable for clinical purposes.

(4) **Frequency.** Almost two-thirds of postnatal growth of the head occurs before the age of 2 and three-fourths before 3; most conditions affecting head size are first seen before the age of 3. Thus, many experts recommend routine measurements at times of routine health care only until that time. No data exist on the yield from measurements of asymptomatic patients.

(5) **Adjustments.** Chronologic age of children who were **premature** should be adjusted as for weight until they are approximately 18 months old, after which time differences become insignificant. Adjustment for parental head size can be carried out before evaluation of asymptomatic, normally developing children with small or large heads.

(6) **Interpretation.** Children with increasing or decreasing percentiles or single measurements greater than the 95th percentile are noteworthy. Risk factors such as prior intracranial bleeding or infection or the presence of neurodevelopmental abnormalities would mandate a higher index of suspicion that small deviations might be important.

2. **Justification**

a. **Test characteristics.** The procedures are simple, reliable, and valid when performed by trained personnel.

b. **Risks and side effects.** Labeling a child as failing to thrive, as having short stature, as being obese, or as having a too small or large head is often a cause of parental and physician anxiety. Workups should be planned based on the individual clinical situation, not in a shotgun approach that would be costly and perhaps harmful to the child. The risk of some so-called abnormalities, such as moderate obesity, may be less than the risks of inappropriate treatments (e.g., crash diets, drugs).

c. **Costs.** The costs involved are small for an individual child, but they become significant from the standpoint of screening a large population. The benefit can be substantial to the individual child and society.

d. **Acceptability.** Measurements of growth parameters are a part of routine health supervision in the published recommendations of every official organization and are standard pediatric tests, although timing and methods may vary. These procedures thus fall into the group of procedures generally accepted as part of adequate health supervision by professionals and by patients.

III. Early intervention

A. **Methods.** The reader is referred to standard texts of neonatology, endocrinology, and pediatrics for discussions of evaluation and treatment of growth disorders.

B. **Justification**

1. **Effectiveness.** Assessment of **size and maturation of the newborn** provides data that are critically important for care in the immediate neonatal period. Differential diagnoses change depending on the size and gestational age of the newborn; a variety of problems may be anticipated and prevented entirely or treated early with a consequent lessening of morbidity and mortality. Independent assessment of either size or maturation is far less useful than a combined appraisal.

   In the infant and child, inapparent disease may be brought to light by periodic growth screening. A British study showed that while 70% of mothers of children whose **heights** were below the third percentile recognized that their children were short, only 10% had sought medical advice regarding that condition. A small percentage of short children will have remediable organic disease, and some children will benefit from improvement of their psychosocial environment. The benefit most frequently seen is the positive psychological effect that may be gained by identifying, evaluating, and discussing a frequent cause of concern among children and parents.

   Poor weight gain or weight loss is the earliest sign of a wide array of conditions that may be ameliorated or cured by intervention.

   For many of these conditions, early intervention may prevent long-term morbidity or even death, which later intervention may not be able to do effectively. **Obesity** is treated very ineffectively late, especially after body image, patterns of social interactions, and habits of exercise and eating are firmly established. Earlier recognition and intervention may improve the outlook.

   Many of the conditions marked by **excessive head growth** cause pathologic changes that may be reversed effectively in early stages but less successfully as time passes. The pathologic causes of **poor head growth** in general are reversed less readily, but early intervention is essential whenever possible since most brain growth has occurred before the age of 3. No quantification of benefits has been published, and it is probably not realistically achievable, due to the wide array of conditions identified, variation in evaluations, vague psychological benefits, and so on.

2. **Risks and side effects.** See Chap. 2.
3. **Costs.** Interventions range from very expensive to insignificant in cost.
4. **Acceptability.** Variable acceptance of evaluation and treatment depends on the condition, the workup indicated, parental understanding and role in the causation, and the specific treatment proposed.

IV. Recommendations

A. **Early assessment**

1. **Newborn**

   a. The gestational age of all newborns should be estimated. The Ballard examination is a good method for general use.

   b. Weight, length, and head circumference measurements should be obtained on all newborns and plotted on percentile charts, such as Lubchenco's, that incorporate gestational age.

2. **Zero to three years**

   a. Length, weight, and head circumference measurements should be obtained at each routine visit for health care supervision; data should be plotted on NCHS graphs, adjusting for duration of prematurity, if any.

   b. The child should be weighed at each health care visit.

B. **Early intervention.** Assessment and treatment must be planned on the basis of past growth patterns, parental size, and other **individual** factors.

References

1. Falkner, F., and Tanner, J. M. (eds.). *Human Growth* (2nd ed.). Vol. 1, *Developmental Biology: Prenatal Growth;* Vol. 2, *Postnatal Growth: Neurobiology;* Vol. 3, *Methodology: Ecological, Genetic, and Nutritional Effects on Growth.* New York: Plenum. 1986. *An excellent compilation of authoritative reviews of selected topics related to human growth.*
2. Rallison, M. L. *Growth Disorders in Infants, Children, and Adolescents.* New York: Wiley, 1986. *A useful, overall review of growth problems seen in clinical practice.*
3. Manser, J. I. Growth in the high-risk infant. *Clin. Perinatol.* 11(1):19, 1984. *A clinically useful review of growth in high-risk infants.*
4. Menkes, J. H. *Textbook of Child Neurology* (3rd ed.). Philadelphia: Lea & Febiger, 1985. pp. 224–234. *Useful reference for conditions affecting head growth.*
5. Battaglia, F. C., and Lubchenco, L. C. A practical classification of newborn infants by weight and gestational age. *J. Pediatr.* 71(2):159, 1967. *Widely used and available through Mead and Johnson Nutritional Division. While underestimating normal growth potential, these articles remain clinically useful.*
6. Usher, R., and McLean, F. Intrauterine growth of live-born Caucasian infants at sea level: Standards obtained from measurements in 7 dimensions of infants born between 25 and 44 weeks of gestation. *J. Pediatr.* 74(6):901, 1969. *An alternative set of neonatal growth standards.*
7. Dubowitz, L. M. S., Dubowitz, V., and Goldberg, C. Clinical assessment of gestational age in the newborn infant. *J. Pediatr.* 77:1, 1970. *A classic description of the Dubowitz exam.*
8. Ballard, J. L., Novak, K. K., and Driver, M. A simplified score for assessment of fetal maturation of newly born infants. *J. Pediatr.* 95(5 part 1):769, 1979. *Gestational age estimation system; also available from Mead Johnson Nutritional Division.*
9. Lubchenco, L. C., Hansman, C., and Boyd, E. Intrauterine growth in length and head circumference as estimated from live births at gestational age from 26 to 42 weeks. *Pediatrics* 37(3):403, 1966. *See reference 5.*
10. Hamill, P. V., et al. Physical growth: National Center for Health Statistics percentiles. *Am. J. Clin. Nutr.* 32(3):607, 1979. *NCHS growth charts, also available from Ross Laboratories and Mead Johnson Nutritional Division, are the best generally applicable American growth curves.*
11. *Nutrition Surveillance.* Atlanta, GA: Centers for Disease Control, 1980. *Design specifications for clinic measuring equipment and some acceptable products available in January 1981.*
12. Himes, J. H., Roche, A. F., and Thissen, D. *Parent-Specific Adjustments for Assessment of Recumbent Length and Stature* Basel, Switzerland: S. Karger, 1981. *Tables for adjustment of length and height based on American data; also available from Ross Laboratories.*

36 Congenital Dislocation of the Hip

George Rab

I. The problem

A. Definition. Congenital dislocation of the hip (CDH) encompasses a continuum of disorders of hip stability, from simple capsular laxity to gross joint dislocation [1]. Terms commonly used include the following:

1. **Dislocation:** the hip joint surfaces are not in contact with each other, and the femoral head lies outside the acetabulum.
2. **Subluxation:** the joint surfaces are in partial contact, and the femoral head lies partially within the acetabulum. This represents a "partial" or "incomplete" dislocation.
3. **Dysplasia:** refers to retarded or abnormal growth, usually in the shape of the femoral head or the acetabulum. Dysplasia usually occurs when the joint surfaces do not mate properly (such as in a chronic subluxation).
4. **Capsular laxity:** hormonal or mechanical factors may play a role in this. Capsular laxity must be present for subluxation or dislocation to occur, and it is responsible for the "dislocatable" but otherwise normal hip in infants.

Much of the difficulty in evaluating studies of CDH prevention is related to the varied and often vague application of these different subsets of patients who clearly have different outcomes.

B. Description. Congenital dislocation of the hip is a serious orthopedic disorder that, if left untreated, can cause major disability. Untreated CDH can result in false acetabulum formation, limb shortening, and degenerative hip changes. In CDH, the femoral head displaces proximally and posteriorly, with ligamentous laxity allowing the capsule of the hip to stretch. This laxity is most pronounced at birth when maternal hormonal factors play a role, although positional factors in the womb are also important.

C. Epidemiology. In the absence of neonatal testing, the incidence of CDH that is first seen when the infant becomes mobile is approximately 1/1000 live births. The prevalence of hip abnormalities detected at birth in screening programs ranges from 2.5 to 31/1000 and averages about 11/1000; one-half to two-thirds of these hip abnormalities have become normal by three weeks of age [1].

1. **Risk groups.** CDH is more common in girls (6 : 1), firstborn children, and breech presentation (hence, caesarean section since breech presentation is a common indication for caesarean). The overall risk for hip instability in females born breech can be as high as 1 in 15. There is also a hereditary component; families with a history of CDH have a significantly increased chance of having children with the disorder. Racial factors are also important; CDH is very rare in blacks, but it is found in very high percentages in some American Indian tribes, including the Cree and Ojibwa populations. CDH often accompanies other musculoskeletal disorders. It is commonly found in conjunction with torticollis, clubfoot, and metatarsus adductus, and frequently accompanies syndromes with multiple areas of skeletal involvement.

II. Secondary prevention

A. Early detection

1. Methods

a. Physical examination of the neonate

(1) Timing. The best time to examine an infant for CDH is in the newborn nursery. There is no one screening test that is diagnostic of the disease, so many examinations have been devised. Careful serial screening is the best method of detection.

(2) Performance and interpretation. Salient features of the examination are shown in Fig. 36-1. The child should be relaxed, perhaps being offered a nipple at the time of the exam. A screaming, excited child will have poor relaxation, and thus frank CHD may not be apparent. It should be noted that the hip may be dislocated at birth or it may be dislocatable. In the dislocatable hip, the femoral head rests within the acetabulum, but there is sufficient ligamentous laxity so that it can be subluxed or displaced posterosuperiorally by the examiner. Children with bilateral dislocations are more difficult to examine, since there is no normal to compare with.

Recommended examination observations and maneuvers are:

(a) **Abnormal gluteal and inguinal skin creases** (Fig. 36-1A). When unilateral, abnormal gluteal and inguinal skin creases may be an obvious sign, due to shortening of the dislocated femur. Many normal children have asymmetric skin creases, however.

(b) **Difference in femoral length (Galeazzi's sign)** (Fig. 36-1B). The child's buttocks are placed on a **firm** surface, carefully making sure that they are even and flat. The hips are flexed 90 degrees. If the hip is dislocated posteriorly, the affected limb will appear shorter and the knee level will be lower. This test is not helpful in bilateral CDH and may be falsely negative with a child under 6 months of age.

(c) **Limitation of abduction with the hips in flexion** (Fig. 36-1C). This is the best single screening test in the newborn nursery and can be done by physicians and nurses as a routine. In the normal newborn the hips can be abducted beyond 70 degrees when flexed. Asymmetry of abduction, or inability to abduct beyond 60 degrees, is highly suggestive of hip dysplasia. The test will not be positive if the hip is dislocatable.

(d) **Ortolani's maneuver** (Fig. 36-1D). In this test, the thigh is grasped with the examiner's hand and the knee is held flexed, to relax the gracilis and the iliotibial band. The thumb is held against the lesser trochanter and the fingers against the greater trochanter. The opposite hand stabilizes the pelvis. As the leg is abducted, the hand gently lifts the hip by pulling up on the greater trochanter. If the hip is dislocated, the examiner may feel a "clunk" as the hip reduces. The sensation of reduction is palpated and usually not audible.

(e) **Barlow's maneuver** (Figs. 36-1D–F). In this test, which is the opposite of Ortolani's maneuver, a dislocatable but reduced hip is felt to slide out of the acetabulum when the leg is brought into adduction. The limb and pelvis is held the same way as described above in Ortolani's. With the hip in flexion and adduction, gentle downward pressure at the knee and outward pressure—using the thumb against the lesser trochanter—forces the located hip to slide over the posterior acetabular rim. The sensation is felt, not heard.

With practice, these tests can be done smoothly. Barlow's and Ortolani's maneuvers are frequently done as a combined abduction-lifting, adduction-pushing maneuver. Models (e.g., "Baby-Hippy") are available to teach the sensation of reduction and subluxation to inexperienced examiners.

b. **Physical examination of the older infant**

(1) **Performance and interpretation.** After the first 2 to 3 months of age, secondary fibrous contracture of the periarticular structure causes the physical findings to change. The ability of the femoral head to be pulled into the acetabulum (the source of a positive Ortolani's test) is lost. **From 3 months to walking age, the main physical findings are those of flexion contracture, adduction contracture, and shortening of the femoral shaft (Galeazzi's sign).**

Detection of flexion contracture can be subtle, but it is a very important physical finding. The normal child can hide a 15- to 20-degree flexion contracture of the hip by simply hyperextending the spine, allowing the pelvis to tilt and the contracted hip to appear to extend normally. This can be avoided by flexing the normal side fully against the chest, forcing the lumbar lordosis to reverse and the pelvis to assume a fully tilted position. The flexion contraction then becomes obvious (Fig. 36-2).

Limitation of abduction remains detectable because the femoral head

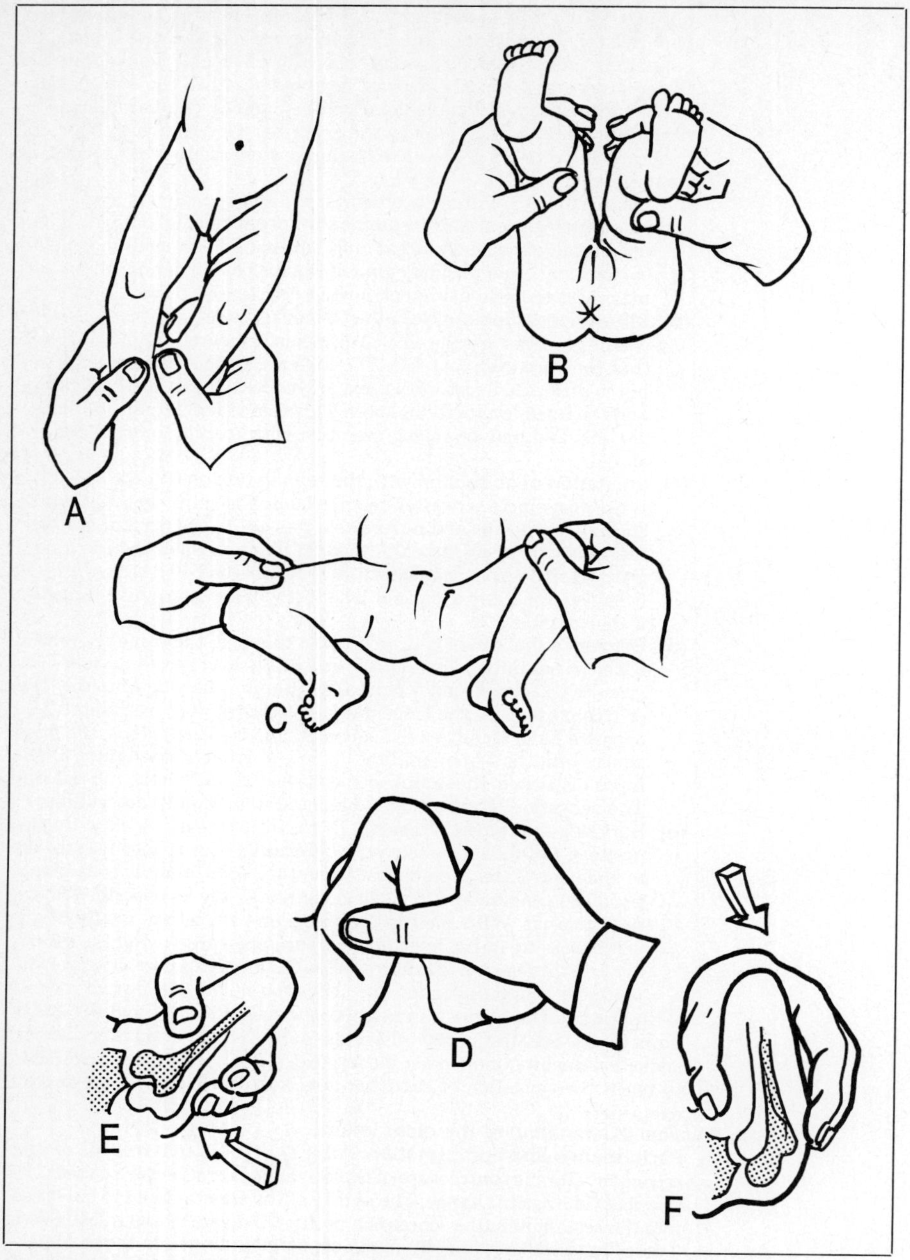

Fig 36-1. Examination maneuvers for congenital hip dislocation. A. Asymmetry for skin folds: Folds may be increased and the hip held in an adducted posture on the dislocated side. B. Galeazzi's sign: The dislocated hip lies posteriorly, making the femur seem short. C. Limitation of abduction. D. Proper method for holding the hlp during Barlow's and Ortolani's maneuvers. E. Barlow's sign: The dislocated hip is lifted into the acetabulum while abducting the femur. F. Barlow's sign: The located hip is dislocated by adducting and pushing posteriorly on the unstable joint. (See text for full description.)

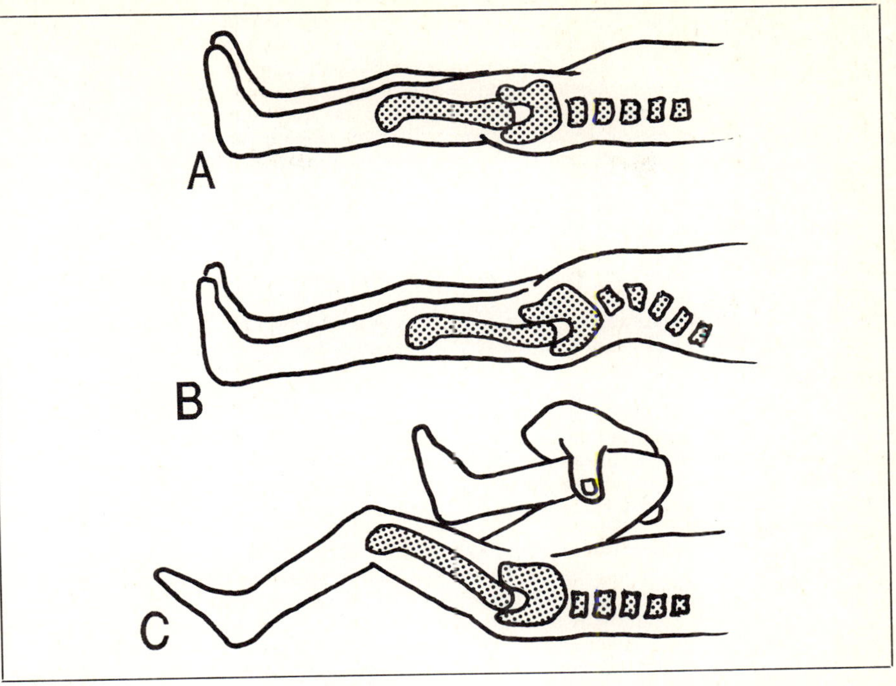

Fig. 36-2. Detection of flexion contracture. A. There is normally a lumbar lordosis in the supine position. B. Hip contractures of up to 30 degrees can be "hidden" by increases in lumbar lordosis. C. By flexing the contralateral hip against the thigh, the lumbar lordosis is flattened out, revealing the underlying hip flexion contraction.

lies posterior and superior to the acetabulum, increasing the lever arm of the adductor muscles and magnifying their influence.

c. **Physical examination of the walking child.** Once the child begins walking, the most obvious physical finding is the presence of a **Trendelenburg limp,** in which the trunk is swung over the affected limb during weightbearing. The gait is frequently described as "waddling." Range of motion may be full, although x-rays at this age will be diagnostic.

d. **Radiologic examination.** It is well known that clinical examination is the best technique for detecting CDH. X-ray films of frankly dislocated or dislocatable hips may appear normal in infants up to 6 months, since the femoral head and acetabulum are cartilaginous at birth. **A questionable exam with normal x-rays therefore should suggest the diagnosis of CDH. A negative radiologic exam does not exclude the disease; abnormal x-rays confirm the disorder,** however.

Radiology examinations are much more useful after the child is 6 months, since at approximately 6 months of age the normal proximal femoral ossific center appears. At this time, radiographic determination of the exact location of the femoral head is much easier. Normal joint development requires physiologic motion with the joint reduced, and there may be retardation of growth if the hip is distorted. This can be seen radiographically by a delay in the appearance of the femoral ossific nucleus on the affected side (after 6 months), or by an increase in the slope of the acetabular roof, which indicates a shallow, dysplastic acetabulum.

2. **Justification**

a. **Test characteristics.** The Centers for Disease Control (CDC) has stated that "the diagnosis of this defect [CHD] lacks clear, reproducible criteria," [2] and many of the positives noted early will revert to negatives within 3 weeks of birth without treatment. With a disease with a prevalence of 0.1% (CDH), using a test with a sensitivity of 99% will generate 91% false positives [3]. Inexperienced examiners may feel a minor click and incorrectly assume it to be a positive Ortolani's sign or Barlow's sign, thus generating a false positive. These two named findings, however, are quite distinctive and different from minor clicks. False negatives are also significant problems [4]. The predictive accuracy of multiple tests over time is difficult to estimate, but there is little doubt that repeated examination of the infant is the best way to detect CDH. Results of individual examinations may be inconclusive, so even experienced observers may miss the diagnosis.

b. **Risks and side effects.** The physical examination tests described have no known risks although radiation may have risks.

c. **Costs** are negligible for the physical examination but are significant for x-rays.

d. **Acceptability.** There appears to be good acceptance, both by the public and the profession, of the physical examination maneuvers.

B. Early intervention

1. **Methods.** In North America, most children with isolated hip clicks are treated by the practitioner who detects them; children with more obvious signs of hip instability are generally referred for orthopedic care.

a. **Isolated clicks with normal examination** are usually benign. Infants with such clicks are placed in double diapers to maintain abduction and reexamined in three weeks. If the hip click is still present, referral to an orthopedic surgeon is wise.

b. **Dislocatable hips in newborns** are normally reduced, so they can be safely held in abduction by any of a number of splints (Frejka pillow, von Rosen splint, Craig splint). Barlow's sign should disappear rapidly, at which time the splint may be discontinued. Follow-up x-rays after appearance of the ossific nucleus of the proximal femur (at 6 months of age) are indicated.

c. **Dislocated hips in newborns.** The Pavlik harness has become the treatment of choice in this group. It is a device that allows the child to actually "kick in" a dislocated hip by limiting extension and adduction (the unstable positions) while allowing active flexion and abduction. Failure of the hip to spontaneously reduce in a properly fitted Pavlik harness is an indication that closed or open reduction of the hip under anesthesia is necessary.

d. **Dislocated hips in older infants.** The Pavlik harness may effect reduction in infants up to 6–9 months of age. If it fails, the child should have preliminary skin traction (to stretch contracted tissues and reduce the chance of avascular necrosis), followed by closed or open reduction.

e. **Dislocated hip in walking child.** Depending on the child's age, he or she may require either closed or open reduction, sometimes preceded by a period in traction. Late reconstructive surgery, usually an osteotomy to reorient the femur or acetabulum because of secondary anatomic changes, is frequently necessary.

2. **Justification**

a. **Effectiveness.** Randomized clinical trials demonstrating the superiority of early detection and intervention over late detection and intervention have not been done and probably are unethical to consider today. Clinical experience holds that when treated early CDH can usually be managed by nonoperative methods, with excellent results. When treated late, multiple operative reconstructive procedures may be required, and the hip may still be abnormal. It is remotely possible that many of the "excellent" results in those cases of CDH detected early would have spontaneously resolved without treatment.

b. **Risks and side effects.** Abduction and immobilization can in rare cases result in aseptic necrosis of the femoral head. However, the risks of nonoperative treatment are far less than those of operative treatment. The real question is whether the risks of nonoperative treatment are small enough to warrant exposure of the many false-positive individuals to them, in order to be certain that intervention was "early enough" in the true positive individuals. Since, as noted earlier, it is difficult to clinically separate false-positive and true-positive individuals, current clinical practice has evolved the stepped approach described in sec. **II.B.1.** With this approach, increasing severity or certainty of a detected condition or diagnosis dictates increased willingness to accept more invasive intervention.

c. **Costs.** The costs of nonoperative intervention are less than the costs of operative intervention.
d. **Acceptability.** Patient acceptance of nonoperative and operative intervention appears to be good but has not been studied.

III. Recommendations

A. Early detection

1. All newborns should be examined for CDH before discharge from the hospital, using the following observations and maneuvers.
   a. Abnormal gluteal and inguinal skin creases.
   b. Difference in femoral length (Galeazzi's sign).
   c. Limitation of abduction with the hips in flexion.
   d. Ortolani's maneuver.
   e. Barlow's maneuver.
2. These tests should be repeated whenever the infant is examined until he or she is 3 months of age.
3. After 3 months of age, the infant should be checked at each health maintenance visit for flexion contracture, adduction contracture, and shortening of the femoral shaft. Ortolani's maneuver and Barlow's maneuver are not helpful after this age.
4. X-rays taken before the infant is 6 months old are not helpful if negative and therefore are not recommended for screening. After 6 months they may be helpful, and certainly, any child who presents with a waddling Trendelenburg limp should be evaluated by radiography.

B. Early intervention

1. Isolated hip clicks found on an otherwise normal examination can be treated, by the primary care provider who detected them, by keeping the infant in double diapers for 3 weeks. If the hip click is still present on re-examination after that time, the infant should be referred to an orthopedist.
2. Dislocatable and dislocated hips of any age should be referred to an orthopedist for evaluation and treatment.

References

1. Hensinger, R. N. Congenital dislocation of the hip. *Clin. Symp.* 31(1):3, 1979. *Excellent review article.*
2. Temporal trends in the incidence of birth defects—United States. *M.M.W.R.* 28(34):401, 1979. *Incidents reported to the CDC.*
3. Frankenburg, W. K. To screen or not to screen: Congenital dislocation of the hip. *Am. J. Public Health* 71(12):1311, 1981. *Commentary on CDH screening by a leader in pediatric screening.*
4. Parkin, D. M. How successful is screening for congenital disease of the hip? *Am. J. Public Health* 71(12):1378, 1981. *Good literature review article.*

37 Hemorrhagic Disease of the Newborn

Sarah Woerner

I. The problem

A. Description. Hemorrhagic disease of the newborn (HDN) is a condition thought to be caused by a vitamin K deficiency. It is most commonly manifested by increased bleeding into the skin, umbilicus, or gastrointestinal tract within one to three days of birth. A late hemorrhagic syndrome, occurring one to three months after birth and affecting breast-fed babies, has also been described [1]. This late syndrome frequently presents as an intracranial hemorrhage.

Vitamin K is necessary for the activity of factors II, VII, IX, and X in blood clotting. It works by modifying the glutamic acid residues on the procoagulant forms of these molecules, allowing them to facilitate the clotting cascade.

Older infants absorb vitamin K through the colon, where it is synthesized by bacteria [2]. In the newborn, however, vitamin K levels are low, presumably because the gut takes several days to weeks to become colonized by bacteria. Additionally, there is poor placental transfer of vitamin K [3]. The newborn infant is therefore almost entirely dependent on extrinsic sources of vitamin K.

B. Epidemiology. Reports of the prevalence of HDN in infants **not** receiving vitamin K at birth show tremendous variation, ranging from none in 6000 babies to 1.7% [4]. Most estimates, however, lie between 0.25% and 0.5% [5].

Breast-fed infants are at increased risk of developing HDN without vitamin K prophylaxis. Vitamin K deficiency has been found to occur at least twice as frequently in breast-fed infants as in those fed cow's milk formulas [4]. Sutherland and associates [4] demonstrated a 5% risk of spontaneous bleeding in unsupplemented breast-fed babies, and a 10% risk of bleeding after circumcision in unsupplemented breast-fed males undergoing that procedure. Recently, there have been several case reports of late HDN in breast-fed babies who did not receive prophylactic vitamin K at birth. The majority of these babies were delivered at home [6, 7, 8]. Breast milk contains 15 μg/liter of vitamin K, while cow's milk contains 60 μg/liter and formulas contain approximately 50 μg/liter.

Other infants at increased risk for HDN include those whose mothers are taking vitamin K antagonists (coumarin, warfarin) or are on anticonvulsant medications (phenytoin, barbiturates); babies with malabsorption (cystic fibrosis, gastroenteritis); and infants receiving antibiotics, which decrease normal gastrointestinal flora.

II. Secondary prevention—early intervention

A. Methods. The current recommendation of the American Academy of Pediatrics is for administration of 1 mg of vitamin K_1 intramuscularly soon after birth (preferably within one hour) [9]. Additional **potential** methods of prevention that have been studied include administering oral vitamin K_1 to the newborn [10], and providing prenatal and postnatal vitamin K supplementation for the mother.

B. Justification.

1. **Effectiveness.** Given intramuscularly at the time of birth, vitamin K decreases the usual decline in vitamin K-dependent clotting factors that occurs during the first three to seven days of life [1]. Sutherland and associates [4] reported a four-fold difference in the incidence of bleeding from all sites between groups of babies given a placebo and those given supplemental vitamin K: 1.7% versus 0.4%, respectively. Prophylactic vitamin K has also been shown to significantly decrease the incidence of bleeding from circumcision in newborn males [4]. The daily requirement for vitamin K in the newborn has been estimated to be 1–5 μg, though 1 mg is generally administered.

   Several authors have investigated the efficacy of **oral**, compared to intramuscular, vitamin K prophylaxis. These studies suggest that oral vitamin K_1 given in doses of 1–2 mg shortly after birth to term, healthy infants does produce therapeutic levels initially, and that it is likely to prevent early HDN [10, 11]. However, no studies on the long-term efficacy of a single oral dose have been conducted.

Studies of mothers receiving oral anticonvulsants during the last months of pregnancy have shown a decreased risk of HDN when mothers were given oral vitamin K supplements before their infants' birth [12].

Some authors have demonstrated that as many as 75% of normal newborns and 33% of their mothers are vitamin K-deficient at the infant's birth [1]. Administration of 20 mg of oral vitamin K to lactating mothers has been shown to produce a 70-fold increase in the amount of vitamin K in breast milk. These and other studies have encouraged some hematologists to recommend that breast-feeding mothers receive vitamin K supplementation [3].

2. **Risks and side effects.** Two forms of vitamin K are available commercially. Vitamin K_1 (phytonadione, Mephyton, AquaMEPHYTON, Konakion) is fat-soluble and causes no known toxicity in doses up to 25 mg. Vitamin K_3 (menadione, Hykinone, Synkayvite) is water-soluble and has caused hemolytic anemia, hyperbilirubinemia, and kernicterus in newborns. For this reason vitamin K_1 is the recommended preparation [1].
3. **Costs.** The cost to the patient of a 1-mg intramuscular dose is \$5–\$10. The cost of a 5-mg tablet purchased from the pharmacy is \$0.05 to \$0.10.
4. **Acceptability.** Some parents express concern about whether the pain of an intramuscular injection is necessary when the oral preparation may be safe and effective. Infants generally tolerate the injection without sequelae.

III. Recommendations

A. **All newborns** should receive 1 mg of vitamin K_1 intramuscularly as soon as possible (within 1 hour) after birth.

B. **Infants whose parents refuse the intramuscular vitamin K** should be given 1–5 mg of oral vitamin K_1 (Mephyton), either in crushed tablet form or liquid form. Although this is **not** the recommended therapy, it is preferable to **no** supplementation.

C. **Breast-fed infants with diarrhea** of more than several days' duration should be given an additional dose of vitamin K_1 (1 mg IM) [1].

D. **Infants with malabsorption** (e.g., cystic fibrosis, biliary atresia) should be supplemented with 50–100 μg orally daily, or 1 mg IM monthly [1].

E. **Other high-risk infants** may benefit from additional measures, and the following guidelines are offered. (These guidelines represent the opinions of respected authors, but because they have not been fully tested yet, they are not discussed in detail in this chapter.)

1. **Infants of mothers receiving anticonvulsants.**
   a. The mother should receive an oral vitamin K supplement during the last several weeks of pregnancy. Oral daily doses of 20 mg have been recommended [10].
   b. Administering 1 mg of vitamin K intravenously to the mother shortly before delivery has been shown to raise the vitamin K levels in cord plasma to detectable amounts and may be of use [8].
   c. If a traumatic delivery is anticipated, cesarean section should be considered to avoid unnecessarily risking hemorrhage in the infant [13].
2. **Infants of mothers receiving oral anticoagulants.** An attempt should be made to switch the mother from oral anticoagulants to heparin therapy from 37 weeks' gestation up until the child is born. Heparin does not cross the placenta and will not affect the infant's coagulation [14].
3. **Breast-fed infants.** Some authors suggest that giving 20 mg of oral vitamin K_1 twice weekly to lactating mothers may prevent late hypoprothrombinemia in breast-fed infants [3].
4. **Other high-risk infants.** In infants with the following risk factors, vitamin K deficiency is likely: infants on antibiotic regimens, infants receiving parenteral nutrition or having decreased dietary intake of vitamin K, and infants with hepatitis [1]. Clotting factor assays and dietary supplementation with vitamin K should be considered in these infants.

References

1. Lane, P. A., and Hathaway, W. E. Vitamin K in infancy. *J. Pediatr.* 106(3):351, 1985. *Excellent up-to-date review of all aspects of vitamin K in infants.*
2. Aballi, A. J., Howard, C. E., and Triplett, R. F. Absorption of vitamin K from the colon in the newborn infant. *J. Pediatr.* 68(2):305, 1966. *These authors demonstrated that vitamin K preparations in newborns were absorbed well rectally.*
3. Shearer, M. J., et al. Plasma vitamin K_1 levels in mothers and their newborn babies. *Lancet* 2:460, 1982. *A good study demonstrating that cord blood levels of vitamin K_1 in newborns are extremely low or nondetectable in those born to mothers who do not receive extra supplementation.*
4. Sutherland, J. M., Glueck, H. I., and Gleser, G. Hemorrhagic disease of the newborn: Breast feeding as a necessary factor in pathogenesis. *Am. J. Dis. Child.* 113:524, 1967. *This important study determined that breast-fed infants have a significantly higher risk of bleeding after birth.*
5. Miller, D. R., and Pearson, H. A. (eds.). *Smith's Blood Diseases of Infancy and Childhood* (4th ed.). St. Louis: Mosby, 1978. *Standard textbook of pediatric hematology.*
6. Chaou, W. T., Chou, M. L., and Eitzman, D. V. Intracranial hemorrhage and vitamin K deficiency in early infancy. *J. Pediatr.* 105(6):880, 1984. *One in a series of articles (see also references 7 and 8) with case reports of late HDN in breast-fed infants who did not receive vitamin K prophylaxis.*
7. Motohara, K., et al. Severe vitamin K deficiency in breast-fed infants. *J. Pediatr.* 105(6):943, 1984. *See annotation for reference 6.*
8. O'Connor, M. E., et al. Vitamin K deficiency and breast-feeding. *Am. J. Dis. Child.* 137(6):601, 1983. *See annotation for reference 6.*
9. Vitamin K compounds and the water-soluble analogues. Use in therapy and prophylaxis in pediatrics (report of Committee on Nutrition). *Pediatrics* 28:501, 1961. *The official Academy of Pediatrics recommendations for vitamin K prophylaxis. The article outlines all the studies serving as a basis for these recommendations.*
10. McNinch, A. W., et al. Plasma concentrations after oral or intramuscular vitamin K_1 in neonates. *Arch. Dis. Child.* 60(9):814, 1985. *This study demonstrates therapeutic vitamin K levels in newborns given oral prophylaxis.*
11. O'Connor, M. E., and Addiego, J. E., Jr. Use of oral vitamin K_1 to prevent hemorrhagic disease of the newborn infant. *J. Pediatr.* 108(4):616, 1986. *Compares oral versus intramuscular vitamin K in breast-fed infants by examining levels of PIVKA in the two groups.*
12. Deblay, M. F., et al. Transplacental vitamin K prevents haemorrhagic disease of infant of epileptic mother. *Lancet* 1(8283):1247, 1982. *A study (cited in a letter) demonstrating that oral vitamin K given prenatally to mothers on anticonvulsants likely leads to a decreased risk of HDN.*
13. Bleyer, W. A., and Skinner, A. L. Fatal neonatal hemorrhage after maternal anticonvulsant therapy. *J.A.M.A.* 235(6):626, 1976. *One of many case reports of hemorrhage in an otherwise healthy infant whose mother had been taking anticonvulsants. The authors give recommendations for preventing other such fatal cases.*
14. Hirsch, J., Cade, J. F., and O'Sullivan, E. F. Clinical experience with anticoagulant therapy during pregnancy. *Br. Med. J.* 1(5691):270, 1970. *The author outlines his regimen, in which he uses heparin rather than oral medications, which has led to decreased risk of bleeding in the neonate.*

38 Ophthalmia Neonatorum

Jay Milstein

I. The problem

A. Description. Ophthalmia neonatorum or neonatal conjunctivitis is a venereal disease manifested by hyperemia, swelling, and discharge from conjunctival surfaces or periorbital tissues during the neonatal period [1, 2]. Prior to routine prophylactic treatment, this disease was a major cause of blindness. However, the frequency of the disease and its complications have decreased dramatically since prophylaxis was introduced. The etiology includes infectious and chemical agents.

1. **Infectious agents.** Two organisms are responsible for most infectious neonatal conjunctivitis.
   a. *Neisseria gonorrhoeae* conjunctivitis usually manifests itself by 2–4 days after birth. With prompt systemic antibiotics and local saline irrigation, clinical response is good [3]. Without treatment, the initial inflammatory response may be followed by the development of a pseudomembrane, keratitis, corneal ulceration, and ultimately visual disability [2].
   b. *Chlamydia trachomatis* or trachomatis inclusion conjunctivitis usually manifests itself by 5–12 days after birth but has been noted as early as 2 days after birth [2]. Clinical response to appropriate topical antibiotic therapy is good if the disease is treated within the first 12 days of life. If definitive therapy is delayed beyond 12 days, membranous conjunctivitis, leading to conjunctival scarring as well as keratitis with superficial corneal vascularization, may develop [4].
   c. Other bacteria, including *Staphylococci, Pneumococci,* B-hemolytic *Streptococci, Proteus, Klebsiella, Pseudomonas,* and *Escherichia coli* have been responsible [2].
2. **Chemical conjunctivitis** usually develops within 24 hours of birth and is frequently seen following ocular prophylaxis, but it is self-limited [5].

B. Epidemiology. Approximately 28% of untreated infants born to mothers with a gonococcal infection will develop gonococcal ophthalmia [3], and from 6–75% of pregnant women may harbor gonorrhea subclinically [6]. Chlamydial infection may be present in 2–20% of pregnant women [7]. According to the Centers for Disease Control (CDC), over 155,000 infants are born to chlamydia-infected mothers each year [8]. Between 18–50% of infants born to infected mothers will develop chlamydia ophthalmia from 1–3 weeks after birth [9]. With the practice of ocular prophylaxis in the United States, the incidence of ophthalmia neonatorum secondary to gonorrhea and chlamydia is approximately 0.04% and 0.4%, respectively [7]. In one study [10] chlamydia ophthalmia occurred more often in black than in white infants, while gonococcal ophthalmia was evenly distributed.

II. Secondary prevention

A. Early assessment. Expectant mothers should be checked closely for possible venereal infections (see Chaps. 15–17). If the mother had premature and/or prolonged rupture of membranes, the newborn infant should be observed more closely for development of conjunctivitis. In general, however, all infants should be observed for such symptoms, since prophylaxis has markedly reduced but not eliminated the disease.

B. Early intervention

1. **Methods**
   a. **All newborns should receive ocular prophylaxis within 1 hour of birth,** with a 0.5- to 1.0-cm strip of 0.5% erythromycin ointment, two drops of 1% silver nitrate, or a 0.5- to 1.0-cm strip of 1% tetracycline ointment placed in each conjunctival sac without rinsing [3]. If chlamydia is endemic in the population served, prophylaxis with erythromycin is preferred.

b. **If the mother has a known gonococcal infection,** a single dose of aqueous crystalline penicillin G should be given IV or IM along with the ocular prophylaxis, since occasional cases of ophthalmia neonatorum have occurred in spite of prophylaxis. The dose is 50,000 units for term infants and 20,000 units for low birth weight infants [3].

c. **If inflammatory changes develop after 24 hours, chemical conjunctivitis is unlikely.** Establishing an etiologic diagnosis is essential for definitive therapy. Eye cultures for gonorrhea, other bacteria, and chlamydia may be warranted, as well as acute Gram's and Giemsa stains to determine if specific treatment is necessary for gonorrheal or chlamydial ophthalmia.

2. **Justification**

a. **Effectiveness.** Ocular prophylaxis has significantly reduced the incidence of ophthalmia neonatorum. Because the incidence of maternal gonorrheal and chlamydia infections is so high, as is the incidence of ophthalmia in the untreated infants, continuation of ocular prophylaxis is warranted. Following the introduction of silver nitrate prophylaxis, Credé reported a reduction in gonorrheal ophthalmia neonatorum, in Leipzig, from an extraordinarily high level of 10% of births to less than 1% [11].

Erythromycin and possibly tetracycline are effective in preventing both gonococcal and chlamydial ophthalmia, while silver nitrate is effective prophylaxis for gonococcal but not chlamydial ophthalmia [12]. The efficacy of tetracycline and erythromycin in the prevention of penicillinase-producing gonococcal ophthalmia is unknown.

b. **Risks and side effects.** The major complication, particularly with silver nitrate prophylaxis, is a chemical conjunctivitis. Although it usually subsides within 24 hours, if it is more sustained, gonococcal or chlamydial infections may have to be considered.

Prophylaxis may be inadequate in infants born to mothers with active gonococcal or chlamydial infections, especially in those whose mothers have premature or prolonged rupture of amniotic membranes, when the duration and magnitude of the infant's exposure to the infective agents may be increased by an ascending infection.

Inadequate prophylaxis for chlamydial ophthalmia may also occur if only silver nitrate and possibly tetracycline are used. Silver nitrate has not been shown to reduce the incidence of chlamydial ophthalmia [7]. Although the Centers for Disease Control consider 1% tetracycline ointment to be effective for chlamydial prophylaxis [12], its efficacy has not been proven and at least several cases of failure in the form of a serious infection have been reported [13].

Another potential hazard of prophylaxis is that the health care provider may falsely assume that ophthalmia neonatorum is no longer a risk in a patient given ocular prophylaxis, and subsequently does not provide adequate follow-up care.

c. **Costs.** The relative costs are $1, $2, and $6 for ocular prophylaxis with silver nitrate, erythromycin, and tetracycline, respectively, based on wholesale prices in 1986. This is relatively inexpensive when compared with the cost of diagnostic tests and the treatment of a case of ophthalmia neonatorum.

d. **Acceptability.** Provider acceptance has been excellent. There has been increasing patient dissatisfaction with silver nitrate, however, because of the chemical conjunctivitis that often ensues.

III. Recommendations

A. All newborns should receive ocular prophylaxis within 1 hour of birth, with a 0.5- to 1-cm strip of 0.5% erythromycin ointment, 2 drops of 1% silver nitrate, or a 0.5- to 1-cm strip of 1% tetracycline ointment in each conjunctival sac without rinsing [3].

B. If chlamydia is highly endemic in the population served, prophylaxis with erythromycin is preferred.

C. If the mother has a known gonococcal infection, a single dose of aqueous crystalline penicillin G should be given IV or IM along with the ocular prophylaxis since occasional cases of ophthalmia neonatorum have occurred with prophylaxis only. The dose is 50,000 units for a term infant and 20,000 units for low birth weight infants [3].

D. Expectant mothers should be assessed closely for possible venereal infections. If the mother had premature or prolonged rupture of membranes, or both, the infant should be observed more closely for development of conjunctivitis. In general, though, all infants should be observed for such symptoms since prophylaxis has reduced but not eliminated the disease.

E. If inflammatory changes develop, particularly after 24 hours, chemical conjunctivitis is unlikely. Establishing a diagnosis is essential for definitive therapy. Eye cultures for gonorrhea, other bacteria, and chlamydia may be warranted, as well as acute Gram's and Giemsa stains to determine if treatment for gonorrheal or chlamydial ophthalmia is necessary. Topical antibiotic therapy is inadequate for gonorrhea.

References

1. Aquavella, J. B. Diseases of the Cornea and Conjunctiva. In H. S. Metz and A. L. Rosenbaum (eds.), *Pediatric Ophthalmology.* Garden City: Medical Examination Publishing, 1982. Pp. 180–234. *This chapter describes the etiology, symptoms, laboratory evaluation, and treatment of ophthalmia neonatorum.*
2. Forster, R. K. Ophthalmia Neonatorum. In L. A. Wilson (ed.), *External Diseases of the Eye.* Hagerstown, MD: Harper & Row, 1979. Pp. 47–55. *This chapter describes etiologic factors, laboratory evaluation, and treatment of ophthalmia neonatorum.*
3. American Academy of Pediatrics Committees. Prophylaxis and treatment of neonatal gonococcal infections. *Pediatrics* 65(5):1047, 1980. *This document contains the American Academy of Pediatrics recommendations regarding prophylaxis and treatment of neonatal gonococcal infections.*
4. Dawson, C. R. Follicular Conjunctivitis. In L. A. Wilson (ed.), *External Diseases of the Eye.* Hagerstown, MD: Harper & Row, 1979. Pp. 57–75. *This chapter describes potential long-term complications of untreated* Chlamydia trachomatis *conjunctivitis.*
5. Nishida, H., and Risemberg, H. M. Silver nitrate ophthalmic solution and chemical conjunctivitis. *Pediatrics* 56(3):368, 1975. *This study is a report on the current nursery routine for prophylaxis against ophthalmia neonatorum based on a 100-nursery survey.*
6. Snowe, R. J., and Wilfert, C. M. Epidemic reappearance of gonococcal ophthalmia neonatorum. *Pediatrics* 51:110, 1973. *This report describes an increase in the incidence of gonococcal ophthalmia neonatorum in North Carolina in 1973. The authors felt that the increased incidence was probably not merely local in scope but national or international.*
7. Hammerschlag, M. R., et al. Erythromycin ointment for ocular prophylaxis of neonatal chlamydial infection. *J.A.M.A.* 244(20):2291, 1980. *This study compares the efficacy of erythromycin ophthalmic ointment and the efficacy of silver nitrate drops for prevention of neonatal conjunctivitis from Chlamydia trachomatis. The efficacy of erythromycin ointment for prevention of respiratory tract infection due to chlamydia was also evaluated.*
8. Chlamydia trachomatis infections. Policy guidelines for prevention and control. *M.M.W.R.* 34(3s):53s, 1985. *This document contains the CDC policy guidelines for prevention and control of Chlamydia trachomatis infections.*
9. Alexander, E. R., and Harrigan, H. R. Role of chlamydia trachomatis in perinatal infections. *Rev. Infec. Dis.* 5(4):713, 1983. *Excellent review article on chlamydia in pregnancy and in newborns.*
10. Armstrong, J. H., Zacarias, F., and Rein, M. F. Ophthalmia neonatorum: A chart review. *Pediatrics* 57(6):884, 1976. *This study presents the results of a 6-year chart review. It describes the etiologies, frequency, clinical features, and therapy of 302 cases of ophthalmia neonatorum.*
11. Prophylaxis of ophthalmia neonatorum. *J. Pediatr.* 41:374, 1952. *This editorial raises the question of whether Credé prophylaxis with silver nitrate should continue to be mandated by statute. The author questions whether the low incidence at the time Credé introduced it was due to successful prophylaxis or to a decreased incidence of gonorrhea.*
12. Prevention of ophthalmia neonatorum. *M.M.W.R.* 34(4s):90s, 1985. *This document contains treatment guidelines for the prevention of ophthalmia neonatorum caused by multiple causative organisms.*
13. Goscienski, P. J. Inclusion conjunctivitis in the newborn infant. *J. Pediatr.* 77:19, 1970. *This is a report of 5 infants being first seen with inclusion conjunctivitis between 3 and 26 days of life. Intracytoplasmic inclusions were identified in each.*

39 Mass Newborn Screening for Inborn Errors of Metabolism

Willard Centerwall
and Linda Greve

I. The problem

A. Definition. The mass screening programs discussed in this chapter are those that screen newborns to detect rare metabolic disorders. The inborn errors of metabolism discussed are mostly recessively inherited disorders of biochemical function that adversely affect the health of the child after birth.

B. Description and epidemiology. There are a number of disorders of newborns that initially are not clinically apparent and are therefore undetectable by even the most perceptive and experienced clinicians. These are metabolic and most often recessively inherited diseases in which normal intrauterine growth and development have been permitted by placental-maternal clearance during pregnancy. After birth, however, when such a child is functioning autonomously, excesses or deficiencies can occur over time to the child's detriment. Most of the disorders included in screening programs result in severe mental retardation if not treated. Disorders that do not result in severe mental retardation and that are included in some screening programs include sickle cell anemia, histidinemia, and congenital adrenogenital syndrome.

For some metabolic errors, early detection will permit control or modification of the abnormal metabolism, thereby preventing damage. These are the diseases that are the target of screening programs.

These diseases also should be sufficiently common to warrant mass newborn screening in an effort to detect all cases occurring in a population. A frequency of one in a million, for example, is too rare to justify testing all newborn infants. Exceptions sometimes are made when the addition of a rare disorder to an existing mass newborn screening program can be accomplished with relatively low additional costs.

Although the primary care provider does not have to acquire great expertise about each condition, it is wise to have at least a modicum of knowledge about the diseases included in his or her state program. Table 39-1 describes the seven diseases that are included, to a greater or lesser extent, in this country's various newborn screening programs [1–3]. Four additional disorders, each included in only one screening program, are named in the footnotes to Tables 39-1 and 39-4.

II. Secondary prevention

A. Early detection

1. **Methods.** Currently, blood is collected from newborn infants to determine if the infant has one or more of the conditions in the screen [4].

   a. **Performance.** In some hospital settings, local health care providers may be involved in the training of personnel and maintenance of good collection techniques. Consideration should be given to the following.

      (1) **Collection of an adequate specimen.** An inadequate specimen is the major reason for needing additional specimens. Figure 39-1 illustrates techniques to enhance optimal blood flow and collection: utilizing the best site to prick, effectively positioning the foot, and using a proper stylette.

      (2) **Prewarming the infant's heel** for several minutes with a hot, moist towel (temperature under 43°C) is done routinely in some nurseries, and in others only with babies with insufficient heel-prick blood flow. In most circumstances, it probably is not necessary.

      (3) **Filter paper products** may differ in absorbency, with resultant difficulty in collection or differences in blood concentration in the paper affecting normal laboratory results. Thus, it is important to have a reliably consistent and uniform source. At least one state had to recall a large batch of collection filter papers.

(4) **Proper technique must be used to avoid injuring the baby.**

(a) Inadequate cleansing of the heel-prick site may cause infections. An application of 70% isopropanol followed by adequate drying (1 or 2 minutes) is the most commonly used satisfactory method.

(b) Not making a prick large enough to ensure an adequate flow of blood may lead to:

(i) Multiple pricks in order to obtain a sufficient specimen. Utilizing the techniques pictured in Fig. 39-1 should minimize this, but even with the most experienced personnel, it is occasionally necessary to make more than one prick. Even so, this is preferable to squeezing the heel to get "the last drop" of blood. Additional pricks should not be done immediately adjacent to a previous puncture site.

(ii) Squeezing or "milking down" or "fingerflicking" (or both) the infant's heel, which may cause tissue injury and hematoma, as well as dilute the blood specimen with tissue fluid.

(c) Pricking too deeply, as might be done by using an oversized stylette or a scalpel blade, may create an unnecessarily large wound and the possibility of striking the bone, with the potential for a complex infection (see Fig. 39-1)

b. **Timing. It is recommended that testing be done between 48 hours after birth and the end of the sixth day of age.** [5, 6]. The screening test should permit detection from samples taken from a population that is readily accessible in its early life. The hospital newborn nursery has provided the "captive audience" and the timing desired. However, more babies are going home earlier from the hospital—at 1 and 2 days of age—and some tests may not pick up an abnormality in some infants until they are 2 or 3 days of age or more. In this respect phenylketonuria (PKU) is the disease creating the greatest concern.

Biological variability in infants is perhaps the major explanation for variability in early test results. The time and content of early oral feedings appears not to be as important as previously thought (Table 39-2).

To minimize missing bonafide cases of PKU, **the American Academy of Pediatrics has recommended retesting all infants discharged home from the hospital under 24 hours of age. This rescreening should be done by 1 week of age** through the local health care providers or public health nurses.

A small percentage of infants may miss initial testing.* Follow-up testing is usually provided by local health care providers and public health nurses. Infants who may be missed include:

(1) Those delivered at home.

(2) Those having an initial illness or marked prematurity, or both, with intensive medical care and concerns causing the routine screening to be inadvertently omitted.

In cases of partial absence of the thyroid gland, inactivity of the residual tissue occurs at various ages. Such cases might be missed by routine mass screening of newborns. The test for galactosemia (transferase enzyme) also bears no relationship to the infant's age at the time of testing.

c. **Interpretation.** A number of variables may affect the interpretation of test results, including the following:

(1) **Prematurity.** Enzyme and hormone production may be reduced due to immaturity of organ systems, thus leading to false-positive test results.

(2) **Atypical and variant conditions, which may give false-positive test results.** The clinical significance of such findings ranges from nil to profound. In the PKU screening, for example, about one-third of the initially positive tests turn out to be "benign hyperphenylalaninemia," a familial tendency toward persistent mild elevation of the blood phenylalanine levels without apparent clinical effects and without spillage of metabolic byproducts in the urine. At the other extreme, very rare cases of atypical PKU have been detected, in which a different metabolic error is involved (dihydropteridine reductase deficiency), and the affected children

*In some states (e.g., California), parents can refuse to have their newborn tested on the basis of a prohibitive religious belief. This accounts for a very small number of missed cases, however.

Table 39-1. Diseases included in mass newborn screening programs in the United States in 1986[a, b, c]

Disease	Incidence and inheritance	Ethnic propensity
Phenylketonuria (PKU)	1:13,000 Autosomal recessive	Irish, English, Polish 1:7,000
Hypothyroidism (cretinism)	1:4,600 Sporadic	No specific ethnic propensity noted
Galactosemia	1:50,000 Autosomal recessive	No specific ethnic propensity noted
Maple syrup urine disease (MSUD)	1:175,000 Autosomal recessive	No specific ethnic propensity noted
Homocystinuria	1:245,000 Autosomal recessive	Irish 1:35,000
Tyrosinemia	<1:1,000,000 Autosomal recessive	French-Canadians 1:12,000
Sickle cell anemia	1:6,000 Autosomal recessive	Blacks 1:500

Key: MR=mental retardation.

[a]For all of the above-listed diseases (with the possible exception of sickle cell anemia) atypical variants have been identified, indicating heterogeneity, i.e., more than one form of the disease. The clinical courses of the variants range from transient metabolic changes and clinically insignificant courses to severe and untreatable disease. Screening results for PKU, for example, reflect this range of extremes.

[b]A 1977 report by the Controller General of the United States [3] gave a **cost-benefit calculation of more than 20 to 1** when the estimated costs of medical-institutional care of the would-be affected cases were compared to the costs of mass newborn screening for seven

Usual untreated clinical course for the classic form of the disease	Therapeutic measures for the classic form of the disease
Delayed mental development by 3–4 mo; moderate to severe **MR** by 2–3 yr. Irritable schizoid behavior; seizures (30%); eczema (25%). Moderate delay in growth; borderline microcephaly. Fairer than normal siblings (skin, hair, eyes); musty odor.	Low-phenylalanine diet started in 2 wk after birth, special milk substitute. Later add low-protein foods. Periodic monitoring of blood phenylalanine levels.
Early signs by 1–6 wk: lethargy, feeding difficulties, constipation, persistent neonatal jaundice, respiratory distress. Classic signs: puffy face, coarse features, enlarged tongue, dry skin and hair, abdominal distention, umbilical hernia, delayed growth, delayed bone age, and delayed dentition, **MR.** Onset and course variable, depends on extent of thyroid deficiency.	Oral thyroid replacement daily, (usually L-thyroxine tablets): initially 10 mg/kg/day, tapering by 4 steps until 3 mg/kg/day at 12 yr. Lifetime maintenance. Monitor clinically and periodic T_4.
Very early onset first few days: jaundice, vomiting, diarrhea, ascites, edema, hepatomegaly, sepsis, bulging anterior fontanelle, bleeding diathesis; 30% die. Later: failure to thrive, cataracts, **MR,** liver cirrhosis, ovarian insufficiency.	Lactose-free diet, usually milk substitute, e.g., soy products, initiate as soon as possible under 1 wk of age. Avoid milk products.
Early onset within days to weeks: poor eating, vomiting, lethargy, convulsions, hypertoxicity, shrill cry, suppressed Moro and deep tendon reflexes, apnea, flaccidity, and death. Odor of maple syrup to urine and body, **severe MR in survivors.**	Early initiation of diet low in leucine, isoleucine, and valine. Even with treatment started before 1 wk old, there is some neurological impairment with moderate MR.
Some do not develop hypermethioninemia until after 1 wk of age. Venous thrombosis, enlarged liver, telangiectases with aging. Kyphoscoliosis, pectus excavation, flat-foot, arachnodactyly. Premature osteoporosis, light complexion, coarse skin. Sublexed lenses by 2–3 yr, growth failure, **MR in 50%.**	Low methionine diet with supplemental cystine. Some respond to pyridoxine (vitamin B_6). Other types are associated with defects in vitamin B_{12} and folate metabolism.
Hepatic and renal disease with normal mentality: cirrhosis, rickets, hyperaminoaciduria, hyperphosphaturia, and glucosuria. **Death** due to liver failure.	Diet low in tyrosine and phenylalanine, with prevention or alleviation in some cases.
Chronic anemia with hemolytic crises: abdominal or bone pain, jaundice, sepsis, thrombosis (early splenomegaly; later, splenic atrophy). **Most die** between 15 and 30 yr of age.	Symptomatic treatment: i.e., blood transfusions, fluids, antibiotics. Prophylactic avoidance of low oxygen tensions or high altitudes.

different diseases, plus preventive management of detected cases. This was based on the test results of 3.2 million babies; cost-benefit rates were $437,185,000 to $18,542,000—23.6 : 1.
[c]Four additional diseases—congenital adrenogenital syndrome, histidinemia, adenosine deaminase deficiency, and biotinidase deficiency—are included in only one state newborn screening program (see Table 39-4).

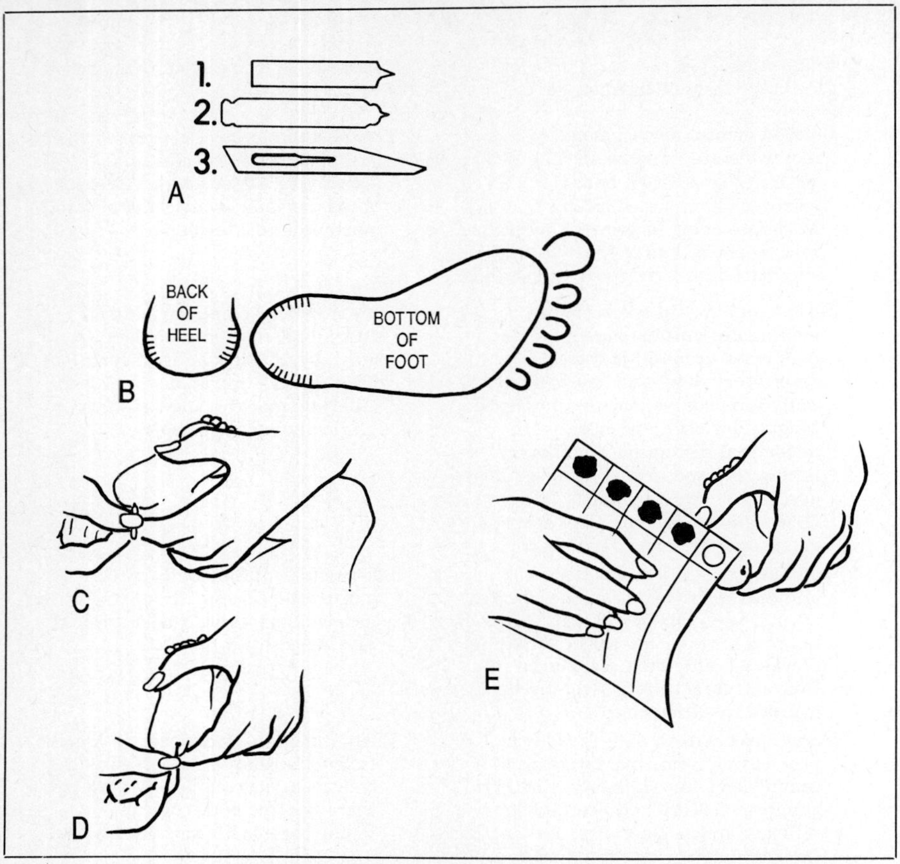

Fig. 39-1. Technique for collection of blood from newborn infant. A. The proper stylettes to be used are one with a 5-mm point for most full-term, plump-footed infants (1) or one with a 2-mm point for most premature and skinny-footed infants (2). Scalpel blades (3) are unacceptable. B. The unacceptable puncture sites are the back of the heel and the bottom of the foot. Acceptable puncture sites are indicated by hash marks. C. Do not puncture through previous site which may be infected. D. Blood flow may be better if the puncture site is held downward with gentle pressure. E. Blotting. It is important to fill each circle completely.

Table 39-2. Influence of time of testing on results of phenylketonuria (PKU) screening*

Age of newborns	Percentage of classic PKU giving false-negative tests
0–24 hr (1 day)	6.3%
25–48 hr (2 days)	1.8%
49–72 hr (3 days)	0.5%
73–96 hr (4 days)	0.2%

*These are conservative upper estimates based on tolerance limits at the 95% level of certainty using a 4 mg/dl blood phenylalanine level cut-off by the fluorometric method. These results are based on approximately 1.24 million infants tested over a 15-year period. Other respected studies report both higher and lower percentages than presented here.

Source: H. N. Kirkman, et al. Fifteen-year experience with screening for phenylketonuria with an automated fluorometric method. *Am. J. Hum. Genet.* 34(5):743, 1982. ©1982 University of Chicago.

Table 39-3. Mass newborn screening: False-positive and false-negative test results[a]

Disease	Range of false-positives[b]	Factors causing false-negatives[c]	Range of incidence of true positives[d]
Phenylketonuria	1+/10,000–25.2/10,000 (1/9,700–1/400)	Sampling < 24 hr of age (biological variability)	1/35,000–1/9,000
Hypothyroidism	11/10,000–130/10,000 (1/900–1/80)	Temporarily functioning ectopic gland [2]	1/6,700–1/3,600
Galactosemia	0.8/10,000–14.6/10,000 (1/12,500–1/700)	Blood transfusions (transferase test)	1/125,000–1/39,000
Maple syrup urine disease	0.4/10,000–2.5/10,000 (1/25,000–1/4,000)	Sampling < 24 hr of age (biological variability)	1/308,000–1/130,000
Homocysturia	2.1/10,000–4.0/10,000 (1/4,800–1/1,500)	Sampling < 1 wk of age [1] (biological variability)	1/242,000–1/116,000
Tyrosinemia[e]	56.6/10,000–71/10,000 (1/180–1/140)	Sampling < 5 days [1] (biological variability)	1/550,000–1/390,000
Sickle cell anemia[f]	128/10,000–430/10,000 (1/70–1/25)	Very rare laboratory error	1/19,000–1/650

[a]Information fitting acceptable criteria (via personal communication) from California, Colorado regional, Georgia, New England regional, New York, and Oregon regional programs was used for the ranges—a total of 16 state newborn screening programs (over 2 million infants tested).
[b]Range of false-positives is largely influenced by different decisions for cut-off levels of lab test values.
[c]The primary factors influencing false-negative results are biological differences relating to timing of samples (see text for details).
[d]The range of disease incidences vary is largely determined by the proportions of ethnic groups being sampled.
[e]Tyrosinemia incidence figures are based only on single-case diagnoses.
[f]About half of the true positive sickle cell cases are SS anemia and half are compound heterozygotes (other hemoglobinopathies). The vast majority of false-positives are sickle cell carriers, AS, verified on primary sample. These are asymptomatic but might benefit from genetic counseling.

are not benefited by the low phenylalanine diet. Variant forms of most of the screened-for diseases have been discovered and, with time, more will be found.

(3) **Laboratory error of technologic or human origin.** It is hoped that these errors will continue to be rare. False-positives are eliminated by performing follow-up confirmation tests. False-negative reporting usually would preclude detection until clinical signs and symptoms prompted additional tests (Table 39-3).

2. **Justification of testing methods**
   a. **Test characteristics.** The tests yield an acceptable minimum of initial false-positive values, which can be eliminated by reasonable confirmatory tests, and a very low to absent number of false-negative screening test results (see Table 39-3).
   b. **Risks and side effects.** Minimal risks exist from these low rates of false-negatives and false-positives. False-positive results require repeated confirmatory tests. Any necessary retesting of an infant, however, is likely to generate some apprehension and anxiety in the parents—even with good, careful, and sensitive handling. Other uncommon complications include local infection, osteomyelitis, and bleeding, all of which are negligible if proper technique is used.
   c. **Costs.** The per capita costs of testing—specimen collection and handling, and laboratory screening of test samples using filter paper collection procedures—are quite low. The costs in 1985 were about $6 per test (i.e., $18 for three tests) and less when more tests done on each sample.

Table 39-4. Mandatory (M) and voluntary (V) mass newborn screening in the United States in 1986[a]

State	Phenyl-ketonuria	Hypo-thyroid	Galacto-semia	Maple syrup urine disease	Homocy-tinuria	Tyrosi-nemia	Sickle cell anemia[b]	Other
Alabama	M	M						
Alaska	M	M						M[d]
Arizona[c]	M	M	M	V	V		V	
Arkansas	M	M						
California	M	M	M					
Colorado	M	M	M	M	M		M	
Connecticut	M	M	M					
Delaware	V	V	V	V	V			
Florida	M	M	M	M				
Georgia	M	M	M	M	M	M		
Hawaii	M	V						
Idaho[c]	M	V	V	V	V	V		
Illinois	M	M						
Indiana	M	M						
Iowa	M	V	V	V				
Kansas	M	M						
Kentucky	M	M	M					
Louisiana	M	M						
Maine	M	M	M	M	M			
Maryland	V	V	V	V	V			
Massachusetts[e]	M	M	M	M	M			
Michigan	M	V						
Minnesota	M	M	M					
Mississippi	V	V						
Missouri	M	M						
Montana	M	M	M	M	M	M		
Nebraska	M	M						
Nevada	M	M	M	M	M	M		
New Hampshire	M	M						
New Jersey	M	M	M					
New Mexico	M	M	M	M	M			

d. Acceptability. Since there is no way to judge clinically which children are at particular risk for being affected, the only satisfactory approach is to routinely check all newborns (or as close to all as possible). For this reason, legislature-required screening of all newborns has been instituted in 45 states, resulting in over 95% of infants being tested. The remaining five states with only voluntary mass screening programs, and other states with mandatory screening for certain disorders and voluntary screening for others, are now testing in excess of 90% of all newborns. Increasing professional and public awareness of the value of early testing and diagnosis has resulted in a much improved utilization of the voluntary programs in recent years. Table 39-4 lists the different diseases being tested for in the various states and regions.

It is anticipated that the list of diseases discussed here will change with time, mainly by the addition of other disorders for which improved tests and treatment have been developed. Also with time, some tests on trial may be dropped. To be certain of the screening required in one's state, it is suggested that inquiries be made through the Department of Health. The reason for the differences between states (as to the extent of involvement with newborn screening efforts) is a matter of differences of philosophy, comprehension, perceived needs, economics, and pressures and politics. It can be anticipated that eventually near consensus and relative uniformity of mandatory testing will be reached throughout the nation, based on the "test of time" regarding so-called tried and true values.

Table 39-4. continued

State	Phenyl-ketonuria	Hypo-thyroid	Galacto-semia	Maple syrup urine disease	Homocy-tinuria	Tyrosi-nemia	Sickle cell anemia[b]	Other
New York	M	M	M	M	M		M	M[f]
North Carolina	V	V						
North Dakota	M	M						
Ohio	M	M	M		M			
Oklahoma	M	M						
Oregon	M	M	M	M	M	M		
Pennsylvania	M	M						
Rhode Island	M	V	V	V	V			
South Carolina	M	M						
South Dakota	M	M						
Tennessee	M	M						
Texas	M	M	M		M		M	
Utah	M	M	M					
Vermont	V	V	V					
Virginia	M	V						M[g]
Washington	M	M						
West Virginia	M	M	M					
Wisconsin	M	M	M	M	V			
Wyoming	M	M	M	M	M		M	
Washington, D.C.	M	M	M	M	M			
Total	51	51	29	19	18	5	5	

[a]None of the United States island territories or Puerto Rico has mass newborn screening programs.
[b]With sickle cell testing, screening is also done for other hemoglobinopathies. Georgia has limited mandatory mass screening, i.e., for only the 60% "ethnically at risk" population. All other states not listed have mechanisms of testing for sickle cell anemia "on request."
[c]All testing in Arizona and Idaho might be mandatory depending on interpretation of laws.
[d]Mandatory screening for adrenogenital syndrome because of relatively high risk in Eskimos (Alaska).
[e]Voluntary urine screening (about 35% of newborns) for amino and organic acid disorders (Massachusetts).
[f]Mandatory screening for histidenemia and adenosinedeaminase; may be discontinued soon (New York).
[g]Mandatory screening for biotinidase deficiency (Virginia); pilot studies in about a dozen other states.

Actually, one could not justify setting up a mass newborn screening program for some of these disorders on an individual basis. Some are too rarely encountered (e.g., homocystinuria, maple syrup urine disease), and others are not consistently sufficiently damaging (e.g., histidinemia). However, because the tests, which utilize the same mailed dried spots of blood at the same laboratories, are so relatively simple and inexpensive, their inclusion has been too inviting for some states to resist, at least on a trial basis.

B. Early intervention

1. Methods (see Table 39-1).

The treatment regimens for classic PKU, galactosemia, maple syrup urine disease (MSUD), and homocystinuria are dietary restrictions of the amino acids or carbohydrates that cannot be metabolized properly due to the lack of the active enzyme. Each disease has variant or atypical forms in which different experimental methods of dietary restrictions, vitamin administration, high cofactor dosages, and/or neurotransmitter precursor supplementations are utilized. Primary hypothyroidism is treated with daily thyroxine replacement. Good results are being reported in these treated hypothyroid children followed since birth who are now reaching 6 to 7 years of age. Homocystinuria, tyrosinemia, and some severe PKU variants are not always successfully treated with current methods. There are benign variants of a number of the above diseases for which no treatment is necessary.

The overall program is essential to the success of the specific medical plan. The logistics and the plans of action for the mass newborn screening programs will differ in different states. It helps to know how the program works and how practitioners become involved in their own states. Specific details for one's own state usually can be obtained from the state's Department of Health, which will also describe responsibilities of the practitioner, the laboratory, and state personnel regarding notification of abnormal results, repeat testing, and treatment.

2. **Justification for early intervention (treatment)**
   a. **Effectiveness.** For a disease to be included in a newborn screening program, there must be practical therapeutic means by which the harmful consequences of the condition can be averted. This limitation explains the failure to include, thus far, such diseases as Tay-Sachs and the limited inclusion of sickle cell anemia. Almost all of the disorders included would progress from an initially normal state to serious neurologic deterioration, but when diagnosed early, may be treated effectively.
   b. **Risks of early treatment methods.** Poor nutrition is a risk for children who are treated with restricted diets, especially if the child is a poor eater or if the mother does not understand the diet. When the diet is a new one and the disease is not perfectly understood, the outcome can be less than optimum, even with good compliance. These children should be followed by a nutritionist or dietician and must be seen frequently until proper intake and growth are assured.

      A pregnant woman with an uncontrolled blood phenylalanine level, called maternal PKU, whether she has been treated to prevent retardation or not, is at high risk of having a retarded child because the high phenylalanine in the mother's blood crosses into the baby's blood and affects the development of the baby's brain. The baby does not have PKU, but microcephaly and developmental delay (mental retardation) are present from birth. Women with PKU should be on a restricted diet before conception so that the blood phenylalanine will be lowered to safe levels. It is important to inform the pregnant adolescent and her family of this risk, and to offer assistance in staying on the diet or reinstituting the diet in the future.
   c. **Costs.** The cost of providing special diets, supplements, and medical supervision over many years is quite high, being in the range of $1000–$2000/year. However, the cost-benefit calculation for the mass newborn screening programs in this country is more than 20 to 1. This means that for every $1 spent, more than $20 are saved when the estimated costs of medical/institutional care of the would-be affected children are measured against the cost of the mass newborn screening programs and preventive management of detected cases.
   d. **Acceptability.** Above and beyond the enormous physical and intellectual benefits to treated patients, there are great psychosocial and emotional benefits to the patients and their families.

III. Recommendations

A. Early detection

1. All newborns, regardless of age, must have a blood sample collected before they are discharged from the nursery.
2. In those infants screened before 24 hours of age there is a slight chance of a false-negative result. Such newborns can be rescreened. Because there is an extremely low chance of the newborn being missed, many state newborn screening programs are discontinuing repeat or second testing. The cost outweighs the benefit. It is therefore sometimes necessary for primary care providers to make private laboratory arrangements in order to comply with the American Academy of Pediatrics' recommendations for repeat testing [5, 6].

B. Early intervention

1. Confirmed abnormal results require rapid consultation and decisions for follow-up care. The primary care provider may be asked to continue to provide direct care within the framework of the usual primary care consultant relationship. The more rare disorders may require hospitalization in order to accurately diagnose and initiate treatment. After discharge, the primary care provider may be asked to provide long-term follow-up, with continued coordination with metabolic specialists.

References

1. Levy, H. L. *Genetic Screening for Inborn Errors of Metabolism.* Rockville, MD: Department of Health, Education, and Welfare, 1975. *This little book provides an excellent, concise, and adequately current review of some 20 metabolic disorders that have been or could be adapted for inclusion in newborn screening programs. Most of the information included in Table 39-1 has been derived from this source.*
2. Mitchell, M. L. *Management of Infants with Congenital Hypothyroidism.* Rockville, MD: Department of Health and Human Services, 1981. *This is an excellent, current review of congenital hypothyroidism, a condition that is now included in the mass newborn screening programs of the vast majority of states. This is the only endocrine and nongenetic condition in such screening programs. It is not included in H. L. Levy's book in reference 1.*
3. U.S. General Accounting Office. *Preventing Mental Retardation: More Can be Done. Report to the Congress.* Washington, DC: U.S. Government Printing Office, 1977. *This unbiased report graphically portrays the marked value of and justification for mass newborn screening programs in this country: the estimated cost-benefit ratio is more than 20 to 1. Included are the basis for such calculations.*
4. Hammond, K. B. Blood specimen collection from infants by skin puncture. *Lab. Med.* 11(1):9, 1980. *This article presents the subject of blood sampling by heel-prick in a comprehensive fashion, including indications, techniques, and precautions.*
5. Kirkman, H. N., et al. Fifteen-year experience with screening for phenylketonuria with an automated fluorometric method. *Am. J. Hum. Genet.* 34(5):743, 1982. *This report comes from North Carolina, a state where 97% of newborn infants are screened in a voluntary program. In the 15½-year period covered, 1,229,635 infants were tested, with 39 cases of PKU detected. By statistical analysis of results, the authors estimate what percentage of infants with PKU might be missed at any given day of age.*
6. Koch, R., Berlow, S., and McCabe, R. B. Neonatal screening for phenylketonuria (letters). *Pediatrics* 73(5):737, 1984. *Missing infants with PKU because of too early testing is a serious issue facing state newborn screening programs. These three letters, with references, explain the current recommendations of the American Academy of Pediatrics, and why there are differences in state policies.*

40 Developmental Disabilities

Peter Michael Miller

I. The problem

A. Definition. Developmental disability (DD) is a legislative term that identifies certain disorders in development. It includes any severe chronic disability attributable to a mental or physical impairment, or combination thereof, that is manifested before the age of 22 years, is likely to continue indefinitely, and will result in substantial limitation in function in three or more of the following areas: (1) self-care, (2) receptive and expressive language, (3) learning, (4) mobility, (5) self-direction, (6) capacity for independent language, (7) economic self-sufficiency, and (8) necessity for special services that are of lifelong or extended duration and are individually planned or coordinated (Developmental Disabilities Assistance and Bill of Rights Act, 1979). There are federal, state, and private agency variations in the definition of specific conditions included or excluded, age limitations, and interpretation of "substantial" handicap.

B. Description. The major conditions generally considered to be the most common and severe developmental disabilities are mental retardation and cerebral palsy. The federal definition also includes learning disabilities. The diagnosis of mental retardation requires consideration of "deficits in adaptive behavior," as well as subaverage intellectual functioning.

A serious effort should also be made to identify any etiologic factors involved. In approximately 20–25% of retarded children there is an identifiable biomedical or single environmental etiology, more likely in the severe to profound group. Other cases are associated with hereditary, environmental, and psychosocial factors.

Cerebral palsy is a nonprogressive, permanent motor impairment caused by a pathologic lesion in the brain of a developing infant or child. It is associated with motor delay, persistent neonatal reflexes, and abnormal specific neurologic features (e.g., in tone and posture).

Cerebral palsy may be classified according to the body part(s) affected (monoplegia, hemiplegia, paraplegia, triplegia, quadriplegia) and/or movement disorder (spasticity, athetosis, dystonia, chorea, ballismus, rigidity, ataxia, tremor, atonia). Some physiologic types have associated clinical findings and etiology—for example, spasticity with prematurity and cerebral trauma, and athetosis with kernicterus. However, mixed clinical forms are not uncommon and etiologic factors frequently overlap categories.

C. Epidemiology. The prevalence of developmental disabilities may vary widely (3–15%) depending on the definition (i.e., conditions included or excluded). Most estimates of the prevalence of mental retardation in the general United States population (i.e., IQ less than 70 with corresponding adaptive levels) are in the 2–3% range. The mild categories (IQ 52–69) comprise approximately 75–89% of that population. Moderately retarded (IQ 36–54) individuals are a smaller group (5–20%), and severe to profound (IQ 20–39) persons occur less frequently (2–5%). Individuals with cerebral palsy are said to number 700,000 (approximately 2–5 per 1000 general population) and 100,000 new cases in young children per year.

A history of certain **risk factors** indicates the need for careful evaluation. Prenatal insults such as maternal illness, infections, and teratogens (e.g., cigarettes, some anticonvulsants or hydantoin, and alcohol) increase the risk of developmental disabilities in the child. Very low birth weight infants (under 1500 gm) have a 10% risk based on weight alone. This risk increases to 30–50% if there were associated problems such as hypoxia, infection, seizures, cerebral bleeding or being small for gestational age. Children in the 1501–2500 gm birth weight group with a history of bronchopulmonary dysplasia, posthypoxic seizures, or meningitis have a 10% risk of a developmental disability occurring. Larger infants who are appropriate weight for gestational age are at increased risk if there is a history of congenital malformation, birth trauma, perinatal hypoxia and seizures, meningitis, or adverse psychosocial factors. Low Apgar scores, especially at 10 or more minutes, may also suggest an increased risk for cerebral palsy.

II. Secondary prevention

A. Early detection

1. Methods

a. Description. General developmental screening should include assessment of motor (gross and fine), social-personal, language, adaptive, and, for older children, school-related, abilities. Studies and experience have demonstrated that standardized, validated, and reliable screening systems are more successful in identifying developmental problems (especially mild ones) than the less accurate method of obtaining a developmental history from the parents and noting only major milestones on examination. Table 40-1 reviews the more useful screening instruments currently available, while Table 40-2 lists the sources for these screening tools. More sophisticated and specific diagnostic tests of a child's current level of development are available and should be provided for all suspect children by a skilled specialist.

b. Performance. Screening tests must be done according to standardized instructions.

c. Interpretation. Screening tests measure only current development and should be used as evidence only of possible developmental delays. Test results are not considered diagnostic and are not necessarily predictive of future abilities or success. They do indicate the need for further careful clinical observation and more specific and thorough developmental evaluations.

d. Timing. The screening tests should be performed at regular intervals, as indicated in Table 40-1. Instructions for individual tests describe the procedure for more frequent screening, depending on initial test results. Children with suspected developmental delays based on clinical examination should also be evaluated as soon as the delay is noted with a screening tool, or be given a more complete evaluation, depending on the degree of suspicion.

Follow-up of high-risk infants may use similar guidelines for developmental screening, with emphasis on testing at 6 and 12 months and 2 and 3 years of age. The preschool exam at 4–6 years should include vision and hearing screening. A few evaluation tools have been developed to measure school readiness, cognitive areas, speech and language skills, and emotional or behavioral problems that may interfere with school performance, especially in children with very low birth weights.

e. Population. Since perinatal incidents are not sufficiently predictive of later developmental disabilities, screening tools are best applied to all children (i.e., both normal and high-risk). Different tools are more appropriate for specific age groups and may be more accurate in certain ranges within the group (see Table 40-1). Socioeconomic and academic abilities of the family are also very important considerations (see population column, Table 40-1).

2. Justification

a. Test characteristics. These screening tests do not result in diagnoses or predictions of future abilities or success. They measure only current development (see Table 40-1 for test characteristics).

b. Risks include mislabeling a child as delayed and causing unnecessary parental anxiety, and not identifying a delay, inappropriately reassuring the parents and missing the opportunity for early intervention. Usually a developmental evaluation by the primary health professional is a positive step toward a constructive and objective monitoring of a child's growth, and support for the family.

c. Costs include the cost of the screening materials and office time, the cost of which can be considerable. Screening procedures managed by skilled, nonphysician health professionals may improve the efficiency of office operations and save the expenditure of time and money on disabilities identified later.

d. Acceptability. Parents are usually delighted to see the health professional's interest in the child's development. Care must be taken to explain the limitations of screenings tools to parents.

Table 40-1. Developmental assessment screening tools

Timing Age	Population	Test	Time (min)	Comments
Neonate	All	Maternal and birth history	5–10	Note potential high-risk conditions (e.g., maternal and neonatal illness and infection, teratogens, blood incompatibility, gestational age, birth trauma, hypoxia, seizures etc.).
Neonate	All	Apgar	1–5–10	To identify immediate condition(s); predictive ability unclear.
Neonate	All	Physical and developmental examination	15–30	See Dubowitz in Selected Readings.
Birth–21yr[a]	All	History, physical developmental examination	20–30	Note parental concerns about growth and development, history of trauma, infection; review child's socioeconomic situation and parents' developmental expectations for child; check for evidence of neglect, abuse. Note height, weight, head circumference; signs and patterns of anomalies.
1 mo–5 yr[a]	All	Rapid Developmental Screening Checklist (RDSC)	5	By Giannini and associates[b]; one-page checklist can be used by an aide.
1 mo–3 yr[a]	All	Guide to Normal Milestones of Development (GNMD-Haynes)	10–15	By Haynes (see Selected Readings); can be used by nurses. Consists of rotating discs that match age with developmental milestones and reflexes.
1 mo–3 yr[a]	High-risk	Developmental Screening Inventory (DSI)	20	By Knobloch; tests adaptive skills, gross and fine motor control, language, personal/social skills; questions for seizures, vision/hearing, parental concerns. Gives Developmental Quotient (DQ). False positive 6%; false negative 2.6% for major abnormality, 10% for minor abnormality.
1 mo–6 yr[a]	High-risk	Denver Developmental Screening Test (DDST)	20–30	By Frankenburg (see Selected Readings); can be given by trained professional; reliability up to 97%. False-positive 3–11%; false-negative 0.4–3%. Less valid for lower socioeconomic population and at older age range; follow up with diagnostic tests if DDST is positive.

Table 40-1. continued

Timing Age	Population	Test	Time (min)	Comments
3 mo–6 yr[c]	All	Prescreening Developmental Questionnaire (PDQ)	5–10	Based on 10 DDST items for given age group; for use with parents of at least high school education; is first stage screening test; if child fails, do second PDQ 2–4 weeks later.
1 mo–6 yr[c]	All	Short DDST	5–10	Based on 3 sample items from each section of DDST; for use with parents with education level less than high school; first stage screen; 25% may fail at least 1 item and need full DDST.
Birth–8 yr	All	Boyd Developmental Progress Scale (BDPS)	5–10	Measures 150 items from observation and parent interview in areas of motor, communication, and self-sufficiency skills; results displayed graphically; is of practical orientation; can be administered by trained paraprofessional.
1–24 mo[d]	All	Milani-Comparetti Motor Development Screening Test (MDST)	4–8	Tests stages of motor development related to presence of "primary motor patterns," including postural control; no equipment needed; can be done by therapists and other health professionals; based on tester observations of child's responses; scored on sheets; good for sequential observation.

[a]Schedule of administration corresponds to schedule of well-child visits according to American Academy of Pediatrics, or Early Periodic Screening, Diagnosis, and Treatment (EPSDT) guidelines.

[b]Developed in conjunction with the American Academy of Pediatrics, Committee on Children with Handicaps, New York Chapter 3, District II, May 1970.

[c]Recommended at 3–6 mo, 9–12 mo, 18–24 mo, 3 yr, 4 yr, and 5 yr.

[d]Recommended at 1½–2 mo, 3½–4 mo, 5½–6 mo, 9–10 mo, 12 mo, 15 mo, 18 mo, 21 mo, and 24 mo.

B. Early intervention

1. **Methods** vary widely depending on the nature of the disability and its etiology but include the following:
   a. **Genetic counseling** to prevent further cases.
   b. **Specific treatment of underlying conditions,** as in congenital hypothyroidism.
   c. **Treatment of specific contributory disabilities,** e.g., hearing, vision.
   d. **Optimizing the functioning of the disabled individual and his or her family** by:
      (1) Identifying and addressing the child's strengths and weaknesses, which will allow achievement of his or her full potential during the most crucial early years.

Table 40-2. Sources for screening tools

Screening tool	Address
Denver Developmental Screening Test (DDST) and Prescreening Developmental Questionnaire (PDQ)	LADOCA Publishing Foundation East 51st Avenue at Lincoln Denver, CO 80216 (303) 295-6379
Milani-Comparetti Motor Development Screening Test (MDST)	Meyer Children's Rehabilitation Institute University of Nebraska Medical Center Omaha, Nebraska 68131 (402) 559-6000
Boyd Developmental Progress Scale (BDPS)	CCD Developmental Progress Scale R. D. Boyd University of Oregon Eugene, Oregon 97403 (503) 686-3111
Knobloch Developmental Screening Inventory (DSI)	(See Selected Readings)
Giannini Rapid Development Screening Checklist (RDSC)	M. Giannini, M.D. 810 Vermont Avenue, N.W. Washington, D.C. 20005 (202) 233-5179

(2) Preventing a single handicap from leading to secondary effects on other areas of development.

(3) Preventing deterioration in development due to inappropriate physical and emotional handling by parents, peers, and society.

(4) Improving interaction with siblings, between the child and parents, and between parents, by lessening parental emotional reactions and promoting greater understanding of the child's needs. This supportive relationship contributes to more successful developmental patterns later.

(5) Helping families focus on the broad needs of the child.

(6) Improving interaction and coordination among health and developmental providers.

(7) Teaching parents how to utilize community resources more effectively and efficiently.

(8) Providing direct supportive service to families in lower socioeconomic levels whose children are at increased risk for continuing developmental problems.

2. Justification

a. Effectiveness. Screening of well or high-risk, or both, children should result in early identification and treatment that either reverses a disease process or slows down its progression. Mass screening of children may identify almost every case of some disabilities that inevitably result in severe disability if untreated, but which can be controlled by total or nearly complete preventive treatments (e.g., newborn metabolic screening of phenylketonuria, congenital hypothyroidism, and galactosemia). For other disabilities early genetic counseling may prevent additional cases (e.g., neurofibromatosis in families). In still others, screening may result in identification of problems that have contributed to developmental retardation (e.g., vision or hearing loss). In all types and degrees of mental retardation, especially mild retardation, early intervention can benefit both the child and family by optimizing the child's functioning.

Interventions by various health professionals (physicians, nurses, occupational and physical therapists, early childhood educators, nutritionists, and social workers) help the family deal with the psychosocial stress and the facilitation of the activities of daily living (e.g., feeding, positioning, toileting, movement).

b. Risks. A family's hopes may sometimes be unrealistically raised by hopeful but unsuccessful efforts to treat the condition or optimize functions.

c. **Costs** vary widely.

d. **Acceptability.** An appropriate combination of medical services and home- or center-based early developmental support can greatly facilitate the parents' abilities to effectively serve as the primary caretakers and "case managers" of the child's needs.

III. Recommendations

A. Early detection

1. All neonates should have high-risk factors identified at birth, with careful scrutiny of Apgar components and physical examination. Those neonates identified as having such factors should be reevaluated by 2 months of age, by means of appropriate neurologic, vision, and hearing (brainstem evoked response [BSER]) testing performed by an adequately trained neurologist or developmental pediatrician, ophthalmologist, and audiologist.
2. Since low-risk as well as high-risk children may later experience developmental disabilities, all children should have histories taken and developmental examinations performed at the periodic stages of care (see Table 40-1). Use of the Rapid Developmental Screening Checklist (RDSC) or the Guide to Normal Milestones of Development (GNMD)-Haynes will facilitate the review.
3. At specific stages of development (see Table 40-1), the Prescreening Developmental Questionnaire (PDQ) or short Denver Developmental Screening Test (DDST) can be utilized, with follow-up of suspect children as described in sec. **II.A.1.**
4. The Developmental Screening Inventory (DSI) is helpful for high-risk infants and for those parents who desire further participation in the developmental monitoring of their children.

B. Early intervention

1. Any child who fails the DSI or DDST should be referred to a pediatric or developmental psychologist for further testing, or to the appropriate medical subspecialist (e.g., neurologist, speech and language pathologist) as indicated by the screening results. Children who pass the screening test should still be observed for later abnormalities in development, and for problems in other areas (e.g., home environment) not specifically checked for in the formal screening process.
2. If follow-up evaluations confirm developmental delays, the primary caretaker and primary physician should discuss the child's and family's needs and the intervention services available in the community.
3. Such services may include individual treatment from occupational and physical therapists, speech therapists, and others. Early infant or toddler developmental programs may present a combination of services in home-based or center-based formats, or both.
4. Public and private agencies should be considered for both direct services and referral assistance. Crippled Children's Services (CCS), Office of Public Education, and Associations for Retarded Citizens, are examples of many such programs.

Selected Readings

Dubowitz, L., and Dubowitz, V. *The neurological assessment of the pre-term and full-term newborn infant.* In *Clinics in Developmental Medicine.* No. 79. Philadelphia: Lippincott, 1981. *Detailed review for all physicians who are involved with neonates.*

Frankenburg, W. K., et al. The newly abbreviated and revised Denver Developmental Screening Test. *J. Pediat.* 99(6):995, 1981. *Describes the short DDST and provides a graphic portrayal of the rate of development with the revised DDST form (DDST-R).*

Frankenburg, W. K., Thornton, S. M., and Cohrs, M. E. (eds.). *Pediatric Developmental Diagnosis.* New York: Thieme-Stratton, 1981. *Well-organized, comprehensive review for primary care physicians of multiple aspects of child development; includes suggestions for school and community interaction; best used with associated videotapes.*

Gabel, S., and Erickson, M. T. (eds.). *Child Development and Developmental Disabilities.* Boston: Little, Brown, 1980. *Aimed at primary care physicians, medical students, and other health and developmental professionals; includes sections on normal development, evaluation, detailed assessment of specific disorders, and a multidisciplinary approach. Also includes more detailed information for readers interested in child development.*

Haynes, U. A Developmental Approach to Case-Finding with Special Reference to Cerebral Palsy, MR and Related Disorders. Washington, DC: United States Government Printing Office, 1967. *Source of the Guide to Normal Milestones of Development (GNMD).*

Holt, K. S. Medical examination of the child with cerebral palsy. *Pediatr. Ann.* 8(10):581, 1979. *Entire issue is an excellent review of most clinical aspects of cerebral palsy.*

Knobloch, H., et al. The validity of parental reporting of infant development. *Pediatrics* 63(6):872, 1979. *Describes developmental screening inventory; discusses DSI reliability and validity and compares it with PDQ.*

Knobloch, H., Pasamanick, B., and Sherard, E. S., Jr. A developmental screening inventory for infants. *Pediatrics* 38(Suppl.):1095, 1966. *The DSI uses selected items from the Gesell Developmental Schedules in adaptive, gross motor, fine motor, language, and personal/social behaviors—between 4 and 56 weeks and 15 and 18 months of age. The article reviews criteria for screening devices, usefulness for prediction and other benefits, and practical implementation of the DSI.*

McCall, R. B. A hard look at stimulating and predicting development: The cases of bonding and screening. *Pediatr. Rev.* 3(7):205, 1982. *An excellent analysis of screening approaches and tools (especially DSI and DDST). McCall comments on the predictive abilities of the tools, and crucial points in the practical implementation of such tests.*

Meier, J. H. *Developmental and Learning Disabilities: Evaluation, Management and Prevention in Children.* Baltimore: University Park Press, 1976. *Very detailed in scope, analysis, resources, and references; directed toward professionals in all fields of child development.*

Milani-Comparetti, A., and Gidoni, E. A. Pattern analysis of motor development and its disorders. *Dev. Med. Child. Neurol.* 9:625, 1967. *Review of MDST screening tool and its applicability.*

41

Child Physical Abuse and Neglect

Jane Gray

I. The problem

A. Definition. Child abuse/neglect is when a caregiver places a child in a situation that may or does endanger his or her life or health (including emotional well-being); abandons, tortures, cruelly confines, or cruelly punishes him or her; deprives a child of necessary food, clothing, or shelter; or exposes a child to the inclemency of the weather.

B. Description. Since 1962 when Dr. C. Henry Kempe's original article, "The Battered Child Syndrome" [1], was published, society has awakened to the multiple problems of the abused/neglected child and his or her family. This increased awareness has led to refinement of the diagnostic criteria for all aspects of childhood maltreatment, including physical abuse, neglect, failure-to-thrive, sexual abuse, and emotional abuse. In addition to the immediate, reportable, medical condition of the child, follow-up data have shown that abused/neglected children also very frequently exhibit nutritional, developmental, and emotional deficits that lead to long-term difficulties. Many individuals in foster care, special educational classes, detention centers, and penal institutions were abused/neglected children. Long-term sequelae are also reflected in the fact that abused and neglected children grow up to be the abusive parents of the next generation, thus perpetuating the cycle of family violence.

C. Epidemiology. Although there are no precise data on the exact incidence of child abuse/neglect, it is estimated that there are one million cases in the United States per year. Every year there has been an increase in the number of reported cases; however, most experts feel that these figures still represent only the "tip of the iceberg."

Originally, physical abuse was the only recognized form of abuse. It is the current experience at the University Hospital of the University of Colorado Health Sciences Center that now sexual and physical abuse are reported about equally. However, other agencies who serve a different geographic area, and thus a different population, have differing incidences. For nonmedical agencies, neglect (including failure-to-thrive) is the most frequently reported form of maltreatment. It is mainly within the past 5 years that the reporting of sexual abuse has increased dramatically.

Abuse/neglect has been found to be more prevalent among infants and children with certain preexisting or **at-risk conditions:** (1) babies born prematurely, (2) infants confined to high-risk nurseries because of neonatal complications, (3) children with handicaps, (4) twins, (5) children of adolescent mothers, and (6) often, but not necessarily, those living in poverty, stressed by a poor environment, and raised by alcohol or drug abusers.

Risk factors for sexual abuse are not as yet specifically determined. Many researchers in the field presently feel there is no such thing as a sexual abuse profile.

II. Primary prevention.

Promoting healthy parenting is essential in preventing child abuse (see Chap. 27).

III. Secondary prevention

A. Early detection

1. Methods

a. Description. At the present time, no screening program has been able to identify specifically those dysfunctional families who will maltreat their children. These programs do involve the evaluation of medical and psychosocial data (whether obtained by direct interviews or by questionnaires [Table 41-1] completed by the parents), and the assessment of observations (made either directly or through review of videotaped interactions) [2].

b. Timing. The timing of the interviews and observations covers the third trimester of pregnancy to the 6-week postpartum checkup. It is generally agreed that assessments done in the immediate perinatal period—including delivery room observations and parent and child interactions—are the most valuable.

c. **Performance** (see Table 41-1)

(1) During the initial interview, **a psychosocial** (as well as medical) **history should be gathered on all prenatal patients.** Often, collection of the psychosocial data is best accomplished over several visits. This is because no one single factor places a family at risk. Rather, it is a complex interplay of positive and negative attributes encompassing a number of factors, the family's emphasis on them, and the family's resistance to change that will influence the outcome of the assessment. Much of this data can be obtained by office or clinic staff, and the physician may only need to clarify and amplify any areas of concern.

(2) **Observations in the delivery room** have proved to be very helpful in assessing parenting potential. Labor and delivery room nurses record their observations on a form designed to elicit the parents' verbal and nonverbal responses, either through the use of a checklist of parental behaviors, or by answering pertinent questions, e.g., how does the mother look, what does she say, what does she do? Such forms take less than 5 minutes of nursing time to complete. If all delivery room interaction forms are placed in a designated area prior to filing with the baby's chart, an appointed person can review the day's delivery room interactions in a matter of minutes.

(3) **Postpartum observations** of interactions of mother and newborn infant, mother and father, and parent and older siblings need to be recorded carefully. Then, prior to discharge, the physician can assess all the medical, psychosocial, and interactional information and decide whether intervention is required.

(4) **Postnatal period observations** include observations of the baby's growth development and social and emotional behaviors, as well as continued observations of the caregiver and child interaction.

d. **Interpretation.** The warning signs in Table 41-1 are **indications** of possible problems. A high-risk situation is created by varying combinations of these signs, the family's degree of emphasis on them, and the family's willingness to change. Warning signs may be balanced by the presence of positive family circumstances (Table 41-2). The interviewer must take into consideration the mother's age, culture, and education, as well as observations of her affect and

Table 41-1. Warning signs of families at risk for child abuse and neglect

Observations during the prenatal period

1. The mother seems overly concerned with the baby's sex or performance.
2. The mother exhibits denial of the pregnancy (not willing to gain weight, no plans for the baby, refusal to talk about the situation).
3. This child could be "one too many."
4. The mother is extremely depressed over the pregnancy.
5. The mother is very frightened and alone, especially in anticipation of delivery. Careful explanations do not seem to dissipate the fears.
6. There is lack of support from the husband or family, or both.
7. The mother or father, or both, formerly wanted an abortion or seriously considered relinquishment and have changed their minds.
8. The parents come from an abusive/neglectful background.
9. The parents' living situation is overcrowded, isolated, or unstable, or is intolerable to them.
10. They do not have a telephone.
11. There are no supportive relatives or friends.

Observations during delivery

1. To accurately note the described risk observations, it is helpful to:
   a. Have a written form, with a baby's chart, of parent('s) reactions at birth:
      How does the mother look?
      What does the mother say?
      What does the mother do?

Table 41-1. continued

b. Record the father's reaction when he attends the delivery.
c. Talk to the nurse and doctor involved with delivery for further information if interaction seems dubious.

2. The following at-risk behavior should be carefully noted:
   a. Passive reaction, either verbal or nonverbal: mother doesn't touch, hold, or examine baby, nor talk in affectionate terms or tones about the baby.
   b. Hostile rejection, either verbal or nonverbal: mother makes inappropriate verbalizations, glances, or disparaging remarks about the physical characteristics of the child.
   c. Disappointment over sex of the baby.
   d. No eye contact.
   e. Nonsupportive interaction between the parents.

Observations during the postpartum period

1. The mother doesn't have fun with the baby.
2. The mother avoids eye contact with the baby and avoids the direct *en face* position.
3. The verbalizations to the infant are negative, demanding, or harsh.
4. Most of the mother's verbalizations to others about the child are negative.
5. The parents remain disappointed over the sex of the child.
6. Negative identification of the child: significance of name, who he or she looks like or acts like, or both.
7. The parents have expectations developmentally far beyond the child's capabilities.
8. The mother is very bothered by the baby's crying; it makes her feel hopeless, helpless, like crying herself, or angry.
9. Feedings: the mother sees the baby as too demanding; she is repulsed by his or her messiness or ignores his or her demands.
10. Changing diapers is seen as a very negative, repulsive task.
11. The mother does not comfort the baby when he or she cries.
12. The reactions of the husband or family, or both, to the baby have been negative or nonsupportive.
13. The mother is receiving little or no meaningful support from anyone.
14. There are sibling rivalry problems or a complete lack of understanding of this possibility.
15. The husband is very jealous of the baby's drain on the mother's time, energy, and affection.
16. The mother lacks control over the situation. She is not involved, or relinquishes control to the doctors and nurses.
17. The mother makes complaints about the baby that cannot be verified.
18. The mother cannot see that attention focused on the baby has any positive value for her.

Source: J. D. Gray, et al. Prediction and prevention of child abuse and neglect. *Child Abuse Negl.* 1(1):45, 1977.

Table 41-2. Positive family circumstances

1. Parents had helpful role models when growing up.
2. Marriage is stable.
3. Parents can have fun together and enjoy personal interests or hobbies.
4. Mother's intelligence and health are good.
5. Father has stable job.
6. Parents have their own home and stable living conditions.
7. Parents have a good friend or relative to turn to, a sound need-meeting system.
8. This baby was planned or wanted.
9. Parents exhibit coping abilities, i.e., capacity to plan and understand need for adjustments because of new baby.
10. Baby is healthy and not too disruptive to parents' lifestyle.
11. Parents see likeable attributes in baby; see baby as separate individual.
12. Either parent can rescue the child or relieve the other in a crisis.
13. Future birth control is planned.
14. Father is supportive to mother and involved in care of baby.

Source: J. D. Gray, et al. Prediction and prevention of child abuse and neglect. *Child Abuse Negl.* 1(1):45, 1977.

the significance of her feelings. Many of these signs can be observed throughout the perinatal period. At present, assessment of parenting potential remains somewhat subjective because of the complex interplay of multiple factors. However, when there is concern or doubt, close follow-up and immediate intervention must be provided.

2. **Justification**

a. **Test characteristics.** Studies on the prediction and prevention of child abuse and neglect are still at a very early stage. Early estimates of the scope of the problem show that approximately 20% of parents will be at risk for dysfunctional parenting, of which child abuse and neglect is an extreme.

Studies done at the University of Colorado Health Sciences Center have shown that families at risk for abnormal parenting practices **can** be identified, and that intervention can prevent nonaccidental injuries requiring hospitalization. A 10% incidence of maltreatment requiring hospitalization was documented in high-risk families who received only routine pediatric and community services. Hunter and associates have studied maltreatment in children who had been admitted to a neonatal intensive care unit [3]. At a one-year follow-up, they found a 3.9% incidence of maltreatment—chiefly neglect since discharge from the neonatal intensive care unit. All these children who had been reported to the Central Registry had been categorized as "high risk" by interview criteria before discharge. No low-risk child had been reported as suffering abuse and neglect [3].

In our experience, assessment of delivery room interactions was 76% accurate in determining families who subsequently had difficulty parenting. The use of a questionnaire [4] alone was 57% accurate, and postpartum interview and observations alone were 54% accurate. Since 1978 the questionnaire has been revised and subjected to field trials. These validation studies show a sensitivity of 83% and a 77% specificity since revision.

b. **Risks and side effects.** Some families will be incorrectly identified as being at risk for abusing their child or children. Without great care, these parents may experience unnecessary guilt, anxiety, and feelings of inadequacy as parents.

c. **Cost.** The costs and time involved in detecting high-risk families has not yet been adequately determined.

d. **Acceptability.** If the screening tools are used routinely for all, there is no discrimination. However, some of those screened may feel that their privacy has been invaded and that such assessment is unacceptable.

B. **Early intervention**

1. **Methods**

a. Most parents make their first contact with the physician during the **prenatal period.** This is not only the time to begin parenting assessments, but also the time to begin intervention. Intervention includes establishing a trusting relationship with the parents, educating them as to the birth process and their options at that time, and for making appropriate referrals. Provision of a positive perinatal experience, which will then positively affect the parents' attachment to the baby, is one of the important goals of the prenatal period.

b. **Immediately after birth,** parents need to be given an opportunity to hold, touch, and explore their baby. This is a time when the baby is very alert, and it thus offers an ideal opportunity to begin parent/child attachment. Many hospitals now offer rooming-in to new mothers; **the importance of this needs emphasis.** These few days in close contact with her baby while still in a secure and supportive setting allows the mother time to focus her full attention on the baby. These rooming-in mothers feel affectionate bonds and gain confidence in caring for the baby more quickly. A supportive staff can also use this time for informal teaching, using the baby as a focus.

c. **Discharge planning** may involve referrals for families at risk; this will be a logical consequence of the perinatal involvement with the family. The referrals will include pediatric well-child care for the infant and postpartum and family planning appointments for the mother. A public health nurse to evaluate, teach, and support the parents in the home is also often indicated. A concept newer to the United States is that of referral to a health visitor [5]. Health visitors have been utilized successfully in Great Britain for many

Table 41-3. Special well-child care for high-risk families

1. Contact the mother by telephone on the second day after discharge.
2. Provide more frequent office visits.
3. Give more attention to the family.
4. Advise discipline only around accident prevention.
5. Use compliments rather than criticism.
6. Accept phone calls at home.
7. Provide regular home visits by a public health nurse or lay health visitor.

years. Each family of a newborn is assigned to a visitor who provides support, education, role-modeling, and concrete aid to the family.

On discharge, a few families will need referrals for specific services. These may include women, infants, and children (WIC) programs, food stamps, housing authorities, or, occasionally, child protective services.

d. Pediatric well-child care in situations of assessed risk for abnormal parenting (Table 41-3) involves close and supportive contact with the family by telephone and in the clinic or office. Building a trusting relationship between parents and health care providers is a priority; families who are experiencing difficulties will thus feel secure using medical personnel as "lifelines" during times of crisis. Because the young infant is particularly vulnerable, well-child visits for those at risk should be scheduled every 1 to 2 weeks. Frequent well-child visits are necessary to provide comprehensive health care, to observe mother/child interactions, to update psychosocial functioning, to provide anticipatory guidance, and to initiate referrals. Because of broader goals, these office visits tend to require more time than do visits of a well-functioning family. Scheduling at least 45 minutes for a high-risk family is not unusual.

Children raised in an environment devoid of good parenting often exhibit multiple problems. Physicians need an especially alert eye for any evidence of physical trauma. On each visit, height, weight, and head circumference need to be recorded and plotted on a growth curve.

Children who lack love and stimulation are not engaged in appropriate adult-child interactions and do not progress developmentally at a satisfactory rate. The at-risk child's development needs to be assessed objectively by the Denver Developmental Screening Test (DDST) or Bayley Scales of Infant Development, rather than the assessment relying solely on the mother's history.

The physician needs to observe the mother/child interaction during the clinic visits. Appropriate interaction with parents will also be reflected in socialization skills (smiling, vocalizations, and so on) in the baby. Then, after the history and physical, the interview should be turned back to the mother. She should be asked how she feels and how things are going for her. She needs to be reassured that parenting an infant is not an easy task and that you are available to offer support or to arrange referrals that may be helpful.

A large segment of the appointment may be spent giving anticipatory guidance. This guidance needs to include the management of illness as well as child care, growth, and development. The mother needs to know what to do if her baby is ill, and she needs to know when to call the doctor. Often, written directions outlining which actions need to be taken and when to call are reassuring to the parents. If a child is ill, it is worthwhile to give the parents a general idea of the expected course of the illness and to warn them of any occurrences of which you wish to be informed. It is also important to call the parents during the course of the disease to check on the medical progress and offer reassurance and support to the parents.

Well-child guidance must meet the immediate needs of the parents and child. Projecting too far ahead will only prove confusing and may overwhelm parents with limited resources. Anticipatory guidance certainly needs to include routine advice on the following: feeding, sleep-waking patterns, stimulation, safety, discipline, independence and exploratory behaviors, and toilet training.

The final step of each visit is to determine if any new referrals to community agencies or other health care providers are necessary. Even if all seems to be functioning well, it is still worthwhile for all those who work with the family to speak together so progress can be assessed and any new treatment options be initiated. A corollary of this is that the physician should not attempt to provide all services to a multiproblem family. These high-risk situations have so many different aspects that no one person can be expected to have all the expertise necessary to benefit these families.

2. **Justification**
   a. **Effectiveness.** In the previously mentioned study done at the University of Colorado Health Sciences Center, one hundred families were assessed to be at high risk for abnormal parenting practices. These families were randomly divided into two groups. Fifty of these families received extra services in the form of continuity of pediatric care, public health nurse visits, and a lay health visitor (intervention group). The other fifty families received routine pediatric care and whatever services the community could offer (nonintervention group). Follow-up occurred when the children were approximately 2 years old. Trauma thought to be nonaccidental that was serious enough to require hospitalization occurred in 10% of children in the nonintervention group. No injury serious enough to require hospitalization occurred in children in the intervention group or in a comparison group of mothers assessed to be at low risk for parenting problems.

      There is also evidence that a strong maternal/infant bond may protect a child from maltreatment. From the work of Kennell, Voos, and Klaus [6], we know that the perinatal period is an important time to support the development of affectionate bonds.

      These preliminary studies demonstrate that appropriate assessments, followed by a sensitive outreach approach to parents perinatally and after discharge, can decrease the incidence and severity of abuse/neglect.
   b. **Risks and side effects.** Aside from the previously mentioned concerns about labeling, the actual support services are enhancements of existing care and probably have negligible risks.
   c. **Costs.** "1980 saw more than 600,000 children born into high risk situations. . . . Over one-half of these children will end up as societal failures. . . . My own estimate is that per annum cost, without inflation, for each societal failure exceeds on the average $10,000 per year. If half of the 600,000 children born each year in America into high-risk families become societal failures, then the cost to our society of failing to cope with this problem will add some $90,000,000 this year alone for children born in 1981" [7]. Preventive services through physicians and nurses already at work in existing facilities add very little to cost. The use of health visitors is also relatively inexpensive. Family Support Services of Denver estimates that it costs an average of $500 per family for 4–6 months' intervention by a lay person.
   d. **Acceptability.** It is too early to be certain, but acceptance of such services by families will probably depend on whether they are perceived as needed, wanted, and nonthreatening.

IV. **Recommendations**
   A. **Primary prevention** (see the recommendations in Chap. 27.)
   B. **Secondary prevention**
      1. **Early detection**
         a. All families who come for prenatal services should be assessed as to their parenting potential.
         b. Evaluations should include medical, psychosocial, and interactional data, and continue from the prenatal into the perinatal and postpartum periods.
      2. **Early intervention**
         a. Intervention with families begins with a sensitive outreach to establish a trusting relationship between parents and health care provider. In this way medical personnel can serve as a lifeline for families in crisis.
         b. Support, education, and appropriate referrals are also important.

References

1. Kempe, C. H., Silverman, F. N., and Steele, B. F. The battered child syndrome. *J.A.M.A.* 181(1):17, 1962. *Excellent basic reference.*
2. Gray, J. D., et al. Prediction and prevention of child abuse and neglect. *Child Abuse Negl.* 1(1):45, 1977. *Early research into prediction of risk and outcome of intervention.*
3. Hunter, R. S., et al. Antecedents of child abuse and neglect in premature infants: A prospective study in a newborn intensive care unit. *Pediatrics* 61(4):629, 1978. *Interview data and observed behaviors in neonatal intensive care unit are predictive of risk.*
4. Helfer, R. E., Hoffmeister, J., and Schneider, C. *MSPP. A Manual for Use of The Michigan Screening Profile of Parenting.* Boulder, CO: Test Analyses and Development Corporation, 1978. *Philosophy, usage, and scoring of questionnaire. Research and statistical data on the use and validity of this questionnaire.*
5. Kempe, C. H., and Helfer, R. E. (eds.). *The Battered Child* (3rd ed.). Chicago: University of Chicago Press, 1980. *A comprehensive overview of child maltreatment.*
6. Kennell, J., Voos, D., and Klaus, M. Parent-Infant Bonding. In R. E. Helfer and C. H. Kempe (eds.), *Child Abuse and Neglect: The Family and The Community.* Cambridge: Ballinger Publishing, 1976. *Basic research data on attachment, coupled with intervention strategies during the perinatal period.*
7. Harris, I. B. Speech at the Governor's Mansion, Denver, Colorado, April, 1981. *Some approximate cost figures.*

42 Visual Problems in Infants and Children

Gordon Smith

I. The problem

A. Description. Our understanding of developmental visual physiology has progressed dramatically in the past 20 years. Coupled with major advances in treatment capabilities (corneal transplant, epikeratophakia, vitrectomy), this understanding enables us to treat a variety of conditions that in the past would have led to blindness. Visual deprivation in infants can cause irreversible anatomic changes; to avoid this, detection must occur early and intervention must be swift.

1. Pathophysiology

a. Amblyopia. The term **amblyopia** traditionally has been used to refer to a state in which there is decreased visual acuity in an eye for which no structural cause exists that can be seen ophthalmoscopically. The Nobel-Prize-winning studies of Wiesel and Hubel [1] clarified the concept of visual deprivation amblyopia. To produce this condition there must be an immature visual system (in a child generally less than 10 years of age) and degradation of the image(s) in one or both eyes. Any cause for degradation of the image (cataract or other opacity of the ocular media, refractive error such as astigmatism, and so on) can cause amblyopia. For the problem to qualify as amblyopia, the vision would remain reduced when the cause of image degradation is corrected. An infant with a cataract, for example, initially cannot see because of the presence of the cataract. Amblyopia, however, quickly follows this mechanical blockade of vision; then, even after the cataract is removed and the image on the retina is made clear, the child still does not see.

b. Binocular vision. Binocularity, commonly demonstrated as the ability to perceive the "3-D" effect (stereopsis), is a physiologic process in which information from both eyes is processed simultaneously. (Binocular, for the purpose of this discussion, refers to simultaneous perception of foveal image.) Wiesel and Hubel [1] showed that binocularity is a visual function separate from, but related to, amblyopia. An infant with crossed eyes may alternately use each eye while suppressing or "ignoring," a cortical function, the image from the other eye. Since the infant never attempts to process information from both eyes simultaneously (to do so would produce double vision, which the infant brain avoids assiduously), there is no binocular vision. In **strabismus** there is often a crude simultaneous perception of peripheral field images. If the centers responsible for binocular vision are not stimulated early in visual development, they may irreversibly atrophy and binocular vision cannot then be recovered. Nonetheless, since each eye is used part of the time (the brain alternately "pays attention" to each while suppressing the image perceived by the other), amblyopia may not develop. It is thus possible to have a visual system with no functional binocularity (stereopsis) but also no amblyopia; or, put another way, absence of binocularity does not necessarily mean presence of amblyopia. However, the reverse—presence of amblyopia—generally means absence of binocularity, since binocularity requires images from both eyes simultaneously.

c. Critical period. Wiesel and Hubel [1] and others have demonstrated that amblyopia and loss of binocularity can become irreversible if allowed to persist through a critical period of infant visual development. The length of the critical period can be estimated based on studies of deprivation amblyopia in animals (cats and primates, among others) and clinical observations in humans. For cases of visual deprivation amblyopia (e.g., cataract) intervention probably needs to occur in the first 2 months of life. Amblyopia will occur

Table 42-1. Opacities of the ocular media

Lid
Ptosis occluding the pupil; hemangioma or other mass of the lid occluding the pupil
Cornea
Developmental anomalies: dermoid, sclerocornea, anterior segment dysgenesis
Infection: chlamydia, bacterial, cytomegalovirus (CMV), herpes
Inflammatory interstitial keratitis
Metabolic: mucopolysaccharidoses type I
Injury: forceps, causing breaks in Descemet's membranes
Iris
Anterior segment dysgenesis
Persistent pupillary membrane
Corectopia (eccentric displacement of the pupil)
Cyst
Aniridia
Lens
Cataract, lenticonus, dislocated lens, microspherophakia
Vitreous
Persistent hyperplastic primary vitreous (PHPV)
Hemorrhage (forceps injury, birth injury)
Persistent hyaloid artery/vascular loops

within weeks of onset of the strabismus if the child always fixates with the same eye. If the child alternates, there may be no amblyopia, but the chance to develop binocular capability drops dramatically if straightening of ocular alignment is not achieved by 24 months of age [2].

2. **Conditions**

   a. **Opacities of the media.** Any opacity that sufficiently degrades the clarity of the image falling on the retina can be amblyogenic. Such opacities might be relatively small, but dense, and located in the central visual axis, nearly filling the pupillary aperture (2–4 mm). It can be difficult to predict whether a given opacity will be amblyogenic, and such decisions need not be made at the primary care level. For specific conditions, see Table 42-1.

   b. **Strabismus.** Misalignment of the visual axes forces the brain to choose which eye will be used and which suppressed. This precludes the binocular state, and, if the same eye is constantly suppressed, may lead to amblyopia. Strabismus can be due to dysfunction of the muscles themselves, or more commonly, due to dysfunction of the neurologic control center for ocular alignment. A constant misalignment is a **tropia.** Misalignment induced by covering one eye that reverts to normal alignment when that eye is uncovered is a **phoria.** The prefix **eso-** means in-turning, **exo-** means out-turning, **hyper-** refers to up-turning, and **hypo-** to down-turning—for example, esophoria or hypophoria.

   c. **Refractive errors.** Refractive errors are really refractive states (or power to bend light rays), the state of which is such that the amount of bending does not focus the light rays on the retina. In myopia (nearsightedness) the light rays come to focus in front of the retina, necessitating a minus power or diverging lens. Because the eye cannot create minus power, an optical aid (spectacle lens or contact lens) is needed to achieve optimum focus.

   In hyperopia (farsightedness) the light rays would come to focus behind the retina (and so are intercepted by the retina while still converging and still unfocused). A plus power or converging lens is needed. A child's healthy eye has the ability to add plus power to the system by contracting the ciliary body muscle (a process called accommodating), which in turn permits the lens to become more spherical, hence more plus-powered. The great majority of children are farsighted; by accommodating they see quite normally and do not need glasses to treat their farsightedness.

   In astigmatism some part of the focusing system (cornea and lens) is not spherical; there is thus more bending power in one meridian (for example, vertically at 90°) than in the opposite (180°). In this case, the eye cannot bring all meridians to focus at once without the aid of a compensating astigmatic (power in one meridian) lens.

Refractive errors are sources of visual problems and are particularly prone to cause amblyopia when one eye has a different refractive state than the fellow eye (anisometropia). Anisometropic amblyopia generally cannot be reversed once a child reaches 8 years of age.

B. Epidemiology

1. **Opacities.** The incidence of opacities of the visual media has not been well studied. Francois reported an incidence of 1/250 live births; however, this must include many opacities not visually significant. The U.S. Department of Health and Human Services, on the other hand, reported an incidence of cataract as 1/6250 live births. The true incidence of all visually significant opacities probably lies somewhere in between.
2. **Strabismus.** The prevalence of strabismus and amblyopia in children under 8 years of age is believed to be about 5%.
3. **Refractive errors.** The prevalence of potentially significant refractive errors in children under 8 years is approximately 20%. Not all such children will need glasses, however, since as the child grows the eye changes shape and some refractive errors disappear.

II. Secondary prevention

A. Early detection

1. Methods

a. **Detection of opacities of the ocular media.** Any condition that degrades the image reaching the retina carries the potential for becoming amblyogenic. A list of types or causes, or both, of such conditions appears in Table 42-1. Once such an opacity is discovered, appropriate referral can be made and therapeutic measures undertaken.

(1) **Ophthalmoscopy.** The best way to rule out a media abnormality is by direct visualization of retinal structures. Examination of the newborn's undilated eyes for opacities and a **red reflex** is a time-honored tradition but in some cases it may be inadequate. This should be performed within the first 2 weeks of life. When an adequate exam cannot be performed on the undilated eye, **dilating** the pupil should be considered. Two acceptable regimens, both of which have been used without problems in premature as well as full-term infants, are listed in **Table 42-2.** We find the placement of an infant lid speculum very helpful [3]. Dilation can be done in the nursery during the discharge physical examination, or in the office during one of the first well-child examinations. Generally, it will take about 20–30 minutes for the drops to take full effect. The dilation itself will last 6–24 hours. Parents should be reassured that the child need not be kept in the dark following dilation and that focusing is normal in 2–4 hours, although the pupils may remain dilated for 24 hours (usually in blonder children). Any opacity of the ocular media, regardless of size, deserves evaluation by an ophthalmologist.

b. **Detection of strabismus.** Intermittent or transient crossing in the first 3–4 months of life is normal. Constant misalignment is never normal. Esotropia (eyes turning in toward the nose) is more common than exotropia (eyes turning out away from each other), especially in infants. If the child always fixates with the same eye, the fellow, misaligned eye will develop amblyopia. The degree of misalignment does not affect this. A small-angle constant deviation is just as amblyogenic as a large one. Checking for strabismus should begin at 4 months and continue until 8 years of age.

(1) **History.** When a parent says the child's eyes turn out, he or she is usually correct. False-positive reports of in-turning are more common because of the phenomenon of pseudostrabismus. The absence of a raised nasal bridge produces prominent epicanthal folds, which, in turn, leaves very little exposed sclera (white) between the canthus and the corneal limbus (dark due to iris behind it). Thus, when a child looks even **slightly** to one side, the white disappears and the eye appears to be crossing. Making the diagnosis of an in-turning eye depends on the assessment of the corneal light reflex or alternate cover test, or both (see below), but it can be difficult and may require confirmatory opinions.

(2) **Corneal light reflex.** One way to detect misalignment is to observe the corneal light reflex. With the room preferably dimmed somewhat, a pen-

Table 42-2. Direct visualization of retinal structures (two regimens)

Brand name		Generic name	Dosage
Cyclomydril		A prepackaged mixture of cyclopentolate 0.2% and phenylephrine 0.5%	1 drop in each eye q5 min twice
Mydriacyl		Tropicamide 0.5%	1 drop of each in each eye q5 min twice
	and		
Neosynephrine		Phenylephrine 0.5%	

light is aimed at the patient. The observer's eye is behind and on line with the light, and the location of the light reflex on the cornea of each eye is noted. If both reflexes bear the same spatial relationship to adjacent landmarks (e.g., both reflexes in the center of the pupil or both reflexes equally nasal or temporal to the center of the pupil) [4], the eye is presumed to be straight.

This test may also be performed using the ophthalmoscope [4]. The observer, after aligning the large circle of light so that it fully encompasses both eyes, brings the cornea and iris into focus using the focusing wheel. The observer can also compare the symmetry of the red reflexes at this time. Color variance of the red reflex is not as important as brightness and the position of the corneal reflexes. The deviating eye will have the brighter red reflex.

(3) Alternate-cover test. A better method is the alternate-cover test. It depends on getting the patient to fixate (on a target), while alternately covering each eye (left, right, left, right) for 1 to 2 seconds thus permitting the uncovered eye to fixate.

Ideally one should do the cover test with the patient fixating both in the distance and at near. Exotropias are more likely to be discovered with distance viewing. Placing a windup music box or attention-getting toy 10–15 ft away is helpful. For near fixation a translucent finger puppet such as one of the Sesame Street characters attached to a penlight works well. Older children can fixate on a target such as letters on the visual acuity chart (distance) and the near card When deviation is present, one can observe the nonfixing eye (covered eye) moving to take up fixation as it is uncovered and the fixing eye is covered. One can cover the eye with three upright fingers or any occluder.

This test does not distinguish between a phoria (crossing occurring only when an eye is occluded) and a tropia (constant crossing). The distinction is not necessary at the primary care level, however, since both conditions need evaluation. Once the child is comfortable with the test, it can be done rapidly (30 seconds for several trials). It should be done beginning at the 4–months' well-child visit, and then each well-child visit thereafter through age 8.

There are several types of strabismus (Brown's syndrome, Duane's syndrome, overaction of obliques, congenital superior oblique palsy) that are best discovered with the eyes in side gaze, at which point the deviation is manifested. Having an attention-getting toy (a colorful toy that makes some noise) is most helpful. One needs to take the toy far enough around the side that the infant runs out of head turn and is forced to move the eyes into a side gaze.

c. Detection of refractive errors is best accomplished by measuring visual acuity and performing the Random Dot E Stereogram [5]. Readers unfamiliar with this new test are referred to the article by Hammond and Schmidt [5].

Visual acuity should be tested at least by age 4 with either the tumbling E (E game) or Lippman test (HOVT). A child should be referred if, as a 3- or 4-year-old, vision is 20/50 or less in either or both eyes; similarly a 5- or 6-year-old with 20/40 or less in either or both eyes should be referred. Also refer any child with an interocular acuity difference of one line with isolated symbols or two lines with linear presentations. Such tests should be performed by age 4 and yearly thereafter until the adult Snellen chart can be used.

2. **Justification**
   a. **Opacities of the ocular media.** It was believed in the past that observation of the red reflex in the newborn would suffice to detect opacities of the ocular media. Unfortunately this is not always the case. While it is certainly true that a difference in the red reflex between the two eyes may herald some problem, similar red reflexes do not rule out a problem. There are cataracts whose optical consistency is such that the amount of light reflected back through them (red reflex) is not substantially diminished, yet no formed image is projectable through them (i.e., they are translucent but not transparent). Such an effect can only be discovered by the examiner's inability to visualize retinal structures such as the optic nerve or major blood vessels. It is extremely difficult, and sometimes impossible, even for the most experienced examiner, to do this through the small undilated pupil of the newborn, especially if the iris is dark. Detection of any opacity of the media in a newborn must occur in the first few weeks of life, however, if time is to be available to intervene effectively.

      Since the cost of pupillary dilation is trivial and the morbidity extremely low (occasional flushing of skin), it may be an acceptable screening approach. Studies remain to be done to demonstrate its sensitivity.
   b. **Detection of strabismus.** Only early detection of strabismus can provide the opportunity to salvage vision.

      The alternate-cover test and corneal light reflex test have not been studied for specificity and sensitivity. Although the corneal light reflex test cannot detect small degrees of misalignment, it is certainly a useful screening device, especially for infants [4]. It is safe to infer that performing the tests will minimize underdetection; the rate of false-positives (unnecessary referrals) is unknown. There are no risks or side effects, and the cost is one's time (30 seconds), excluding referrals for false-positives.
   c. **Detection of refractive errors.** Our current knowledge of the sensitivity and specificity of vision screening methods is imperfect. Friendly [6] has shown that the test/retest reliability for the HOTV test is less than that of the E game. Both tests tend to overrefer (HOTV greater than the E game), minimizing false-negatives. It is felt that the cost to society of the overreferrals is less than the alternative cost of a missed diagnosis and attendant visual loss.

      The Random Dot Stereo E test appears very promising in that it has a high sensitivity (perhaps 98%) to detection of vision disorders, with no risk and a cost of only 2 minutes of a nonprofessional's time.

B. Early intervention

1. **Methods**
   a. **Opacities of the ocular media.** Corneal, lens and vitreous opacities are now all approachable surgically if ophthalmologic assessment concludes that the opacity is amblyogenic and that no other factors are present to prevent development of vision. This assessment might include a visual evoked response (VER; also called visual evoked potential [VEP]) or the forced preferential looking test, to estimate the amount of amblyopia when visual acuity cannot be measured. Management will continue at least until the child is age 9; parents need to understand that they are embarking on a long-term project.
   b. In **strabismus,** the amblyopia, if present, is treated first by patching or glasses, or both. Sometimes glasses will control the crossing as well (accommodative esotropia). When the amblyopia has been treated, one then attempts to achieve alignment with surgery.
   c. **Refractive errors** are of course compensated for (not corrected) by optical devices (spectacles or contact lenses).
2. **Justification**
   a. **Opacities of the ocular media.** Surgical removal of ocular media opacities can be highly effective. The risks associated with general anesthesia in healthy infants are extremely small [2]. A good prognosis demands early discovery and treatment.
   b. **Strabismus.** Misalignment, if treatable, is treated by glasses (accommodative esotropia) or surgery. Success can be defined at several levels. At the highest level, the eyes are straight and binocular vision is attained. At the next level the eyes are straight but binocular vision is not attained. Lastly, the eyes would be straighter but not perfectly aligned.

c. **Refractive errors.** Optical aids are extremely effective in compensating for refractive errors, if the treatment is applied early in the course of the condition. The younger the child the quicker the response to treatment.

The cost of these various treatment regimes has not been well studied, but the alternative of an amblyopic eye and the cost if the patient loses the good eye has been considered unacceptable.

III. Recommendations

A. Early detection

1. Ophthalmoscopy

a. An ophthalmoscopic view of retinal structures, sometimes requiring pupillary dilation, should be performed on all infants in the first 2 weeks of life.

b. The red reflex should be assessed, and an attempt to view retinal structures should be made at 2 months and at subsequent well-child visits until age 8.

2. **Strabismus evaluation.** Corneal light reflex should be assessed and an alternate cover test should be done at near and far at each well-child visit, beginning at 4 months and continuing to 8 years.

3. **Vision assessment.** Measurement of visual acuity should be accomplished by the time a child is 4 years of age. Useful tests include the E game, the HOTV, the Random Dot E Stereogram, STYCAR, and Allen Picture Card tests. For older children, the Snellen chart and Titmus or Telebinocular machines are effective screening devices.

   Assessment of vision is the definitive defense against amblyopia, and it is worthwhile for primary care practitioners to expend the effort to make the appropriate assessments.

B. Early intervention

1. Vision-threatening media opacities are treated surgically.
2. Strabismus is referred for evaluation. Eyeglasses or surgery, or both, may be used to correct alignment. If amblyopia is present, it may be treated first with patching.
3. Refractive errors are treated with optical devices (spectacles or contact lenses). Anisometropic amblyopia may require patching as well.
4. If it is believed that abnormalities are present or questions exist, referral should be made to an ophthalmologist.

References

1. Wiesel, T. N., and Hubel, D. M. Effects of visual deprivation on morphology and physiology of cells in the cat's lateral geniculate body. *J. Neurophysiol.* 26 978, 1963. *One of a series of Nobel-Prize-winning studies demonstrating the complexity of the issue.*
2. Ing, M. R. Early Surgical Alignment for Congenital Esotropia. In R. D. Reinecke (ed.), *Strabismus II. Proceedings of the 4th Meeting of the International Strabismological Association.* Orlando FL: Grune & Stratton, 1984. P. 4. *A large retrospective study that demonstrated the importance of intervention before a child reaches 24 months of age.*
3. Harley, R. D. Pediatric Ophthalmology. In J. Flynn (ed.), *Examination of the Infant Eye* (2nd ed.). Philadelphia: Saunders, 1983. P. 12. *Good summary of infant eye examination techniques.*
4. Cibis, G. W., and Waeltermann, J. M. Rapid strabismus screening for the pediatrician. *Clin. Pediatr.* 25(6)304, 1986. *An excellent description of how to perform the corneal light reflex test, with clarifying diagrams and photos of different conditions.*
5. Hammond, R. S., and Schmidt, P. P. A Random Dot E stereogram for the vision screening of children. *Arch. Opthalmol.* 104(1)54, 1986. *A good description of how to perform the test and where to obtain it.*
6. Friendly, D. S. Preschool visual acuity screening test. *Trans. Am. Ophthalmol. Soc.* 76:383, 1978. *Review of preschool vision screening tests.*

Selected Reading

Nelson, L. B., Brown, G. C., and Arentsen, J. J. *Recognizing Patterns of Ocular Childhood Diseases.* Thorofare, NJ: Slack, 1985 *An excellent, succinct atlas-format coverage of the majority of childhood eye abnormalities and diseases.*

43 Childhood Hearing Loss

Richard Chole

I. The problem. While as many as 10% of children below the age of 5 are affected by significant hearing loss, its recognition and treatment are often delayed until the child reaches school age and undergoes hearing testing [1]. Childhood hearing loss may vary from a minor conductive hearing loss to profound or complete loss of auditory perception. Since the development of speech and language is based on auditory perception, a delay in the diagnosis and treatment of hearing loss in children may result in speech and language difficulties that could persist into later life. The early recognition and prompt treatment of childhood hearing loss may lead to a more normalized acquisition of speech and language skills [2]. Children with hearing loss can be divided into two major groups: (1) mild to moderate hearing loss, usually due to middle ear disease; and (2) severe to profound hearing loss due to congenital or acquired abnormalities of neurosensory pathways.

A. Description

1. **Moderate hearing loss (conductive).** Hearing loss in children in the first group is usually due to persistent otitis media with effusion (OME). These children have a 10–40-dB hearing loss, and an average of about 27-dB loss in the speech frequencies [3]. An astute parent or teacher may notice periods of inattention. Children in the 1- to 5-year-old age group with persistent OME tend to have delayed speech development. Although many children will develop persistent OME after a bout of acute otitis media, its diagnosis in these children is often delayed until they are near school age when prekindergarten audiometry shows a moderate hearing loss. If such a hearing loss is undetected during the first years of life, when speech acquisition is occurring, the child may have delayed speech and poor language skills that could persist through adult life.
2. **Severe hearing loss (neurosensory).** Severe to profound hearing loss in infants may be due to congenital abnormalities of the inner ear, perinatal toxic substance exposure, or perinatal infections of the central nervous system (CNS) [4].

B. Epidemiology

1. It is estimated that 30–50% of children between the ages of 1 and 5 have middle ear effusions; however, only 1–3% develop middle ear effusions that persist for months to years. While it is true that many children with persistent OME also have bouts of acute otitis media, most children with persistent OME have no symptoms. Some children with persistent OME may exhibit delayed speech acquisition, while others may exhibit inattentiveness and delayed learning. Although middle ear disorders other than persistent OME do occur in children, they are relatively uncommon. Children at **high risk** for OME include children with cleft palate and Down's syndrome, American Indians and Eskimos, and children intubated during the neonatal period.
2. **Severe hearing loss (sensorineural).** Severe to profound congenital hearing loss of the neurosensory type occurs in 1 in every 7000 live births. In many cases the definite cause of the hearing loss cannot be determined.

   The majority of children with congenital sensorineural hearing loss have suffered *in utero* viral infections. The toxoplasmosis, rubella, cytomegalovirus, and herpes simplex virus (TORCH) syndrome includes the most frequent causes of congenital hearing loss: rubella and cytomegalovirus. Other causes of severe sensorineural hearing loss in children include bacterial and viral meningitis and a great number of hereditary defects. Hereditary hearing loss may be associated with retinitis pigmentosa (Refsum's disease), cardiac arrhythmias (Jervell-Lang-Nielsen syndrome), goiter (Pendred's syndrome), and over two hundred other syndromes. Neonatal hyperbilirubinemia and aminoglycosides have also been associated with sensorineural hearing loss.

Several **risk factors** have been identified; these have been used to compile a high-risk registry for sensorineural deafness [5]. These risk factors include the following:

- **a.** Family history of childhood hearing loss.
- **b.** History of congenital infection.
- **c.** Malformation of the head and neck (dysmorphic syndromes and nonsyndromal abnormalities, overt or submucous cleft palate, morphologic abnormalities of the pinna).
- **d.** Low birth weight (< 1500 gm).
- **e.** Hyperbilirubinemia at a level exceeding indications for exchange transfusion.
- **f.** CNS infection.
- **g.** Severe asphyxia, with the infant having an Apgar score of 0–3 and failing to have spontaneous respiration by 10 minutes or hypotonia beyond 2 hours.

II. Secondary prevention

A. Early detection

1. Methods

a. Otoscopy

(1) Description. Careful otoscopic examination with pneumatic otoscopy should be performed at each periodic health examination. It will reveal most of the abnormalities causing **conductive** hearing loss in children.

(2) Performance. The diagnosis of middle ear effusion can usually be made with the closed head, pneumatic otoscope. The speculum of the otoscope is placed into the ear canal, to a point where an airtight seal is created. The bulb attached to the pneumatic otoscope is first compressed slowly, then released rapidly while the observer visualizes the light reflection.

(3) Interpretation. A tympanic membrane in a child with a middle ear effusion may appear quite normal on otoscopic examination [6]. There is usually little discoloration of the tympanic membrane, and the light reflection is usually in its normal position. In some cases, the tympanic membrane may appear retracted and somewhat darker in color. As a middle ear effusion persists over months to years, the fluid in the middle ear tends to thicken and become mucoid. Mucoid fluid behind a tympanic membrane usually has a darker appearance, sometimes to the point at which it appears a dark blue (erroneously called idiopathic hemotympanum). A normal tympanic membrane with an air-containing middle ear will have excellent mobility, while a middle ear filled with fluid is less compressible and the tympanic membrane is less mobile.

b. Tympanometry

(1) Description. Tympanometry is the single most valuable diagnostic tool in assessing middle ear effusion.

(2) Performance. Tympanometry is a simple procedure that can be performed by a nonphysician in a few minutes. A sealed probe is placed into the ear canal. The end of the probe has three openings: a continuous tone (usually 400 Hz) is placed into one opening; through the second opening, a positive and negative pressure can be exerted in the ear canal, and consequently on the tympanic membrane; reflected sound can then be measured through the third opening. The absorption of sound by the tympanic membrane and middle ear can thereby be measured. The compliance of the tympanic membrane is maximal when the pressure in the external canal equals pressure in the middle ear.

(3) Interpretation. By varying the pressure in the external auditory canal from −200 to 200 cm of water, a graphic representation of the compliance of the tympanic membrane and middle ear with respect to changing pressures can be obtained (Fig. 43-1). The type A tympanogram is seen in normal ears. A Type B tympanogram, in which the tympanic membrane changes little in compliance with changing ear canal pressure, has a high correlation with OME. In the Type C tympanogram, one finds negative middle ear pressure, consistent with eustachian tube dysfunction with or without OME. False-positives (estimated at 5%) may occur due to difficult or improper probe placement. False-negatives are not a problem.

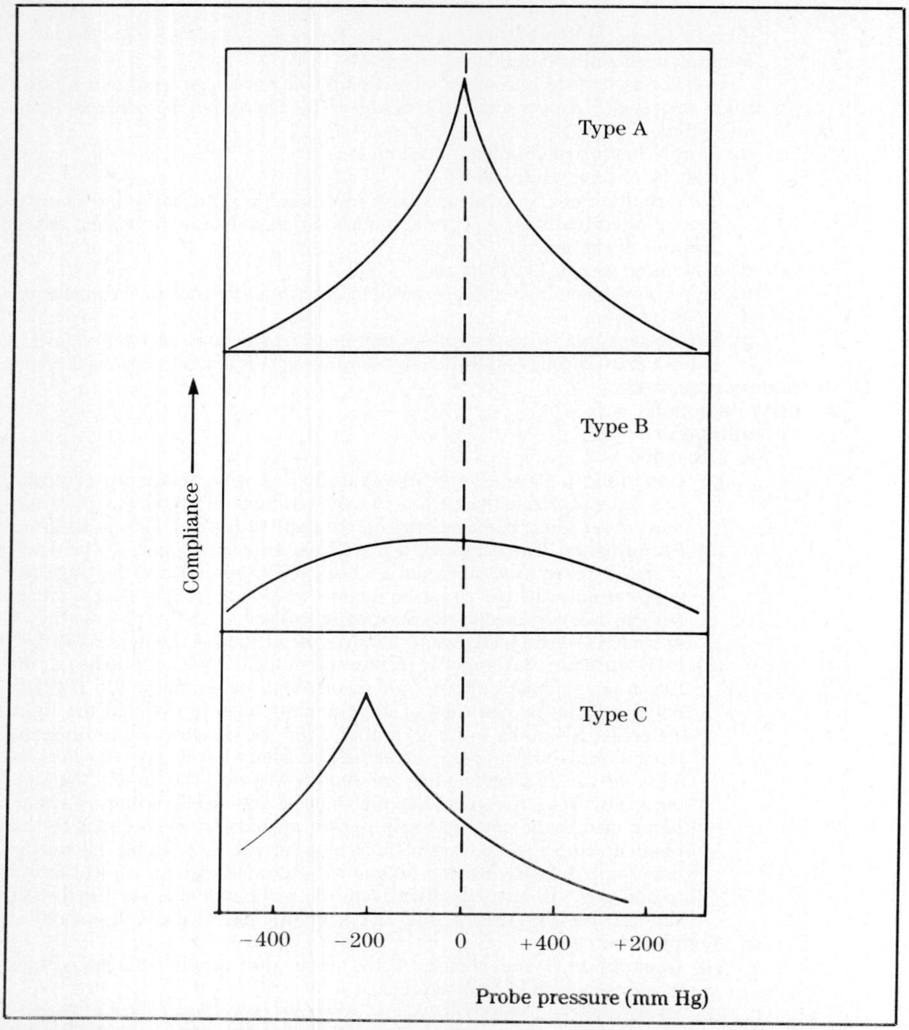

Fig. 43-1. Tympanogram types representative of tympanograms seen in children. Type A is the normal configuration. Type B shows a relatively flat response, which has a high correlation with middle ear effusion. Type C illustrates a negative pressure of approximately 200 mm Hg, which is seen in individuals with eustachian tube dysfunction.

c. Auditory brainstem responses

(1) Description. Another means of detecting hearing loss at birth or in the infant is the use of auditory brainstem responses (ABR).

(2) Performance. A microphone is placed over one ear of the newborn to be tested and clicks are administered at a rate of 11/second. Evoked responses are obtained from scalp electrodes and averaged in an averaging computer. This method, however, takes 30–45 minutes of skilled technician time.

(3) Interpretation. The ABR thresholds are determined by the audiologist performing the test. They are usually 5–15 dB higher than behavioral thresholds.

d. Behavioral hearing testing

(1) Description. Behavioral hearing testing includes several types of hearing assessment, each appropriate at different ages: startle responses,

Table 43-1. Hearing test characteristics

Tests	Sensitivity	Specificity	Predictive value*	Cost	Appropriate age
Neurosensory					
Auditory brainstem responses (ABR)	High	Good*	Excellent	$50	Any age
Audiometry	High	High	Excellent	$30	2 and over
Conductive					
Pneumatoscopy	Good	Good	Good		Any age
Tympanometry	High	High	Excellent	$5–$15	Any age
Audiometry	Good	High	Good	$30	2 and over

*Cannot differentiate between conductive and neurosensory losses.

sound field audiometry, play audiometry, behavior audiometry, pure-tone audiometry, and speech reception thresholds.

(2) **Performance.** In children under 6 months of age, one may be able to detect **startle responses.** Between 6 and 18 months, **sound field audiometry** and **play audiometry** can be performed. The 1-year-old child will usually be able to localize sound and turn toward that sound. As language skills begin after the age of 18 months, more sophisticated **behavior audiometry** can be used, including the type that detects speech sounds. For example, the child can be asked to identify or point to body parts. **Pure-tone audiometry** and **speech reception thresholds** can be obtained in many children after the age of 30 months. Office screening with pure-tone audiometry is performed at 250, 500, 1000, and 2000 Hz.

(3) **Interpretation.** Audiometric evaluation usually reveals a 10–40-dB conductive hearing loss in the ear affected with OME. Thin serous fluid in the middle ear, especially with the presence of air bubbles, leads to a small conductive hearing loss; very thick mucoid fluid, on the other hand, further impedes the mobility of the tympanic membrane and leads to a larger hearing loss. Recent studies, however, have shown that volume is a more important determinant of conductive hearing loss than viscosity. Tympanometry and pure-tone audiometry should be a part of routine health maintenance in preschool children. If hearing loss of more than 20 dB is detected, the patient should be referred for complete audiometry.

2. Justification

a. Test characteristics (Table 43-1). Under ideal conditions, the diagnosis of severe hearing loss in a newborn can be made shortly after birth. Some astute parents may make the diagnosis shortly after birth and commonly do so before the child's physician does. Unfortunately, though, many children with severe neurosensory hearing loss are not identified until delayed speech development occurs. Because of (1) lack of physician and parent awareness of the methods of diagnosing neonatal hearing loss, (2) denial, or (3) inattention, diagnosis of this disorder is often delayed until the child is over 2 years of age. Early detection of neurosensory hearing loss is important, since the early use of hearing aids leads to better language and speech development.

b. Risks and side effects

(1) **Tympanometry.** False-positives and false-negatives frequently occur with tympanometry (about 10% each). Tympanometric results must be correlated with otoscopic findings [7].

(2) **ABR.** False-negatives occur rarely with ABR testing. Children with cortical dysfunction may be hearing-impaired but respond normally to ABR testing. False-positives are common (about 10%) in infants; positive ABR results must be documented with behavioral tests as the child grows.

(3) **Behavioral audiometry.** There is no risk of false-negatives in behavioral audiometry done by a skilled audiologist. False-positives are common in very young children, but repeat testing, as the children mature, yields reliable results.

c. **Costs** (see Table 43-1). Some automatic tympanometers can be purchased for as little as $2000. The cost of a pure-tone hearing test is $15–$30; the cost of tympanometry is $5–$15.

d. **Acceptability.** Otoscopy, tympanometry, brainstem audiometry (ABR), and behavioral audiometry, are atraumatic and well accepted by children.

B. Early intervention

1. Neurosensory hearing loss

a. **Methods.** If severe hearing loss is detected in the early months of life, **hearing aids** can be fitted to a child as young as 3 or 4 months of age.

b. **Justification**

(1) **Effectiveness.** The potential for acquisition of normal speech and language in such a child is enormously improved over the child with undetected hearing loss. Many children will be eager hearing aid wearers by the time they are 8 to 9 months old. Failure to recognize and treat severe hearing loss during the first year of life will lead to a measurable delay in speech and language development.

(2) **Risks and side effects** are negligible.

(3) **Costs.** Hearing aids cost approximately $400 plus regular battery replacement.

(4) **Acceptability.** A hearing aid is acceptable to parents and children with severe hearing loss, since both the child and parent recognize the benefits of amplification.

2. Conductive hearing loss—OME [8]

a. **Methods**

(1) **Antibiotics** may be prescribed: trimethoprim-sulfamethoxazole [9]—bid for 6–8 weeks, or erythromycin [10] 20–30 mg/kg bid.

(2) **Antibiotics plus steroids** are currently being evaluated, but results so far are inconsistent.

(3) **Myringotomy** with tympanostomy tubes [11]. After a 6- to 8-week trial of antibiotics, myringotomy is indicated. This should be done under general anesthesia in small children. Middle ear fluid should be aspirated and a tube inserted to maintain aeration.

(4) **Adenoidectomy** may decrease the incidence of persistent OME [12], but this is usually reserved for more severe cases.

b. **Justification.** The detection and treatment of childhood hearing loss is of great importance. Early detection of conductive hearing loss and its prompt treatment can allow children to acquire normal speech and language, whereas some of the children who continue to be hearing-impaired during crucial periods of speech and language development may have long-term learning disabilities. It has been shown that children whose hearing loss is first detected when they start school continue to have language development problems throughout adult life. These "slow learners" have a disability due to early childhood auditory deprivation [13].

(1) **Antibiotics.** Trimethoprim (TMP)-sulfamethoxazole (SMZ) for 6 weeks is one currently accepted regimen.

(a) **Effectiveness.** In children with OME, Marks and associates [9] found that after 6 weeks of TMP-SMZ, the effusions in 64% had cleared up, while in the placebo group the infection had cleared up in only 27%. Maynard [14] found a 47% reduction in OME with ampicillin, 125–250 mg given daily for 1 year. Combinations of decongestants and antihistamines have not been shown to be effective by themselves for OME. However, use in combination with antibiotics for acute otitis may enhance the effectiveness of antibiotics [15, 16].

(b) **Risks** include sensitivity to sulfas and rare idiosyncratic bone marrow depression.

(c) **Costs** of antibiotic treatment are $20–$40 for antibiotics and $20–$50 for follow-up visits.

(d) **Acceptability** is good.

(2) **Myringotomy with tympanostomy tubes**

(a) **Effectiveness.** Myringotomy with tube insertion completely reverses the conductive loss in 95% of cases.

(b) **Risks.** After myringotomy, 1–5% of children have intermittent or persistent otorrhea. The incidence of perforation or cholesteatoma is unknown, since the disease process itself may result in these complications. The risk of life-threatening complications from general anesthesia in healthy children is 1 in 40,000 children.

(c) **Costs.** Myringotomy costs approximately $500–$1000.

(d) **Acceptability** is good. Children with myringostomy tubes may have bouts of otitis with otorrhea. Parents and children may find it difficult to avoid contamination of the middle ear by water during bathing or swimming.

(3) **Adenoidectomy**

(a) **Effectiveness.** Maw [12] showed that adenoidectomy significantly decreased the incidence of OME when compared to a control (no surgery) group. Adenotonsillectomy offered no improvement over adenoidectomy alone.

(b) **Risks.** Adenoidectomy requires a general anesthetic. Risk of significant postoperative bleeding is 1%. Velopharyngeal incompetence, either temporary or permanent, may occur.

(c) **Costs.** Adenoidectomy costs $500–$1000.

III. Recommendations

A. Early detection

1. Neurosensory hearing loss

a. All newborn infants should be assessed for **high-risk registry** categories. These include:

(1) Family history of childhood hearing loss.
(2) Congenital infection.
(3) Head and neck malformations.
(4) Birth weight < 1500 gm.
(5) Hyperbilirubinemia.
(6) CNS infection.
(7) Severe asphyxia.

b. High-risk registry infants should be tested with **auditory brainstem responses** by 3 months of age.

c. **Acoustic testing (auditory brainstem responses) of all newborn infants is not universally recommended** because of the high incidence of false-positives and the cost of the test ($50–$75).

2. Conductive hearing loss.

a. **Pneumatic otoscopy** should be performed on all infants and children at each regularly scheduled periodic health examination.

b. Primary care providers should note whether **speech and language skills** are progressing normally, and whether the parents feel their child hears normally. If not, investigate the suspected hearing impairment.

c. **Tympanometry** is not justified as a routine screen for all preschool children. If a provider elects to include this test, however, testing at 6, 12, 24, and 36 months is reasonable. Children with persistent effusions and Type B tympanograms on two occasions, 2 weeks apart, should be treated (see sec. **III.B.2**).

d. **Pure-tone audiometry** should be performed on all children before entering elementary school. Individuals with over 15-dB loss in speech frequencies should be referred for formal audiologic evaluation.

B. Early intervention

1. Neurosensory hearing loss

a. Diagnostic services should be completed and management begun by 6 months of age.

b. The services should include the following.

(1) **Medical services.** Reevaluation, treatment, and genetic evaluation and counseling, if indicated.

(2) **Audiologic services.** Assessment, selection of hearing aid(s), family counseling.

(3) **Psychoeducational management.** Individualized educational plan, information about implications of hearing impairment.

2. Conductive hearing loss

a. Diagnosis should be sought in children who have just had a bout of acute otitis media and in children with speech and language delay.

b. The services should include the following.

(1) **Medical services.** Pneumatic otoscopy at intervals; tuning fork tests in older children.

(2) **Audiologic services.** Tympanometry and pure-tone and speech audiometry.

(3) **Medical and surgical management.**

References

1. Jaffe, B. F. (ed.). *Hearing Loss in Children: A Comprehensive Text.* Baltimore: University Park Press, 1977. *A compendium dealing with all aspects of childhood hearing loss.*
2. Paradise, J. L. Otitis media during early life: How hazardous to development? A critical review of the evidence. *Pediatrics* 68(6):869, 1981. *Discussion of the controversies surrounding early intervention for OME.*
3. Bluestone, C. D., et al. Workshop on effects of otitis media on the child. *Pediatrics* 71(4):639, 1983. *Excellent review of effects of otitis media.*
4. Konigsmark, B. W., and Gorlin, R. J. *Genetic and Metabolic Deafness.* Philadelphia: Saunders, 1976. *An authoritative compendium of known causes of genetic deafness that may occur in children.*
5. American Academy of Pediatrics, Joint Committee on Infant Hearing. Position statement, 1982. *Pediatrics* 70(3):496, 1982. *Official American Academy of Pediatrics statement.*
6. Chole, R. A. *A Color Atlas of Ear Disease.* Norwalk, CT: Appleton-Century-Crofts, 1982. *Demonstrates the appearance of most ear diseases as seen with the otoscope.*
7. Paradise, J. L. Editorial retrospective: Tympanometry (editorial). *N. Engl. J. Med.* 307(17):1074, 1982. *Good overview of controversy concerning benefits and weaknesses of tympanometry.*
8. Chole, R. A. Acute and Chronic Infection of the Temporal bone Including Otitis Media with Effusion. In C. W. Cummings (ed.), *Otolaryngology: Head and Neck Surgery.* St. Louis: Mosby, 1986. Vol. 4, pp. 2963–2988. *Comprehensive summary of OME and its complications.*
9. Marks, N. J., Mills, R. P., and Shaheen, O. H. A controlled trial of cotrimoxazole therapy in serous otitis media. *J. Laryngol. Otol.* 95(10):1003, 1981. *A study of the benefit of TMP-SMZ in OME.*
10. Ernston, S., and Sundberg, L. Erythromycin in the treatment of otitis media with effusion (OME). *J. Laryngol. Otol.* 98(8):767, 1984. *Evidence for the efficacy of long-term antibiotic treatment of OME.*
11. Meyerhoff, W. L. Use of tympanostomy tubes in otitis media. *Ann. Otol. Rhinol. Laryngol.* 90(6 Pt 1):537, 1981. *An overview of the theory and practice of tympanostomy tubes for OME.*
12. Maw, A. R. Chronic Otitis Media with Effusion and Adenotonsillectomy: A Prospective Randomized Controlled Study. In D. J. Lim, et al. (eds.), *Recent Advances in Otitis Media with Effusion.* Philadelphia: Decker, 1984. Pp. 299–302. *A study of the efficacy of tonsillectomy and adenoidectomy in OME.*
13. Klein, J. O., et al. Otitis Media with Effusion During the First Three Years of Life and Development of Speech and Language. In D. J. Lim, et al. (eds.), *Recent Advances in Otitis Media with Effusion.* Philadelphia: Decker, 1984. Pp. 332–334. *An overview of speech problems in young children with OME.*
14. Maynard, J. E., Fleshman, J. K., and Tschopp, C. F. Otitis media in Alaskan Eskimo children: Prospective evaluation of chemoprophylaxis. *J.A.M.A.* 219(5):597, 1972. *Early trial of antibiotic prophylaxis.*
15. Moran, D. M., et al. The use of an antihistamine-decongestant in conjunction with an anti-infective drug in the treatment of acute otitis media. *J. Pediatr.* 101(1):132, 1982. *Small trial showing significantly less persistent effusion after acute otitis media when an antihistamine-decongestant is added to antibiotic treatment.*
16. Cantekin, E. I., et al. Lack of efficacy of a decongestant-antihistamine combination for otitis media with effusion ("secretory" otitis media) in children. Results of a double-blind, randomized trial. *N. Engl. J. Med.* 308(6):297, 1983. *Large, well-designed trial showing the lack of efficacy of decongestants in otitis media with effusion.*

44 Communication Disorders in Childhood

Rebecca Leonard

I. The problem

A. Definitions

1. **Speech/language disorders** affect the perception, comprehension, or production of sounds, words, or sentences.
2. **Fluency disorders** affect the rhythm and flow of speech.
3. **Voice disorders** affect normal pitch, loudness, or quality of voice production.

B. Description

1. **Speech/language impairment.** The process of mastering speech/language skills may take from birth to the age of 7 or 8 years. The typical end result represents one of the most complex of human behaviors. Development of speech/language skills parallels cognitive development toward differentiation of function and differentiation of perceptions or ideas. Thus, "Mama" may initially be used by the child to represent several ideas, such as "Mama, I'm hungry," "Mama, I'm wet," or "Mama, I'm tired." Later, the child will learn to use more complex sentences to elaborate his or her thoughts. Speech sound development may proceed along similar lines, as when the child initially uses a "th" sound to stand for other fricative sounds—for example substituting "th" for "s"(thithter/sister); "th" for "f" (thire/fire); or "th" for "sh" (thoe/shoe). In time, the fricative class of speech sounds should be more completely differentiated.

   Significant delays or deviations in normal speech/language acquisition constitute impairment. Problems are usually manifested as difficulty in one (or more) of the following linguistic areas.

   a. **Semantics**: problems in comprehending meanings or understanding concepts, and difficulty in symbolizing, i.e., assigning an arbitrary verbal referent (word) to an object or idea.

   b. **Grammar:** problems in organizing the basic units of language (words) into appropriate syntactic structures such as phrases and sentences, and difficulty with the use of morphemes (smallest units of meaning, as "-ed" for past tense, or "-s" for plural).

   c. **Phonology:** problems in understanding or producing, or both, i.e., "articulating," the sound patterns of language. If the problem here is principally one of **articulation,** the sounds in error may reflect the cause. For example, hearing loss may be associated with errors in high frequency or low intensity sounds (f, th, s), while cleft palate may interfere with sounds requiring high oral airflows and pressures (p, t, k, s). An error of **deletion,** in which a sound is omitted, may be more serious than a **substitution,** in which one sound is used for another. A **distortion,** representing an approximation of the appropriate sound, probably interferes least with the speaker's intelligibility.

   d. **Pragmatics:** difficulty using language to communicate in social, interactive contexts.

2. **Fluency disorders.** Children with emerging speech/language skills are typically disfluent, often repeating words, phrases, or entire sentences during their conversational speech. The differentiation between "normal" disfluencies and stuttering is not always apparent. Similarly, there appears to be no uniform agreement on the etiology of childhood stuttering. Of children who are actually judged to be stutterers, perhaps 80% recover without treatment, half of these by puberty and the remaining 30% by high school [1–3].

   Three subtypes of fluency disorder have been described in children, including the following [2]:

a. **Developmental stuttering.** Children who may be called developmental stutterers experience brief periods of stuttering between the ages of 1 and 5. By 5 fluency has typically increased to normal.

b. **Benign stuttering.** Children exhibiting this type of disfluency experience a prolonged period of stuttering—for perhaps two years—sometime between the ages of 3 and 11, then spontaneously recover.

c. **Persistent stuttering.** Onset of stuttering is also during childhood for this group, but the frequency and severity of the disorder become worse with age, persisting into adulthood.

3. **Voice disorders.** Voice disorders may be seen in children who have experienced congenital laryngeal anomalies, e.g., laryngeal webs or papillomas. Voice quality may also be detrimentally influenced in children who have undergone frequent or prolonged periods of intubation. Other vocal fold lesions are the result of hyperfunctional voice. In children, this type of disorder is most frequently associated with vocal nodules [4].

C. **Epidemiology.** Recent estimates indicate that 5–6% of all noninstitutionalized, school-age children in the United States experience communication disorders serious enough to interfere with their education [5]. Additional evidence suggests that this figure may increase to 10% if only elementary or preschool-age children are considered. Rates of specific disorders are as follows [5]:

1. **Speech/language impairments** account for about 75–80% of all communication disorders in children.
2. **Fluency disorders,** or **stuttering,** which occur in about 1% of the adult population, may have a prevalence five times greater in young children. There is general agreement that stuttering occurs three to four times more often in males than in females, and that it tends to recur in families, though not necessarily in the immediate family.
3. **Voice disorders** occur in about 3% of school-age children.

Certain populations of children are **at risk** for communication impairment. All types of communication disorders appear to occur more frequently in boys than in girls. Various reports indicate that between 20–40% of children with repaired cleft palate may experience residual speech/language problems. Prevalence figures of 90% for children who are mentally retarded and 50–70% for children who have neurogenic disorders, have also been reported [5]. Children with hearing loss—even a mild, recurrent conductive loss, if experienced during critical language learning stages—may be vulnerable to communication impairment [6]. Similarly, children with serious psychological or emotional disability and children reared in extreme environmental deprivation, or perhaps in multilingual environments, may also be subject to a communication handicap. In other cases, communication disorders occur with no strong evidence to suggest specific etiologic or related factors.

II. Secondary prevention

A. Early detection

1. Language/speech disorders

a. Methods

(1) **Description.** A diagnosis of speech/language disorder is made when the child's verbal skills can be shown—by direct testing or observation, or both, and parent report—to be either deviant or, as is more often the case, significantly delayed. Some screening instruments, and a large number of more comprehensive diagnostic tests, are available for use with children.

(2) **Performance.** A summary of expressive language items taken from three screening instruments and one diagnostic test [7–10] are presented in Table 44-1. Staging of the items at 6-month intervals appears to account for slight variations among the tests in order and time of appearance of skills. In very young children, test information is obtained by observation and parent report. For older children more direct testing methods are desirable. In general, screening instruments can be easily and quickly administered with no specialized training, while diagnostic testing requires greater expenditures of time and training. (Refer to cited articles [7–10] for details of administration of each test.)

(3) **Interpretation.** Screening instruments identify children who may not be performing in an expected manner in terms of speech/language abilities, and who should be referred for further evaluation. Diagnostic tests

Table 44-1. Expressive language development screening instruments

	(80%)[a] Birth to Three Developmental Scale[b] (137 subjects)	(75%)[a] Sequenced Inventory of Communication Development[c] (252 subjects)	(75%)[a] Early Language Milestones[d] (191 subjects)	(75%)[a] Denver Developmental Screening Test[e] (>1000 subjects)
0–6 mo	Vocalizes Squeals Laughs	Vocalizes in response to imitation of his own voice "Talks" to people Laughs	Coos Reciprocal vocalization Laughs	Vocalizes with 2 identical vowels Vocalizes in response to adult imitation of him Laughs
6–12 mo	2 identifiable consonants Vowel combinations	Uses vowels Uses consonant-vowel combinations Uses consonants Intonational patterns	Monosyllabic babbling Polysyllabic babbling "Mama"/"dada" initially, nonspecific	"Mama"/"dada" initially, nonspecific Imitates speech sounds
12–18 mo	Vocabulary of 2–3 words Jargon Imitates adult vocal play	Sound combinations Sound-like words Imitates sounds Question inflection Sentence-like intonation pattern	First word beyond "mama"	3 words other than "mama" and "dada"
18–24 mo	Vocabulary of 20+ words 2 words plus combinations	2- to 3-word combinations Combines consonant sounds Imitates intonation Uses consistent sound combinations as words	Vocabulary up to 50 words 2-word combinations Tells 2 or more wants	Combines 2 words Names 1 picture
24–30 mo	Asks questions Recites portions of nursery rhymes, songs Names 5 pictures	Asks questions Names 3 pictures Uses verb phrases Uses pronouns as subjects Uses plurals Relates experiences	Uses "me," "you"	Uses plurals
30–36 mo	Carries on conversation	Uses adjectives Uses prepositional phrases	Uses prepositions Brief conversation Names, describes uses of 2 objects	Comprehends prepositions Gives first and last name

[a]The percentage of individuals who are able to demonstrate those language skills at the ages indicated.
[b]From T. Bangs and S. Dodson. *Birth to Three Developmental Scale.* Hingham, MA: Teaching Resources Corporation, 1979.
[c]From D. Hedrich, E. Prather, and A. Tobin. *Sequenced Inventory of Communication Development.* Seattle: University of Washington Press, 1975.
[d]From J. Coplan, et al. Validation of an early language milestone scale in a high risk population. *Pediatrics* 70(5):677, 1982.
[e]From W. Frankenburg, et al. *Denver Developmental Screening Test: Manual/Workbook for Nursing and Paramedical Personnel* (revised ed.). Denver: LADOCA Project and Publishing Foundation, 1975.

are designed to indicate the specific strengths and deficits of a child's speech/language repertoire.

(4) **Interval/timing.** Routine screening should be conducted at 6-month intervals between the ages of 1 and 3 years. This interval is recommended because it accounts for (1) changes expected in normal development and (2) standard deviations associated with many screening items.

(5) **Population.** Children known to be at risk for communication disorders should be of particular concern. A large percentage of speech/language disorders, however, occur in children not previously known to be at risk for communication handicaps. For this reason this aspect of development should not be overlooked in any child.

b. **Justification**

(1) **Test characteristics.** It is generally accepted that early detection of suspected speech/language disorders may minimize the degree of potential impairment. For example, language development in the profoundly hard-of-hearing child whose hearing loss is identified and treated early is likely to more closely approximate normal language development than the child whose hearing loss is not recognized until he or she is 3 or 4 years old. On the other hand, there are probably no test instruments currently available that allow an examiner to predict with 100% accuracy whether a young child with a suspected speech/language disorder will indeed be "disordered" by a given age, with or without intervention. One exception may be the child with severe speech/language impairment and associated cognitive or physical difficulties that are apparent at a very early age.

(2) **Risks or side effects or both.** A primary problem with testing in young children is failing to identify a child in jeopardy due to: (1) reliance on subjective testing methods, i.e., parent report and observation of only a small sample of behavior; and, (2) wide variability in time (not order) of appearance of individual skills.

It should also be remembered—particularly in view of the difficulties often associated with identifying a communication disorder in a very young child—that the purpose of testing is not to label the child as disordered, but simply to identify a need for further evaluation or intervention.

(3) **Costs.** Diagnostic evaluation costs vary widely according to geographic region and test site, and usually to amount of time required.

(4) **Acceptability.** For screening purposes, tests that have been standardized on large numbers of children and that require no special training to administer are recommended for non–speech/language professionals.

There is no standard test battery that speech/language pathologists use to assess language skills in children. Initial tests assess general language function, while subsequent measures evaluate specific abilities, such as articulation of speech sounds, auditory perceptual skills, pragmatics, or vocabulary. Depending on the individual child and problem, many eclectic combinations would be considered appropriate.

2. **Fluency disorders.** The differentiation between disfluencies that will be outgrown and those that will persist into adulthood is not clear; however, prognosis is influenced by the following [1–3]:

a. **Frequency of disfluencies.** Disfluency on 7% of syllables occurring in connected speech is excessive; less than 3% is within normal limits.

b. **Type of disfluencies.** Part-word or sound repetitions, and sound prolongations, are viewed more seriously than repetitions of words, phrases, or sentences.

c. **Tension or struggle.** Prognosis is less favorable when speech is produced with tension or struggle than when even disfluencies are produced in an easy, effortless manner.

Concern by a parent or professional is sufficient cause for referral to a speech/language pathologist. This professional will observe the child's speech in a variety of situations and will analyze both number and type of disfluencies occurring in each situation.

Environmental or other factors that appear to precipitate disfluency will be noted. A complete speech/language evaluation may also be done to examine a possible relationship between emerging language skills and disfluencies. Given the prevailing view that disfluency may be exacerbated (if not caused) by an individual's response to his or her own lack of fluency, or to other people's reactions to his or her disfluency, early referral deserves serious consideration.

3. **Voice disorders.** Symptoms of congenital or acquired voice disorders may include persistent hoarseness or other quality aberrations, or unusual pitch or loudness. If a disorder is suspected, referrals to an otolaryngologist and speech/language pathologist may be indicated. Evaluation by the speech/language pathologist will involve a complete description of physical and perceptual characteristics of the child's voice, as well as specific vocal behaviors that may have precipitated the disorder.

B. Early intervention

1. Speech/language disorders

a. Methods

(1) Description. Intervention, which is tailored to a child's specific needs, may range from a few sessions of parent counseling, to intensive therapy. In young children, general stimulation and facilitation of speech/language development is often a primary objective. In older children, treatment may focus on specific deficits—for example, discrimination of speech sounds, elaboration of vocabulary, or establishing appropriate motor patterns of sound or word production.

b. Justification

(1) Effectiveness. Clinical experience suggests that subjective judgments about prognosis in a young child with a possible speech/language disorder are favorably influenced by the following circumstances or observations.

(a) Other developmental skills are within normal limits. This is particularly true of motor skills, which appear to be highly correlated with language development [6].

(b) A discrepancy exists between receptive and expressive language abilities. Emerging language skills typically lag behind receptive language skills by about 6 months. When the discrepancy is larger than this—e.g., when receptive skills appear normal for age but expressive skills are delayed beyond 6 months—the prognosis is more favorable than when both receptive and expressive skills are delayed.

(c) Social skills appear generally adequate, i.e., the child demonstrates an interest in his or her environment and in interacting or communicating with others in his environment.

(d) Social environment is appropriate.

(e) Vocabulary skills are not severely depressed, i.e., the child knows the names of many things, even though the words may be unintelligible or not used generatively as parts of phrases or sentences. Behavior of this type is viewed more optimistically than evidence that the child does not know, or does not remember, the names of things.

(f) The child is very vocal, even if vocalizations are unintelligible, as opposed to the child who is extremely quiet (at home, in the test situation, and so on).

(g) Intonation of vocal output is appropriate, i.e., utterances sound like questions, or statements, or exclamations, even though content may not be intelligible, as opposed to vocalizations that are lacking in affect or are very stereotyped.

(h) A child is able in general, though not always, to directly imitate at least some features of an adult's communication (particularly sounds or words, intonation, or phrasing).

Growing evidence in the speech/language literature [1, 3] supports treatment effectiveness. Perhaps the best studies have utilized rigorous single-subject designs that have carefully separated treatment effects from normal growth and development. On the other hand, the effects of early versus later treatment, or different responses to different treatments, have not often been investigated. In part, this is related to difficulties in controlling for subject variability in large group comparisons.

Ethical considerations have also precluded some studies that would critically examine prediction factors and effectiveness of treatment by age. A common view in communication disorders is that there are certain maturational periods of the nervous system when the development of verbal skills is most facilitated. These periods may differ to some extent among children; however, once the so-called prime time is missed, the child's ability to fully achieve his or her linguistic potential—whatever this may be—is diminished. This is why a great deal of emphasis is placed on early identification of, and early intervention in, the child with a speech/language disorder.

(2) **Risks and side effects.** Other than intervention for a problem that might spontaneously resolve, there would seem to be minimal risks associated with early intervention for speech/language disorders. Possible risks of later intervention include the following: (1) inappropriate behavior patterns are more long-standing and more resistant to change; (2) prime times for speech/language acquisition may have passed; and (3) a school-age child may miss academic experiences to attend therapy, since the primary service delivery program for this age group, at least in the United States, is the public schools. In addition, there may be some stigma associated with leaving the classroom to attend treatment sessions.

(3) **Acceptability.** Behavioral and physiological treatments may draw heavily from various learning theories and psychosocial theoretic perspectives, as well as from linguistics and speech sciences. There is no standardized approach used by all clinicians in the treatment of speech/language disorders.

2. **Fluency disorders.** It is not clear that early intervention can prevent adult stuttering. In fact, as noted, there is some concern that calling a young child's attention to disfluencies may be detrimental. On the other hand, there is broad clinical evidence that parent counseling can be useful in educating parents about typical or expected disfluency, and ways of promoting more fluent verbalization in a child [1–3]. These efforts may alleviate anxiety in both parent and child and perhaps minimize a more serious problem.

   Increasing research evidence supports the value of therapy in individual children who stutter [3]. Strategies of direct intervention in older children often involve establishing fluency—perhaps by rate control or delayed auditory feedback—supplemented with behavior modification techniques for shaping and reinforcing fluency, or decreasing disfluencies. Anxiety reduction through counseling may also be an integral feature of therapy.

3. **Voice disorders.** Treatment of hyperfunctional voice disorders in children typically involves (1) identifying and eliminating abusive vocal behaviors, and (2) identifying and maintaining voice use patterns that reflect the greatest efficiency and economy. Although there is a lack of solid objective evidence regarding treatment success in this area, clinical evidence indicates that even moderate cooperation in achieving treatment objectives may be sufficient, in children, to reduce lesion size and improve voice. Since vocal nodules in children often regress with growth of the larynx (at puberty) and since, possibly, vocal behaviors improve with age, such partial effectiveness may be sufficient. Early reeducation in voice use may also be important in prevention of a later recurrence.

III. Recommendations

A. Early detection. The identification and elaboration of a speech/language disorder in a young child with newly emerging skills may not be an easy task. The primary care provider should do the following:

1. Identify children **at risk** for this type of disorder and anticipate and provide for their special needs. Those at risk include children with:
   a. Cleft palate.
   b. Mental retardation.
   c. Hearing loss.
   d. Psychological disability.
   e. Environmental deprivation.
   f. Sensorimotor impairment.
2. Monitor the speech/language development of all children between the ages of 1 and 3 years via observation, parent report, and screening testing. The screening would use an instrument standardized on a large number of children and requiring no specialized training, as the Birth to Three Developmental [7] or Early Language Milestone [9] scales.
3. In general, when there is doubt about either the normalcy or adequacy of a child's speech/language capabilities, a thorough diagnostic evaluation is indicated.

   If fluency is in question, an immediate referral to a speech/language pathologist is recommended. If a voice disorder is suspected, referrals to an otolaryngologist and speech/language pathologist would be appropriate.

B. Early intervention. Communication disorders in children are particularly serious because they can adversely affect so many other aspects of a child's intellectual and social development [6]. Thus, early intervention for children in jeopardy is strongly recommended. The primary care provider is urged to:

1. Assist in resolving any medical problems that may be contributing to a patient's communication disorder.
2. Assist in seeking immediate and appropriate treatment by a speech/language pathologist when a communication disorder has been identified or is suspected. It is particularly important to remember that this professional can become effectively involved in treating patients as young as 1 year old or younger.
3. Assist in educating both parents and professionals regarding the need for early detection and intervention in children with communication disorders.

References

1. Perkins, W. H. *Speech Pathology: An Applied Behavioral Science* (2nd ed.). St. Louis: Mosby, 1977. *Excellent introductory text on normal and disordered communication.*
2. Cooper, E. B. Etiology and treatment of stuttering. *Ear Nose Throat J.* 59(2):60, 1980. *Brief review of etiologies of stuttering.*
3. Guitar, B. Stuttering. In J. K. Darby, Jr. (ed.), *Speech Evaluation in Medicine.* New York: Grune & Stratton, 1981. Pp. 295–307. *Concise summary of developmental stuttering.*
4. Wilson, K. *Voice Problems of Children.* Baltimore: Williams & Wilkins, 1972. *Types and features of voice disorders in children.*
5. Leske, M. C. Prevalence estimates of communicative disorders in the U.S. Speech disorders. *A.S.H.A.* 23(3):217, 1981. *Extensive review of prevalence statistics for communication disorders.*
6. Paradise, J. L. Otitis media during early life: How hazardous to development. A critical review of the evidence. *Pediatrics* 68(6):869, 1981. *Review of controversy over chronic conductive hearing loss as a cause of communication disorders.*
7. Bangs, T., and Dodson, S. *Birth to Three Developmental Scale.* Hingham, MA: Teaching Resources Corporation, 1979. *Screening instrument.*
8. Hedrich, D., Prather, E., and Tobin, A. *Sequenced Inventory of Communication Development.* Seattle: University of Washington Press, 1975. *Diagnostic test used by speech/language professionals.*
9. Coplan, J., et al. Validation of an early language milestone scale in a high risk population. *Pediatrics* 70(5):677, 1982. *Screening instrument.*
10. Frankenburg, W., et al. *Denver Developmental Screening Test: Manual/Workbook for Nursing and Paramedical Personnel* (revised edition). Denver: LADOCA Project and Publishing Foundation, 1975. *Screening instrument for general developmental skills.*

45 Dental Caries

Stephen M. Blain
and Philip A. Trask

I. The problem

A. Description. The annual expenditure for dental care is over $4.8 billion per year [1]. Most of this cost is due to the ravages of dental caries. Caries cause pain and infection, with possible bacteremia, and loss of masticatory ability; are esthetically unappealing; and require restorative treatment. Orthodontic problems often arise from caries as a result of space loss between teeth; caries can require immediate and long-term orthodontics.

1. **Etiology.** Dental caries are felt to be caused by acid decalcification of the tooth enamel by streptococci, lactobacilli, and gram-positive filamentous rods. These cariogenic microbes metabolize monosaccharides and disaccharides and secrete into the plaque a strong acid that dissolves the enamel, thus initiating the caries process.

   Dental plaque provides the ideal environment for caries formation. Certain plaque bacteria, especially *Streptococcus mutans*, possess a mechanism for adhesion by which they initially colonize smooth surfaces; this is done through the production of water-insoluable glucans from sucrose. These glucans increase plaque tenacity and limit acid diffusion away from the tooth. Other organisms can later cohere to enlarge the plaque and contribute to the production of nutrient storage polysaccharides. Once cavitation has occurred, microoganisms not possessing adhesion properties (e.g., lactobacilli) may be a factor in the progressive destruction of the tooth.

   Irregular tooth morphology and enamel defects can facilitate the caries process, as can crowded or irregular teeth that make cleaning difficult. Lastly, although hereditary factors are often blamed for excessive caries, environmental factors, especially poor diet and lack of proper oral hygiene habits, are the major contributing factors to dental caries.

2. **Classification.** Carious lesions may be clinically diagnosed by an opaque whitening of the enamel (decalcification) or a brown discoloration of the enamel surface, or both. The basic types of lesions include the following:
   a. **Occlusal** lesions occur in the pits and grooves of the biting surface of the tooth. This area has a high propensity to decay because it is not self-cleansing.
   b. **Smooth surface** lesions occur on the vertical sides of the teeth adjacent to the tongue or cheek and usually near the gum line.
   c. **Interproximal** lesions develop between the teeth and are most often diagnosed by radiographs.
   d. **Rampant caries** occur suddenly in teeth that were for many years relatively immune to decay. Rampant caries usually involve the interproximal surfaces of the lower anterior teeth and have a predilection for early teenagers.
   e. **Nursing bottle caries** involve the deciduous maxillary anterior teeth and first primary molars and are usually a result of prolonged bottle feeding, during which time the child is put to bed with a bottle of milk or juice. Excessively prolonged breast-feeding can also cause nursing caries [2, 3]. The length of time carbohydrates are applied to the teeth, not the quantity, is directly related to the caries activity. During sucking, the lip and tongue protect the lower incisors and the substrate pools around the upper incisors. Thus caries of the maxillary and not the mandicular incisors are pathognomonic for nursing caries in infants and small children.

3. **Epidemiology.** Surveys conducted between 1961 and 1980 in the United States indicate a substantial decrease in caries prevalence and an increase in the number of caries-free children 5–7 years of age [4]. Current estimates of the num-

ber of carious teeth have ranged from 0.60 for the average 2-year-old to 4.75 for the average 12-year-old. Levels of treatment have ranged from 3–39% for the same age group [5].

Studies from the American midwest in the 1930s showed that caries are negatively correlated with fluoride concentration in the drinking water, while mottling of tooth enamel (fluorosis) is positively correlated with fluoride concentration [6]. The fluoride concentration at which caries protection is greatest and fluorosis is avoided is approximately 1 part per million (1ppm).

a. Risk of caries varies among different groups and in different geographic regions. Children in the middle socioeconomic group have significantly fewer caries than their poorer urban and rural counterparts. Rural children and blacks have significantly greater caries experience and significantly less treatment than urban children and whites, respectively. Caries prevalence tends to be higher in females than males. The general pattern of caries increments shows tapering off after adolescence; the peak incidence of carious lesions for any tooth or surface tends to occur within the first few years after eruption of the tooth [7]. Newly erupted enamel is more susceptible to caries. The longer the enamel is exposed to various salivary and dietary ions, the more mature or dense the surface enamel becomes, making it less soluble and more resistant to acid/caries processes.

II. Primary prevention

A. Methods

1. Fluoride

a. Drinking water fluoridation. When fluoride is available systemically during tooth calcification, it will be incorporated into the enamel matrix. Infants and children should receive oral fluoride in recommended amounts from birth through 12 years of age [8]. The fluoride may be present in the water supply in adequate amounts, in which case the child needs no supplemental fluoride.

It is important to assess the fluoride content in the drinking water of individual families because in many communities the fluoride content is not homogeneous. The city water department can usually provide the amount of flouride naturally present in the water, so supplements of the correct dose can be prescribed to bring the total fluoride intake to the optimal level.

In some areas, (e.g., those in which families use local well water,) it may be necessary to test the patient's drinking water for fluoride content.

b. Supplemental fluoride

(1) Systemic. If the amount of fluoride in the family's water is not sufficient, fluoride drops or chewable tablets should be prescribed. Fluoride supplementation is not currently recommended for breast-fed infants of mothers living in fluoridated areas, although fluoride supplementation is recommended for formula-fed infants, depending on the fluoride content of the local water supply [9]. The manufacturers of infant formula now make their products with defluoridated water so that the included fluoride is less than 0.3 ppm. This simplifies the calculation of the infant's total intake of fluoride [8].

Possible prescriptions for fluoride based on Table 45-1 should also take into account other sources of fluoride, e.g., vitamins, self-applications, and topical treatment by dentists [10]. When children are given supplemental fluoride, it is important to reassess the dose and need—taking into account age and water supply—and to reinforce its continued use when indicated.

The benefits of systemic fluoride supplements—liquid or chewable tablets—can be greatly enhanced if they are taken before evening bedtime after brushing the teeth. Clean teeth allow for closer contact between enamel and fluoride. In addition, during sleep oral clearance is vastly diminished, thus allowing the maximum topical enamel uptake of the fluoride in the oral environment.

It is better not to prescribe fluoridated vitamins because the benefits mentioned just above would be lost and parents may not be consistent in administering the vitamins. However, if vitamins are the vehicle for the fluoride supplement, they should be taken with meals, due to fat- and water-soluble characteristics of vitamins.

(2) Topical fluoride. Topical fluoride uptake by the enamel occurs each time

Table 45-1. Recommended dosage levels in supplemental fluoride

	Drinking water fluoride concentration (ppm)		
Age (yr)	0.0–0.3 (mg/day)	0.3–0.7 (mg/day)	0.7+ (mg/day)
0–2	0.25	0.0	0.0
2–3	0.50	0.25	0.0
3–13	1.00	0.50	0.0

the surface enamel is exposed to fluoride, i.e., by means of fluoridated drinking water, fluoridated toothpaste, chewable fluoride tablets, or fluoride drops. Controlled topical fluoride treatments by the dentist provide for even greater enamel absorption of fluoride. Topical fluoride applications can also facilitate the remineralization of an initial demineralized carious lesion.

Fluoride treatments administered in the dental office are recommended every 6 months, beginning when the child is mature enough to cooperate, and continuing throughout adolescence.

2. **Anticipatory guidance.** The prevention of dental caries should begin by counseling the parents of newborns. Information should be included regarding normal dental development. Emphasis should be placed on the fact that caries are related more to the duration and frequency of carbohydrates available to dental plaque than to the total amount of carbohydrates ingested. For example, nibbling on a few candies for a few hours is much more cariogenic than eating all of the candy at one time. A small amount of juice or milk in a nursing bottle suckled slowly during the day or while sleeping provides a continuous "sugar-bath." If this occurs every day, nursing caries will result. Parents should also be cautioned about giving their children dried fruits, especially raisins, and honey. These foods are considered natural but are extremely cariogenic.

With the eruption of the deciduous teeth, the parents should be cautioned about nursing bottle caries and the need for a balanced diet (to include the four basic food groups) and a low sucrose intake. In instances when it is difficult to stop the bottle habit, a bottle with pure water or one that is empty can be used. Sweets and desserts should be consumed during mealtime when the self-cleansing action and saliva content are optimal. This is the time to implement oral hygiene procedures—using a soft, toddler toothbrush and very small amount or no fluoridated toothpaste—at a regularly scheduled time and with the assistance of the parent(s).

Toothpaste is not necessary for infants. Many do not like the taste and the foaming action may prevent good visualization of the teeth. In addition, the ingestion of fluoride-containing toothpaste should be minimal, if given at all. The mechanical disruption of the plaque by brushing is most important. Flossing should commence whenever the space between teeth closes. Thorough brushing and flossing once per day (prior to bed is ideal) is adequate. Due to decreased salivation and oral movements during sleep, any retained carbohydrates will remain for prolonged periods of time, increasing potential caries activity.

At approximately 2–3 years of age, the child can be referred to a dentist. Follow-through on referrals is often incomplete, however, so it behooves the primary medical care provider to continue to encourage routine preventive dental care.

As the child matures, oral hygiene as well as proper nutrition should be reinforced. By 8 years of age, the child should have the manual dexterity and coordination to perform the oral hygiene procedures by himself or herself. Until then, a parent or older sibling must assume total responsibility for the oral hygiene. For children under 8, brushing helps initiate responsibility for their own oral health.

B. Justification

1. Fluoride

a. **Effectiveness.** The decline in dental caries is mainly attributed to an increase in the use of fluoride in the various forms described. Fluoridated enamel is much more resistant to the acid-solubility of the caries process. Also, fluoride, when in contact with the plaque, tends to be bactericidal to the microbes in the plaque, thus reducing their virulence.

(1) **Drinking water fluoridation.** Studies by Dean [6] in the 1930s showed that people in communities with drinking water naturally fluoridated to a level of 1 ppm had maximal protection from caries and very little fluorosis. Subsequent studies have confirmed the efficacy of fluoridation at 0.7–1.2 ppm, depending on ambient temperatures and humidity. The reduction in caries from optimal drinking water fluoridation is about 30–60% [11, 12].

(2) **Supplemental fluoride**

(a) **Systemic fluoride.** Dietary fluoride supplementation in drop, tablet, or lozenge form for children in communities with unfluoridated or suboptimally fluoridated water has been shown to reduce dental caries by about 55% [12].

(b) **Topical fluoride.** Topical fluoride applied by dentists reduces caries about 15%, and use of fluoridated toothpaste will reduce caries 3–5% [13].

b. **Risks.** Present data suggests that the current fluoride dosages would not be sufficient to cause fluorosis [8]. In contrast, 10 years ago, fluoride-containing vitamin preparations were not available with today's smaller fluoride concentrations. In addition, the small amounts of naturally occurring fluoride in water and foods were not considered in the dosage scheme. At that time a small amount of cosmetically acceptable fluorosis (white specks on an ivory background) was reported, and the suggested dosage was then revised downward [14].

There is some concern that children 2–4 years of age who are using fluoride-containing dentifrices or mouth rinses may swallow them instead of expectorate them. Ingestion could lead to excess fluoride intake, resulting in mild fluorosis [15]. However, despite the increased use of fluoride toothpastes and rinses, there appear to be no significant changes in the prevalence of dental fluorosis in the past 40 years [16].

The Safely Tolerated Dose (STD) and Certainly Lethal Dose (CLD) for fluoride have been conservatively set at 8 and 32 mg/kg, respectively [17]. Fluoride and fluoridation have been studied extensively and shown to be very safe. An excellent single source reference is the text by Newbrun [18].

c. **Costs.** Fluoridation of community water is the most effective, safe, convenient, and economical method of preventing caries [14]. Water fluoridation provides constant topical as well as systemic benefits. Each dollar spent on fluoridation saves $50 on dental treatment.

d. **Acceptability.** Most major cities in the United States have fluoridated water. Fluoride has been accepted by parents and dentists as the single most potent aid in preventing caries. Virtually all professional organizations involved with medical, dental, public, and child health or preventive medicine have endorsed fluoridation. In spite of these endorsements and the large volume of studies and literature that support the use of fluoride, small vocal groups of antifluoridationists have mounted campaigns against artificial fluoridation, using political intimidation and presentations of distorted and emotion-laden information [19].

III. Secondary prevention

A. Early detection

1. Methods

a. **Description.** The intraoral exam by the primary care provider should include the following:

(1) **History, oral hygiene, and diet assessment:** evaluation of the parents' oral hygiene practices with their child, nursing and feeding routines, complaints of oral-dental symptoms, accidents, and oral habits.

(2) **Caries assessment:** identification of opaque, whitish, chalky, or brown lesions; mobile teeth; and fistulous tracts emanating from the gums.

(3) **Orthodontic assessment:** identification of missing teeth, crowded teeth, and irregularly shaped dental arch, and determination of the occlusion or bite.

b. **Performance.** Intraoral examinations are best performed with the child in a reclining position. If the child is less than 4 years of age, the parent can cradle the child on his or her lap with the child's head on the physician's knees. The parent can also restrain the child's arms and legs. A high-intensity light and a tongue blade are necessary. A mouth mirror may be helpful for visualizing inaccessible areas and retracting the soft tissues.

The mouth is a vulnerable area for most children so the examination should be performed slowly and gently. Children will usually keep their mouths open once an object is in it and will rarely bite intentionally. An open mouth in a crying infant or toddler can be an advantage when examining this age group.

c. **Interpretation.** Obvious plaque and gingival inflammation secondary to poor oral hygiene are indications for counseling the parents regarding the quality and frequency of oral hygiene. If any discolorations, caries, soft tissue lesions, or bite discrepancies are noted, the child should be referred to a pediatric dentist.

d. **Timing.** The primary care provider should begin intraoral exams postnatally, and they should be included on each well-baby visit. Examining the intraoral structures, including the dentition, gingiva, and vestibular and lingual tissues, can be incorporated into the ENT examination routine. At approximately 2 or 3 years of age, the child can be referred to a dentist for a more thorough evaluation and the initiation of topical fluoride treatments. Follow-through on referrals is often incomplete, so it behooves the primary medical care provider to continue routine oral/dental examinations, as well as diet and oral hygiene counseling.

2. **Justification**

a. **Test characteristics.** Physicians can effectively screen for obvious caries and malocclusions, identify detrimental feeding patterns and habits, and motivate parents toward routine dental health care.

b. **Risks** are negligible.

c. **Costs.** Because examination of the oral cavity, including teeth and bite, involves very little additional time, it can be done during examination of the throat at each well-baby visit.

d. **Acceptability.** Most pediatricians take histories and perform intraoral examinations routinely, especially for evaluation of pharyngeal area.

B. **Early intervention**

1. **Methods.** Counsel parents to eliminate caries-producing behavior and reinforce oral hygiene. Refer them to a children's dentist for treatment of caries and orthodontic evaluation.

2. **Justification**

a. **Effectiveness.** Dental caries is a preventable and repairable disease. Early examination and early restoration of caries is better than later restorations or extraction. Fluoride, diet, and oral hygiene counseling can result in a caries-free childhood.

The main benefit of early involvement in oral health care for infants and children is the opportunity to intercept behaviors that are potentially damaging, and at the same time provide valuable preventive information to parents that is structured to meet the individual needs of each family situation [20]. Bite discrepancies and thumb- or finger-sucking habits can cause orthodontic problems.

b. **Risks** are minimal.

c. **Costs** are little or none.

d. **Acceptability** is good.

IV. **Recommendations**

A. **Primary prevention**

1. The primary care provider should determine whether a newborn infant's drinking water has optimal or suboptimal fluoride concentration. This should be recorded and reassessed if the family moves.
2. Infants and children should receive oral fluoride supplementation in recommended amounts from birth through 12 years of age, according to their age and the fluoride content of their drinking water.
3. Fluoride supplementation is not currently recommended for breast-fed infants of mothers living in fluoridated areas. Formula-fed infants should receive fluoride according to the fluoride content of their drinking water.
4. Systemic fluoride supplements should be taken in a manner that also enhances topical uptake for the teeth already calcified and erupted—"After brushing and flossing and before bed, chew, swish, and swallow one tab."

5. Fluoride dosage should be reassessed at ages 2 and 3 years. To maintain compliance, parents should be reminded to continue fluoride drops or tablets on an ongoing basis.
6. Primary care providers should participate in the activities that encourage their communities to fluoridate their water supplies.
7. Topical application of fluoride twice each year in the dentist's office is recommended, along with the daily use of a fluoridated toothpaste.
8. When the deciduous teeth erupt, the parents should be cautioned about nursing bottle caries and the need for a balanced diet (to include the four basic food groups) and a low sucrose intake.
9. This is also an excellent time to begin oral hygiene procedures—preferably with a soft, toddler toothbrush and small amounts of fluoridated toothpaste—at a regularly scheduled time and with the assistance of the parents. Flossing may commence whenever the space between teeth cannot be cleansed by the toothbrush. Thorough brushing and flossing once per day is adequate; before bed is ideal. These oral hygiene messages need continual reinforcement.

B. Secondary prevention

1. **Early detection**
   a. An oral/dental examination should be performed by the physician during well-baby or well-child visits.
2. **Early intervention**
   a. If any hard or soft tissue pathology is noted, the child should be referred to a pediatric dentist. After 2 years of age, the child should be referred to the pediatric dentist for routine 6-month examinations, prophylaxis, and fluoride applications.

References

1. Wycoff, S. J. Community Dentistry and Public Health. In B. L. Braham and M. E. Morris (eds.), *Textbook of Pediatric Dentistry*. Baltimore: Williams & Wilkins, 1980. Pp. 529–531. *Cost factors in preventive dentistry.*
2. Kotlow, L. A. Breast feeding: A cause of dental caries in children. *J. Dent. Child.* 44(3):192, 1977. *Documents that dental caries do occur with prolonged breast-feeding.*
3. Gardner, D. E., Norwood, J. R., and Eisenson, J. E. At-will breast feeding and dental caries: Four case reports. *J. Dent. Child.* 44(3):186, 1977. *See annotation for reference 2.*
4. Leverett, D. H. Fluorides and the changing prevalence of dental caries. *Science* 217(4554):26, 1982. *Effectiveness of fluoride on caries and oral health.*
5. Brunelle, J. A., and Carlos, J. P. Changes in the prevalence of dental caries in U.S. school children, 1961–1980. *J. Dent. Res.* 61:1346, 1982. *Epidemiologic reference.*
6. Dean, H. T. Endemic fluorosis and its relation to dental caries. *Public Health Rep.* 53:1443, 1938. *Study of naturally occurring fluoride in water supplies.*
7. McDonald, R. E., and Avery, D. R. *Dentistry for the Child and Adolescent* (3rd ed.). St. Louis: Mosby, 1978. Pp. 115–117. *Comprehensive pediatric dentistry text.*
8. American Academy of Pediatrics, Committee on Nutrition. Fluoride supplementation. *Pediatrics* 77(5):758, 1986. *Official fluoride supplement recommendation.*
9. Schusterman, S. More on fluoride in breast milk. *Pediatr. Alert* 5:99, 1980. *Fluoride availability in human milk.*
10. Margolis, F. J., et al. Fluoride supplements for children. A survey for physician prescription practices. *Am. J. Dis. Child.* 134(9):865, 1980. *Survey of what physicians' actual fluoride prescribing practices are.*
11. Hastreiter, R. J. Fluoridation conflict: A history and conceptual synthesis. *J. Am. Dent. Assoc.* 106(4):486, 1983. *Good overview of fluoridation supplement controversy.*
12. Margolis, F. J., et al. Fluoride: Ten-year prospective study of deciduous and permanent dentition. *Am. J. Dis. Child.* 129(7):794, 1975. *See annotation for reference 4.*
13. Swango, P. A. The use of topical fluorides to prevent dental caries in adults: A review of the literature. *J. Am. Dent. Assoc.* 107(3):447, 1983. *Good reference on topical effectiveness of fluoride.*
14. Trask, P. A. Fluoride dosage update. *J. Calif. Dent. Assoc.* 6(3):50, 1978. *Fluoride dosages relevant to existing fluoridation water content.*
15. Heifetz, S. B., and Horowitz, H. S. Amounts of fluoride in self-administered dental products: Safety considerations for children. *Pediatrics* 77(6):876, 1986. *Safety aspects of fluoride products.*

16. Driscoll, W. S., et al. Prevalence of dental caries and dental fluorosis in areas with optimal and above optimal water fluoride concentrations. *J. Am. Dent. Assoc.* 107(1):42, 1983. *Epidemiologic study of dental health and fluoride in the water.*
17. Heifetz, S. B., and Horowitz, H. S. The amounts of fluoride in current fluoride therapies: Safety considerations for children. *A.S.D.C. J. Dent. Child.* 51(4):257, 1984. *See annotation for reference 15.*
18. Newbrun, E. (ed.). *Fluorides and Dental Caries* (3rd ed.). Springfield IL: Thomas, 1986. *Good text on research and utilization of fluoride.*
19. Margolis, F. J., and Cohen, S. N. Successful and unsuccessful experiences in combating the antifluoridationists. *Pediatrics* 76(1):113, 1985. *Good reference for responding to antifluoridationists.*
20. Goepferd, S. J. Infant oral health: A rationale. *A.S.D.C. J. Dent. Child.* 53(4):257, 1986. *Guide to infant health counseling.*

46 Anemia in Children

Sarah Woerner

I. The problem

A. Definition. Anemia is defined as a reduction in red cell mass or blood hemoglobin concentration [1].

B. Description. Anemia can occur via three mechanisms: (1) failure to produce red cells, (2) failure of maturation of red cells, or (3) increased destruction of red cells. Table 46-1 lists the types and prevalences of childhood anemias in each of these categories.

This chapter discusses iron deficiency and sickle cell anemias, as these are two conditions that the primary care physician is likely to encounter in daily practice and for which acceptable preventive measures exist.

Iron-Deficiency Anemia

I. The problem

A. Description. Iron-deficiency anemia is caused by inadequate intake of dietary iron or excess iron loss through blood loss. If untreated, children may experience signs and symptoms directly attributable to anemia (pallor, easy fatigability, tachycardia, and possible congestive heart failure), as well as effects secondary to iron deficiency without anemia (decreased growth, intestinal malabsorption, occult gastrointestinal bleeding, decreased muscle performance, and behavioral changes) [2].

B. Epidemiology. This anemia is most often encountered in children between 6 months and 2 years of age and in adolescents. In the United States, it is estimated that up to 24% of the 6-month to 2-year-old children have iron-deficiency anemia, and that 24–68% have iron deficiency without anemia. The prevalence of anemia in the adolescent female population is estimated at 11–27% [3]. **Groups at particular risk** are premature infants and children of lower socioeconomic classes.

II. Primary prevention

A. Methods. Primary prevention of most iron-deficiency anemia is handled by assuring adequate dietary intake of iron. Parents should be informed of the following recommendations of the Committee on Nutrition of the American Academy of Pediatrics [4] (see also Chaps. 29 and 30).

1. **Premature infants.** All premature infants need iron supplementation by 2 months of age. The dose is 2 mg/kg/day of elemental iron, which can be supplied by iron-fortified formulas that contain 12 mg of elemental iron per liter, or by use of ferrous sulfate drops (containing 15 mg of elemental iron per 0.3 cc).
2. **Breast-fed term infants** require no supplementation until 4–6 months of age, at which time iron-fortified cereal should be introduced. (Rice cereal contains 1 mg of elemental iron per tablespoon.)
3. **Formula-fed term infants** require supplemental iron by 4 months of age at a dose of 1 mg/kg/day (15 mg/day maximum). This can be provided in the form of iron-containing formula and cereals.
4. **If cow's milk is introduced into the diet, it should be after 6 months of age.** Intake should be limited to 750 cc/day to encourage intake of other iron-containing foods and to diminish the risk of intestinal bleeding aggravated by milk proteins.
5. **Older children and adolescents** should be informed of the merits of good nutrition and cautioned against fad diets. Adolescent females in particular should be observed for excessive weight loss or unusual eating patterns. Iron supplements should be considered if eating habits are poor or if adolescent females have excessive menstrual blood loss.

B. Justification (see Chaps. 29 and 30).

1. **Effectiveness.** Giving iron-fortified formula or cereal is an effective means of preventing iron deficiency [4].

Table 46-1. Classification and prevalence of childhood anemias[a]

A. Disorders of red cell production
  1. Marrow failure
    a. Aplastic anemia (rare: 2–13 cases/million population)[b]
    b. Pure red cell aplasia (rare)
    c. Marrow replacement
      (1) Malignancy
      (2) Osteopetrosis (rare)
      (3) Myelofibrosis (rare, except in chronic renal failure)
    d. Pancreatic insufficiency with marrow failure (rare)
  2. Impaired erythropoietin production
    a. Chronic renal failure
    b. Hypothyroidism/hypopituitarism
    c. Chronic inflammation
    d. Protein malnutrition
B. Disorders of red cell maturation
  1. Abnormalities of cytoplasmic maturation
    a. Iron deficiency (3–24% of American children under 3 years) [3]
    b. Thalassemia (3–10% of Greek- or Italian-Americans and 0.5% American blacks carry beta genes)[c]
    c. Lead toxicity (rare)
  2. Abnormalities of nuclear maturation
    a. Vitamin B_{12} deficiency (rare, except in strict vegetarians)
    b. Folate deficiency (rare, except in infants fed goat's milk)
    c. Primary dyserythropoietic anemias (rare)
    d. Erythropoietic protoporphyria (rare)
C. Disorders involving increased destruction of red cells
  1. Defects of hemoglobin—sickle cell (8% American blacks with sickle trait; 0.2% American blacks with SS disease; rare in other races)
  2. Defects of red cell membrane—spherocytosis (rare; 220 cases per million population)[c]
  3. Defects of red cell metabolism (13% of American black males and 2% American black females; increased incidence in Greek- and Italian-Americans.)[c]
  4. Antibody-mediated
  5. Mechanical injury
  6. Thermal injury
  7. Oxidant-induced injury—vitamin E deficiency (increased in premature infants)
  8. Infectious-agent-induced injury
  9. Paroxysmal nocturnal hemoglobinuria (rare)

[a]Adapted from D. G. Nathan and F. A. Oski (eds). *Hematology of Infancy and Childhood* (2nd ed.). Philadelphia: Saunders, 1981. Prevalences taken from referenced texts.
[b]From F. A. Oski and J. A. Stockman III. Anemia due to inadequate iron sources or poor iron utilization. *Pediatr. Clin. North Am.* 27(2):237, 1980.
[c]From R. Behrman and V. Vaughn. In W. Nelson (ed.), *Nelson Textbook of Pediatrics.* Philadelphia: Saunders, 1987.

2. **Side effects.** Some mothers claim that formulas with iron cause gastrointestinal upset or constipation in their infant; available data do not support this.
3. **Cost.** Iron-fortified and non-iron-fortified formula ($2 per liter, premixed; $1.60 per liter, concentrate) are more expensive than cow's milk ($1 per liter).
4. **Acceptability.** In the younger age group dietary measures are generally accepted. To some families, however, the higher cost of iron-fortified formulas may make them less acceptable than regular milk. In the older (adolescent) age group compliance with modification of diet habits or taking supplements may not be high.

III. Secondary prevention (screening)

A. Methods. Methods to screen for iron-deficiency anemia include testing of hemoglobin and hematocrit (an office procedure), or more sophisticated measurements of serum iron, total iron bonding capacity, serum ferritin, or erythrocyte protoporphyrin.

A helpful screening test for iron deficiency is the red cell distribution width (RDW) test, which is a measurement of variation of red cell size calculated by most modern-

Table 46-2. Tests used to detect iron-deficiency anemia

Type of test	Procedure	Availability	Sensitivity	Specificity	Costs $	Costs Time	Risks	Interpretation
Hematocrit	Mechanical centrifugation or calculation on Coulter counter, using capillary or venous blood	Office or lab procedure	Good	Poor	$.50–$15	Mins	Minor pain from blood-drawing	Not specific for iron-deficiency anemia
Hemoglobin	Optical densitormetry of hemolyzed capillary or venous sample	Office or lab procedure	Good	Poor	$.50–$15	Mins	Minor pain from blood-drawing	Same as above
Mean corpuscular volume	Read directly by a Coulter counter	Clinical lab	Good	Fair	$11–$15	Mins	Minor pain from blood-drawing	Decreased MCV may be seen in thalassemia and lead toxicity as well as iron deficiency
RDW [5]	Calculated by Coulter counter	Clinical lab	100%	66%	$11–$15	Mins	Minor pain from blood-drawing	Very sensitive screening tool; specificity may be increased by using in conjunction with MCV [14]
Free erythrocyte protoporphyrin	The amount of protoporphyrin unbound to iron is measured by fluorescent antibody, either as a rapid capillary test or a more elaborate procedure on venous blood	"Rapid Test" is not readily available as office procedure; labs usually send it out to larger labs	Good	Fair	$21	Mins or hrs	Minor pain from blood-drawing	Increased levels may be seen with lead toxicity as well as iron deficiency
Serum ferritin	Radioimmunoassay of venous serum	Most large labs	Excellent	Good	$25–$30	Hrs	Minor pain from blood-drawing	May be falsely elevated with inflammatory or liver disease
% iron saturation	Serum iron is measured and divided by total iron binding capacity	Most labs	Good	Good	$13–$16	Hrs	Minor pain from blood-drawing	% saturation may be inaccurate in many conditions that alter TIBC, e.g., thyroid disease, pregnancy, malnutrition
Therapeutic trial of iron	3 mg/kg/day of elemental iron given orally (see text)	Anywhere	Good	Excellent	$5–$6*	1 mo	Risks: (1) may delay diagnosis of other forms of anemia; (2) large amounts of iron may cause overload in patients with homozygous thalassemia	

*Calculated for administration of ferrous sulfate to a 10-kg child for 1 month.

day Coulter counters. A higher than normal RDW value is a very sensitive and fairly specific means of detecting iron deficiency, even before changes in hematocrit, hemoglobin, and mean corpuscular volume (MCV) occur [5].

One of the easiest and most cost-effective methods of diagnosis is the therapeutic trial of iron therapy [6]. Table 46-2 is a comparative listing of tests, including the therapeutic trial, used to detect iron-deficiency anemia.

B. Justification

1. **Effectiveness.** When treatment is instituted early, before symptoms appear, the child remains healthy and may actually improve in some parameters, such as attention span and cooperativeness [7].

   If treatment is begun after symptoms have occurred, there is often a very rapid increase in the child's vigor and appetite; this may precede the rise in hemoglobin by weeks. Cardiovascular status, if previously compromised, may also improve more rapidly than the anemia, presumably due to iron's role in enzyme activation in muscle and other metabolically active tissues [2].
2. **Risks and side effects.** The risks of obtaining blood are minimal. A potential risk of a therapeutic trial of iron therapy would be the missing of another underlying cause of the anemia. In patients with homozygous thalassemia, iron therapy is not indicated and could potentially contribute to iron overload.
3. **Cost.** The cost of a 3-month therapeutic trial of iron for a 10-kg child is approximately $2 (100 ml of ferrous sulfate).
4. **Acceptability.** Screening involves only minor discomfort and cost to the patient/parent. Compliance with iron therapy is variable.

IV. Recommendations

A. Primary preventions: prevention with nutritional measures [4] (see also sec. **II.A.** above)

1. Premature infants need iron supplementation by 2 months of age.
2. Breast-fed term infants require no supplementation until 4–6 months, when iron-fortified cereal should be introduced.
3. Formula-fed term infants require supplemental iron by 4 months.
4. If cow's milk is introduced into the diet, it should be after 6 months.
5. Older children and adolescents should be informed of the merits of good nutrition and cautioned against fad diets. Iron supplementation should be considered for children or adolescents with poor eating habits or excessive menstrual blood loss.

B. Secondary prevention

1. **Early detection (screening)**
   a. Hemoglobin or hematocrit measurements should be performed on all children during periods of high risk: 4–9 months (premature infants), 9–15 months (term infants), 3–5 years (preschool), and 12–14 years (adolescent females). Fig. 46-1 illustrates a suggested procedure for diagnosing iron-deficiency anemia.
2. **Early detection (therapeutic trial)**
   a. If the hemoglobin/hematocrit is low (Table 46-3) in a child older than 3 months, and if the history suggests iron deficiency, a therapeutic trial of iron should be started, at a dose of 3 mg/kg/day elemental iron (see Fig. 46-1).
   b. Hemoglobin/hematocrit should be measured after 1 month of therapy. If a response is seen, therapy should be continued for a total of 3 months. If no response is seen and compliance was good, a further diagnostic search is indicated.
   c. In any child less than 3 months or older than 3 years, blood loss and other causes of anemia should be ruled out before diagnosing nutritional iron deficiency.

Sickle Cell Anemia

I. The problem

A. Description. Sickle cell anemia is transmitted by an autosomal dominant gene that causes substitution of an "S" hemoglobin chain for a normal "A" chain. This substitution results in severe changes in the hemoglobin molecule, leading to "sickling" of red blood cells, obstruction of tiny blood vessels, and numerous other effects.

1. **Heterozygous sickle cell disease,** or "sickle trait," does not usually produce severe morbidity or mortality. However, several conditions are known to be definitely correlated with sickle trait. These include idiopathic hematuria, pulmonary embolism with antecedent thrombophlebitis, splenic infarction at high altitudes (greater than

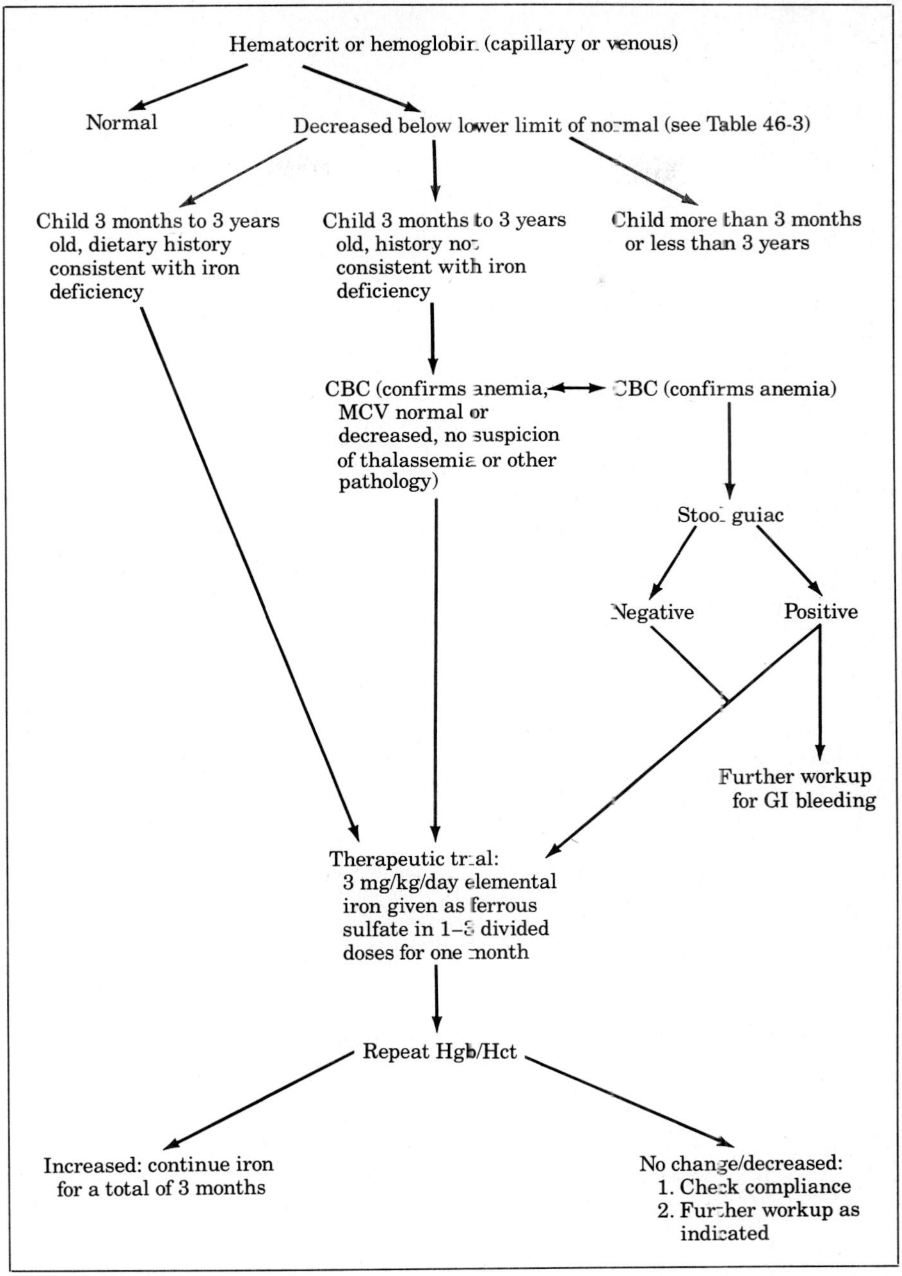

Fig. 46-1. Recommended screening procedure for iron-deficiency anemia. (CBC=complete blood count; MCV=mean corpuscular volume; GI=gastrointestinal.)

Table 46-3. Normal values for hemoglobin/hematocrit*

Age	Hemoglobin*	Hematocrit*	Mean corpuscular volume*
Preterm infants			
Birth	18		
2–3 wk	14.5		
5–6 wk	10.5		
10 wk	9.5		
Term infants			
Birth	19.0 (16.8)	61 (53.6)	119 (109.6)
2–3 wk	15.6 (13.0)	46 (38.7)	111 (102.8)
5–6 wk	11.9 (10.4)	36 (29.8)	102 (91.8)
12 wk	11.3 (10.4)	33 (29.7)	88 (80.1)
Children			
6mo–2 yr	12.5 (11.0)	37 (33)	77 (70)
2–4 yr	12.5 (11.0)	38 (34)	79 (73)
5–7 yr	13.0 (11.5)	39 (35)	81 (75)
8–11 yr	13.5 (12.0)	40 (36)	83 (78)
12–14 yr			
female	13.5 (12.0)	41 (36)	85 (78)
male	14.0 (12.5)	43 (37)	84 (77)
15–17 yr			
female	14.0 (12.0)	41 (36)	87 (79)
male	15.0 (13.0)	46 (38)	86 (78)
Adults			
18–19 yr			
female	14.0 (12.0)	42 (35)	90 (80)
male	16.0 (14.0)	47 (40)	90 (80)

*Numbers without parentheses represent the mean; numbers in parentheses represent lower limits of normal. The normal values are from venous blood samples, but capillary samples have been proved to correlate highly enough to be used for screening purposes [6].
Source: Adapted from tables in D. G. Nathan and F. A. Oski (eds.), *Hematology of Infancy and Childhood,* (2nd ed.). Saunders, Philadelphia, 1981.

10,000 ft above sea level), and bacteriuria in pregnancy (without measurable effect on pregnancy complications or birth weight) [8]. In addition, a study of military recruits showed that men with sickle trait had a 30- to 40-fold increased risk of sudden unexplained death under conditions of extreme physical exertion. This finding may have important implications for screening [9].

2. **Homozygous sickle cell disease** (SS disease) is a much more severe condition generally, but with variations in severity that are still poorly understood. If untreated, complications affecting almost any organ system may arise. These include stroke, sensorineural hearing loss, proliferative retinopathy, pulmonary infarction and chronic pulmonary disease, renal papillary necrosis, infections (sepsis, meningitis, osteomyelitis, pneumonia), severe pain from bone infarction, pancytopenia from "aplastic crises," delayed growth, and leg ulcers.

   Infants with sickle cell disease may be asymptomatic for the first several months to a year of life because of their increased levels of fetal hemoglobin. If these babies are not diagnosed early, the first symptom of the disease may be overwhelming sepsis, splenic sequestration of red cells leading to life-threatening acute anemia, or even sudden death.

II. Primary prevention

Primary prevention of sickle cell anemia can be achieved (1) through genetic counseling of persons with the gene so that they are aware of the risks of having an affected child, and (2) through prenatal diagnosis in pregnant women at risk, some of whom may wish an abortion if the baby has homozygous sickle cell disease (see Chaps. 13 and 14).

III. Secondary prevention

A. Early detection

1. **Methods.** Table 46-4 lists the current tests available to diagnose sickle cell hemoglobinopathy.

   a. **Cord blood testing** should employ citrate agar electrophoresis at a pH of 6.2, since ordinary electrophoresis or "sickle prep" tests will not distinguish fetal from sickle hemoglobin [9].

b. **Sickle prep.** The sickle prep slide test can be done in the office setting. It utilizes the patient's capillary blood, which is incubated for 15 minutes on a slide or in a test tube with the reducing agent sodium metabisulfite. A positive prep occurs when red cells show sickling, as measured either by observation under the microscope or by change in optical density in a test tube. This is an easy, quick test to perform, but **positive results should always be confirmed by hemoglobin electrophoresis,** since false-positive tests may occur.

c. **Hemoglobin electrophoresis** is a routine test that separates hemoglobin A from hemoglobin S.

2. **Justification**

a. **Test characteristics.** See Table 46-4.

b. **Risks and side effects.** The physical risks of post-natal screening (using cord blood or venous sampling) are minimal. There is some concern, however, about the potential psychological risks to patients, particularly those diagnosed as having sickle cell trait who are unlikely to have any unusual health problems. In some instances, appropriate follow-up and counseling may not be available to the families whose child is "labeled" as having a sickle gene; in these cases misconceptions regarding the significance of the positive screen may occur. It is difficult to find studies examining these nonmedical risks of screening, and more research needs to be done.

c. **Costs** (see Table 46-4). Cord blood screening is more expensive than office or routine screening because of the special techniques required.

d. **Acceptability.** There is little information available on parent acceptability of early screening. Presumably, most educated parents would want to know as early as possible if their child was affected.

B. Early intervention

1. **Methods**

a. **Education.** When a diagnosis of sickle cell anemia is made in the neonatal period, education of the family should begin immediately. The importance of early evaluation of fevers and irritability in the infant should be stressed.

b. **Penicillin prophylaxis.** A recent double-blind, controlled study has demonstrated the efficacy of daily prophylactic penicillin in the prevention of pneumococcal septicemia in patients with sickle cell disease [10]. The authors recommend beginning such prophylaxis at the age of 4 months.

2. **Justification**

a. **Effectiveness and benefits.** A NIH consensus report concluded that morbidity and mortality rates are significantly reduced by newborn screening programs, provided that they are linked to a system that can provide comprehensive clinical follow-up [12]. Early screening allows for more aggressive management of involved children, including the use of penicillin prophylaxis as mentioned above. An additional claimed benefit is that screening of newborns permits detection of couples at risk and gives them the opportunity to receive education and genetic counseling before future pregnancies [13].

In one short-term controlled study it was found that newborn screening did increase parental awareness of complications [14]. Finally, given evidence that sickle trait seems to be linked to unexplained sudden death under certain rare conditions, screening may prove beneficial in identifying individuals at risk for this complication.

b. **Risks and side effects.** Patient (parent) education carries no risks. Since penicillin is a relatively safe drug, the risks of giving it as prophylaxis are minimal. Theoretical risks might include potential development of resistant organisms, development of a penicillin allergy, predisposition to *Candida* infections, and parental delay in seeking evaluation for illness because the child is already taking medication.

c. **Costs.** The cost of 125 mg of penicillin V given twice daily for a month is $8.

d. **Acceptability.** Some families may be resistant to educational programs. In addition, acceptability of taking medication on a long-term basis may vary.

IV. Recommendations

A. Primary prevention (see Chaps. 14 and 15)

1. Genetic counseling should be offered to all patients with sickle cell trait or disease.
2. Prenatal diagnosis should be discussed with all parents at risk of having a child with sickle cell disease.

Table 46-4. Postnatal tests to detect sickle hemoglobinopathy*

Age	Procedure	Availability	Risks	Sensitivity	Specificity	Costs		Patient acceptability
						$	Time	
Newborn	Cord blood screening using citrate agar electrophoresis	Most large centers; not routinely done in small labs	Labeling	Good	Good, but results should be confirmed at 4–6 wks	$25–50	Hrs	Good
More than 6 mos	"Sickle prep" test (using sodium metabisulfite) (see text)	Kits widely available to be used in office	Minor (capillary sample)	Good (99% accurate in some trials)	Good (confirmatory electrophoresis should always be done if results are positive)	$2–5	Mins	Good
	Hemoglobin electrophoresis	Most large clinical labs	Minor (venous blood)	Good	Good (some abnormal hemoglobins may be confused with sickle cell)	$20–30	Hrs	Good

*See also Chap. 14.

B. Secondary prevention

1. Early detection

a. Ideally, mass screening of all newborns (in conjunction with other mandatory newborn tests) should be performed [12].

b. In areas where statewide mass screening is not in place, cord blood of all black infants should be screened using citrate agar electrophoresis. (Infants who have undergone prenatal diagnosis may be excepted.)

c. All infants with positive newborn tests should be rescreened with hemoglobin electrophoresis at 4–6 weeks of age for definitive diagnosis.

d. All children with a positive family history of sickle cell disease, or black children whose family sickle status is unknown, should be screened using the sickle prep test or by electrophoresis.

e. Any positive sickle prep should be confirmed by hemoglobin electrophoresis.

2. Early intervention

a. The physician following a patient with sickle trait or disease should work in conjunction with a national sickle cell center in order to provide the best long-term care for the patient and his or her family [15].

b. Counseling and education of patients and their families regarding all aspects of sickle cell disease should be **ongoing.**

c. The physician should advise the family to seek attention as early as possible for problems such as pain and fever that might indicate serious disease.

d. Based on current information, penicillin V should be administered prophylactically to all children by the age of 4 months who have sickle cell disease (standard dose is 125 mg of penicillin V potassium bid). This may need to be modified according to age [9].

References

1. Nathan, D. G., and Oski, F. A. (eds.). *Hematology of Infancy and Childhood* (2nd ed.). Philadelphia: Saunders, 1981. *Probably the most up-to-date authoritative textbook on pediatric hematology. Excellent reference.*
2. Oski, F. A. The nonhematologic manifestations of iron deficiency. *Am. J. Dis. Child.* 133(3):315, 1979. *A good review of the manifestations of iron deficiency independent of anemia.*
3. Oski, F. A., and Stockman, J. A., III. Anemia due to inadequate iron sources or poor iron utilization. *Pediatr. Clin. North Am.* 27(2):237, 1980. *A review article of iron metabolism and utilization.*
4. American Academy of Pediatrics, Committee on Nutrition. *Pediatric Nutrition Handbook* (2nd ed.). Elk Grove Village, IL: American Academy of Pediatrics, 1985. *American Academy of Pediatrics' recommendations on nutrition.*
5. McClure, S., Custer, E., and Bessman, J. D. Improved detection of early iron deficiency in nonanemic subjects. *J.A.M.A.* 253(7):1021, 1985. *Examines the use of red cell distribution width (RDW) in screening.*
6. Reeves, J. D., et al. Screening for iron deficiency anemia in one-year-old infants: Hemoglobin alone or hemoglobin and mean corpuscular volume as predictors of response to iron treatment. *J. Pediatr.* 98(6):894, 1981. *An article describing a screening program in which all 1-year-olds with hemoglobins less than 11.5 were given therapeutic trials of iron.*
7. Walter, T., Kovalskys, J., and Stekel, A. Effect of mild iron deficiency on infant mental development scores. *J. Pediatr.* 102(4):519, 1983. *A study concluding that treatment of iron deficiency improves attention span.*
8. Knasel, A. Is sickle cell trait a health hazard? Medical problems: A brief review. *Am. J. Pediatr. Hematol. Oncol.* 4(2):179, 1982. *A good review of the health problems of patients with sickle trait.*
9. Kark, J. A., et al. Sickle cell trait as a risk factor for sudden death in physical training. *N. Engl. J. Med.* 317:781, 1987. *A study of 2 million military recruits demonstrating a death rate of 32.2 per 100,000 for blacks with sickle trait compared to 1.2 per 100,000 for blacks without sickle trait.*
10. Gaston, M. H., et al. Prophylaxis with oral penicillin in children with sickle cell anemia. A randomized trial. *N. Engl. J. Med.* 314(25):1593, 1986. *A double-blind, controlled study demonstrating an 84% reduction in pneumococcal septicemia in children with sickle cell who were given penicillin prophylaxis, versus those children not given such prophylaxis (control group). There were no deaths in the treated group and three in the control group.*

11. Scott, R. B., and Harrison, D. L. Screening of the umbilical cord blood for sickle cell disease: Utilization and implementation. *Am. J. Pediatr. Hematol. Oncol.* 4(2):202, 1982. *A description of the most effective methods of cord blood screening.*
12. Consensus Conference: Newborn screening for sickle cell disease and other hemoglobinopathies. *J. A. M. A.* 258(9):1205, 1987. *A detailed report recommending that states implement mandatory newborn screening (using filter paper disc and citrate agar electrophoresis) of all newborn infants.*
13. Rucknagel, D. L. A decade of screening in the hemoglobinopathies: Is a national program to prevent sickle cell anemia possible? *Am. J. Pediatr. Hematol. Oncol.* 5(4):373, 1983. *A commentary on the effectiveness of prenatal and postnatal screening.*
14. Nussbaum, R. L., et al. Newborn screening for sickling hemoglobinopathies: Houston, 1976 to 1980. *Am. J. Dis. Child.* 138(1):44, 1984. *Controlled study of screening effectiveness; shows that it did increase parental awareness of complications.*
15. Gaston, M., and Rosse, W. F. The cooperative study of sickle cell disease: Review of study design and objectives. *Am. J. Pediatr. Hematol. Oncol.* 4(2):197, 1982. *A review of the current studies of sickle cell disease, with a comprehensive list of national sickle centers.*

47 Lead Poisoning

Lynn R. Goldman and John Harris

I. Lead poisoning

A. Definition. The problem of lead poisoning in children has been identified since the nineteenth century. Originally this disease was defined by the presence of high lead levels, with severe encephalopathy, seizures, coma, mental retardation, or death.

By the current Centers for Disease Control (CDC) definition, a child with lead poisoning may or may not be asymptomatic. Lead toxicity, according to the CDC, is defined as existing whenever a child has:

1. Two successive blood lead levels ≥25 μg/dl, with or without symptoms; and
2. Erythrocyte protoporphyrin (EP) levels ≥35 μg/dl whole blood [1, 2].

B. Description. The effects of lead toxicity are nonspecific and not readily identifiable. Some effects, such as neurologic and renal damage, may result in chronic impairment. Listed below are symptoms and signs for different clinical states.

1. **Subclinical lead toxicity.** The child is asymptomatic except that he or she may show altered behavior such as attention disorders or learning disabilities. Because the dose-response for these effects is not well understood, laboratory examinations may show a blood lead level of anywhere between 25 and 70 μg/dl, and an EP level between 35 and 109 [1, 3].

   Children with lead levels ≥ 25 are at greater risk for neurologic, psychologic, behavioral, and learning disturbances [4–8]. Children exposed to maternal lead levels < 25 in utero may have subtle developmental delays [9]. Growth is diminished in children with slight elevations in lead levels [10].

2. **Moderate lead toxicity.** The child may have fatigue, pallor, anorexia, abdominal pain, sporadic vomiting, constipation, malaise, irritability, sleep disturbances, and developmental regression [1, 3]. Blood lead is usually >70 μg/dl, but occasionally may be as low as 50 μg/dl. EP is >35 [3].

3. **Lead encephalopathy.** The child may have the above symptoms plus coma, seizures, bizarre behavior, atasia, apathy, incoordination, vomiting, and alteration in state of consciousness. Blood lead is usually ≥100 μg/dl, but these symptoms may be seen at levels as low as 70 [3].

C. Epidemiology. Screening under the Lead-based Paint Poisoning Prevention Act began in mid-1971. From 1972–1980, programs located in all sections of the United States reported screening 3,350,000 children ages 1–5; 6.6% were reported as having a blood lead of >30 μg/dl, the level considered abnormal by the CDC at that time [11].

Furthermore, in a random United States sample of American children aged 6 months–5 years, the National Center for Health Statistics showed that 4% of children had lead levels ≥30 μg/dl. In this sample, the incidence of lead levels >30 μg/dl ranged from 2.1% in rural areas to 11.6% in inner cities [12]. In 1980, 2400 children out of 502,925 screened (incidence of 0.5% among high-risk screened populations) were admitted to hospitals for treatment of lead poisoning, and 1.2% of those screened had lead poisoning according to the definition used at that time [11].

Though children of low socioeconomic status are at most risk for lead poisoning, children from all races and socioeconomic classes may be affected. Preschool-age children are at highest risk, and lead poisoning is most common in the summer months [13]. In the 1960s, most cases of lead poisoning were described as occurring in children eating lead-based paint chips. However, it is now understood that excess lead ingestion can occur in dust-contaminated environments with normal childhood hand-to-mouth behavior. While this hand-to-mouth behavior is still the most important route of exposure, particularly in the old sections of eastern United States cities, clinicians should suspect lead poisoning in a child in any of the following situations: (1) existence of pica behavior; (2) father working in lead smelter or automobile battery plant; (3) family living near lead smelters or other point sources of exposure; and (4) sibling or parent with lead poisoning. Besides dust, other common environmental sources of lead include some glazed pottery, cosmetics, printed matter, toys, and canned goods [14]. In addition, children with nutritional deficiencies of iron, calcium, or zinc, are also at increased risk because of increased gastrointestinal absorption of the lead [14].

II. Primary prevention

A. Methods. Primary prevention involves eliminating or isolating sources of lead in the environment. Examples from the past include the 1977 ruling by the Consumer Product Safety Commission (CPSC) limiting lead in household paints and the phased reduction of lead in gasoline, which began in 1976. There are still millions of housing units with lead-containing paint. Those that are deteriorating, along with contaminated soils and other environmental sources, continue to present a threat to children, and measures should be taken to prevent exposure. An additional source is through parents who are exposed at work or in hobbies [1]. Prevention of occupational exposure and industrial hygiene measures such as changing clothes and bathing prior to contact with the child will decrease exposure.

B. Justification. Because even subtle neurologic deficits resulting from lead absorption are probably permanent, it is desirable to identify and reduce or eliminate sources of lead to which other children may be exposed and to prevent further lead exposure in children with lead absorption.

1. **Effectiveness.** Primary prevention is the most effective way of eliminating childhood lead exposure and its consequences. Reductions in environmental lead are associated with a fall in average blood lead levels [15]. Presence of lead in the environment has been found to be the most significant factor contributing to increases in blood lead levels [16].
2. **Risks.** In removing lead sources from the environment, care must be taken to avoid exposing workers or children in the area.
3. **Costs** vary by source. A cost/benefit analysis performed by the Environmental Protection Agency for removal of lead from gasoline showed net savings even without considering the cost of low-level lead exposure [17]. The costs of lead removal from homes are not well known, but a cost/benefit analysis showed significant savings in the prevention of childhood exposure [18].

III. Secondary prevention

A. Early detection

1. **Methods.** The need is to identify and follow up children with undue lead burden before severe neurologic sequelae occur. The most useful screening tests are the erythrocyte protoporphyrin (EP) and blood lead tests [1]. These tests represent different parameters of an assessment of lead burden. Blood lead represents lead absorption, while EP measures the adverse metabolic effects of lead on heme synthesis.

   a. **Erythrocyte protoporphyrin** may be done on either a venous or capillary specimen; for mass screening, capillary specimens are used. Assessment of protoporphyrin in blood is based on the direct fluorescence of zinc protoporphyrin in whole blood as measured by a hematofluorometer [19]. Hematofluorometric analyses can be done cheaply and rapidly, so a result is immediately available at the time of screening.

   The acid extraction technique for measuring EP is the standard method used in many hospital labs. Although the acid extraction technique is considered to be more accurate than the hematofluorometric methods, the agreement between the two procedures is very high [20]. EP elevations occur primarily only in three conditions: iron-deficiency anemia, undue lead burden, and erythropoietic protoporphyria [19].

   b. **Blood lead measurement** is also used in conjunction with EP for lead screening. This technique can also be done on either a capillary or venous specimen, but blood from venous specimens is definitely preferable because of the possibility of contamination of capillary blood with ambient lead dust [19]. Measurement of blood lead is usually done by one of four techniques [19] and requires care and experience for accurate results. Precautions must always be taken to avoid contamination of the skin, blood, or test tube with lead dust.

   c. **Population.** Screening should be performed annually on children between the ages of 1–6 with suspected exposures to lead. This includes children living in pre-1977, deteriorating housing, children living near other environmental sources, children whose parents or siblings have histories of lead exposure, and children with pica behavior.

Table 47-1. Risk categories for lead poisoning in asymptomatic children[a]

Blood lead (μg/dl)	Erythrocyte protoporphyrin (EP) by extraction (μg/dl whole blood) <35	35–109	110–249	>250
Test not done	I	b	b	b
≤24	I	Ia	Ia	EPP[c]
25–49	Ib	II	III	III
50–60	d	III	III	IV
>70	d	d	IV	IV

[a]Reflects priority for medical evaluation from the screening results; not to be used for diagnostic purposes. See the text for explanation of risk categories.
[b]Blood lead level necessary to estimate risk.
[c]EPP=erythropoietic protoporphyria; although rarely from iron deficiency, it may cause EP elevations to 300 μg/dl.
[d]Combination of results not generally observed in practice; if observed, retest with venous blood immediately.
Source: Centers for Disease Control. *Preventing Lead Poisoning in Young Children: A Statement.* Atlanta: U.S. Department of Health and Human Services, 1985.

d. **Further evaluation.** Based on the EP and lead results, the CDC classifies asymptomatic children into risk categories I to IV (Table 47-1). Category I represents a child at no risk from undue lead burden at the times of testing, and category IV represents children with urgent need for medical attention. These classifications do not indicate whether or not treatment is necessary. In fact, treatment is only instituted after confirmatory tests and clinical evaluation. It is common practice to refer any child in categories III and IV to a physician and to do periodic follow-up lead and EP measurements on any child in category II, III, or IV [1].

The diagnostic tests that a physician should consider when a child is in categories III and IV include: (1) confirmatory EP and blood lead; (2) complete history and physical; (3) measurement of iron, iron-binding capacity, and hemoglobin; (4) flat plate of abdomen and x-ray of long bones; (5) 8-hour calcium EDTA mobilization test; (6) measurement of urine for increased excretion of aminolevolinic acid (ALA-U) and coprophyrin (CPU); and (7) assay of inhibition of aminolevulate dehydratase (ALA-D) activity in in vitro circulating erythrocytes.

In children with blood levels of lead in excess of 55 μg/dl or who are symptomatic, the calcium EDTA mobilization test should not be done; instead chelation therapy should be started [3]. Examination of red cells for basophilic stippling and tests of hair and fingernails are not considered useful diagnostic tests [1].

2. **Justification**

a. **Test characteristics.** Although the combination of elevated EP (≥ 35 μg/dl) and elevated serum lead (≥ 25 μg/dl) is required for a diagnosis of lead toxicity, either test may be used as an initial screen. The EP is almost 100% sensitive, but not specific, as mentioned previously. Use of hematofluorometric measurement is slightly less specific than the acid extraction technique because it can give falsely high readings when the serum bilirubin is slightly elevated [19]. It is only recommended for use in screening in the field because it is inaccurate in stored blood [19].

Measurement of blood lead is a very sensitive indicator of lead toxicity, but it is nonspecific. False-negatives may occur during the early stages of lead poisoning [19]. False-positives are found in capillary determinations, where small amounts of lead from the skin can cause spuriously high values [19]. It is therefore necessary to confirm high capillary blood leads with venous determinations prior to instituting chelation therapy [19]. For the National Health and Nutrition Examination Study (NHANES) II, only 26% of children with elevated blood lead levels had high EP levels as well [1].

b. **Risks.** The only risks are those associated with phlebotomy or capillary blood sampling.

c. **Costs.** The costs of an EP and blood lead test in hospital labs usually range from \$10–\$20 each. County health departments often provide EP (hematofluorometric method) and blood lead at no cost or only a minimal charge.
d. **Acceptability.** The ideal initial screening test for lead toxicity is the EP. It will detect virtually 100% of those with lead toxicity, and, in addition, it will identify children with iron-deficiency anemia and other treatable conditions.

B. Early intervention

1. **Methods.** Children with lead poisoning should see a doctor for evaluation and for consideration of chelation therapy according to existing protocols [3]. Public health authorities should be notified to ensure that housemates are tested and that appropriate environmental follow-up is instituted. Nutritional deficiencies such as iron or calcium deficiencies should be identified and corrected. Symptomatic children are treated with BAL and $CaNa_2$ EDTA. Asymptomatic children are treated when blood lead is 56–69 μg/dl, or when the $CaNa_2$ EDTA challenge test is positive. If blood lead is <70, they are treated with $CaNa_2$ EDTA alone [3].
2. **Justification**
   a. **Effectiveness.** Treatment will reverse acute symptoms, prevent progression of chronic neurologic damage, and in severe cases prevent death.
   b. **Risks.** $CaNa_2$ EDTA is associated with renal and hepatic toxicity. Urine output, urinanalysis, blood urea nitrogen, creatinine, and liver function must be monitored carefully during its use. It can also cause depletion of zinc and symptoms of zinc deficiency. BAL causes minor symptoms, liver enzyme elevations, and hemolysis in individuals deficient in glucose 6-phosphate dehydrogenase [3].
   c. **Costs.** Chelation therapy is usually done on an inpatient basis; cost is related to total body burden of lead to be chelated. Long-term follow-up is necessary, and a second course of $CaNa_2$ EDTA therapy is required if blood lead concentrations rise above 50 μg/dl within 5–7 days after treatment. In that case further hospitalization is necessary [3].
   d. **Acceptability.** Treatment of lead poisoning is essential but futile in the absence of environmental follow-up to prevent further episodes in the same child.

IV. Recommendations. The following recommendations are based on the CDC monograph, *Preventing Lead Poisoning in Young Children: A Statement* [1].

The goal of screening is to prevent undue lead exposure and absorption and lead poisoning. This goal is best achieved with adherence to the following principles.

A. Primary prevention

1. Physicians should continue to be involved in and support efforts to reduce environmental lead levels and exposures.
2. Physicians taking care of children at risk for lead poisoning should educate the children's parents about the potential environmental sources of lead.

B. Secondary prevention

1. **Early detection**
   a. Screening for lead poisoning should be done with EP and blood lead determination.
   b. Children with suspected exposures to lead are the primary target population. These include the following groups:
      (1) Children aged 1–6 living in or frequenting pre-1977, and especially pre-World War II, dilapidated housing.
      (2) Children living near lead smelters, highways with heavy traffic, or hazardous waste sites where lead is a major pollutant.
      (3) Children whose parent(s) are exposed to lead at work or in a hobby.
      (4) Children aged 12–36 months with a history of pica behavior.
      (5) Children with siblings or housemates with lead levels ≥ 25 μg/dl of whole blood.
   c. Children with suspected exposures to lead should be screened at least once a year, beginning when they are 9–12 months of age. Screening should be done between May and October.
2. **Later assessment.** Any child with abnormally high lead and EP levels, or with symptoms that the physician suspects are due to lead poisoning, should receive a diagnostic evaluation including the following:
   a. Detailed history and physical examination.
   b. Nutritional status workup and hematologic evaluation for iron deficiency.
   c. Confirmatory diagnostic tests that should include repeat EP and blood lead tests and other tests already discussed in this chapter.

3. Early intervention

a. Children in category III or IV should be referred to a physician or medical center experienced in handling lead poisoning.

b. County public health departments should be notified whenever lead levels of ≥ 25 μg/dl are found so that an environmental investigation can begin.

References

1. Centers for Disease Control. *Preventing Lead Poisoning in Young Children: A Statement.* Atlanta, Ga: U.S. Department of Health and Human Services, 1985. *Most current recommendations from the CDC.*
2. *Lead.* Geneva: World Health Organization, 1977. *WHO consensus document on lead exposure.*
3. Piomelli, S., et al. Management of childhood lead poisoning. *J. Pediatr.* 105:523, 1984. *Good review of clinical aspects and medical treatment issues.*
4. Needleman, H. L., et al. Deficits in psychologic and classroom performance of children with elevated dentine lead levels. *N. Engl. J. Med.* 300:689, 1979. *Study of subclinical psychologic effects.*
5. Rutter, M. Low Level Lead Exposure: Sources, Effects, and Implications. In M. Rutter and R. R. Jones (eds.), *Lead Versus Health.* New York: Wiley, 1983. Pp. 333–370. *Good review of sources of exposure.*
6. Ernhart, C. B., Landa, B., and Schell, N. B. Subclinical levels of lead and developmental deficit—a multivariate follow-up reassessment. *Pediatrics* 67:911, 1981. *Study of subclinical psychologic effects.*
7. Bellinger, D. C., and Needleman, H. L. Lead and the relationship between maternal and child intelligence. *J. Pediatr.* 102(4):523, 1983. *Study of subclinical psychologic effects.*
8. Winneke, G., Hrdina, K. G., and Brockhaus, A. Neuropsychological studies in children with elevated tooth lead concentrations. I. Pilot study. *Int. Arch. Occup. Environ. Health* 51(2):169, 1982. *Study of subclinical psychologic effects.*
9. Bellinger, D. C., et al. Longitudinal analyses of prenatal and postnatal lead exposure and early cognitive development. *N. Engl. J. Med.* 316(17):1037, 1987. *Longitudinal study of prenatal and early childhood lead exposure in middle class children.*
10. Schwartz, J., Angle, C., and Pitcher, H. Relationship between childhood blood lead levels and stature. *Pediatrics* 77(3):281, 1986. *National Health and Nutrition Examination Survey data on lead and growth.*
11. Surveillance of childhood lead poisoning. *M.M.W.R.* 31(9):118, 1982. *Statistics on prevalence.*
12. Mahaffey, K. R., et al. National estimates of blood lead levels. United States, 1976–1980: Association with selected demographic and socioeconomic factors. *N. Engl. J. Med.* 307(10):573, 1982. *Statistics on risk factors.*
13. Lin-Fu, J. S. Lead Poisoning and Undue Lead Exposure in Children: History and Current Status. In H. L. Needleman (ed.), *Low Level Lead Exposure: The Clinical Implications of Current Research.* New York: Raven Press, 1980. Pp. 5–16. *Good review of history and risk factors.*
14. Mahaffey, K. R. Nutritional factors in lead poisoning. *Nutr. Rev.* 39(10):353, 1981. *Good review of nutritional interactions.*
15. Annest, J. L., et al. Chronological trend in blood lead levels between 1976 and 1980. *N. Engl. J. Med.* 308(23):1373, 1983. *Trends over time in average population lead levels.*
16. Bellinger, D., et al. Correlates of low-level exposure in urban children at 2 years of age. *Pediatrics* 77(6):826, 1986. *Good cohort study and multivariate analysis.*
17. Schwartz, J. *Costs and Benefits of Reducing Lead in Gasoline. Draft Final Report.* Washington, DC: U.S. Environmental Protection Agency, 1984. *Cost/benefit analysis for phase-out of gasoline lead.*
18. Provenzano, G. The Social Costs of Excessive Lead Exposure During Childhood. In H. L. Needleman (ed.), *Low Level Lead Exposure: The Clinical Implications of Current Research.* New York: Raven Press, 1980. Pp. 299–315. *Analysis of benefits and costs of preventing lead exposure.*
19. Piomelli, S., and Graziano, J. Laboratory diagnosis of lead poisoning. *Pediatr. Clin. North Am.* 27(4):843, 1980. *Good review of laboratory procedures.*
20. Karacic, V., Prpic-Majic, D., and Telisman, S. The relationship between zinc protoporphyrin (ZPP) and "free" erythrocyte protoporphyrin (FEP) in lead-exposed individuals. *Int. Arch. Occup. Environ. Health* 47(2):165, 1980. *Compares tests for protoporphyrin.*

48 Asymptomatic Bacteriuria in Children

Israel Zelikovic and
Raymond Adelman

I. The problem

A. Definitions [1, 2]

1. **Asymptomatic (covert) bacteriuria (ABU)** is found in an asymptomatic child with two properly obtained, clean-voided urine cultures growing 10^5 colonies or more per milliliter of a single organism; a catheterized urine growing more than 10^3 colonies per milliliter; or a suprapubic tap growing any colonies.
2. **Urinary tract infection (UTI)** is found in a symptomatic child with a properly obtained, clean-voided urine culture growing 10^5 colonies or more per milliliter of a single organism; a catheterized urine growing more than 10^3 colonies per milliliter; or a suprapubic tap growing any colonies.

B. Description.
The spectrum of UTI in children includes asymptomatic bacteriuria, uncomplicated UTI (lower tract infection), and complicated UTI (upper tract infection) [1, 2].

ABU in children is common; often recurrent, it may lead to symptomatic UTI and may be the first clue to an underlying urinary tract abnormality [2, 3]. However, most of the children with ABU show no sequelae, and hypertension or end-stage renal disease are uncommon consequences.

1. **Etiology.** Gram-negative enteric bacteria are the most common organisms causing bacteriuria [3, 4], with *Escherichia coli* accounting for 80% [3]. Other organisms, seen especially in neonates and in children with urinary tract abnormalities, are *Proteus* (common in boys), *Klebsiella, Pseudomonas, Enterobacter, Staphylococcus aureus* and *albus, Streptococcus viridans, Enterococcus,* and *Candida* [3, 4]. Although ABU is usually caused by a single organism, multiple organisms may be present in children with urinary tract abnormalities.
2. **Pathophysiology.** Bacteria usually ascend the urinary tract following perineal colonization; neonatal bacteriuria is often hematogenous [1, 3].

   The short female urethra and its proximity to fecal flora may in part explain the increased susceptibility of girls to bacteriuria [1, 4]. Sexual intercourse increases the risk of bacteriuria in adolescent girls [1]. Instrumentation of the urinary tract, prolonged catheter drainage, obstruction, and urinary stasis predispose to bacteriuria [1, 3].

   Defense mechanisms protecting against bacterial growth in the urinary tract include low and high urinary pH, high urinary osmolality, complete bladder emptying, phagocytosis, and secretory IgA secretion by the bladder mucosa [3, 5].

   Bacterial adherence through attachment of bacterial fimbriae to glycolipids on the surface of uroepithelial cells is of great importance in the genesis and severity of UTI [5, 6]. Fimbriated strains of *E. coli* are present in 94% of children with pyelonephritis versus 14% of children with ABU [6].

C. Epidemiology.
The incidence of ABU varies with age, sex, and diagnostic criteria employed. The prevalence of ABU in the neonate ranges from 1% in the full-term infant to 3% in the premature infant [3]. In the neonatal age group males predominate, whereas females predominate afterward.

The prevalence of ABU is 1% of preschool children, 1.2–1.8% of schoolgirls, and 0.03% of schoolboys [2, 3]. In girls the risk of acquiring bacteriuria is 5–10% during the school years [2].

Bacteriuria is much more common in children with urinary tract abnormalities, renal stones, and indwelling catheters.

D. Sequelae.
Bacteriuria in schoolgirls is associated with increased risk of recurrent symptomatic infections [7], in which renal parenchymal infection and renal scarring are well established complications [2, 5]. Hypertension or renal insufficiency, however, are unusual [7]. In 20–30% of school-age girls with ABU, radiologic evaluation will demon-

strate upper urinary tract damage or vesicoureteral reflux, or both [7, 8]. However, most of the kidney damage occurs before 5 years of age [8]. Prospective studies of schoolgirls over 5 years of age with ABU have failed to demonstrate reduced glomerular filtration rate (GFR), impaired renal growth, or progressive kidney damage in kidneys that are normal at the outset, even when vesicoureteral reflux is present and bacteriuria is left untreated [8, 10].

About 50% of neonates and infants with ABU will have evidence of urinary tract abnormality [2, 11]. Neonatal bacteriuria, particularly if associated with anatomic defects, may result in renal scarring, rapidly developing renal atrophy, and renal insufficiency [2, 5]. To reduce the risk of renal damage, diagnosis and treatment of bacteriuria in neonates and infants must be prompt. Bacteriuria in males beyond infancy is also associated with a very high incidence of urinary tract abnormalities [12].

E. Risk groups. The children who are at risk of bacteriuria and subsequent renal damage are premature infants discharged from the neonatal intensive care unit; females under the age of 5 years with a history of bacteriuria; children with constipation [13]; children with a family history of urinary tract infections or anomalies; and children with urinary tract abnormalities.

II. Secondary prevention

A. Early detection

1. Methods

a. Proteinuria, hematuria, and pyuria may occur with bacteriuria but are not diagnostic.

b. Bacteriuria. The presence of bacteria, when an unspun, air-dried, gram-stained urine sample is examined under oil immersion and high-power microscopy, highly correlates with significant bacteriuria.

c. Chemical screening tests. Several simple, nonexpensive, and rapid methods have been developed for the screening and detection of bacteriuria [14]. The "Chemstrip" is a chemical test that combines the determination of nitrite and leucocyte esterase found in the presence of bacteria in the urine, but it has the disadvantage of low specificity [15].

d. Slide cultures. The most suitable and recommended method for office and home use is the "Dipslide:" this culture technique, consisting of an agar-coated slide, is an excellent alternative to the standard culture, yielding high rates of sensitivity and specificity [14].

e. Standard cultures. In every suspected case, a positive standard urine culture that is properly obtained is essential for the diagnosis of bacteriuria [1]. A positive culture (more than 10^5 colonies per milliliter of a single organism) has an 80% diagnostic reliability in a female and a 95% reliability in a male (less contamination). Two positive cultures in a female carry 95% diagnostic reliability [1, 2]. In infants and toddlers the confidence level for a single positive culture from a specimen collected in a plastic bag is low [16], unless careful attention is given to technique. With a catheterized urine specimen, significant bacterial counts generally exceed 10^3 colonies per milliliter, and with a suprapubic tap, any number of colonies is diagnostic [1].

False-positive urine cultures occur with poor collection of urine, vaginal discharge (especially in the adolescent female), and storage of urine at room temperature. False-negative cultures or cultures yielding low colony counts are due to dilute urines (afternoon specimen or postdiuretics), partial treatment with antibiotics, extremely acid urine contamination of the collection jar with cleaning solution, and complete ureteral obstruction. Growth of mixed bacteria in urine culture, in the absence of urologic abnormality, usually indicates contamination.

A urine culture should be obtained to detect possible bacteriuria in every child with fever of unknown origin, particularly those under 2 years of age.

f. Renal ultrasound and voiding cystourethrogram. Every child under 5 years of age with bacteriuria should have a renal ultrasound and voiding cystourethrogram (VCUG) performed to evaluate for possible anatomic abnormalities. An intravenous pyelogram (IVP) is usually indicated if the ultrasound or VCUG are abnormal. Bacteriuria in male children after infancy is very uncommon. Bacteriuria detected in a male child at any age may signify a structural urinary tract abnormality and calls for prompt treatment and radiologic evaluation [17]. Special attention should be paid to premature infants in whom bacteriuria and urinary tract abnormalities are common.

Children in whom radiologic evaluation reveals mild-to-moderate reflux need no further workup, whereas children with massive reflux or obstruction should be referred for further urological evaluation.

2. **Justification.** Screening for ABU in children is very controversial. Although bacteriuria in schoolgirls rarely leads to end-stage renal disease or hypertension, it is not an entirely benign condition and may signify an underlying urinary tract abnormality or may result in recurrent symptomatic UTIs [7]. The main drawbacks to screening schoolgirls for bacteriuria, however, are: (1) the large population that must be screened to detect 1–2% with persistent bacteriuria; (2) the observation that in 0.2–0.5% of the schoolgirl population with a radiologically demonstrable anatomic abnormality, most of the kidney damage has already occurred before the age of 5 years and does not progress afterward; and (3) the uncertainty about the need for treatment of schoolgirls with ABU [8, 10].

   Bacteriuria in infancy is often associated with urinary tract abnormality and carries a high risk of intrarenal damage [2, 5]. However, screening infants for ABU is not recommended, mainly because of the difficulties of obtaining an adequate urine specimen in this age group. The only group of children that should be screened (with an annual or semiannual Dipslide test or standard urine culture) are the children at risk to have bacteriuria or renal damage (see sec. **I.E**). Mass screening of children for bacteriuria is unwarranted until an accurate and noninvasive method is devised to detect those with urinary tract abnormalities or renal scarring.

B. Early intervention

1. **Methods.** The approach to treatment of bacteriuria in children depends on age, presence of urinary tract abnormalities, and the patient's compliance. We treat children with ABU if they are less than 5 years of age, have a urinary tract abnormality, or tend to develop symptomatic UTIs.

   a. **Antibiotics.** The antibiotics usually used in the treatment of bacteriuria are amoxicillin or ampicillin, nitrofurantoin, sulfisoxazole, trimethoprim-sulfamethoxazole (Bactrim), and cephalosporins. Bacteriuria usually responds to treatment within 24–48 hours, as evidenced by a negative Gram's stain of the uncentrifuged urine specimen, a negative Dipslide, and a sterile urine. Pyuria may persist for a few days and does not indicate failure of response. Failure of the patient to respond suggests noncompliance, poor absorption of drugs, bacterial resistance, improper dosage, or underlying structural defect, indicating the need for prompt radiologic evaluation [3].

      Bacteriuria is usually treated for 7–10 days. Successful treatment of ABU and uncomplicated UTI has been reported with single-dose or 3-day therapy with amoxicillin (50 mg/kg), trimethoprim-sulfamethoxazole (50 mg/kg), or nitrofurantoin [3, 18], although recurrence rates may be higher [2]. The advantages of short-course therapy are: better compliance, fewer side effects, and cost savings. However, the efficacy of short-course therapy in children with bacteriuria has not been fully established, and we reserve it for children with low compliance.

      A urine culture should be taken 3–7 days after completion of therapy to detect a relapse. In addition, in children at risk with ABU, two to three urine cultures per year should be obtained in order to detect recurrences, which are common.

      Recurrent episodes of symptomatic or asymptomatic bacteriuria can be prevented by the prophylactic use of trimethoprim-sulfamethoxazole (10 mg/kg/day), or nitrofurantoin (1–2 mg/kg/day), both of which are effective and have few side effects [2, 19]. Antibiotic prophylaxis may be continued anywhere from 6 months to 2 years, or longer if necessary. However, prophylactic therapy should be reserved for children under 5 years of age with vesicoureteral reflux, scarring, or other urinary tract abnormalities, and for children at any age with more than three documented bacteriuria episodes per year.

   b. **General measures.** Other suggested therapeutic maneuvers for treatment of bacteriuria include increased fluid intake, complete bladder emptying, and proper hygiene.

   c. **Surgery.** Since mild-to-moderate reflux usually disappears with increasing age, surgery is not indicated if repeat urine cultures, ultrasound of kidneys every 1–2 years to detect hydronephrosis or impaired kidney growth, and long-term prophylactic therapy can be maintained [20]. Ureteral reimplantation may be indicated with more severe vesicoureteral reflux, uncontrolled infection, and progressive scarring. There is no evidence that urethral dilatation, meatotomy, or urethrostomy reduces the incidence of bacteriuria [3].

2. **Justification.** Prompt treatment of bacteriuria, especially in infants and young children with reflux or other urologic abnormalities, is extremely important since delay increases the risk of renal parenchymal scarring [5].

Several investigations have questioned the need for the treatment of ABU in schoolgirls. The objections raised were: (1) treatment only reduces the duration of bacteriuria and has no effect on the emergence of symptoms, clearance of vesicoureteral reflux, kidney function, kidney growth, or the progression of renal scars [8–10]; (2) short-course therapy may eliminate organisms of low virulence, but it may precipitate, rather than prevent, symptomatic infections from more virulent bacteria [17]; and (3) there is the possibility of side effects associated with long-term antibiotic administration.

III. Recommendations

A. Early detection

1. Early diagnosis and radiologic evaluation for urinary tract abnormalities, and treatment of ABU in infants and young children is of crucial importance.
2. Routine screening of most children for bacteriuria is not recommended until a noninvasive method can be developed to detect those with urinary tract abnormalities or renal scarring.
3. Screening for ABU using a semiannual or annual Dipslide or standard urine culture should be performed on children at high risk for bacteriuria and subsequent renal damage (see sec. **I.E**).
4. Bacteriuria can be tentatively diagnosed by examining a clean, uncentrifuged urine specimen under high-power microscopy for the presence of bacteria, with or without Gram's staining.
5. At least two properly obtained cultures should be obtained to confirm the diagnosis of ABU. The urine should be a clean-voided midstream specimen from a properly prepped child.
6. The diagnosis of bacteriuria in infants should not be based only on a urine culture collected in a plastic bag, the confidence level of which is low, especially if improperly obtained.
7. Suprapubic aspiration of urine is a safe procedure even in neonates and is the most accurate method for the diagnosis of bacteriuria. Sterile bladder catheterization is also a reliable method.
8. If a urine specimen cannot be plated within a short time, it should be refrigerated at 5 °C and plated within 48 hours.
9. Indications for renal ultrasound and VCUG are: first bacteriuria in any male child, first bacteriuria in any child less than 5 years of age, first bacteriuria in a child with a family history of UTI or anomalies, and recurrent bacteriuria in any female child.

B. Prevention/treatment

1. Antibiotic therapy should be given to children with ABU if they are less than 5 years of age, have a urinary tract abnormality, or tend to develop symptomatic UTIs.
2. Antibiotic therapy of bacteriuria is usually of 7–10 days' duration. Short-course therapy can occasionally be used in children with low compliance.
3. Every child at risk with a history of bacteriuria should be followed up by performing two to three urine cultures per year.
4. Surgical intervention is not indicated in a child with mild-to-moderate vesicoureteral reflux if repeat urine cultures, ultrasound of the kidneys every 1–2 years, and prophylactic therapy can be maintained.
5. The child with bacteriuria and massive reflux should be referred for further urologic evaluation. Ureteral reimplantation may be indicated.
6. Urethral dilatation, meatotomy, or urethrostomy, are of no benefit in reducing the incidence of bacteriuria.
7. Prophylactic antibiotic therapy is recommended for children under 5 years of age with vesicoureteral reflux, scarring, or other urinary tract abnormalities; and for children with three or more documented bacteriuria episodes in 1 year.

References

1. Kunin, C. M. *Detection, Prevention and Management of Urinary Tract Infections* (4th ed.). Philadelphia: Lea & Febiger, 1987. *A comprehensive book on UTI.*

2. Ogra, P. L., and Faden, H. S. Urinary tract infections in childhood: An update. *J. Pediatr.* 106(6):1023, 1985. *An updated analysis of UTI in children.*
3. Adelman, R. D. Urinary Tract Infections in Children. In B. M. Tune and S. A. Mendoza (eds.). *Pediatric Nephrology.* New York: Churchill Livingstone, 1984. P. 155. *A comprehensive review of UTI in childhood.*
4. Naylor, G. R. A 16-month analysis of urinary tract infection in children. *J. Med. Microbiol.* 17(1):31, 1984. *A bacteriologic study of UTI in children.*
5. Winberg, J., et al. Clinical pyelonephritis and focal renal scarring. A selected review of pathogenesis, prevention and prognosis. *Pediatr. Clin. North Am.* 29(4):801, 1982. *A review of pathogenesis, prevention, and prognosis of UTI in children.*
6. Harber, M. J., and Asscher, A. W. Virulence of urinary pathogens. *Kidney Int.* 28(5):717, 1985. *A review of bacterial pathogenic factors in UTI.*
7. Gillenwater, J. Y., Harrison, R. B., and Kunin, C. M. Natural history of bacteriuria in schoolgirls. A long-term case-control study. *N. Engl. J. Med.* 301(8):396, 1979. *A prospective study of the natural history of bacteriuria in schoolgirls.*
8. Sequelae of covert bacteriuria in schoolgirls. A four-year follow-up study. Cardiff-Oxford Bacteriuria Study Group. *Lancet* 1(8070):889, 1978. *A prospective study of the sequelae of ABU in schoolgirls.*
9. Covert bacteriuria in schoolgirls in Newcastle upon Tyne: A 5-year followup. *Arch. Dis. Child.* 56(8):585, 1981. *A prospective study of the natural history of ABU in schoolgirls.*
10. Jones, K. V., et al. Renal functional changes in schoolgirls with covert asymptomatic bacteriuria. *Contrib. Nephrol.* 39:152, 1984. *A prospective study of renal function in schoolgirls with ABU.*
11. Siegel, S. R., et al. Urinary infections in infants and preschool children: Five-year followup. *Am. J. Dis. Child.* 134(4):369, 1980. *A prospective epidemiologic study of UTI in preschool children.*
12. Cohen, M. The first urinary tract infection in male children. *Am. J. Dis. Child.* 130(8):810, 1976. A prospective epidemiologic study of UTI in boys.
13. Regan, S., Yazbeck, S., and Schick, E. Constipation, bladder instability, and urinary tract infection syndrome. *Clin. Nephrol.* 23(3):152, 1985. *A study of the association of constipation with urinary tract infection.*
14. Durbin, W. A., Jr, and Peter, G. Management of urinary tract infections in infants and children. *Pediatr. Infect. Dis.* 3(6):564, 1984. *A review of diagnosis and management of UTIs in children.*
15. Barlett, R. C., O'Neill, D., and McLaughlin, J. C. Detection of bacteriuria by leucocyte esterase, nitrite and the automicrobic system. *Am. J. Clin. Pathol.* 82(6):683, 1984. *A study of chemical screening tests of bacteriuria.*
16. Aronson, A. S., Gustafson, B., and Svenningsen, N. W. Combined suprapubic aspiration and clear-voided urine examination in infants and children. *Acta Paediatr. Scand.* 62(4):396, 1973. *A comparative study of the diagnosis of UTI in children.*
17. Dodge, W. F. Cost effectiveness of renal disease screening. *Am. J. Dis. Child.* 131(11):1274, 1977. *A comprehensive review of screening of renal disease.*
18. Fine, J. S., and Jacobson, M. S. Single-dose versus conventional therapy of urinary tract infections in female adolescents. *Pediatrics* 75(5):916, 1985. *A study and a review of the literature on single-dose therapy of UTI in children.*
19. Stamey, T. A., Condy, M., and Mihara, G. Prophylactic efficacy of nitrofurantoin macrocrystals and trimethoprim-sulfamethoxazole in urinary infections. Biologic effects on the vaginal and rectal flora. *N. Engl. J. Med.* 296(14):780, 1977. *A study of prophylactic antibiotic therapy in UTI.*
20. Aladjem, M., et al. The conservative management of vesicoureteric reflux: A review of 121 children. *Pediatrics* 65(1):78, 1980. *A report on the natural history of conservatively managed reflux in children.*

49 Hypertension in Children

Israel Zelikovic and
Raymond Adelman

I. The problem

A. Definition. Hypertension is the presence of systolic and/or diastolic blood pressure levels persistently above the 90–95th percentile for any given age [1, 2] (Figs. 49-1, 49-2, and 49-3).

B. Description. Hypertension is an important problem in childhood and infancy. Although a secondary cause is found in most hypertensive children, essential hypertension does occur, especially after puberty [3, 4]. As in the adult, abnormalities in the renin-angiotensin system, the sympathetic nervous system, or extracellular fluid, or all three, are the major pathophysiologic factors underlying childhood hypertension [5]. The important causes of acute and chronic hypertension in children are listed in Tables 49-1 and 49-2.

Chronic renal disease accounts for nearly 80% of secondary hypertension in children [6]. Chronic pyelonephritis, obstructive uropathy, and glomerulonephritis are the most common causes. In acute childhood hypertension, the most common renal diseases are acute poststreptococcal glomerulonephritis, hemolytic-uremic syndrome, and Henoch-Schönlein purpura [7].

Renal vascular disease causes 5–20% of secondary hypertension [7, 8]. In children, renal artery stenosis due to fibromuscular dysplasia is the most common cause; in neonates it is renal artery thrombosis secondary to the use of umbilical artery catheters [9]. Coarctation of the aorta is the most common surgically correctable vascular cause of hypertension in children.

Drugs associated with elevated blood pressure include tobacco, sympathomimetics, oral contraceptives, amphetamines, glucocorticoids, and cyclosporine. Endocrine and metabolic causes of hypertension are uncommon but should be considered. Although little is known about the etiology and pathophysiology of childhood essential hypertension and its evolution into adult hypertension, genetic predisposition, obesity, and high sodium and low potassium intake appear important [3, 4].

C. Epidemiology. The incidence of hypertension in the pediatric age group is roughly 1% [10], depending on the methods of the study and the definition of hypertension selected. Blood pressure rises with chronologic age, but it is better correlated with body mass, height, or degree of sexual maturation [10, 11]. A heavier, taller, and more sexually mature child is more likely to have a higher blood pressure. A higher incidence of hypertension is noted in black children [11].

The younger the child and the higher the blood pressure, the more likely a secondary cause will be found [4, 12]. Neonates discharged from neonatal intensive care units, especially those with a history of umbilical artery catheterization or bronchopulmonary dysplasia, have a high incidence of hypertension [9, 13]. Other risk groups for developing secondary hypertension are children with renal disease, those who have undergone organ transplantation [14], and those receiving drugs that may elevate blood pressure. Essential hypertension is more commonly recognized in adolescence, although it may begin earlier [3]. At risk for developing essential hypertension are children who are obese, have a family history of essential hypertension, and "track" at the upper quartile or quintile. A clear correlation exists between high blood pressure readings in adolescence and adult hypertension [15].

Most hypertensive children are asymptomatic. The child with severe hypertension may present with headaches, visual disturbances, malaise, Bell's palsy, convulsions, abdominal pain, or vomiting. Failure to thrive, irritability, personality changes, and poor performance in school have also been attributed to hypertension [10]. The consequences of severe hypertension in children are similar to those observed in adults: cerebrovascular accidents, renal damage, and congestive heart failure. Left ventricular hypertrophy and fundoscopic vascular changes may be seen.

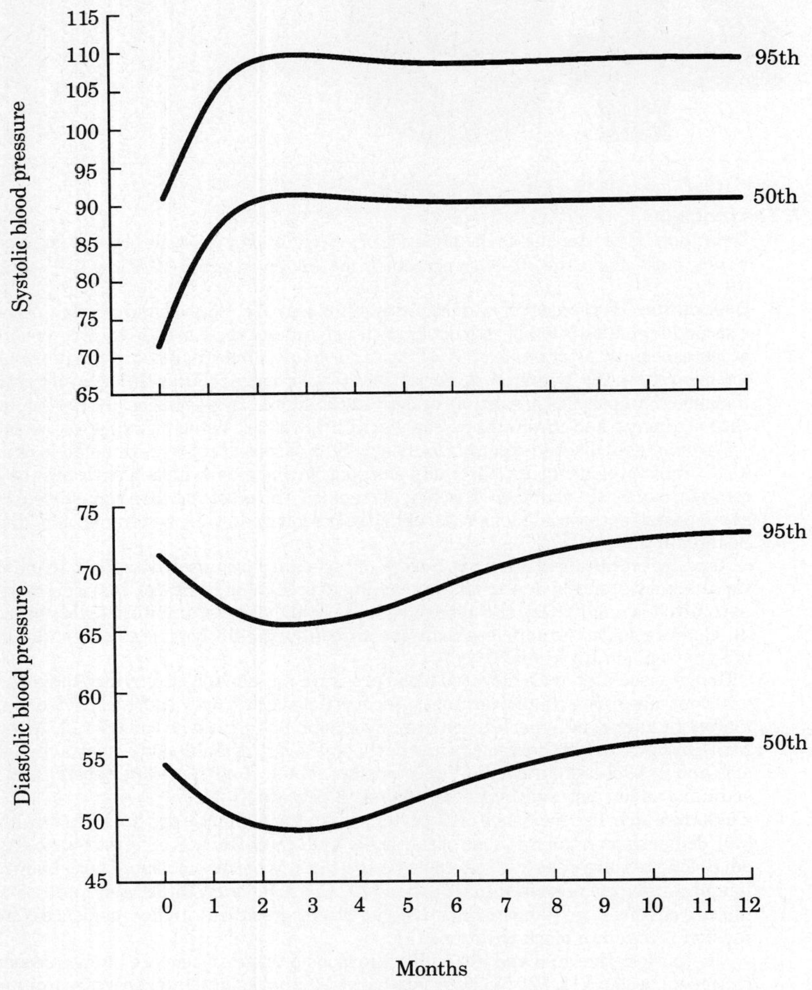

Fig. 49-1. Blood pressure percentiles for boys and girls from birth to 12 months. Korotkoff phase IV is used for diastolic blood pressure. (Adapted from Report of the Second Task Force on Blood Pressure Control in Children. *Pediatrics* 79(1):1, 1987.)

Fig. 49-2. A. Blood pressure percentiles for boys, 1-13 years of age. B. Blood pressure percentiles for girls, 1–13 years of age. Korotkoff phase IV is used for diastolic blood pressure. (Adapted from Report of the Second Task Force on Blood Pressure Control in Children. *Pediatrics* 79(1):1, 1987.)

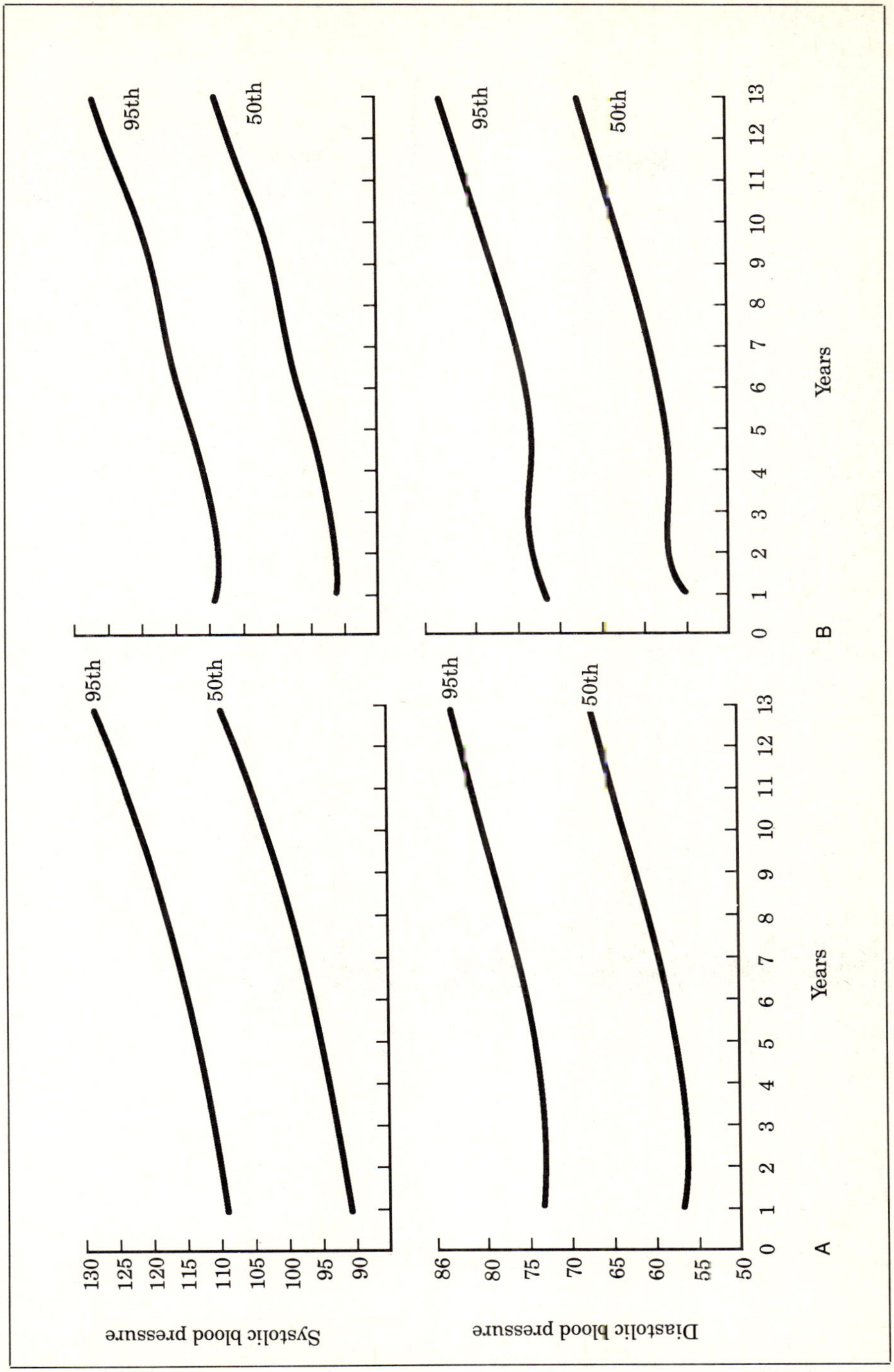
Systolic blood pressure
Diastolic blood pressure
95th
50th
Years
A
B

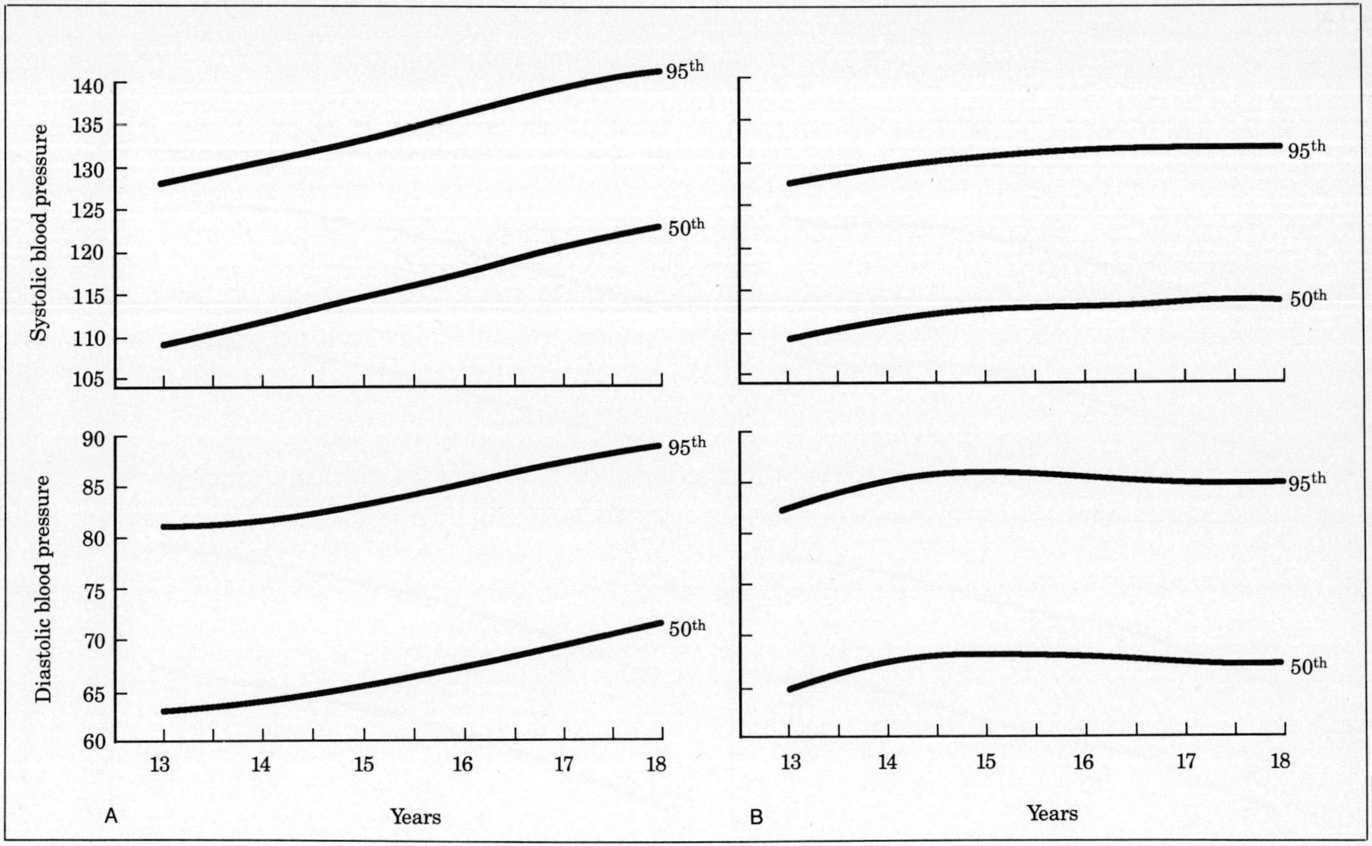

Fig. 49-3. A. Blood pressure percentiles for boys, 13–18 years of age. B. Blood pressure percentiles for girls, 13–18 of age. Korotkoff phase V is used for diastolic blood pressure. (Adapted from Report of the Second Task Force on Blood Pressure Control in Children. *Pediatrics* 79(1):1, 1987.)

Table 49-1. Causes of chronic hypertension in infants and children

Etiology	Common	Uncommon
Renal	Chronic pyelonephritis Chronic glomerulonephritis Obstructive uropathy Post-renal transplantation Nephrocalcinosis	Alport's disease Neoplasm Radiation Collagen vascular disease
Renovascular	Renal artery stenosis Renal artery thrombosis	Renal vein thrombosis Neurofibromatosis
Cardiovascular	Coarctation of the aorta	
Endocrine		Pheochromocytoma Neuroblastoma Primary hyperadrenalism Ovarian tumors Adrenogenital syndrome
Metabolic		Hypercalcemia Hypernatremia
Drugs and toxins	Steroids Oral contraceptives Theophylline Amphetamines Sympathomimetics (ephedrine, etc.) Tobacco Cyclosporine	Heavy metals (mercury, lead)
Neurologic	Increased intracranial pressure (any cause)	Guillain-Barré Dysautonomia (Riley-Day)
Miscellaneous	Essential	Turner syndrome

Table 49-2. Causes of acute hypertension in infants and children

Renal
- Acute postinfectious glomerulonephritis
- Hemolytic uremic syndrome
- Henoch-Schönlein purpura
- Systemic lupus erythematosus
- Membranoproliferative glomerulonephritis
- Chronic pyelonephritis
- After genitourinary surgery
- After renal transplantation
- After blood transfusion to child with azotemia
- Renovascular disease

Nonrenal
- Elevated intracranial pressure (any cause)
- Blood pressure-elevating drugs and toxins
- Burns
- Guillain-Barré syndrome
- Familial dysautonomia
- Essential hypertension
- Traction

II. Secondary prevention

A. Early detection

1. **Methods.** Indirect auscultation sphygmomanometry is the most common method for measuring blood pressure in children. Appropriate cuff selection is essential [16]. The width of the bladder within the cuff should cover at least two-thirds of the length of the upper arm, and the length of the bladder should encircle at least three-fourths of the upper arm. A small cuff results in spuriously high blood pressure measurements. In a sitting child, the elbow should be at the level of the heart; blood pressure readings are higher when measured on a dependent arm.

   The fourth Korotkoff phase (muffling of sounds) is regarded as the best index of diastolic blood pressure in children.

   Other methods for blood pressure measurement in children are: Doppler ultrasound, oscillometry, and direct recording through an arterial line, as commonly used in intensive care units. The palpation and the flush technique are only rough estimates of blood pressure and are not widely used. Hypertension is diagnosed only when repeated blood pressure measurements in a resting child are elevated.

   Diagnostic evaluation of the hypertensive child should start with a complete patient and family history and a careful physical examination (including auscultation for abdominal bruit and blood pressure readings in all four limbs to rule out coarctation of the aorta). Initial laboratory tests include urinalysis and culture, complete blood count, serum creatinine, blood urea nitrogen, electrolytes, calcium, phosphorus, chest x-ray, electrocardiogram, and renal ultrasonography. The best cardiac marker of the effect of chronic hypertension in children is the presence of left ventricular hypertrophy on echocardiogram [16].

   Additional studies are individualized [4, 12] and may include renal radionuclide scan, intravenous pyelogram, voiding cystogram, plasma renin activity, urinary catecholamine and steroid metabolites, renal vein renin, renal biopsy, and renal arteriography or digital subtraction angiography.

B. Early intervention.

There is no doubt that severe hypertension in children requires prompt treatment. However, it is not always clear at the outset whether mild-to-moderate hypertension will have serious consequences later in life and whether such consequences will be mitigated by early intervention [10]. Moreover, the long-term effects of antihypertensive drugs on the growth and development of children have not been clearly established.

Generally, treatment of childhood hypertension should be approached in phases [4, 11]. An asymptomatic child with mild hypertension is initially treated with salt restriction and a program for weight loss and controlled exercise.

Pharmacologic therapy in mild hypertension should be initiated with chlorothiazide (10–40 mg/kg/day) or hydrochlorothiazide (2–4 mg/kg/day). A potent loop diuretic like furosemide should be administered only in the presence of reduced renal function or volume overload, or both. The next step is the addition of a vasodilator like hydralazine (1–5 mg/kg/day) or a beta-blocker like propranolol (1–5 mg/kg/day). Captopril (0.3–5 mg/kg/day), an angiotensin I converting enzyme inhibitor, is an effective hypotensive agent in hyperreninemic states, but may cause a reversible decline in renal function [17].

Vasodilators like minoxidil and prazosin, central-acting drugs like clonidine, and sympathetic inhibitors like reserpine and guanethidine should be reserved for severe resistant hypertension.

Acute elevation of blood pressure can be successfully treated with sublingual nifedipine 0.25–0.50 mg/kg; IV hydralazine 0.1–1.0 mg/kg; IV diazoxide 3–5 mg/kg; IM reserpine 0.07 mg/kg; or sodium nitroprusside infusion [7]. One must avoid acute and profound falls in blood pressure by initially employing the lower range of drug dosage.

Children with unilateral renovascular disease may be treated with percutaneous transluminal angioplasty, surgical correction [8], or medical management. Neonatal hypertension due to renal artery thrombosis usually responds to conservative medical management.

III. Recommendations

A. Early detection

1. Blood pressure should be routinely measured in high-risk infants from birth, and in all children from age 3 years onward.
2. Measurement of blood pressure should be performed by a trained person on a quiet, relaxed child, using an appropriate-size cuff, and, if the child is in a sitting position, with the arm at the heart level.

3. The fourth Korotkoff phase (muffling) should be used for determination of diastolic blood pressure.
4. Repeated blood pressure measurements in the office and at home are necessary to confirm the diagnosis of systemic hypertension
5. Blood pressure of children at risk of developing hypertension (see sec. **I.C.**,) should be measured at least every 6 months.
6. The work-up of the hypertensive child should be rational, sequential, and as noninvasive as possible.
7. The young child with severe hypertension should have earlier and more extensive evaluation for a secondary cause than an adolescent with mild hypertension in whom essential hypertension is more common.

B. Intervention/treatment

1. Severe hypertension should be promptly treated, pharmacologically or later, if indicated, surgically. Blood pressure should not be normalized immediately but initially lowered to a safe level.
2. Mild or moderate hypertension should be treated in a stepwise approach that includes (in order) weight loss, change in diet, exercise, diuretics, and finally, more potent antihypertensive drugs.
3. The hypertensive child and his or her family should be instructed and encouraged to monitor the blood pressure at home.
4. Hypertensive children and adolescents should avoid isometric exercise like weight lifting. If a stress test is normal, a controlled exercise program and even competitive sports can be recommended, under proper medical supervision.

References

1. Report of the Second Task Force on Blood Pressure Control in Children. *Pediatrics* 79(1):1, 1987. *A comprehensive review of pediatric hypertension, including blood pressure standards in children.*
2. DeSwiet, M., Fayers, P., and Shinebourne, E. A. Systolic blood pressure in a population of infants in the first year of life: The Brompton study. *Pediatrics* 65(5):1028, 1980. *Systolic blood pressure standards in infants in the first year of life*
3. Berenson, G. S., Cresanter, J. L., and Webber, L. S. High blood pressure in the young. *Annu. Rev. Med.* 35:535, 1984. *A focus on essential hypertension in children.*
4. Ingelfinger, J. R. *Pediatric Hypertension.* Philadelphia: Saunders, 1982. *A comprehensive text on pediatric hypertension.*
5. Bailie, M. D., and Mattioli, L. F. Hypertension: Relationships between pathophysiology and therapy. *J. Pediatr.* 96(5):789, 1980. *Review of pathophysiology and therapy of childhood hypertension.*
6. Londe, S. Causes of hypertension in the young. *Pediatr. Clin. North Am.* 25(1):55, 1978. *Reviews the etiologies of childhood hypertension.*
7. Balfe, J. W., and Rance, C. P. Recognition and management of hypertensive crises in childhood. *Pediatr. Clin. North Am.* 25(1):159, 1978. *Review of acute hypertension in children.*
8. Watson, A. R., Balfe, J. W., and Hardy, B. E. Renovascular hypertension in childhood: A changing perspective in management. *J. Pediatr.* 106(3):366, 1985. *Review of renovascular hypertension in children.*
9. Adelman, R. D. Neonatal hypertension. *Pediatr. Clin. North Am.* 25(1):99, 1978. *Review of neonatal hypertension.*
10. Portman, R. J., and Robson, A. M. Controversies in Pediatric Hypertension. In B. M. Tune and S. A. Mendoza (eds.), *Pediatric Nephrology.* New York: Churchill-Livingstone, 1984. Pp. 265–296. *Review of childhood hypertension.*
11. Voors, A. W., et al. Studies of blood pressures in children, ages 5–14 years, in a total biracial community: The Bogalusa heart study. *Circulation* 54(2):319, 1976. *Standards of blood pressure in children and determinants of blood pressure values.*
12. Mentser, M. Diagnosis and treatment of hypertension in children. *Pediatr. Clin. North Am.* 29(4):933, 1982. *Review of diagnosis and treatment of pediatric hypertension.*
13. Sheftel, D. N., Hustead, V., and Friedman, A. Hypertension screening in the follow-up of premature infants. *Pediatrics* 71(5):763, 1983. *Hypertension screening in premature infants.*
14. Waltzer, W. C., et al. Etiology and pathogenesis of hypertension following renal transplantation. *Nephron* 42(2):102, 1986. *A detailed review of hypertension after renal transplantation.*

15. Gruskin, A. B. The adolescent with essential hypertension. *Am. J. Kidney Dis.* 6(2):86, 1985. *Review of adolescent hypertension.*
16. Bailie, M. D., et al. A symposium: Hypertension: More than ever, a pediatric concern. *Contemp. Pediatr.* 2:30, 1985. *A discussion about clinical management of pediatric hypertension.*
17. Colavita, R. D., Gaudio, K. M., and Siegel, N. J. Reversible reduction in renal function during treatment with captopril. *Pediatrics* 71(5):839, 1983. *A report of side effects of captopril.*

50 Coronary Artery Disease Prevention in Infancy, Childhood, and Adolescence

Thomas A. Riemenschneider

I. The problem

A. Definition. Arteriosclerosis is a disease process involving the large- and medium-sized blood vessels throughout the body. Cholesterol and lipids are deposited in the intimal layer of the vessels in a progressive fashion, leading to the development of fibrous plaques that may eventually progress to cause obstruction of blood flow. Obstruction of coronary arteries may lead to myocardial infarction and chronic disability or death.

B. Description. Pathologic studies have demonstrated a progressive sequence of involvement of the coronary arteries, with onset early in life. Nonelevated deposits of fat (fatty streaks) are found in the aorta of many children by the age of 3 years, and the number of these lesions increases with age. Fatty streaks begin to appear in the coronary arteries during the second decade and are present in nearly everyone by the age of 20. The presence of these lesions has been correlated with the development of clinical coronary artery disease. Raised arterial lesions (fibrous plaques) are found during the second decade and have increased significantly both in number and size by the fourth decade of life. Studies now are defining the natural history of coronary artery disease in childhood as well. Postmortem studies on young adult males, casualties of battle in Korea and Vietnam, have demonstrated the presence of advanced coronary arteriosclerosis in a significant number of them. In later adult life, the plaques become complicated lesions—with ulceration, calcification, hemorrhage, and thrombosis—that have the potential to narrow the arterial lumen and cause obstruction of blood flow.

C. Epidemiology. Coronary artery disease is the leading cause of mortality in the United States, occurring more frequently than deaths from cancer and accidents (the second and third leading causes of death) combined. Each year, approximately 1 million people in the United States experience myocardial infarction or sudden coronary-artery-related death, or both. One out of five male children in the United States will develop clinical evidence of coronary heart disease before age 60. Approximately $65 billion was spent in the United States in 1986 for medical services, hospitalization, medications, and lost work output related to coronary artery disease.

1. **Risk factors.** Certain factors have been shown in adult epidemiologic studies to be associated with an increased risk of coronary artery disease. The risk increases significantly as the number of risk factors increases. These factors include the following.

   a. **Major risk factors**

   (1) **Hypercholesterolemia.** As in adults, data in children suggest a continuum of risk for the probability of developing coronary heart disease with increasing cholesterol levels, suggesting that the lowering of serum lipids may diminish this risk. For most children, the cholesterol level is affected primarily by environmental factors—of which dietary intake of cholesterol and saturated fats is a major component—and to a lesser degree by genetic factors. Only a small percentage of cases of hypercholesterolemia result from inherited hyperlipidemias, of which type II familial hypercholesterolemia is of greatest importance in the pediatric population. The Bogalusa study suggests that serum cholesterol levels are relatively stable during childhood, with a gradual increase occurring after 17 years of age [1]. Children with hypercholesterolemia have more relatives with an elevated serum cholesterol level and coronary mortality than children with normal cholesterol levels [2].

   (2) **Hypertension.** Adult studies confirm an increased risk of coronary heart disease in the presence of hypertension, which is reduced if the hypertension is controlled. The risk appears to be continuous, with higher blood pressures associated with increased coronary mortality. Recent studies in children have established normal values for blood pressure by age and sex

[3], and suggested a true frequency of 1–3% of primary hypertension [4, 5]. Blood pressure in children undergoes a rather continuous rise with growth, with some acceleration of this rise during adolescence.

(3) **Smoking.** Smoking has been shown to be a major independent risk factor for coronary artery disease, with both the duration and quantity of smoking contributing to the risk. The highest risk is found in those who began smoking before the age of 20. Initiation of smoking in children and adolescents appears to be related to the smoking habits of parents and siblings and to the peer pressure encountered in school and social settings.

b. Minor risk factors

(1) **Sedentary living habits.** The effect of regular exercise, leading to physical conditioning, is not clearly established, but it may exert a beneficial effect on major risk factors, thus indirectly impacting on the incidence of coronary heart disease. Our society encourages a sedentary lifestyle, with increasing use of the automobile and viewing of television. The Saskatchewan Child Health Study has demonstrated a decrease in parameters of physical fitness with increasing age—coincident with entry into school [6].

(2) **Obesity.** A weak association has been demonstrated between obesity and coronary artery disease—overweight individuals tend to have higher serum cholesterol, hypertension, and carbohydrate intolerance, and to lead a sedentary life. Once a particular weight range is achieved in childhood, it is difficult to alter; childhood obesity is thus likely to become adult obesity [7].

(3) **Hyperglycemia.** A relationship has been demonstrated between diabetes and premature arteriosclerosis. Unfortunately, preliminary data do not suggest that control of the diabetes diminishes the risk of coronary heart disease.

(4) **Psychosocial tension.** Some studies indicate a relationship between individual response to stress and the risk of coronary artery disease, with those exhibiting classic type A behavior said to be at special risk. We are aware also that adult behavior patterns are established in infancy and childhood and are influenced by parental attitudes.

(5) **Family history.** Individuals with a positive family history of premature (occurring at less than 50 years of age) coronary heart disease are at increased risk to develop coronary artery disease. The risk is greatest when the disease is present in first-order relatives. This relationship may represent familial patterns of other risk factors—hypercholesterolemia, smoking, hypertension, and obesity, as well as genetic differences in anatomy and metabolism of coronary arteries.

II. Primary prevention and health promotion

A. Methods. The primary care providers should be outspoken advocates for the principles of a healthy life-style for all, with emphasis on proper nutrition and eating patterns, regular physical activity, and discouragement of smoking. Primary care providers are viewed by the community as important sources of information about health and thus can do much to influence public opinion about life-styles and behaviors in many different settings, including the office practice, the school system, the home, and the community. The primary care provider should be aware that he or she serves as a role model to patients, families, and the community; thus the practice of a healthy life-style by the provider has a profound influence on all those with whom he or she comes in contact.

1. **Office practice.** In the office, the primary care provider can take advantage of many opportunities to provide health education, influence the development of healthy life-styles, and prevent the development of risk factors. As part of history-taking and the physical examination of all patients, the primary care provider and the nurse can explain why he or she is asking about family history, why bood pressure determination is important, and what the relationship of nutrition and obesity are as height and weight are checked. Increasing numbers of health-related pamphlets, brochures, charts, posters, videotapes, and even computerized information are available from public organizations such as the American Heart Association, American Dietetic Association, American Cancer Society, U.S. Government Printing Office, and so on. Most of these materials are free or of minimal expense and can be made available in the office setting.

The primary care provider should begin to educate new mothers—since they will have the earliest influence on the development of health habits in children—at the time of or even before the infant's birth. Health information should include the effect of smoking on the fetus and the newborn; proper nutrition and relationship to obesity (caloric intake); prevention of hypertension (salt intake); prevention of heart disease (cholesterol and saturated fat intake); and importance of establishing a lifelong physically active life-style. The provider should emphasize repeatedly how important the parents' influence is in the establishment of healthy life-styles in their children.

The primary care provider should begin to direct efforts at health education to the child as well as the mother. Areas of importance include making personal choices of healthy life-styles, dealing with peer pressure, need for an active life-style, proper nutrition, and avoidance of smoking. Some excellent commercially available programs are successfully educating preschoolers about heart health (e.g., *The Heart Treasure Chest,* American Heart Association, 1985).

2. **School education programs.** Within the school system, the primary care provider should advocate the introduction of principles of preventive cardiology into the curriculum. Excellent prepared resources geared to children of specific ages are available through the American Heart Association. These materials can be presented by the teacher, with assistance from the school nurse. The primary care provider can also participate in these programs, emphasizing important points and supplementing the materials. The provider can urge, through PTA groups and school administrators, that proper nutrition be taught in the lunchroom through: (1) provision of nutritionally balanced meals; (2) labeling the nutritional value of foods; and (3) removal or reduction of "junk" foods in vending machines and replacing them with fruits, fruit juices, and other nutritional snacks.

   The primary care provider and the school system should emphasize the negative long-term consequences of smoking. Because the effects of smoking are delayed, the adolescent may feel little concern for their impact and have the misconception that smoking can be stopped at any time. An alarming development is the rapid increase in teenage female smokers. Unfortunately, studies suggest that only 20–40% of smokers who try to stop smoking do so successfully. Thus, efforts to prevent adolescents from taking up the habit are of major importance. Parental, sibling, and peer pressures are the most important factors in the decision to start smoking. Thus, antismoking programs in the schools that emphasize positive peer pressure to enhance the nonsmoking image, and negative peer pressure to discourage smoking, appear to be particularly beneficial.

   An article in *Sports Illustrated* emphasized the poor physical condition of our youth despite the "fitness boom"; this boom is being enjoyed largely by middle class adults [8]. Recent cutbacks in educational funding have compromised physical education programs in the school system. The primary care provider should advocate programs of regular physical activity in the school system, with emphasis on activities that develop physical and cardiovascular fitness and teach individual sports activities that may be continued throughout a lifetime.

   The impact of Title IX legislation on the physical activity pattern of females has been profound, and the primary care provider should advocate increasing the participation of girls in school physical education activities. In addition to the direct effect on the generation of females participating, we can anticipate additional benefits to future generations, since the increased physical activity of mothers in the family will promote increased activity in their offspring.

3. **Community education programs.** In the general community, the primary care provider occupies a position of respect and influence, and he or she will have many opportunities to speak out to educate the public regarding coronary artery disease and risk factors. Through participation in activities of groups such as the American Heart Association and speaking at public forums, on television, on radio, and through the newspapers, the provider can bring the message of heart disease prevention to the lay public. The provider and his or her family can also educate the community by becoming advocates of a healthy life-style, and by demonstrating principles of proper nutrition, nonsmoking behavior, weight control, and vigorous physical activity.

B. Justification

1. **Cost to the primary care provider** for his or her role in education consists of a commitment of time devoted to organization, teacher training, and participation. The costs are balanced by the satisfaction of participation. We are presently in a period of great interest and public awareness of the concepts of a healthy life-style and a desire for further knowledge. Thus, the chances of public acceptance of principles of prevention are great.
2. **School and community education programs.** Follow-up analyses of community

and school education programs, such as the Chicago Heart Association's Body Power Program [9], demonstrate both an increase in knowledge regarding prevention and a change in attitudes and behaviors. Costs to the school are minimal, including time for teacher training and a minimal charge to cover the cost of printing of materials by the Heart Association. While demands on teacher time are constantly increasing, we have found great enthusiasm among educators for well-organized programs in prevention of heart disease that are supported by in-service teacher training and well-developed resources.

III. Secondary prevention

A. Early detection of those at high risk

1. Methods

a. Community screening programs. While mass screening of children for risk factors for coronary heart disease has been advocated by some, the benefits of such programs in this author's opinion are outweighed by the costs in time, personnel, and logistics of implementation. Furthermore, depending on the ages and circumstances of the population to be screened, the incidence of risk factors may be minimal. For example, the identification of children with abnormally elevated blood pressure will finally be as low as 1–3% [4], after multiple determinations of pressure have been obtained. Additional problems arise related to the determination of which children need follow-up and in assuring that follow-up evaluation is accomplished.

b. Screening in the practice setting. A more efficient and effective method of "screening" can be achieved in the office practice setting as part of a program of prevention and health-promoting education of children and their parents. Under these circumstances, the primary care provider can have a significant impact on families, with a minimum of expense in time and money. Through the use of posters, printed handouts, and videotapes, supplemented by nurse and primary care provider counseling, the concepts of proper nutrition and exercise and the discouragement of smoking can be related to the prevention of coronary artery disease. Within the framework of a heightened awareness of risk factors, the physician should seek to identify children who will be at increased risk for the development of coronary artery disease.

Effective screening in the office setting should include the following steps.

(1) Family history. At the first well-baby visit, the primary care provider should take a careful family history, with emphasis on the occurrence of coronary artery disease, myocardial infarction, stroke, hypertension, obesity, diabetes, and familiar hyperlipidemias. In addition, the provider should explore maternal and family knowledge, attitudes, and behaviors regarding coronary risk factors, diet and nutrition, physical activity, and smoking. Of great importance is the updating of this history at yearly intervals to reflect changes in the family health background.

The family history is the most important screening tool that the provider can use: when the family history indicates the presence of risk factors, they will be more likely to be found in the child.

(2) Blood pressure determination. Beginning at the age of 3 years, children should have yearly measurement of blood pressure. This may be time-consuming in the small, uncooperative child, and must be done with proper cuff size and by personnel trained to obtain accurate readings. The Second Task Force on Blood Pressure Control in Children [3] has published "normal values" for children 2–18 years of age; graphs of these values are commercially available for comparison. An elevated blood pressure (above the 95th percentile) should be rechecked on several occasions. Londe [4] has shown a tracking phenomenon of blood pressure measurements, demonstrating that the blood pressure in two-thirds of children in whom repeated measurements are above the 95th percentile will remain elevated for 3–9 years. Furthermore, half of these children had a hypertensive parent and slightly more than half were considered obese.

(3) Obesity. The pattern of height and weight of the child should be plotted on each visit and reviewed with the parent. A disproportionate increase in weight compared to height should alert the primary care provider to the possibility of obesity.

(4) Physical activity. The physical activity profile of the child should be monitored by the primary care provider; an active life-style with participation in exercise should be advocated for all children.

(5) **Nutrition.** The primary care provider should inquire into the child's nutritional pattern—eating habits and intake of calories, saturated fats, simple sugars, and salt. Parental and patient education regarding proper nutrition can be incorporated into the history-taking at this point. A diet appropriate in calories for age and low in sugar, with no added salt, and limited amounts of saturated fats and cholesterol should be advocated.

(6) **Serum cholesterol.** A cholesterol determination should be performed on all children whenever coronary heart disease risk factors, particularly a family history of coronary heart disease occurring before the age of 50, have been identified. It has also been recommended that the serum cholesterol be obtained routinely at the time of entry into school, and again during adolescence [10]. The National Institute of Health Cholesterol Consensus Conference [11] has advocated that cholesterol levels in children of between 170–185 mg/dl should be considered high normal, and that these children should receive counseling about diet modification and other cardiovascular risk factors. A serum cholesterol over 185 mg/dl should be considered elevated, and children having such levels should receive special dietary and risk factor instructions and be followed up at yearly intervals. When an abnormal value is obtained, measurement should be repeated on at least two more occasions. If the elevation persists on multiple determinations, a lipid profile to include cholesterol, triglycerides, and lipoprotein electrophoresis, should be obtained.

(7) **Smoking.** As the child approaches adolescence, the primary care provider should begin to inquire about smoking habits. This history can also be used to discourage the activity. In a family with smokers, sibling and peer history of smoking should alert the primary care provider to more strongly emphasize this area.

B. Justification. It is clear that coronary artery disease begins in early childhood, although it may not manifest itself until the person reaches his or her forties or fifties. The clinical manifestations may become apparent suddenly and without prior warning, resulting in loss of life or disability, disruption of families, and considerable economic cost to individuals, families, and our nation. Epidemiologic studies have demonstrated the existence of a coronary risk profile in adults and have confirmed that risk factors may become apparent during childhood. Thus, it seems logical to identify individuals at risk as early in life as possible—before morbidity and mortality occur.

With the exception of family history, sex, and age, the risk factors identified are to a large degree the result of environmental influences and learned behaviors that are established during infancy and childhood. In a recent important report from the Bogalusa Heart Study, the first documentation of an early, direct correlation is provided between total and low-density lipoprotein (LDL) cholesterol levels, systolic blood pressure, and the presence of fatty streaks and fibrous plaques in 35 children and young adults (ages 7–24 years) dying since 1978 [12]. This study supports the link between risk factors and anatomic changes in the aorta and argues strongly that prevention of cardiovascular disease should begin early in life. Only by modifying the child's environment early in life can we ensure the formation of life-styles that will prevent or modify the disease process.

While there is a lack of longitudinal data necessary to provide absolute proof of the efficacy of such an approach, most epidemiologic research supports reasonable modification of nutritional, physical activity, and smoking patterns. Conversely, it can be argued that no one has demonstrated the benefits of an excess of dietary cholesterol, saturated fat, salt, simple sugars, or calories. Similarly, we know of no benefits of a sedentary life-style or smoking.

Primary care providers who care for children have long advocated the concept of health maintenance and preventive medicine to ensure both the quality and quantity of life. Thus, it is particularly appropriate for us to also play a major role in the prevention of coronary heart disease through community and patient education, institution of general preventive measures, and early identification of individuals at high risk.

C. Early intervention for those at high risk

1. Methods

a. Nutrition. If the serum cholesterol level is elevated, dietary evaluation should be performed, with appropriate modification outlined for the child. Change will be more easily complied with if the primary care provider can affect the eating pattern of the entire family. A diet that is low in saturated fats and cholesterol, simple sugars, and salts, but of adequate calories for growth, should be advocated. While decreases in serum cholesterol of 20–40 mg/dl may be achieved with dietary intervention, the absolute cholesterol level achieved may be less important than the modification in lifetime eating habits. Because of concern regarding myelinization of the central nervous system by fatty acids, and immaturity of the renal system to increased solute and sodium loads, interventions to lower serum cholesterol and decrease salt intake are generally contraindicated in patients younger than 2 years of age.

b. **Type II hypercholesterolemia.** When identified in children, early, vigorous intervention is essential. Dietary modification should be instituted and will result in maximal response if instituted before the child is 2 years old. When the child is unresponsive to dietary alterations, cholestyramine may be added to produce a reduction in cholesterol and LDL to near normal levels [13].

c. **Physical activity.** Regular exercise has been shown to affect weight and obesity, high-density lipoprotein (HDL) cholesterol and triglycerides, and hypertension. Furthermore, regular exercise promotes physical and cardiovascular fitness and a general sense of well-being, which allows a more effective response to stress. Children should be encouraged to develop lifelong habits of regular exercise, which may have a positive effect on several risk factors. This pattern may be hard to achieve in our mechanized, "televised" society but should be advocated by the primary care provider for all of his or her patients, particularly those at risk. Involvement of the entire family in physical activity is a more effective means of achieving this goal in the individual patient.

d. **Smoking.** The primary care provider should strongly discourage smoking in all patients, and especially in those at risk. This effort can be carried out in the office setting as described previously, but it is perhaps best accomplished through school programs that include peer pressure and support [14].

e. **Hypertension.** When a child demonstrates elevated blood pressure (above the 95th percentile) on repeated determinations, initial intervention should include control of obesity, elimination of added salt in the diet, encouragement of regular exercise, and cessation of smoking. When marked elevation in blood pressure or lack of response to initial measures are encountered, medical intervention may be indicated as outlined by the Second Task Force on Blood Pressure Control in Children [3].

f. **Obesity.** Successful attempts to modify obesity must include two components: modification of dietary intake and ongoing increase in physical activity [15]. All recent evidence suggests that diet alone will ultimately be unsuccessful, since decreased caloric intake leads to a decrease in metabolic rate and an eventual regaining of the weight transiently lost. When altered dietary intake is accompanied by an increase in daily physical activity, metabolic rate increases, more calories are burned, weight is successfully lost, and there is a greater chance for maintenance of the newer weight level when the diet is discontinued.

2. **Justification of intervention.** The risk factors for coronary artery disease are largely the result of learned behaviors and life-style patterns set in early childhood [16]. Thus, the advocacy of a healthy life-style with proper nutrition, regular exercise, and nonsmoking may result in modification of "coronary-prone" behavior, with alteration or prevention of the development of coronary artery disease [17]. Efforts by the primary care provider should be directed toward community education and to identification and education of those at risk within his or her practice. The costs of such an approach are minimal, consisting largely of primary care provider time and commitment. Risk factor screening can be integrated into the framework of the regular practice with little additional effort. Teaching materials for school, community, and office setting are available through organizations such as the American Heart Association without charge or at nominal cost. The performance of a serum cholesterol determination is approximately $15–$25, while a lipoprotein electrophoresis determination is $35–$50. Early identification and modification of risk factors may delay or prevent the onset of coronary artery disease.

IV. Recommendations

A. Primary prevention

1. The primary care provider should be an advocate in his or her community of a healthy life-style that promotes cardiovascular health.
2. The primary care provider should participate in community education in the school system, in community service organizations, and in his or her practice.
3. The primary care provider and his or her family can serve as effective role models of a healthy cardiovascular life-style in the community.

4. The primary care provider should develop and implement a comprehensive program of health education and health promotion, one that includes knowledge about nutrition, exercise, nonsmoking, and prevention of heart disease. This program should be integrated into daily practice activities and should include communication by the primary care provider and nurse, as well as the use of prepared materials.

B. Early detection

1. A detailed family history, with emphasis on cardiovascular diseases; risk factors; and family knowledge, attitudes, and behaviors related to risk factors, should be obtained at the first office visit and updated on at least a yearly basis.
2. Blood pressure should be carefully measured yearly from the age of 3 years and be compared to standards for children based on age and sex. Blood pressures above the 95th percentile should be confirmed by repeat measurements.
3. Growth parameters should be monitored carefully to identify early patterns of obesity.
4. A family and patient nutritional history should be taken at intervals and be combined with counseling on proper diet and nutrition.
5. Serum cholesterol measurements should be obtained (1) whenever a family history of premature coronary heart disease or risk factors, or both, are encountered, (2) routinely at the time of entry to school, and (3) once again during adolescence. Lipid electrophoresis should be obtained whenever repeat determinations of cholesterol are abnormal, or whenever a family history of inherited hyperlipidemia is encountered.
6. Smoking should be discussed with children and the long-term effects emphasized.

C. Early intervention

1. In the presence of an elevated serum cholesterol or obesity, or both, dietary evaluation and modification should be carried out.
2. In children with type II hyperlipidemia, dietary restriction may be supplemented with medication in an attempt to lower serum cholesterol.
3. All children with identified risk factors, and especially those who are obese, should be encouraged to develop habits of regular physical activity.
4. A particular effort should be made to discourage children with identified risk factors from beginning or continuing the habit of smoking.
5. Children with elevated blood pressure should be counseled regarding control of weight, elimination of added salt in the diet, patterns of regular physical activity, and cessation of smoking.

References

1. Frank, G. C., Berenson, G. S., and Webber, L. S. Dietary studies and the relationship of diet to cardiovascular disease risk factor variables in 10-year-old children—The Bogalusa heart study. *Am. J. Clin. Nutr.* 31(2):328, 1978. *Correlation of diet and serum cholesterol in children.*
2. Schrott, H. G., et al. Increased coronary mortality in relatives of hypercholesterolemic school children: The Muscatine study. *Circulation* 59(2):320, 1979. *Increased incidence of death from heart disease in relatives of children with elevated cholesterol.*
3. Report of the Second Task Force on Blood Pressure Control in Children. *Pediatrics* 79(1):1, 1987. *Best source of information on methods of blood pressure measurement, classification, and treatment in children.*
4. Londe, S. Blood pressure standards for normal children as determined under office conditions. *Clin. Pediatr.* 7(7):400, 1968. *Classic study of blood pressures in children obtained in the office setting.*
5. Voors, A. W., Webber, L. S., and Berenson, G. S. Time course studies of blood pressure in children—The Bogalusa heart study. *Am. J. Epidemiol.* 109(3):320, 1979. *Moderational changes in blood pressure in a carefully studied pediatric population.*
6. Bailey, D. A. *Exercise, Fitness and Physical Education for the Growing Child—A Concern* (a presentation). National Conference of Fitness and Health; Ottawa, Canada, December 4, 1972. *Report of declining physical fitness in Canadian children.*
7. Charney, E., et al. Childhood antecedents of adult obesity. Do chubby infants become obese adults? *N. Engl. J. Med.* 295(1):6, 1976. *Correlation study of childhood and adult obesity.*
8. Kirshenbaum, J., and Sullivan, R. Hold on there, America. *Sports Illustrated* 58(5):69, 1983. *Documents the poor physical fitness of American children.*

9. Sunseri, A. J., et al. *The Chicago Heart Health Curriculum Program.* Chicago: Chicago Heart Association, 1980. *Excellent, comprehensive, interactive curriculum for fifth- and sixth-grade children.*
10. Strong, W. B. (ed). *Atherosclerosis: Its Pediatric Aspects.* New York: Grune & Stratton, 1978. *Excellent review of natural history, risk factors, and pediatric aspects.*
11. National Institute of Health Consensus Conference. Lowering blood cholesterol to prevent heart disease. *J.A.M.A.* 253(14):2080, 1985. *NIH Consensus Conference establishes lower limits for normal and abnormal cholesterol levels.*
12. Newman, W. P., III, et al. Relationship of serum lipoprotein levels and systolic blood pressure to early atherosclerosis. *N. Engl. J. Med.* 314(3):138, 1986. *Landmark study demonstrating progressive atherosclerosis in children studied postmortem who had premortem elevated cholesterol and blood pressure.*
13. Glueck, C. J., Fallat, R., and Tsang, R. Pediatric familial type II hyperlipoproteinemia, therapy with diet and cholestyramine resin. *Pediatrics* 52(5):669, 1973. *Results of pharmacologic treatment of hyperlipidemia in children.*
14. Evans, R. I. Smoking in children: Developing a social psychological strategy of deterrence. *Prev. Med.* 5(1):122, 1976. *Strategies for preventing smoking in children.*
15. Brownell, K. D. *The LEARN Program for Weight Control.* Philadelphia: University of Pennsylvania Press, 1985. *Excellent manual with a comprehensive approach to achievement of optimal weight.*
16. Lauer, R. M., and Shekelle, R. B. (eds.). *Childhood Prevention of Atherosclerosis and Hypertension.* New York: Raven Press, 1980. *Excellent review of pathogenesis, risk factors, and intervention.*
17. Voller, R. D., and Strong, W. B. Pediatric aspects of atherosclerosis. *Am. Heart J.* 101(6):815, 1981. *Excellent concise review of pediatric risk factors and strategies for intervention.*

51 Adolescent Idiopathic Scoliosis

Daniel R. Benson

I. The problem

A. Definition. The vertebral column when viewed from the front or back is normally straight. Any deviation to the side represents the pathologic condition known as scoliosis. Although there are many different types of scoliosis, by far the most common is idiopathic in etiology. By definition, this means that we do not yet understand what causes this condition in otherwise normal children.

B. Description. Idiopathic scoliosis can occur at any point during the growth cycle (infancy to vertebral maturity) but is most likely to occur during the rapid adolescent growth. Adolescent idiopathic scoliosis is the most common type of spinal deformity seen in the United States (70% of the total).

When scoliosis is present in the skeletally immature child, there is a chance that the curvature will become worse with further growth. It is therefore incumbent that this condition be diagnosed early and followed carefully with periodic examinations. If this is not done, a small, easily treatable curve may develop into severe scoliosis, which in turn may need surgery.

Not all idiopathic scoliotic curves are progressive. The chance of a curve increasing is greatest in children who have considerable growth remaining. For example, the curve in a premenstrual girl in whom a mildly severe idiopathic scoliosis (5–19° by Cobb measurement) is diagnosed has a 20% chance of progressing. The same curve, occurring one year after menarche has occurred, has a 1.6% chance of progression. Larger curves (20–29°) have a much greater chance of progression; in a premenstrual female there will be a 68% chance of progression in these curves [2]. Unfortunately, because we do not know which curves will increase, all have to be clinically—and sometimes roentgenographically—followed.

When spinal growth is complete, most small or moderate curves will cease to increase, even if they were previously progressive. Large curves (greater than 50°) will become worse, even in the adult, creating cosmetic disfigurement, back pain, and in some cases, pulmonary compromise and right heart failure [3,4]. Curves of 60° have a 70% chance of progression in the adult.

C. Epidemiology [5, 6]. Idiopathic scoliosis is generally reported as being much more common in girls, although recent school surveys have shown more small spinal curves in boys than had previously been suspected. The reported ratio of female predominence (3.6 : 1) probably reflects the lesser risk of progression of comparable curves in males (about one-tenth).

Prevalence studies have varied, depending on differences in the criteria for diagnosis (e.g., degree of curvature). Using 10° of spinal curvature as a minimum for diagnosis, most studies reveal that scoliosis is present in 1.6% of adolescents between the ages of 12 and 17 (1.2% of boys and 2.1% of girls).

Depending on the remaining growth, degree of curve, and sex, some are progressive (10% of all detected cases) and will need treatment. Only a small number (0.6% of the overall adolescent population) actually will need to be treated (1.0% of females and 0.1% of males). Of those who require treatment, one out of three will require surgery, while the other two can be successfully treated with a brace.

II. Secondary prevention

A. Early detection

1. Methods

a. School screening programs. Scoliosis screening programs have been advocated to detect scoliosis earlier and to prevent the medical and social problems that result from untreated, progressive scoliosis. The usual site for widespread screening programs has been the school. Only a brief examination (less than one minute) is needed to visually inspect the child's back for abnormal curves. This is usually done during the most rapid growth period (10–12 for girls; 11–13 for boys) and involves examination of the back in both standing and bending positions. With the shirt or blouse removed (girls may be examined wearing a bra), the thoracic and lumbar spine are evaluated for excessive kyphosis or lordosis by observing the child from the side. The spine is then examined from the back with special note being made of an elevated shoulder, prominent scapula, or asymmetrical waistline. However, the most effective method of diagnosing scoliosis is the forward bend test (Fig. 51-1). Because the vertebrae and their attached ribs rotate into the convexity of the scoliosis curvature, the rib cage will be prominent on that side (Fig. 51-2). Very small amounts of curvature can be detected by this method.

Other methods of more effectively screening large numbers of school children have been studied. Moire topography, a method that produces a three-dimensional image of the trunk shape (similar to a relief map), can be photographed and studied for asymmetry. To date, this has not proved to be technically or financially feasible on a widespread basis.

The referred child with a significant curvature is the fruit of all these labors. It is the feeling of the Scoliosis Research Society and the American Academy of Orthopaedic Surgeons that finding 6 children in 1000 who need treatment is worthwhile. For this reason, both of these organizations support, in particular, the screening of children for scoliosis in the school.

b. Office screening. To complement school screening programs the spine should be included in each general physical examination done by the primary care provider. Checks for scoliosis should start at the postnatal exam and continue through the adolescent growth spurt.

Examination of the spine for deformity should include the entire torso and lower extremities. While the child is standing erect, the back is examined for elevation of the shoulders or scapula, lateral shift of the thorax (decompensation), loss of waistline symmetry, and abnormal posture. To best examine for thoracic or lumbar prominence, the child should bend forward at the waist, allowing the arms to fall forward so they hang away from the body. The rib or flank humps become more prominent as the bending increases (see Fig. 51-2). The range of motion of the spine is also checked by using this maneuver combined with side bending and extension. Any painful areas should be located and evaluated.

The pelvis is normally level. If there is a difference in height, the patient may have a leg length difference. This can present as scoliosis. The legs are measured from anterior iliac crest to the tip of the medial malleolus. A difference of greater than one-half is significant. A more accurate check can be made roentgenographically using the scanogram technique. Neurologic examination of the lower extremities is done to rule out spinal cord or root pathology as a cause of the spinal deformity.

c. Roentgenographic examination. When scoliosis is noted, it must be quantitated, since treatment is based on the degree of the curvature. A standing (posterior/anterior) roentgenogram of the spine is taken to allow for the maximum effect of gravity. The posterior/anterior (PA) roentgenogram is selected to avoid unnecessary breast radiation. If a lateral or anterior/posterior (AP) roentgenogram is required, the breasts are protected with a lead shield. The pelvic organs (ovaries or testicles) are protected with a lead apron applied just below the pelvic crests. Any lateral curvature is regarded as being abnormal. When a curve is seen, it is measured using the Cobb-Lippman method (more commonly called the Cobb angle). The end vertebra of each curve is selected and lines are constructed over the superior body and under the inferior body. Because this intersection usually takes place well beyond the extent of the x-ray film, perpendiculars are constructed to each line to create an identical angle near the spine (Fig. 51-3).

2. Justification

a. Test characteristics

(1) School screening programs. The test, although in itself inexpensive and sensitive, has been criticized for not being specific enough. Screening programs, depending on the experience of the screening nurse or physician examiner, refer from 1–20% of the examinees for a diagnostic evaluation. The number referred can be minimized by effective training programs in the art of examination for spinal deformity. Large numbers of referrals are a problem because they may result in a medical appointment and a roent-

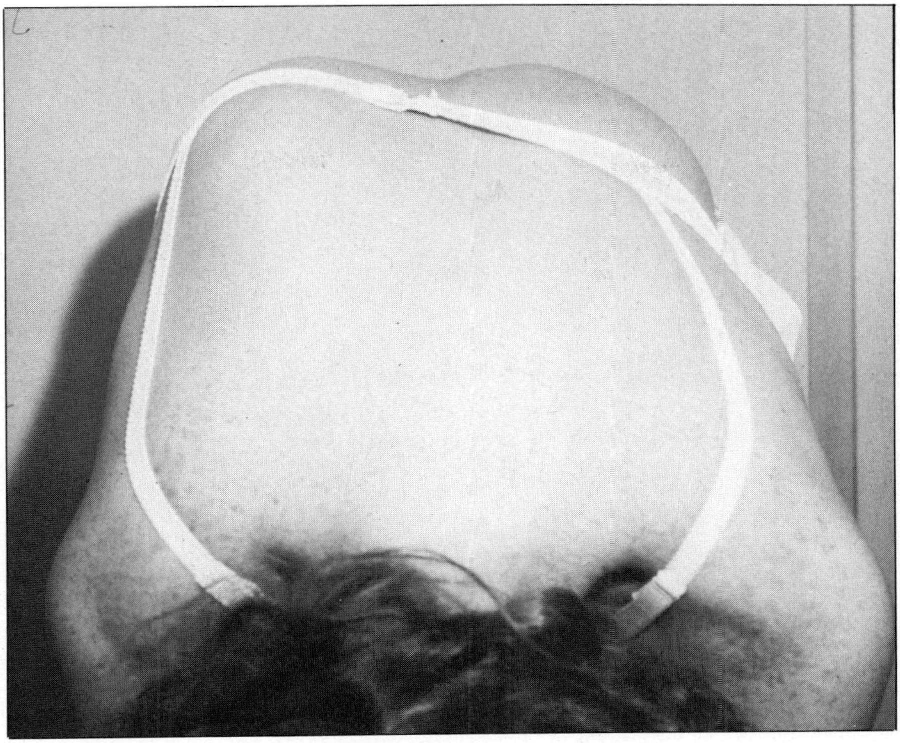

Fig. 51-1. The degree of scoliosis can be estimated by the forward bend test This adolescent girl demonstrates a right thoracic curve that is represented by the elevation of the ribs on that side. The back can be examined from the front of the patient (as in this case) or from the back (see Fig. 51-2).

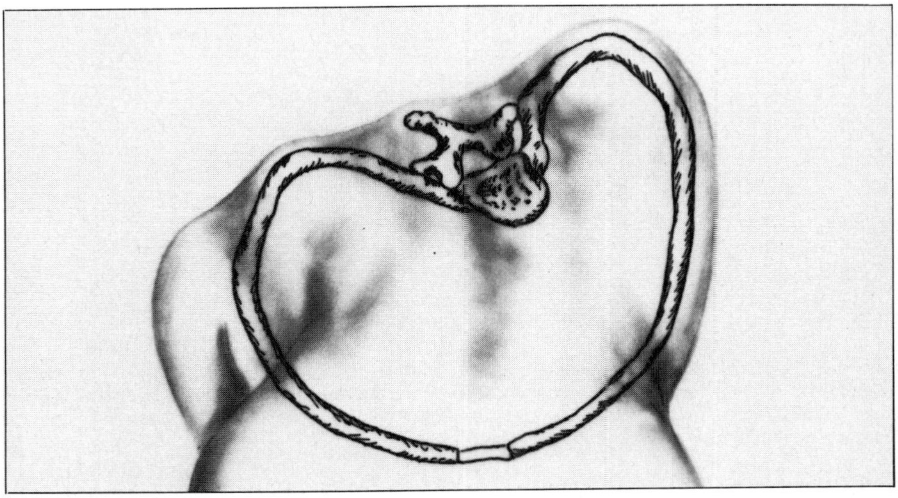

Fig. 51-2. The diagnosis of scoliosis can be made fairly accurately with the forward bend test. Because the vertebrae and their attached ribs rotate with the convexity of the curve, a rib hump is raised. This can be the first clinical sign of a curve. In this case, the drawing demonstrates a right thoracic spinal curve, which is the usual in adolescent idiopathic scoliosis.

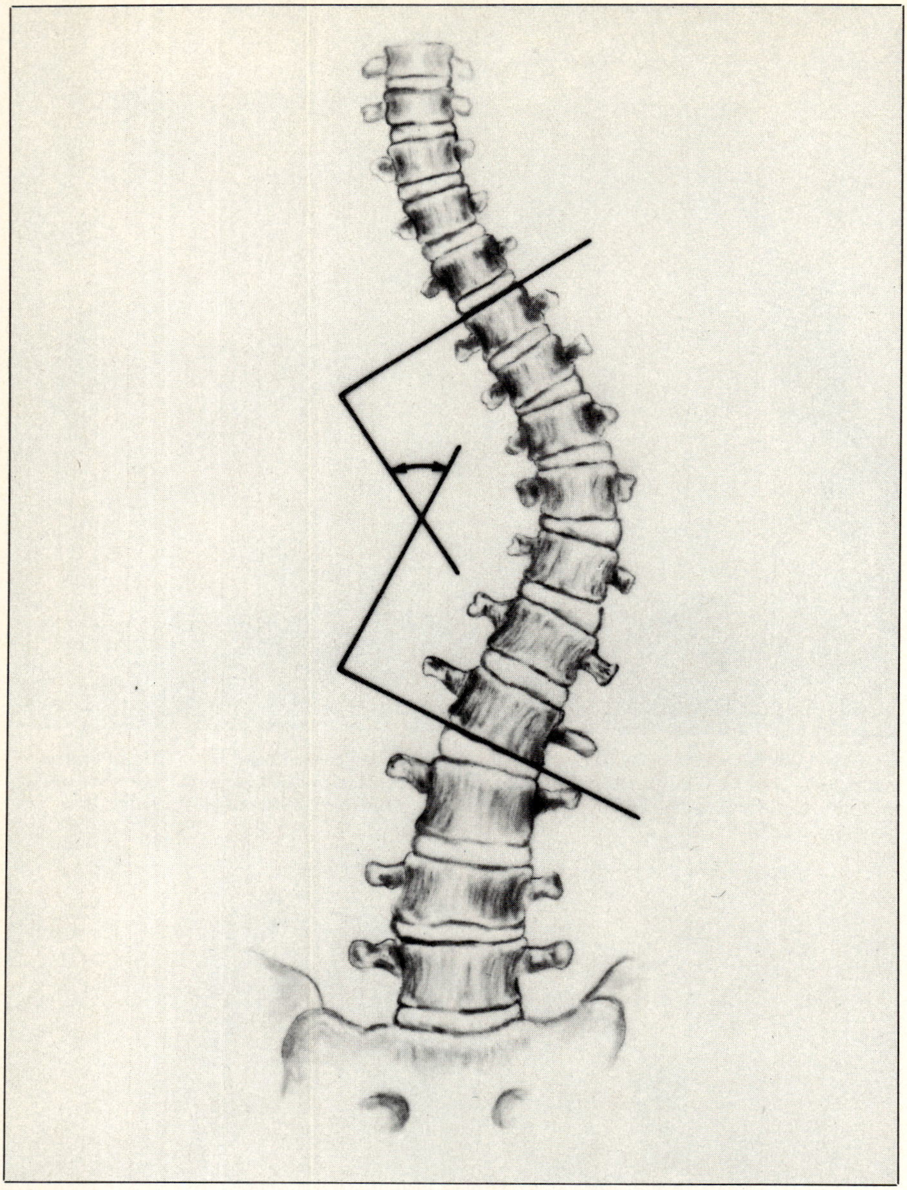

Fig. 51-3. The Cobb-Lippman method is used to quantitatively measure scoliotic curvature. The top and bottom vertebrae in a curve are determined and lines constructed parallel to their bodies. Perpendiculars to these lines intersect and can be measured on the x-ray. This drawing demonstrates a typical curve measurement.

Table 51-1. Costs of scoliosis screening

Examination	Time	Cost
School	½ min	$1–2
Office	15 min	$35
X-ray	15 min	$40–50

genogram, since the latter is the usual diagnostic test for scoliosis. Obviously, this increases the cost to both the family and society and creates unnecessary anxiety and radiation. It has been estimated that between 15–18% of referrals have **no** curve, and only 10% of all those referred will actually need any treatment. On the other hand, some curves may be missed by this simple screening examination and the children will go on to develop significant deformity [1].

(2) **Office screening.** The posture and bending characteristics of the vertebral column are examined for symmetry. The neurologic examination of the lower extremities should also be done.

(3) **Roentgenographic examination.** If scoliosis is suspected, a standing PA x-ray of the spine is taken (see sec. **II.1.b**). Kyphosis is evaluated by taking a standing lateral x-ray of the spine.

b. **Risks and side effects.** In addition to those risks already mentioned, the office examination that results in a roentgenographic examination results in radiation exposure.

c. **Costs.** See Table 51-1.

B. Early intervention

1. Methods

a. **Observation.** The treatment of idiopathic scoliosis depends on the degree of curvature. Treatment does not start until the curve has been proved to be progressive. If the first roentgenographic examination reveals a 10–19° curvature, treatment is delayed until 10° of progression is seen (i.e., 15–25° curvature). If the first curve measurement is over 20° but less than 29°, only 5° of progression is allowed before initiation of treatment. Curves greater than 30° in a skeletally immature child are treated immediately, since the chance of progression is greater. Following the curve for progression means that periodic examination and roentgenograms are necessary, usually at 4-month intervals. If the child is a member of a family with proved curvature, then he or she might be taken more often. These examinations should be continued until the child completes growth (15–16 years for girls and 17–18 years for boys).

If significant progression is proved, then specific treatment is considered. It is at this point that a specialist who treats spinal deformity should be consulted; in most cases, this will be an orthopedic surgeon.

b. **Nonoperative intervention.** The usual treatment for the progressing curve is one of several bracing systems. These include the Milwaukee, Boston, and Lyon braces and a variety of other similar braces. Selection of the appropriate brace is based on the degree of curvature, age of the child, and area of the spine that needs treatment. For thoracic curves, the Milwaukee brace has been the standard treatment. For lower curves, the Boston brace system (or a modified [extended] Boston brace), or another of the low-profile braces, has frequently been used. An alternative for thoracic curves is the Lyon brace. Electrostimulation of the muscles on the convexity of the curve has been tried. Most investigators of this technique have not been satisfied with the results and have abandoned its use.

All of the above bracing programs are combined with appropriately designed exercises. The exercise program is directed by a physical therapist. The exercises include muscle strengthening and, if necessary, stretching. Abdominal strengthening exercises are emphasized, as well as exercises designed to correct torso shift or asymmetry. The exercises provide stimulus to the brace-supporting body muscles. In the end, when bracing has been completed, the strong muscles will function to support the spine. The goal in bracing programs is to prevent increase in curve size. Although correction of the curve may occur, more usually the original curvature of the spine is not significantly improved at the end of the treatment.

c. **Operative intervention.** When the patient either has a curve too severe for bracing (50° or larger) or is too old to be treated with a brace (i.e., has passed spinal maturity), then surgery is considered. Depending on the degree of curve, a variety of surgical procedures can be performed. These include anterior and/or posterior surgical instrumentation and fusion. Even the most severe curvature can be corrected at almost any age.

2. **Justification**

a. **Effectiveness.** Early diagnosis and treatment can prevent late, significant problems. These problems include decrease in pulmonary function and right heart failure (with severe curves of 100–200°), which increase the risk of morbidity and mortality. Cosmetic disfigurement with its attendant psychosocial problems and back pain are other difficulties in untreated progressive scoliosis. On the other hand, a small progressive curve can be effectively controlled until spinal maturity, using a variety of bracing techniques. More pronounced curves can be surgically corrected and fused.

In several states and countries (Delaware, Minnesota, Great Britain, Sweden) where screening programs are widespread, operative treatment for idiopathic scoliosis has virtually disappeared. The goal is not to have to perform these serious, complicated operations, but to treat the patient before they are needed, with bracing or some other mode of therapy.

If the brace is used as directed until spinal maturity, almost all of these curves can be maintained at the diagnosed level and some can even be improved. With effective treatment, the late complications mentioned earlier can be avoided.

b. **Risks and side effects.** The major risk of scoliosis screening is overreferral. If the examination is not done accurately, more children than necessary will be referred for further examination, and possibly an x-ray [1]. This can be costly to the family and can create unnecessary anxiety. Physicians who see these normal spines may become disenchanted with the screening system and will then not support it.

c. **Costs.** The cost of an office visit to evaluate spinal deformity is approximately $35, plus $40–$50 if an x-ray is taken. Follow-up examinations, which should occur each 4 months in the growing adolescent, cost only slightly less (a total of $255 per year of remaining growth). Purchase of an orthosis (i.e., Milwaukee brace) differs depending on the local economy, but it is almost $1500 in our community. In a small child with a lot of remaining growth, one or even two brace replacements may be needed over the course of treatment. Surgical correction and fusion require 10 days of hospitalization, and there should be follow-up outpatient care over several years. The total cost—including surgery, anesthesia, and hospital fees—approximates $20,000. The cost will vary according to the cost-of-living in a given area (large cities tend to be more expensive).

d. **Acceptability.** Bracing requires good rapport between the patient, parents, and the doctor. If the course of treatment is well outlined and the patient accepts that the responsibility is hers or his, then acceptability is not a problem. A good clinic, where the nurses and doctor understand the problems of bracing and can deal with them, helps immeasurably. If other children in braces also attend the same clinic, communication develops. Family problems, or a lack of the patient acceptance of responsibility, inevitably lead to difficulties. There are some children who cannot withstand the peer pressures when they have to wear a brace. In these cases, bracing is probably more detrimental than helpful.

III. Recommendations

A. Early detection

1. Examine the back and spine for deformity at the time of any physical examination. This examination should be started as soon after birth as possible.
2. School screening is most productive, in terms of identification of spinal curvature, during the adolescent period. Girls should be examined at least once, and if possible, twice (one year apart) during the premenarchal period (10–12 years); boys, who mature slower, should be checked slightly later (11–13 years).
3. Any child with positive physical evidence of possible curvature should be referred to his or her primary doctor for further evaluation and possibly roentgenographic examination (a standing PA of the spine).

B. Early intervention

1. Any curve greater than 10° but less than 20° (Cobb-Lippman method) should be followed carefully with clinical or roentgenographic, or both, examination (each 4–6 months) until spinal maturity (15–16 in females and 17–18 in males). Increasing

curvature of 10° in curves initially measured between 10° and 19°, or 5° in curves initially measured between 20° and 29°, indicates significant progression. These patients need to be referred to a specialist who treats spinal curvature.

2. Curves over 30° in a skeletally immature child, or those that are progressive, should be referred to a specialist who treats spinal curvature.

References

1. Howell, J. M., Craig, P. M., and Dawe, B. G. Problems in scoliosis screening. *Can. J. Public Health* 69(4):293, 301, 1978. *The problems of overreferral or missed diagnosis are discussed. Cost of screening in the schools can be a problem.*
2. Lonstein, J. E., and Carlson, J. M. The prediction of curve progression in untreated idiopathic scoliosis during growth. *J. Bone Joint Surg. [Am.]* 66(7):1061, 1984. *Statistics on the potential for curve progression have been carefully gathered. This article provides a basis for offering prognostic advice to an adolescent with idiopathic scoliosis.*
3. Nachemson, A. A long-term follow-up study of non-treated scoliosis. *Acta Orthop. Scand.* 39:466, 1968. *The morbidity and mortality of untreated scoliosis is graphically presented.*
4. Nilsonne, U., and Lundgren, K. D. Long-term prognosis in idiopathic scoliosis. *Acta Orthop. Scand.* 39:456, 1968. *See reference 3.*
5. Rogala, E. J., Drummond, D. S., and Gurr, J. Scoliosis: Incidence and natural history. A prospective epidemiological study. *J. Bone Joint Surg. [Am.]* 60(2):173, 1978. *This article discusses the actual incidence of adolescent idiopathic scoliosis in the population.*
6. Rinsky, L. A., and Gamble, J. G. Adolescent idiopathic scoliosis. *West J. Med.* 148:182, 1988. *Excellent recent review.*

52 Routine Pediatric Immunizations: Structuring a Program

Chinh Le

Active immunization programs probably represent the most significant contribution of medical science in the prevention of crippling and fatal diseases. The worldwide eradication of smallpox since 1977 is an outstanding example. Unfortunately, despite vaccine availability, only 20% of the developing world's children are adequately immunized. According to World Health Organization data, preventable childhood diseases kill 5 million each year and leave 5 million others with serious disabilities. In the United States the incidence of many communicable diseases has dramatically decreased as a result of improved standards of living and routine childhood immunizations. This, however, does not justify a casual attitude of the public or health care providers toward compliance with routine immunizations.

Although there are currently more than 50 vaccines licensed for use in the United States, this chapter mainly addresses the practical aspects of **routine immunization programs.**

I. The problem

A. Description. Infectious illnesses for which routine immunization of the general population is targeted include **diphtheria, tetanus, pertussis, poliomyelitis, measles, rubella, mumps,** and ***Haemophilus influenzae*** type b. These illnesses are briefly discussed under their respective sections.

B. Epidemiology. Despite the dramatic decrease in the incidence of these preventable diseases since the 1950s and 1960s, sporadic and epidemic cases continue to occur in the United States. This is because of (1) low immunization rates in certain disadvantaged urban and rural populations or in individuals or groups apathetic to immunization programs; (2) inadvertent importation of communicable diseases from immigrants and visitors; and (3) increased traveling of United States citizens to countries where many infections are still endemic or epidemic.

II. Primary prevention

A. Methods. In **active immunization,** immunity is obtained by production of antibody or antitoxin following administration of an antigen (vaccine or toxoid). **Passive immunization** is the use of preformed circulating antibodies to provide temporary protection against a specific microbial agent.

1. **Nature and efficacy of active immunobiologic agents** [1]. Vaccines are bacterial or viral antigens altered to eliminate or modify the pathogenicity of the microbial agents. Table 52-1 describes the **types of antigen** used for some available and investigational vaccines. In general, **inactivated** vaccines made from killed organisms, whether used whole or fractionated, required frequent doses to achieve or maintain protective antibody levels. By contrast, **attenuated live** viral vaccines usually produce longer-lasting immunity.

   Toxoids are bacterial toxins modified by formaldehyde treatment to remove their toxic effects, but they retain their ability to induce antibody (antitoxin) formation. Adjuvants, such as aluminum salts, are sometimes used to enhance the immunogenicity of vaccines. Current vaccines used in routine childhood immunization have an **efficacy rate** of 70–95% (Table 52-2). Although vaccine-induced titers are generally lower than those stimulated by natural infection, vaccine-induced immunity protects against both clinical illness and viremia after natural exposure.

2. Just as there are individual biologic variations in the response to illness, there are variations in the immune response to, and in adverse reactions to, vaccines. These variations may be due to certain microbial characteristics, the age of the host, other concurrent illnesses, nutritional status, or genetic or other unidentified factors.

B. Justification. A program of immunoprophylaxis must be soundly based on biologic and epidemiologic concepts. Recovery from an infectious process, whether subclinical or symptomatic, usually results in natural, specific, and long-lasting immunity. The **objectives of immunoprophylaxis** are: (1) for the individual, to obtain protection without

Table 52-1. Nature of active immunizing agents

Type	Available vaccines
Whole, inactivated (killed) organisms	Pertussis[a], typhoid, plague, trivalent inactivated poliomyelitis (Salk), typhus, cholera, influenza, rabies, Rocky Mountain spotted fever, *Mycoplasma pneumoniae*[b]
Purified fractions of whole killed organisms	Pneumococcus, meningococcus, hepatitis B, *Haemophilus influenzae* Type b, Group A Beta-hemolytic streptococcus[b]
Inactivated toxins (toxoids)	Tetanus[a], diphtheria[a], anthrax
Live attenuated organisms	Measles[a], mumps[a], rubella[a], trivalent oral poliomyelitis (Sabin), yellow fever, tularemia[b], adenovirus[b], varicella[b], cytomegalovirus[b], rotavirus[b], shigella[b], cholera[b], and salmonella typhi[b]
Cross-reactive organisms	Smallpox; bacille Calmette-Guérin (BCG)

[a]Available in monovalent form and in combination with other vaccines.
[b]Investigational products at the time of this writing.

undergoing clinical illness; and (2) for society, to eliminate communicable diseases and their complications in those vaccinated, and to protect the susceptible by breaking the chain of transmission of infectious agents ("herd immunity").

An analysis of the incidence of vaccine-preventable diseases during prevaccine years and during current years when immunization levels of school-age children approach 90–95% clearly demonstrates the benefits of present immunization programs [2] (Table 52-3).

Reduced incidence and morbidity of diseases should lead to significant cost savings for society in terms of medical care cost and productivity gains, even after the cost of vaccination programs and cost of treating vaccine complications are computed. Presented in Table 52-4 are the 1981 estimates for 4 vaccines using an analysis of 1 million cohort for each vaccine (adapted from the work of J. S Willems and C. R. Sanders [3]). An analysis of 1983 determined a benefit/cost ratio of 14:4 for an immunization program using a combined measles-mumps-rubella (MMR) vaccine [4].

III. Recommendations

A. General recommendations (see Tables 52-5, 52-6, 52-7)

1. **Recommendations on immunization practices represent a balancing of scientific evidence of benefits and costs** in order to achieve optimal levels of protection by the safest and most efficient means. One should therefore consider: (1) the actual risk of the disease; (2) the cost/benefit to the individual and society in preventing the disease; (3) the safety, cost-effectiveness, and feasibility of the immunization program; (4) the alternatives to vaccine in preventing the disease; (5) the special characteristics and needs of the populations or individuals to be immunized; and (6) the means of getting effective vaccines to the target population. In many cases, this last problem can be a major deficiency of immunization programs. All of these factors need to be reevaluated from time to time in the changing epidemiology of diseases and health care priorities.
2. **Effective legislation** must be enacted to (1) offer a fair compensation for individuals who suffer from vaccine-associated illness; (2) limit the medicolegal liability of vaccine manufacturers and health care providers; and (3) ensure adequate funding and support for public health programs, surveillance of disease and control of outbreak, and research and development of safer and more effective vaccines.
3. In many settings, voluntary vaccination programs are not as effective as **mandatory programs.** In all states legislation is in effect for mandatory vaccination for school entry, raising immunization levels to 95% in school-age children. In view of current immunization gaps for toddlers and young adults, and the persistent prevalence of vaccine-preventable diseases in these age groups, efforts should be now put in requiring mandatory proof of immunity (most effectively done by adequate immunizations records) for entry in day-care centers and colleges or places of employment.
4. Routine or random surveys of immunization levels, adequate surveillance of dis-

Table 52-2. Routine childhood immunization efficacy and adverse reactions

Immunobiologic agents	Vaccine efficacy[a] (after primary immunization)	Duration of immunity	Side effects and adverse reactions[b]
DTP (diphtheria, tetanus, pertussis)	Diphtheria: 80–90% Pertussis: 70–90%	10 yrs 6 yrs	Mild and self-limited: local erythema, induration, and/or tenderness (40–70%), fever of 38.0–40.4 °C (50%), drowsiness, fretfulness (30–50%), anorexia (20%), sterile abscess or nodule
DT (diphtheria, tetanus, child's type	Tetanus: >95%	10 yrs	Rare severe systemic reactions (see text), (lower frequency with Td and DT than with DTP)
Td (tetanus, diptheria, adult type)[c]			Td: local swelling (1–2%), fever (7%)
TOPV (trivalent oral polio vaccine, Sabin	Greater than 95%; most recipients are protected after a single dose	Lifetime	Paralytic reaction (see Chap. 57)
IPV (trivalent inactivated polio vaccine, Salk)	Greater than 95%	?5 yrs. Better with new vaccine	No serious effects
Measles	95%	Lifetime	Fever, mild morbilliform rash (10–20%) within 6–10 days and lasting up to 5 days; encephalitis and encephalopathy (1 per 1 million doses)
Mumps	Greater than 90%	Lifetime	Fever (1%); parotitis (rare); rash; central nervous system involvement (febrile seizure, deafness, encephalitis) within 30 days, very rare and usually self-limited
Rubella	95%	Lifetime	Fever (1–4%), rash (1–10%), lymphadenopathy (10–14%), arthralgia (3–40%), arthritis (1%) within 7–25 days persisting 1–11 days and rarely recurring; more common in older vaccinees
Haemophilus influenzae Type B	40–80% in children 2 years or older 60% in children between 18 and 23 months Not immunogenic for children <18 months	Under investigation	Minor febrile (2%) and local reactions in 10% of vaccinees (see Chap. 61)

[a]Vaccine efficacy, for adequately vaccinated individuals, as measured by disease protection in epidemiology studies or by adequacy of antibody titers, or both.
[b]Percentage represents the frequency of side effects and adverse reactions per 100 vaccine recipients.
[c]DT (child's type) and Td (adult type) differ in their content of diphtheria toxoid per dose: DT and DTP contain 7–25 Lf units; Td contains 2 Lf units.

Table 52-3. Comparison of maximal and current morbidity of vaccine-preventable diseases

Disease	Maximal cases (year)	1983 (provisional)	Percent change
Diphtheria	206,939 (1921)	5	−100.00
Measles	894,134 (1941)	1436	− 99.84
Mumps[a]	152,209 (1968)	3285	− 97.84
Pertussis	265,269 (1934)	2258	− 99.15
Poliomyelitis (paralytic)	21,269 (1952)	8	− 99.96
Rubella[b]	57,686 (1969)	953	− 98.35
Congenital rubella syndrome	20,000 (1964–1965)	20	− 99.20
Tetanus[c]	601 (1948)	75	− 87.52

[a]First reportable in 1968.
[b]First reportable in 1966.
[c]First reportable in 1947.
Source: Data are from Dr. Alan Hinman of the Centers for Disease Control.

Table 52-4. Vaccination program costs and gains (1981)

Vaccine	Net medical care costs	Net costs (including productivity gains)
Pertussis	Decrease of $1.1 million	Decrease of $1.4 million
Poliomyelitis	Decrease of $0.2 million	Decrease of $0.9 million
Measles	Decrease of $4.6 million	Decrease of $11.3 million
Rubella	Decrease of $9.8 million	Decrease of $17.2 million

Sources: J. S. Willems and C. R. Sanders. Cost-effectiveness and cost-benefit analyses of vaccines. *J. Infect. Dis.* 144:486, 1981; C. C. White, J. P. Koplan, and W. A. Orenstein. Benefits, risks and costs of immunization for measles, mumps and rubella. *Am J. Public Health* 75:739, 1985.

ease, and **prompt reporting of vaccine-preventable infections** to the local public health department must be maintained to ensure eradication of these diseases.

The practitioner should take every opportunity on medical visits to review the immunization levels and needs of every patient; to reemphasize to parents the importance of keeping on schedule with recommended immunizations; and to administer needed vaccines when there are no absolute contraindications.

5. **Parent and patient information and record-keeping.** Despite the overall beneficial effect of routine immunization programs, many vaccine-preventable illnesses continue to occur epidemically or sporadically even among children within reach of our health care system. Parental and physician hesitancy and concerns continue to result in failure to fully immunize many individuals. The reasons for these public concerns are multiple: (1) wide airing of legitimate scientific disagreements and controversies, leading to public confusion and misinformation; (2) mistrust of vaccination unjustly enhanced by regarding an unrelated problem—such as symptoms of a concurrent disease—as a vaccine reaction; and (3) apathy fueled by religious or naturopathic beliefs that "shots" are unnatural, unnecessary, and unsafe. The public's confidence in national health policies can be quite tenuous, and the balance between acceptance of and rejection of immunization programs can be quite fragile. **It is the responsibility of the physician and other primary health care providers to (1) constantly emphasize to the parents and older patients that vaccine-preventable illnesses still occur in this country and worldwide; (2) clarify realistic expectations of vaccine efficacy and side effects;** (3) dismiss any myth unjustly linked to immunization; and (4) emphasize the importance of keeping up with the recommended vaccination schedule **at the times indicated.**

Table 52-5. Recommended schedule for active immunization of normal infants and children

Recommended age[a]	Vaccine(s)[b]	Comments
2 mo	DTP-1, OPV-1	Can be given earlier in areas of high endemicity
4 mo	DTP-2, OPV-2	6-wk–2-mo interval between OPV doses desired to avoid interference
6 mo	DTP-3	An additional dose of OPV at this time is optional for use in areas with a high risk of polio exposure
15 mo[c]	MMR, DTP-4, OPV-3	Completion of primary series
18 mo	Conjugate Hib	See Chap. 61
4–6 yrs[e]	DTP-5, OPV-4	Preferably at or before school entry
14–16 yrs	Td	Repeat every 10 years throughout life

[a]These recommended ages should not be construed as absolute, i.e., 2 mo can be 6–10 weeks.
[b]For all products used, consult manufacturer's package enclosure for instructions for storage, handling, and administration. Immunobiologics prepared by different manufacturers may vary, and those of the same manufacturer may change from time to time. The package insert should be followed for a specific product. Abbreviations given are those in Table 52-2.
[c]Provide at least 6 months between DTP-3 and DTP-4, or if fewer than 3 DTPs have been received, at least 6 weeks since the previous dose. A tuberculin skin test should be done at 12 months, or it may be given simultaneously with MMR at 15 months.
[d]Up to fifth birthday.
[e]Up to the seventh birthday.

In a busy clinical practice, it is often useful to supplement verbal advice with a handout to the parents. Figure 52-1 is an example of such a handout on immunization. If a child is exempt from specific immunization, the health care provider should sign a statement explaining the medical contraindications, which immunization the child cannot receive, and if the medical exemption is temporary or permanent.

Prior to immunization, parents and older patients should be questioned about concurrent illnesses and past immunization history, including any adverse reactions to previously administered vaccines. They should be advised of possible side effects and given simple instructions for dealing with them. Severe and unusual reactions reported should be noted in the patient's records, and this information should be passed along to the local or federal public health authority and to the manufacturer. A careful record of immunization should be retained by the parents (or older patients). It is best that the physician's records denote the vaccine by name, manufacturer, lot number, dose, site, and route used.

As practical knowledge about vaccines continues to develop, and as biologic and epidemiologic determinants of various infections continue to evolve, the practitioner must be prepared to keep up with current recommendations of immunization programs as they are revised by public health and infectious disease experts [1, 2, 5–12]. Specific questions may be addressed to the Chapter Chairman, Committee on Infectious Diseases of the American Academy of Pediatrics*; the Division of Immunization Services of the Centers for Disease Control†; or through consultations with infectious disease physicians or local health authorities.

*141 Northwest Point Boulevard, Elk Grove Village, IL 60007; (312) 228-5005 or (800) 433-9016.
†Centers for Disease Control, Atlanta, GA 30333; (404) 329-1860.

Table 52-6. Recommended immunization schedule for infants and children up to seventh birthday who were not immunized at the recommended time in early infancy[a]

Timing	Vaccine(s)[b]	Comments
First visit	DTP-1, OPV-1 (if child is 15 mo of age or older, MMR)	DTP, OPV, and MMR can be administered simultaneously to children 15 mo of age or older (also administer tuberculin skin test at first visit)
2 mo after first DTP, OPV	DTP-2, OPV-2	
2 mo after second DTP	DTP-3	An additional dose of OPV at this time is optional for use in areas with a high risk of polio exposure
6–12 mo after third DTP	DTP-4, OPV-3	
18 mo of age[c]	Conjugate Hib	
Preschool[d] (4–6 yr)	DTP-5, OPV-4	Preferably at or before school entry
14–16 yr	Td	Repeat every 10 years throughout life

[a]If initiated in the first year of life, give DTP-1, 2, and 3, OPV-1 and 2, according to this schedule; give MMR when the child is 15 months old.
[b]Abbreviations given are those in Table 52-2.
[c]*Haemophilus influenzae*'s vaccine should be administered when child is 18 months of age up to the fifth birthday; it can be given simultaneously with other vaccines at separate anatomic sites (see Chap. 61 for more details).
[d]The preschool dose is not necessary if the fourth dose of DTP and the third dose of OPV are administered after the fourth birthday.

Table 52-7. Recommended immunization schedule for persons 7 years of age or older

Timing	Vaccine(s)[a]	Comments
First visit	Td-1, OPV-1, MMR[b]	OPV not routinely administered to those 18 years of age or older. Use IPV. Also administer tuberculin skin test at first visit
2 mo after first Td, OPV	Td-2, OPV-2	
6–12 mo after second Td, OPV	Td-3, OPV-3	OPV-3 may be given as soon as 6 weeks after OPV-2
10 years after Td-3	Td	Repeat every 10 years throughout life

[a]Abbreviations given are those in Table 52-2.
[b]Persons born before 1957 can generally be considered immune to measles and mumps and need not be immunized. Rubella vaccine may be given to persons of any age, particularly to women of childbearing age. MMR may be used since administration of vaccine to persons already immune is not deleterious. See specific chapters for more details.

INFORMATION AND CONSENT FOR IMMUNIZATION

	(Doses)		(Doses)		IMPRINT AREA
____ /DPT	____	____ /Tri polio	____	____ /MMR	
____ /DT	____	____ /TB screen		____ /Measles	
____ /Td	____	____ /HIB		____ /Mumps	
____ /Other	____			____ /Rubella	

Date given ______________________ Given by ______________________

Physician's signature ______________________________, M.D.

Benefits and Reactions from Immunization of Children

Immunization can prevent crippling or fatal disease. Outlined below are the dangers of these diseases and the benefits and side effects of immunization. Please review this information carefully; if you have questions, please ask them. The American Academy of Pediatrics recommends that all normal, healthy children in the United States receive these vaccines. In addition, these immunizations are required for school entry, by California state law.

DISEASE

Diphtheria
- Occurs primarily in children
- Attacks the throat
- Interferes with breathing
- Produces poison that damages heart, kidneys, and nerves
- 10% of cases are fatal

Tetanus ("Lockjaw")
- Caused by dirt getting into wounds
- Causes painful muscular contractions
- 50% of cases are fatal

Pertussis ("Whooping Cough")
- Most severe in young infants
- Can cause pneumonia in 20% of cases and causes convulsions in 2 in 100 cases
- Rarely fatal in older children, but one in every 100 babies with whooping cough dies
- Brain damage may occur in 1 in 1000 cases

Polio
- Causes paralysis of muscles of arms, legs, respiratory system
- 10% of cases die

VACCINE

Diphtheria and Pertussis and Tetanus Toxoids (DTP)
- Given to children under age 6 years
- Almost all children will be protected after completing three doses and booster
- Common reactions include soreness, mild fussiness, sleepiness, a lump at injection site, and fever for 12 to 14 hours after vaccinations
- Convulsion or collapse reactions may occur once in 2000 doses
- Brain damage may occur once in 300,000 doses

Diphtheria, Tetanus, Toxoid (Td or DT)
- Td given to persons over 6 years old
- DT given to persons less than 6 years old
- Reactions include soreness and swelling in the injection site and mild fever
- Severe reactions are very rare

Oral Polio Vaccine (OPV, Live, Sabin)
- 95% of persons receiving primary series and booster will be protected
- Given by drops (no shots)
- No common reactions
- A paralytic reaction to the vaccine occurs in the person vaccinated once in 8 million doses; it may occur in an unimmunized close contact once in 6 million doses

Fig. 52-1. Parents' form for information and consent for immunization.

DISEASE	VACCINE
Measles Serious common childhood disease Always causes high fever (103°–105°) and rash; usually lasts 10 days May cause pneumonia or ear infection Causes deafness, blindness, convulsions, brain disorders in 1 of every 1000 children who get the disease Of children who develop a brain disorder from measles, 1 in 10 dies	Measles Vaccine 95% of persons receiving one dose of the vaccine will be protected 10–20% of children immunized may have mild fever and rash within 10 days 1 person in 1 million vaccinated may develop a brain disorder
Mumps Usually causes fever and swelling of salivary glands May cause inflammation of testicles in adolescent and adult males (20%) May cause inflammation of pancreas May cause a temporary brain disorder Can result in permanent deafness	Mumps Vaccine 90% of persons receiving one dose will be protected Very rarely fever and swelling of salivary glands may occur after vaccination
Rubella ("German Measles") When contracted by pregnant women can cause miscarriage, stillbirth, or multiple birth defects, including deafness and heart disease Usually a mild disease with mild fever, rash, and swollen glands	Rubella Vaccine 95% of persons receiving one dose will be protected About 1% of young children and 5–10% of teenagers may develop temporary arm, leg, or joint pains Very rarely vaccine may cause rash Children of pregnant women can be vaccinated without risk to their mother
HIB (Hemophilus Influenza Type B) Attacks 1 in 1000 children before age 5 and is leading cause of childhood meningitis and epiglottitis 5% of cases are fatal Risk of infection is increased for children attending day-care centers	HIB Vaccine 60–80% of children age 18 months to 5 years will be protected after one dose 2–10% have mild side effects, redness and swelling at injection site; fever to 101°F lasting < 24 hours and occurring about 24 hours after vaccination
	MMR Vaccine Combined measles, mumps, and rubella vaccine Protection as good as vaccines given separately Reactions are not increased over separate vaccines

SCHEDULE OF IMMUNIZATIONS

In the first year your child will receive 3 DTPs and 2 or 3 polio vaccines; in the second year MMR, DTP, polio boosters, and Hib vaccination at 18 months; between 4 and 6 years of age another polio booster and a DTP or DT booster.

Special Notes

1. Children who have diseases that lower the body's resistance to infection and those who have cancer or take chemotherapy drugs or cortisone should not receive measles, mumps, or rubella vaccines. Live polio vaccine should not be given to those children or to a child who lives in a household with a person with such problems.
2. Children under medical care for any acute or chronic medical condition should not be given vaccines in a school immunization program without their physician's approval.
3. Measles, mumps, and rubella vaccines can be given in combination (MMR) as one shot. Children who have had one of the diseases or vaccines can still be given the combination vaccine to complete their immunization, or they may receive individual vaccines.
4. Women who are pregnant or who may become pregnant within the next three months should not receive measles, mumps, or rubella, or the combined MMR vaccines.
5. If either parent or other adult living in the household never received the oral live polio vaccine, that person should consider receiving Salk polio vaccine protection. The risk of contracting paralytic polio from the vaccinated child is 1 in 6 million.
6. Keep a record of your child's immunizations where you can find it. You will need it when you enroll your child in day-care or school.
7. Administration of acetaminophen (15 mg/kg/dose) at the time of DTP vaccination and 4 hours later significantly decreases the incidence of local side effects and febrile reactions.

CONSENT: I have reviewed the information provided above. I understand the benefits and risks of these immunizations and wish my child to receive them as outlined in the schedule above.

____________________ (Witness)

____________________ (Parent's signature)

____________________ (Date)

Fig. 52-1 (continued).

6. **Routine childhood immunization schedules (see Tables 52-5, 52-6, 52-7).** The recommendations of the Advisory Committee on Immunization Practices (ACIP) of the United States Public Health Services, circulated in the *Morbidity and Mortality Weekly Reports* [5–10, 13], should be followed. These recommendations usually parallel those of the American Academy of Pediatrics (AAP), published in the *Report of the Committee on Infectious Diseases*, 1986 (commonly referred to as the "Red Book") [11]. Where they differ, discussion is provided in the chapters on specific diseases.

   Because the type and concentration of antigen vary in different products, the manufacturer's package insert should be consulted regarding the **route, volume** of individual doses of immunizing agents, and recommended **site** of administration. **Inactivation** of vaccines can occur from inappropriate **handling or storage** and can result in immunization failure. Therefore, the manufacturer's recommendations for optimal storage conditions (temperature, light, and shelf life) must be carefully followed. Table 52-8 provides a succinct summary of these recommendations, but it is not a substitute for the package insert of each vaccine.

B. **Specific recommendations**

1. **Age at and intervals between administration of various immunobiologic agents.** In general, immunization can be started at any age, although response may be suboptimal for some vaccines if they are given too early. This may be due to interference with maternal antibodies, e.g., as with the measles, mumps, and rubella

vaccines, or to the inherent inability of infants less than 18–24 months of age to respond to some antigens, e.g., to the pneumococcal or *Haemophilus influenzae* polysaccharide antigens.

Premature infants are able to produce IgM and IgG antibodies to various antigens. Diphtheria, tetanus, pertussis (DTP) and oral polio vaccine (OPV) can be administered in full regular doses at the appropriate chronological age, i.e., starting at 2 months of age. If the infant remains in the hospital, OPV probably should be delayed until discharge, to avoid in the nursery cross-infection with OPV to more immunocompromised patients.

For vaccines requiring successive doses to complete a primary immunization, it is best to adhere to the recommended intervals between doses. Giving OPV or toxoid vaccines at less than recommended intervals may lessen the antibody response. Live virus vaccines not administered on the same day should be given at least one month apart. On the other hand, **interruption of the routine** immunization schedule, regardless of duration, **does not** interfere with the adequacy of final immunity and does not necessitate additional doses of vaccine.

Under special circumstances, such as a concurrent epidemic in the community or a person who is traveling to highly endemic areas routine recommendations can be altered. For example, in measles outbreaks, the measles vaccine may be given to infants between 6 and 15 months of age; those infants then should be reimmunized after 15 months of age. **Vaccination after exposure to natural disease** is safe and potentially protective and can usually control an epidemic in progress. There appears to be no contraindication to immunization of an individual incubating natural infections.

2. Unless supported by a written statement from a physician or by serologic tests, **parental recollection of the child's past history of natural infection by vaccine-preventable agents is generally not accurate** and should **not** preclude the administration of routine childhood vaccines when otherwise indicated. **Children whose immunization records are lost** should be fully (re-)immunized appropriately for their age under the assumption that they have received no prior adequate immunizations. This is usually more cost-effective than assessing their immunity status by serologic testing. There is no known harm in repeat doses of commonly used live virus vaccines to persons who are already immune by virtue of prior immunization or infection. The side effects might be slightly increased with killed vaccines or toxoids because of exaggerated Arthus's reactions. Side effects, however, are usually transient and not severe.
3. **Simultaneous administration of vaccines.** While potentially accentuating vaccine side effects (this is especially true with cholera, typhoid, and plague vaccines), administration of several vaccines at separate anatomic sites usually does not result in reduced immunologic response. Children whose compliance with medical care recommendations cannot be assured would benefit from this approach at the appropriate age for vaccine administration.
4. **Administration of immune globulin (IG)** may interfere with antibody response to live attenuated vaccines. Therefore, measles, mumps, and rubella vaccines should not be given for at least 6 weeks, or preferably 3 months, after receiving IG. If administration of IG becomes necessary within 14 days after a live vaccine has been given, the vaccine probably should be repeated 6 weeks, or preferably 3 months, after the IG was given. By contrast, the IG interference is of little practical importance with OPV and inactivated products because of the large antigen mass in such preparations. These can therefore be given anytime after IG use.
5. **General contraindications for immunization include:**
   a. **An acute febrile illness.** However, it is not necessary nor advisable to postpone routine immunization because of concurrent minor upper respiratory infections.
   b. **Immunodeficiency diseases, generalized malignancies, and systemic immunosuppressive therapy.** These patients should **not** receive currently available **live** attenuated vaccines, smallpox vaccines, or bacille Calmette-Guérin (BCG) vaccines. (Varicella vaccine is an exception, however.) There is no contraindication for these patients to receive killed vaccines, toxoids, or polysaccharide vaccines, although it may be best to offer them during periods of least immunosuppression. Except for OPV, which can be transmissible to contacts, the use of live virus vaccines (such as MMR, varicella vaccines) is not contraindicated in household contacts of immunosuppressed patients. The risk to these patients of being exposed to a wild virus and natural infection may be reduced by vaccinating their close susceptible contacts.

Table 52-8. Recommendations for handling and storage of biologicals

Biological	Shipping requirements	Condition on arrival	Storage requirements	Shelf life expiration
DTP (diphtheria, tetanus, pertussis)	Without refrigeration if deliverable in 4 days. May use refrigerant.	May be out of refrigeration for up to 4 days.	Refrigerate immediately upon arrival—store at 2–8 °C (35–46 °F). DO NOT FREEZE—this reduces potency.	Up to 18 months; check date on vial or container.
TD—adult tetanus-diphtheria, Tetanus toxoid	Without refrigeration if deliverable in 4 days. May use refrigerant.	May be out of refrigeration for up to 4 days.	Refrigerate immediately upon arrival—store at 2–8 °C (35–46 °F). DO NOT FREEZE—this reduces potency.	Up to 2 years; check date on container or vial.
Rubella virus; measles virus; measles/rubella—combined virus; Measles/mumps/rubella—combined virus; Mumps	Must use refrigeration. Maintain at 10 °C (50 °F) or less. DO NOT USE DRY ICE. See special instructions on shipments of live virus vaccines.	Should be below 10 °C (50 °F). If above this temperature, refuse shipment or return to shipper. DO NOT USE WARM VACCINE.	If possible, separate vaccine from diluent. Store as follows. Vaccine: refrigerate immediately upon arrival. Store at 2–8 °C (35–46 °F). PROTECT FROM LIGHT AT ALL TIMES, since such exposure may inactivate virus. Diluent: do not refrigerate. Store at 15–30 °C (59–86 °F), room temperature.	Vaccine—Up to 2 years; check date on container or vial. Diluent—Indefinite.
Poliovirus	Shipped in dry ice by bus or air.	Should be frozen. If thawed but still cold—below 8 °C (46 °F)—refreeze immediately. If thawed and warm—above 8 °C (46 °F)—or vaccine cloudy, refuse shipment or return to shipper. DO NOT USE THAWED, WARM, OR CLOUDY VACCINE.	Maintain continuously if in frozen state—10 °C (14 °F) or lower. Vaccine may be refrozen—if not opened; maximum of 10 freeze/thaw cycles permissible, provided total cumulative duration of thaw does not exceed 24 hrs and temp. does not exceed 8 °C (46 °F) during period of thaw.	Up to 1 year; check date on container or vial.
Haemophilis b	Insulated container not frozen.	Should not be frozen.	Refrigerate (2–8 °C). DO NOT FREEZE.	Up to 2 years.

Instructions for reconstitution or use	Shelf life after reconstitution, thawing, or opening	Special instructions
Shake vigorously before withdrawing each dose.	Until outdated, if not contaminated.	Rotate stock so that most current expiration-dated stock is used first.
Shake vial vigorously before withdrawing each dose. When used in jet injector gun, shake vial before each injection.	Until outdated, if not contaminated. If using multidose vials for jet injector, discard remainder of contents on day of use.	Rotate stock so that most current expiration-dated stock is used first. Multidose vials for jet injector use should not be utilized in the needle/syringe method of immunization.
RECONSTITUTE JUST BEFORE USE. Singles: inject into vial of lyophilized vaccine and agitate to ensure thorough mixing. Withdraw entire contents into syringe and inject total volume of vaccine subcutaneously. Multidose vials: withdraw ALL diluent from ampule into syringe, inject into vial of lyophilized vaccine and agitate to ensure thorough mixing. 10-dose vial: withdraw 0.5 cc of reconstituted vaccine into separate syringe and needle for each immunization. 50-dose vial: place on jet injector gun with dosage of 0.5 cc.	After reconstitution, use immediately or store in dark place at 2–8 °C (35–46 °F). DISCARD IF NOT USED WITHIN 8 HOURS.	Rotate stock so that most current expiration-dated stock is used first. Use only the diluent supplied to reconstitute vaccine. DO NOT use diluents from other vaccines or manufacturers. 50-dose vials: for jet injector use should not be utilized in needle/syringe method of immunization. 10-dose vials: may be used for both jet injector and needle/syringe methods of immunization.
Thaw before using—may be rubbed between hands for rapid thawing.	Vaccine in a liquid state in unopened vials may be used for up to 30 days, provided it has been stored at 2–8 °C (35–46 °F). Once the vial is opened, it must be refrigerated at 2–8 °C (35–46 °F) and used within 7 days.	If the dropper becomes contaminated from touching the mouth, do not reuse dropper or reintroduce into the vial. Sterilize dropper by boiling in water (cool before replacing dropper in vial), or use new dropper, before continuing administration. USE ONLY DROPPER SUPPLIED IN PACKAGE.
Use only diluent supplied.	Multiple vials stable for 30 days at 2–8 °C. Single dose vial: discard unused reconstituted vials after 8 hours.	

Table 52-8 (continued).

Biological	Shipping requirements	Condition on arrival	Storage requirements	Shelf life expiration
Typhoid	Without refrigeration if deliverable in 4 days. May use refrigerant.	May be out of refrigeration for up to 4 days.	Refrigerate immediately upon arrival. Store at 2–8 °C (35–46 °F). DO NOT FREEZE—reduces potency.	Up to 18 months; check date on vial or container.
Influenza	Same as typhoid	Same as typhoid	Same as typhoid	Same as typhoid
Tuberculin purified protein derivative (PPD) stabilized solution	Without refrigeration if deliverable in 3 days.	May be out of refrigeration for up to 3 days.	Refrigerate immediately upon arrival at 2–8 °C (35–46 °F). Should not be exposed to heat, sunlight, or daylight.	Up to 1 year; check vial or container date and manufacturer's instructions.

[a]All materials used for administering live virus vaccines should be burned, boiled, or autoclaved prior to disposal.

[b]These recommendations are not a substitute for the package insert included with each different biologic.
Source: State of California, Department of Health Services, August 1979.

c. **An evolving neurologic disorder.** Immunizations likely to cause fever or possible adverse neurologic reactions should be temporarily avoided until the primary disease is under control or has become static. This is particularly true with administering pertussis vaccine in infancy.

d. **Prior anaphylactic reaction** to the same or a related vaccine or to additive components of the vaccine (i.e., trace amounts of the antibiotics neomycin or streptomycin; preservatives such as mercury). In clinical practice, the history of "allergic reactions" is often vague and ill-documented and does not constitute a contraindication, unless these reactions were anaphylactic in nature. Since the current influenza, yellow fever, measles, and mumps vaccines are prepared from chick embryo tissue cultures, these vaccines should be used with caution in patients with known anaphylactic reactions to eggs. On the other hand, varicella, rubella, and oral polio vaccines are prepared in nonavian systems, and egg allergy is not contraindicated.

6. **Pregnancy.** The risk of fetal infection precludes the administration of live virus vaccine (except for oral polio vaccine) to females who might be pregnant or who might become pregnant shortly after vaccination. However, there is no good evidence that currently used live, attenuated virus vaccines cause congenital malformations in humans.

   Administration of MMR to children of pregnant mothers is not contraindicated. The risk of a susceptible woman of childbearing age to exposure to wild viruses would actually be reduced by vaccinating her close susceptible contacts.

   When any vaccine or toxoid is to be given during pregnancy, waiting to do so until the second or third trimester, when possible, is a reasonable precaution in order to minimize concern about adverse effects on pregnancy.

References

1. Anderson, D. C. Prevention of Infectious Diseases: Active Immunizing Agents. In R. D. Feigin and J. D. Cherry (eds.), *Textbook of Pediatric Infectious Diseases*. Philadelphia: Saunders, 1981. Pp. 1731–1756. *Comprehensive review of immunizing agents used in routine pediatric immunizations.*

Instructions for reconstitution or use	Shelf life after reconstitution, thawing, or opening	Special instructions
Shake vial vigorously before withdrawing each dose.	Until outdated, if not contaminated.	Rotate stock so that the most current expiration-dated stock is used first.
Shake vial vigorously before withdrawing each dose.	Until outdated, if not contaminated.	Rotate stock so that the most current expiration-dated stock is used first.
Loaded syringes should not be held. Use as soon as possible.	Until outdated.	

2. Hilleman, M. R. Newer directions in vaccine development and utilization. *J. Infect. Dis.* 151(3):407, 1985. *Discussion of current issues in routine childhood and adult immunizations programs, with emphasis on cost/benefits.*
3. Willems, J. D., and Sanders, C. R. Cost-effectiveness and cost-benefit analyses of vaccines. *J. Infect. Dis.* 144(5):486, 1981. *Review of studies on cost/benefits of immunization programs.*
4. White, C. C., Koplan, J. P., and Orenstein, W. A. Benefits, risks and costs of immunization for measles, mumps and rubella. *Am. J. Public Health* 75(7):739, 1985. *Cost analysis of current MMR immunization policy, when compared to the actual and estimated costs attributed to diseases.*
5. Advisory Committee on Immunization Practices (ACIP). General recommendations on immunization. *M. M. W. R* 32(1):1, 1983. *Current recommendations by the Centers for Disease Control.*
6. Advisory Committee on Immunization Practices (ACIP). Diphtheria, tetanus and pertussis: Guidelines for vaccine prophylaxis and other preventive measures. *M.M.W.R.* 34(27):405, 1985.
7. Advisory Committee on Immunization Practices (ACIP). Poliomyelitis prevention. *M.M.W.R.* 31(3):22, 1982.
8. Advisory Committee on Immunization Practices (ACIP). Measles prevention. *M.M.W.R.* 31(17):217,229, 1982.
9. Advisory Committee on Immunization Practices (ACIP). Mumps vaccine. *M.M.W.R.* 31(46):617, 625, 1982.
10. Advisory Committee on Immunization Practices (ACIP). Rubella prevention. *M.M.W.R.* 33(22):301, 1984.
11. American Academy of Pediatrics, Committee on Infectious Diseases. *Report of the Committee on Infectious Diseases* (20th ed.). Evanston, IL: American Academy of Pediatrics, 1986. Pp. 1–53. *Succinct reviews of infectious diseases and recommendations for their treatment and prevention by infectious disease experts from the American Academy of Pediatrics.*
12. Fulginiti, V. A. Immunizations: Current controversies. *J. Pediatr.* 101(4):487, 1982. *Discussion of current controversies in childhood immunization programs.*
13. Advisory Committee on Immunization Practices (ACIP). New recommended schedule for active immunization of normal infants and children. *M. M. W. R.* 35(37):577, 1986. *New CDC schedule recommending DTP at 15 months.*

53 Tuberculosis in Children

Chinh Le

I. The problem

A. Description. Tuberculosis (TB) is an acute or chronic infection caused by *Mycobacterium tuberculosis*, and rarely by *M. bovis*. More than 95% of primary infections are in the lungs, but severe infections can occur in any organ, with varying signs and symptoms. Childhood tuberculosis is most often asymptomatic. Pulmonary or extrapulmonary foci of infection may reactivate at any time, often after long periods of latency [1].

Tuberculosis is usually acquired by inhalation of respiratory droplets from an infected person, usually an adult with chronic or cavitary disease. Children are rarely infectious because of minimal pulmonary lesions and little or no productive cough. Young children and adolescents are at increased risk for dissemination of disease. Transplacental or perinatal transmission of tubercle bacilli can also occur from a mother with active tuberculosis to her infant. About 50% of untreated children born to mothers with active pulmonary TB will develop the disease during the first year of life. Household contacts under 15 years old of adults with active tuberculosis have the highest rate of disease—up to 67% in an earlier study. However, recent reports in the United States indicate that only 22% of household contacts of all ages are now infected. By far the most important determinant of transmission is the severity of the disease in the adult case; degree of crowding and intimacy of exposure are also important factors [2].

B. Epidemiology[2, 3]. In 1985, approximately 5.6% of the tuberculosis cases reported in the United States occurred in children and adolescents. The incidence was 3 cases per 100,000 population in the pediatric age groups, and 9.3 cases per 100,000 in the United States general population [4].

In 1985, 11.4% and 34.5% of all cases of tuberculosis in the United States were from Asian and black populations, respectively. For children, however, tuberculosis takes its heaviest toll on minorities and the socioeconomically disadvantaged. In 1984, 53% of reported cases in children under 15 years of age occurred in nonwhites, and another 25% in Hispanics. Foreignborn individuals in these ethnic groups have a seven-fold or greater rate of tuberculin skin test reactivity when compared to those born in the United States, independent of the length of stay in the United States or a history of bacille Calmette-Guérin (BCG) vaccination.

II. Prevention

A. Early detection

1. Methods

a. Screening methods. The **tuberculin skin test** is the most appropriate tool for case-finding and one of the main criteria for diagnosing tuberculosis infections.

(1) The **Purified Protein Derivative,** or Mantoux-PPD, at a 5-tuberculin unit concentration (5TU) given intradermally is the standard skin test (Table 53-1) [5].

Dosages other than 5TU have not been standardized and have limited demonstrable usefulness in ordinary practice.

(2) **Multiple puncture devices,** which are more convenient, include the tine test, Aplitest, Sterneedle, Heaf test, Slavotest-PPD, and Mono-Vac test. All of these tests share the disadvantage of not being able to control exactly the dose of antigen injected. These screening devices therefore have variable accuracy (75–98.6%). When compared with the Mantoux-PPD-5TU, these tests have a false-positivity rate of 3–10%, and a false-negativity rate of 6–35%. Usually, tests using liquid antigens are better than those using dry agents. To some experts, the Mono-Vac test is the preferred agent at this time because of its low (1.5%) rate of false-negative reaction. However, all multiple puncture-type devices must be regarded only as screening tools. The Mantoux-PPD test should be utilized for retesting reactors, for diagnosis

Table 53-1. Standards for administration and reading of purified protein derivative (PPD) skin tests

Recommended antigen PPD tuberculin, stabilized with Tween® 80 and standardized by biologic assay to 5 tuberculin units (TU).
Administration 0.1-ml dose, with a short (one-half in.) bluntly beveled platinum (26-gauge) or steel (27-gauge) needle with a glass or plastic tuberculin syringe. Preferred site: volar or dorsal site of forearm. Injection should be intradermal, producing a discrete 6–10-mm diameter wheal.
Reading Read at 48–72 hours after injection in good light, with forearm slightly flexed at elbow; extent of induration (not erythema) should be measured transversely across the reaction. Size of induration is recorded in millimeters.
Interpretation 10 mm or more of induration signifies tuberculous infections. However, when evaluating suspects or close contacts of individuals with tuberculosis, a reaction of 5 mm or more is considered significant. A converter is defined as an individual whose tuberculin reaction has increased by at least 6 mm, from less than 10 mm to 10 mm or more in induration, within 24 months

of suspected cases in contacts, and for periodic surveillance programs of high-risk groups, e.g., hospital personnel.

(3) Test modifiers

(a) An incubation period of 2–10 weeks occurs between infection and development of a positive skin test.

(b) Temporary anergy to tuberculin can result from severe infection, malnutrition, concurrent or recent viral (e.g., measles, influenza, varicella) or mycoplasmal infections, or immunosuppression.

(c) The **booster phenomenon** in serial tuberculin testing is found in all age groups but increases with age (1% in children, 7–8% in persons 50 years or older), particularly in areas endemic for mycobacteria other than *M. tuberculosis*.

(d) It is usually not possible to differentiate between a tuberculin skin test reaction caused by a **BCG vaccination** and a natural tuberculous infection in a person who had received BCG vaccine, unless the reaction is very large. Furthermore, protection from BCG can vary from 0–80%. The American Thoracic Society and the American Lung Association therefore recommend that the history of BCG vaccination not alter the guidelines for interpretation of the skin test reaction [4, 5, 6].

b. Indications for tuberculin testing include:

(1) Screening of infants, children, and adolescents. **Routine** tuberculin skin testing should be done at the time of, or before, measles immunization, and sometime during the preteen and adolescent years. There is, however, some disagreement about the frequency of repeated tuberculosis screening in normal children. Of new cases of tuberculosis, 80% are discovered by diagnostic workup or by evaluation of contacts of index cases rather than by routine screening. Even among urban poor populations in the United States, routine tuberculin testing would only yield 2–3 cases of unsuspected tuberculosis per 1000 individuals screened. The American Lung Association and the Centers for Disease Control, having in mind the goal of eliminating tuberculosis as a public health problem while considering cost-effective data, recommend that repeated routine screening should be done only in areas where the case detection rate is at least 1% (1 case found per 100 screened). The American Academy of Pediatrics, on the other hand, seeing tuberculosis as a problem of the individual person, still recommends routine tuberculin skin testing on an annual or biennial basis. Until more data are available to determine the role and frequency of tuberculin screening tests, practitioners may use the tuberculosis prevalence in their communities and individual risks of their patients as guidelines.

(2) Contacts of patients with active tuberculosis. In such an instance, if the initial tuberculin reaction is negative, the test should be repeated 8–10 weeks after removal or effective treatment of the index case; if the child remains in contact with an adult with active tuberculosis, the tuberculin test should be repeated at 3-month intervals.

(3) Immigrants or migrant individuals from areas of high endemicity of tuberculosis (such as people from developing countries and Native Americans and Eskimos) and their close contacts.

(4) Individuals with unexplained lower respiratory infections or pulmonary lesions, or those with systemic symptoms compatible with tuberculosis.

(5) Preparation for instituting therapies that may suppress cell-mediated immunity. With long-term corticosteroid treatment, immunosuppressive agents, and radiation, it may prove prudent to obtain a baseline tuberculin skin test, since immunosuppression can induce anergy, reactivation of tuberculosis can occur under these circumstances, and chemoprophylaxis is indicated for patients who react positively to tuberculin and are on immunosuppressive therapy.

2. **Justification.** Despite the decline in the incidence of tuberculosis in the United States, early detection and prevention of this disease in the pediatric population cannot be overemphasized.

   a. Primary tuberculosis tends to occur in infancy and childhood and is generally asymptomatic. A recent converter has a 1–5% risk of developing active tuberculosis during the first year after acquisition of the tubercle bacilli. The lifetime risk of disease reactivation is about 0.5% per year [5].

   b. Detection of a case of tuberculosis in a child should lead to an index case and other infected contacts, usually adult. Thus both the individuals (for treatment) and the community (for interrupting the spread of disease) are benefitted.

B. Early intervention

1. **Methods.** Individuals with a positive Mantoux test should be evaluated for clinical symptoms, and radiologic or bacteriologic findings of tuberculosis, or both. Appropriate treatment should be initiated for patients with active disease. Their contacts should be rapidly and carefully investigated, especially all household members and children, without waiting for bacteriologic confirmation of the diagnosis, which may take weeks [2].

   a. **Chemoprophylaxis.** For preventive therapy, **isoniazid** (INH) is used at a dose of 10/mg/kg body weight given as a single daily dose (maximum 300 mg) over a period of 12 months [5]. **It should be given to all skin-test converters and to skin-test reactors in the pediatric and adolescent age groups.** Tuberculin-negative children who are household or close contacts (i.e., common babysitting arrangements) of individuals with recently diagnosed active tuberculosis should receive INH and should be skin-tested again in 2–3 months. If the skin test is positive and the chest x-rays are negative, therapy should be continued for a total period of 12 months. If the skin test is negative and exposure has ended (or the index case is receiving adequate therapy), INH may be discontinued.

   b. **Isoniazid hepatotoxicity** has been rarely reported in the pediatric age groups. Elevated liver function tests occur in 6.8–10% of children and adolescents during the first 3 months of INH prophylaxis. These abnormalities usually improve despite continuance of therapy. Routine monitoring of liver function tests is not recommended. Children who are taking other drugs that might interfere with INH metabolism (such as phenytoin [Dilantin]) should be closely monitored for drug toxicity. INH is contraindicated in individuals with acute liver disease of any etiology.

   c. The care of the **infant born to a tuberculous mother** has to be individualized. If the tuberculin-reactive mother has no clinical or radiologic evidence of tuberculosis, the infant does not need prophylaxis, but he or she should be followed carefully with regular skin testing while the mother is given INH prophylaxis. If the mother has active tuberculosis, the infant should be carefully evaluated for congenital tuberculosis. The mother should be treated and separated from the infant until she is noncontagious (i.e., shows negative sputum smears). The other individuals in the infant's environment also should be investigated and treated appropriately. If tuberculosis infection has been ruled out in the infant, he or she should be given INH prophylaxis and closely followed. BCG vaccine should be given to the skin-test negative infant if there is any question about the family's reliability and compliance with medical treatment and follow-up.

The skin test should be performed again 6–8 weeks after BCG vaccination to document a "take"; if it is negative, another dose of BCG must be given.

d. BCG vaccines are used in many areas of the world where tuberculosis is prevalent, with an efficacy range from 20–80% in controlled studies [5]. Although BCG can confer a high degree of protection against severe tuberculosis, the efficacy of BCG vaccines available in the United States is unknown, and their indications in this country are rare.

2. Justification. A recent converter has a 1–5% risk of developing active tuberculosis during the first year following acquisition of the tubercle bacilli. The lifetime risk of disease reactivation is about 0.5% per year [4].

Chemoprophylaxis can reduce the rate of developing active tuberculosis by 70% and reduce its complications (meningitis, dissemination) by 90% for many years, perhaps lifelong.

III. Recommendations

A. Early detection

1. Children should be routinely tested for tuberculosis before or at the time of the measles/mumps/rubella vaccination (15 months of age) and perhaps biennially.
2. Any child exposed to an adult with active tuberculosis should also be tested and closely followed.
3. Multiple puncture devices are adequate screening tools for tuberculosis, but a 5TU-PPD Mantoux should be used for diagnostic workup of an individual exposed to tuberculosis or who gives a positive result to multiple puncture skin-testing.

B. Early intervention

1. Asymptomatic children and adolescents with a positive 5TU-PPD and a negative chest x-ray should receive a year of isoniazid prophylaxis (10 mg/kg/day, with maximum dose of 300 mg). Routine monitoring for liver function test abnormalities is not recommended, but the patient should be evaluated and the drug stopped if signs and symptoms of hepatoxicity develop.
2. **BCG vaccine.** Routine BCG vaccination is not recommended for the American population, although it may be considered in infants and children in high-risk populations, such as Native Americans. It is contraindicated in persons with immunodeficiency or immunosuppression and in pregnant women.

   Some authorities recommend BCG vaccines for: (1) infants and children whose families are unlikely to return for regular follow-up visits and who may thus become infected by continuous exposure to active tuberculosis; (2) groups in which an excessive rate of new infections is found (skin test conversion $\geq$ 1% annually); and (3) health workers who may be at an increased risk of repeated exposure.

References

1. Smith, M. H. D., and Marqui, J. R. Tuberculosis and Other Mycobacterial Infections. In R. D. Feigin and J. D. Cherry (eds.), *Textbook of Pediatric Infectious Disease* (2nd ed.). Philadelphia: Saunders, 1987. Pp. 1342–1387. *Comprehensive review of epidemiology, pathogenesis, and clinical aspects of tuberculosis in children.*
2. Bloch, A. B., and Snider, D. E. How much tuberculosis in children must we accept? *Am. J. Public Health* 76(1):14, 1986. *Excellent editorial on the epidemiology and prevention of tuberculosis in children.*
3. Powell, K. E., Meador, M. P., and Farer, L. S. Recent trends in tuberculosis in children. *J.A.M.A.* 251(10):1289, 1984. *Review of epidemiology of tuberculosis in the United States from 1976 to 1981.*
4. Snider, J. E., Jr. Bacille Calmette-Guérin vaccinations and tuberculin skin tests. *J.A.M.A.* 253(23):3438, 1985. *Discusses the difficulty in interpreting skin tests in patients with a past history of BCG vaccination; also gives specific recommendations.*
5. American Thoracic Society, Medical Section of the American Lung Association. Treatment of tuberculosis and tuberculosis infection in adults and children. *Am. Rev. Respir. Dis.* 134:355, 1986. *Joint statement by the American Thoracic Society and the CDC on prophylaxis treatment of tuberculosis.*
6. Clemens, J. D., Chuong, J. J., and Feinstein, A.R. The BCG controversy: A methodological and statistical reappraisal. *J.A.M.A.* 249(17):2362, 1983. *A scholarly analysis of BCG vaccine efficacy data from eight major controlled trials.*

54 Diphtheria in Children

Chinh Le

I. The problem

A. Description [1]. Diphtheria is an acute, contagious disease caused by *Corynebacterium diphtheriae* and characterized by membraneous nasopharyngitis or obstructive laryngotracheitis, or both. Cutaneous, rarely vaginal, and conjunctival or otic infection can also occur. Myocarditis, neural damage leading to paralysis, and interstitial nephritis may occur secondary to an exotoxin. Five to ten percent of cases are fatal, but mortality in those with severe cases with myocarditis may exceed 50%. Humans are the sole reservoir of *C. diphtheriae*, which is spread chiefly by the secretions of infected persons or asymptomatic carriers, directly or via contaminated articles, including food. Infection and carrier state can rarely occur in immunized persons, but the disease is severe in those unimmunized or inadequately immunized.

B. Epidemiology [2, 3]. During 1971–1981, the overall United States incidence rate of diphtheria continued to decline to only rare cases (0.01 case per million), with more cases in children less than 15 years and in Native Americans (22.6 cases per million). Persons immunized with three or more doses of diphtheria toxoid had a lower fatality rate (1.3%) than totally unimmunized persons (13.4%). It has been postulated that the decline of diphtheria may be due to the loss of the gene for producing diphtheria toxin in a highly immunized population.

II. Primary prevention

A. Methods. The only effective control is by a community program of active immunization with diphtheria toxoid. It is administered as a triple antigen along with tetanus toxoid and pertussis vaccine (DTP). Combined diphtheria and tetanus toxoids (DT) are available for children less than 7 years of age in whom pertussis vaccine is contraindicated. An adult form (Td) is available for immunization of persons 7 years of age or older. Complete primary immunization for diphtheria consists of four doses of DTP or DT, and for previously immunized persons 7 years of age and older, 3 doses of Td. A single-antigen product is available but rarely indicated.

Because of decreasing antibody levels with age, active protections should be maintained by administering a dose of Td every 10 years after the completion of the primary immunization schedule.

Contraindications and side effects of DTP, DT, and Td vaccines are discussed in Chap. 52 and in Table 52-2.

B. Justification. The current rarity of diphtheria (1–5 cases per year) in the United States is due to the high immunization levels among children. Toxigenic strains of *C. diphtheriae* still circulate in the United States and around the world, and immunization does not eliminate their carriage in the pharynx, nose, or skin. The morbidity and mortality of this infection remain high; and the efficacy of chemoprophylaxis has not been firmly established. Therefore, the only effective control measure for diphtheria is active immunization on a community or worldwide basis. Vaccine efficacy is greater than 90%.

III. Recommendations [4]

A. Specific immunization schedule for diphtheria, in combination of tetanus and pertussis, is given in Chap. 52 and Tables 52-5, 52-6, and 52-7.

B. A booster dose of Td should be given every 10 years after primary immunization.

C. Diphtheria infection is not always followed by lasting immunity. Therefore, active immunization should be initiated or completed during convalescence.

References

1. Benenson, A. S. (ed.) *Control of Communicable Diseases in Man. An Official Report of the American Public Health Association* (14th ed.). Washington, DC: American Public Health Association, 1981. *Concise review of pathogenesis, epidemiology, and control of diphtheria.*
2. English, P. C. Diphtheria and theories of infectious disease: Centennial appreciation of the critical role of diphtheria in the history of medicine. *Pediatrics* 76(1):1, 1985. *Historical perspective on the control of diphtheria.*
3. Chen, R. T. et al. Diphtheria in the United States, 1971–1981. *Am. J. Public Health* 75(12):1393, 1985. *Current epidemiology of diphtheria in the United States population.*
4. Immunization Practices Advisory Committee. Diphtheria, tetanus and pertussis: Guidelines for vaccine prophylaxis and other preventive measures. *M.M.W.R.* 34(27):405, 1985. *Updated recommendation by the CDC.*

55 Pertussis in Children

Chinh Le

I. The problem

A. Description. Pertussis is an acute, highly contagious infection caused by *Bordetella pertussis;* it is characterized by a paroxysmal or spasmodic cough that usually ends with an inspiratory whoop. Atypical forms of the illness may occur in young infants and partially immune individuals.

Humans are the only hosts of *B. pertussis*, and actively infected individuals are the only sources. Whether a carrier state exists or not is unknown, but it is unlikely. Transmission occurs via large, airborne droplets during the catarrhal stage of the disease. Up to 90% of nonimmune household contacts acquire the disease. Inadequately immunized school-age children and adults with waning immunity may have a mild atypical infection, which constitutes a major reservoir of infection.

The importance of preventing pertussis is measured by its complications; hospitalization is required in 75% of infected children less than 1 year of age. The most severe complications are bronchopneumonia (22%), seizure (2%), and encephalopathy (0.4%). Mortality is about 0.5–1% before age 1.

B. Epidemiology. Approximately 2000–3000 cases of pertussis are reported a year in the United States, with many more cases unrecognized and unreported. Infants less than 1 year of age are most severely affected. In 1984–1985, 42.5% of reported cases occurred in infants less than 1 year of age, and 16.5% in persons older than 15 years. Of these, 55% had received less than three doses of diphtheria, tetanus, and pertussis vaccine (DTP), and 31% had received none.

II. Primary prevention

A. Method. Pertussis vaccine is a suspension of inactivated *B. pertussis* cells. Potency is assayed by comparison with the United States Standard Pertussis Vaccine in the intracerebral mouse protection test. Routine primary immunization against pertussis is administered in combination with diphtheria and tetanus toxoids (DTP). Each 0.5 ml of DTP contains 4 protective units of pertussis antigen. A total dose of at least 12 units (or 3 doses) is the minimum number considered necessary for adequate vaccine protection. Routine booster doses should be given about 1 year after completion of the initial series and before school entry [1].

Mild and self-limited adverse reactions are common with DTP vaccinations (see Table 52-2). Rarely severe systemic reactions—anaphylaxis and peripheral neuropathy—have been reported, although a causal relationship cannot always by established. However, because of adverse media publicity, no vaccine has evoked as much fear and controversy as the pertussis vaccine. Severe reactions attributed to this vaccine include: collapse and shocklike state (0.6%); persistent screaming episodes (greater than or equal to a 3-hour duration, 1%); temperature greater than 40.5 °C (0.3%); isolated convulsion with or without fever (0.6%); acute encephalopathy (1 in 110,000 doses); and, permanent neurologic deficit (1 in 310,000 doses). There has been no scientific evidence linking pertussis vaccine to sudden infant death or infantile spasm; occurrence of these two conditions coincides with the DTP immunization schedule and can be expected to be related by chance alone [2].

An acellular pertussis vaccine is being evaluated in the United States following its successful preliminary use in Japan. The incidence of common side effects is reduced by this vaccine, but whether the incidence of severe adverse reactions and vaccine efficacy are comparable with those of the present vaccine awaits further investigation.

B. Justification [1, 2, 3,]. Specific antibiotic treatment has little or no impact on the further course of clinical illness after the paroxysmal cough has begun. Pertussis vaccine efficacy in protecting children in household contact with an adult or child with pertussis ranges from 70–95%. A high degree of protection persists for 3 years, declining thereafter over the following 6–12 years.

There is no question that the current low rate and morbidity of pertussis in the United States is largely the result of widespread active immunization since the 1940s. It has been reported that with a homogeneous vaccination coverage of 80% or greater, herd immunity exists. In countries where the use of DTP vaccine dropped in the mid-1970s, from 80% to 15–30% (Japan and several European countries, for example), there was a following 5- to 16-fold increase in pertussis, at epidemic levels. In the United States, recent county- or statewide outbreaks have also been associated with low immunization levels.

The risk of permanent neurologic disability from pertussis infection would be 13 times greater than now associated with DTP vaccination; the risk of pneumonia would be 89 times greater; and hospitalization for pertussis would be 62 times more likely than it is for vaccine-related complications [3]. An analysis of disease-related costs and costs associated with vaccine and vaccine reactions gave a benefit/cost ratio of 11.1:1 in favor of continuing the present pertussis immunization program [4].

Thus, using the best available estimates on frequency of complications of both the vaccine and the disease, routine pertussis immunization with the present vaccine should continue. A less reactogenic and safer vaccine may be available within this decade.

III. Recommendations

A. General recommendations

1. Pertussis vaccine should be given in combination with DTP starting at 6–8 weeks of age in the standard, single-dose volume of 0.5 ml. The **recommended schedules** for primary booster doses are given in Tables 52-5 and 52-6. In epidemic situations, immunization may be started as early as 2 weeks of age, and the first three doses can be given as frequently as 4 weeks apart.
2. If specific contraindications exist to the administration of pertussis vaccine, combined diphtheria and tetanus toxoids (DT) should be used. It is **not** recommended to reduce the volume of DTP administered to less than 0.5 ml per dose, or to use an increased number of reduced-volume doses to equal the total volume of the five recommended doses in an attempt to reduce side effects. Neither the efficacy of such practices in reducing the frequency of associated serious adverse effects, nor the resulting protection against disease have been determined.
3. Occurrence of **any** of the following reactions after administration of a pertussis-containing vaccine is a **contraindication** to further doses of pertussis vaccine.
   a. Fever of 40.5 °C (105 °F) or greater within 48 hours that is unexplained by another cause.
   b. Collapse or shocklike state (hypotonic-hyporesponsive episode) within 48 hours.
   c. Persistent, inconsolable crying lasting 3 hours or more, or an unusual, high-pitched cry occurring within 48 hours.
   d. Convulsion(s) with or without fever, occurring within 3 days, or encephalopathy occurring within 7 days, even though cause and effect may not be established.
   e. Allergic hypersensitivity to the vaccine.
4. Because the incidence rate and severity of pertussis decrease with age and because of potential adverse reactions, pertussis immunization is not recommended for persons 7 years of age and older. In exceptional cases, such as persons with chronic pulmonary disease or health care personnel exposed to pertussis outbreaks, a booster dose of 0.25 ml of adsorbed pertussis vaccine may be considered.*
5. **Education** of the public, and particularly parents of infants, to the dangers of pertussis and to the benefits of initiating immunization on time and adhering to the immunization schedule is important. Effective legislation must be enacted to protect the vaccine supply and contain the cost of the immunization program.

B. Specific recommendations

1. **Immunization of infants and young children who have underlying neurologic disorders**
   a. Administration of DTP in the **presence of an undiagnosed or changing, uncontrolled neurological disease** (such as infantile spasms, progressive encephalopathy, uncontrolled epilepsy) may result in confusion about causation or even aggravate manifestation of the disease. Therefore, the decision to immunize must be made on an individual basis; both the American Academy

*Available from Biologic Products Division, Michigan Department of Health, P.O. Box 30035, Lansing, MI 48909.

of Pediatrics (AAP) and the Advisory Committee on Immunization Practices (ACIP) recommend that where the risk of disease is low, pertussis immunization should be deferred until the neurologic disorder is stable. DT should then be given in lieu of DTP. If immunization is deferred, then the decision whether to commence immunization with DTP or DT should be made no later than the child's first birthday. Reassessment of children for whom immunization was deferred should be made at each office or clinic visit, and pertussis vaccination should be started as soon as feasible.

b. Parents of children with a history of convulsions should be made aware of the slightly increased chance of postimmunization seizures. However, the following conditions are **not** considered contraindications to pertussis vaccination.

(1) Stable neurologic conditions, such as cerebral palsy or simple seizures that can be satisfactorily explained and controlled.

(2) Resolved or corrected neurologic disorders (such as neonatal hypoglycemia or hypocalcemic seizure and corrected hydrocephalus).

(3) Family history of convulsion, or if a sibling has had a seizure following receipt of a pertussis-containing vaccine (although there is a small increase in neurologic events in these children following DTP vaccinations [5]).

2. Children who have recovered from culture-proved pertussis need not receive further doses of pertussis vaccine. Lacking culture confirmation of the diagnosis, however, DTP immunization should be completed, since a pertussislike syndrome may have been caused by other respiratory agents.

References

1. Advisory Committee on Immunization Practices (ACIP). Diphtheria, tetanus and pertussis: Guidelines for vaccine prophylaxis and other preventive measures. *M.M.W.R.* 34(27):405, 1985. *Revised, standard CDC recommendations, with specific discussion on side effects and contraindications.*
2. American Academy of Pediatrics, Committee on Infectious Diseases. Pertussis vaccine. *Pediatrics* 74(2):303, 1984. *Official AAP position on pertussis vaccine, with specific recommendations.*
3. Cherry, J. D. The controversy about pertussis vaccine. *Topics in Clinical Infectious Disease* 6:216, 1986. *Scholarly review of the health care benefits and risks of pertussis immunization programs.*
4. Hinman, A. R., and Koplan, J. P. Pertussis and pertussis vaccine: Reanalysis of benefits, risks and costs. *J.A.M.A.* 251(23):3109, 1984. *Current review supporting continuation of present pertussis vaccination strategy.*
5. American Academy of Pediatrics, Committee on Infectious Diseases. Family history of convulsions in candidates for immunization with pertussis-containing vaccines (diphtheria, tetanus, pertussis). *Pediatrics* 80(5):743, 1987.

56 Tetanus in Children

Chinh Le

I. The problem

A. Description [1]. Tetanus ("lockjaw") is caused by an exotoxin (tetanospasmin) produced by *Clostridium tetani.* It is characterized by severe intermittent tonic spasms of voluntary muscles that are painful. Fatal asphyxia may occur.

Tetanus is a serious disease, with a case fatality rate of 26% (52% for patients 60 years of age and older) in recent years.

B. Epidemiology. *C. tetani* is a normal inhabitant of animal and human intestines, and its spores are ubiquitous in the environment. The organisms can multiply and elaborate toxin in trivial as well as overtly contaminated wounds; devitalized wounds are at greatest risk. Neonatal tetanus occurs among infants born under unhygienic conditions to inadequately immunized mothers. Except for tetanus neonatorum, tetanus is not communicable.

Approximately 70–100 cases of tetanus a year were reported in the United States in the early 1980s, and only 4% of these occurred in persons less than 20 years of age. This reflects the success of childhood vaccination programs and standards of hygiene. During 1982–1984, of those with tetanus reported in the United States, 95% had not received a primary series of tetanus toxoid [2].

II. Primary prevention

A. Methods

1. **Tetanus toxoid** is prepared by formaldehyde treatment of tetanus toxin. It is available in combined adsorbed preparations with diptheria toxoid and pertussis vaccine (DTP, DT [for children under 7 years old] and Td [for persons 7 years and older]). Although tetanus toxoid is available as a single immunizing agent, persons requiring tetanus booster immunization should be given Td (or DT) to also enhance immunity against diphtheria. Available data do not indicate more reactions following receipt of Td than following receipt of single antigen tetanus toxoid.

   The only contraindication to DT or Td is a history of a neurologic or severe hypersensitivity reaction following a previous dose. Intradermal skin testing with appropriate dilute tetanus toxoid, or measurement of serum tetanus antitoxins levels, may be useful in determining the safety of further tetanus toxoid doses in patients with a previous history of severe reactions to diphtheria or tetanus toxoids, or both.

   Prevention of neopatal tetanus can be only ensured by adequate immunization levels in pregnant women.

2. **Tetanus immune globulin (TIG).** TIG of human source is the preferred product for passive immunization since equine antitoxin carries a higher risk of adverse reactions.

B. Justification. Naturally acquired immunity to tetanus toxin does not occur in the United States population. A completed primary series generally induces protective levels of serum antitoxin that persist for 10 or more years. Tetanus toxoid given as prophylaxis in wound management does not prevent the development of tetanus in 25% of cases. Thus, universal primary and booster immunization is necessary to protect persons in all age groups.

III. Recommendations [3]

A. Primary immunization should be started between 6–8 weeks of age using the combined DTP vaccine (or DT if pertussis vaccine is contraindicated) (see Tables 52-5, 52-6, and 52-7). Vaccine side effects are discussed in Table 52-2.

B. Neonatal tetanus prevention. There is no evidence that tetanus and diphtheria toxoids are teratogenic. A previously unimmunized pregnant woman should receive two doses of Td spaced 4–8 weeks apart, preferably during the last two trimesters, then a third dose 6–12 months after the second dose. Incompletely immunized pregnant women

Table 56-1. Recommended tetanus prophylaxis in wound management

History of tetanus immunization	Type of wound[a]	Immunization schedule
Uncertain, unimmunized, or incomplete (less than three doses of tetanus toxoid)	Low-risk	Td or DT or DTP, followed by complete immunization schedule
	High-risk	Td or DT or DTP plus TIG[b], followed by complete immunization schedule
Full primary series[c] plus booster dose within 10 years	Low-risk	None
	High-risk	None if less than 5 years since last dose; Td if more than 5 years
Full primary series[c] with no booster, or last booster more than 10 years ago	Low-Risk	Td
	High-risk	Td

[a]Low-risk wounds are minor, clean wounds; high-risk wounds are wounds that yield anaerobic conditions or are incurred under conditions in which tetanus exposure is probable (such as, but not limited to, contamination with dirt, feces, soil, saliva; puncture wounds; avulsions; wounds resulting from missiles; crushing; burns; and frostbite).
[b]TIG=human tetanus immune globulin; 250–500 units are given intramuscularly at separate site from Td or DT injection.
[c]Full primary series means primary immunization schedule consisting of four doses in children, or three doses in persons 7 years of age and older.

should complete the three-dose series, and a booster dose should be given to those immunized more than 10 years previously.

C. **Booster immunization.** Surveys indicate that the proportion of the population lacking protective levels of circulating antitoxin against tetanus increases with increasing age. To ensure continued adequate immunity, a Td dose should be given routinely every 10 years.

D. **Tetanus prophylaxis in routine wound management.** Wound cleaning, debridement when indicated, and proper immunization are important. Patients with unknown or uncertain previous immunization histories should be considered to have had no previous tetanus toxoid doses. Td (or DT, or DPT for children younger than 7 years of age) is the preferred preparation to concurrently enhance diphtheria protection (Table 56-1).

References

1. Schofield, F. Selective primary health care: Strategies for control of disease in the developing world. XXII. Tetanus: A preventable problem. *Rev. Infect. Dis.* 8(1):144, 1986. *Review of tetanus infection, epidemiology, and modes of prevention.*
2. Tetanus—United States, 1982–1984. *M.M.W.R.* 34(39):602, 607, 1985. *Current status of the epidemiology of tetanus in the United States.*
3. Advisory Committee on Immunization Practices (ACIP). Diphtheria, tetanus and pertussis: Guidelines for vaccine prophylaxis and other preventive measures. *M.M.W.R.* 34(27):405, 1985. *Current recommendations from the CDC.*

57 Poliomyelitis in Children

Chinh Le

I. The problem

A. Description. Poliomyelitis—caused by poliovirus types 1, 2, and 3—is an acute, highly contagious enteroviral infection with a wide range of manifestations—from inapparent illness to minor clinical cases, aseptic meningitis (nonparalytic) and flaccid asymmetric paralysis.

Although 95% of poliovirus infections are inapparent or mild, prognosis can be grave in those with paralytic poliomyelitis. Mortality is 1–4%, but up to 10% in adults or those with bulbar disease; 10–20% may have severe permanent disability. There is no specific treatment.

B. Epidemiology [1]. Poliovirus infection occurs only in humans and is spread by the oropharyngeal-fecal route. Maternal-to-newborn transmission can occur. Infection is more common in infants and young children, and it occurs earlier under conditions of poor sanitation and hygiene. While paralytic poliomyelitis is still prevalent in many underdeveloped countries, it is now rare in the United States; 8–10 cases are reported yearly, and 76% are temporally associated with the use of the oral polio vaccine. In the United States in recent years, outbreaks of wild disease have occurred in groups who have rejected immunizations, because of foreign importation, and in sporadic endemic areas.

II. Primary prevention

A. Method. While both the live attenuated trivalent oral vaccine (OPV) and the inactivated poliovaccine (IPV) are highly effective in reducing the incidence of poliomyelitis, heated disagreement continues among experts regarding their relative safety and efficacy. However, when the benefits and risks for the entire population are considered, the Advisory Committee on Immunization Practices (ACIP), the American Academy of Pediatrics (AAP), and the National Academy of Sciences have renewed their recommendations that the OPV remain the vaccine of choice for primary routine immunization of children in the United States for the following reasons: OPV is simpler and cheaper to administer, it stimulates natural infection, and it induces both systemic and intestinal immunity. It is also excreted in the stools of vaccine recipients and may induce immunization of unvaccinated contacts. However, OPV is not without problems [2]. Controversies, both scientific and medicolegal, surround the association of OPV and paralytic disease in OPV recipients or their close contacts (the incidence is estimated at 1 case in approximately 2.64 million doses distributed; for vaccine recipients, 1 case per 8.7 million doses; for contacts of vaccinees, 1 per 5.5 million doses). Although immunodeficient patients and adults are at higher risk for this paralytic reaction, about 90% of the cases occur in previously healthy individuals. Another concern is the potential reversion of the live attenuated OPV virus to a "wild" virus with greater neurovirulence. (Type 3 has in particular been noted to have a tendency to mutate during the viral replication that occurs during immunization.) Furthermore, respose to OPV in some tropical countries has been less than optimal because of vaccine instability and interference from other infecting enteric viruses [3].

For the above reasons, a return to IPV has been suggested. However, IPV has its own theoretical disadvantages. It requires subcutaneous injections, probably offers a shorter duration of immunity unless booster doses are given, and it may induce only low levels of antibodies to poliovirus type 3 (Finland epidemic, 1984–1985 [4]. These concerns may be allayed now that an improved IPV product with higher potency has been licensed [5].

B. Justification. Poliovirus vaccines are highly effective: two doses of OPV or four doses of IPV are effective and produce protective antibody responses to all three serotypes in excess of 90–95% of vaccines. The use of both live and killed virus vaccines has resulted in a marked decrease in the worldwide incidence of paralytic disease. However, outbreaks can still occur in areas with circulating wild strains of polio virus despite high overall community vaccination levels (Taiwan, 1982; Finland, 1984–1985) [6].

III. Recommendations

A. OPV is the vaccine currently used for routine immunization of normal children in the United States (up to age 18). The schedule is given in Tables 52-5, 52-6, and 52-7. The primary series consists of three doses; the first two doses should be separated by at least 6, and preferably 8, weeks. The third dose is given at least 6 weeks and customarily 8–12 months after the second dose. In high-risk areas, an additional dose of OPV should be given at 6 months of age. Before school entry, all children who previously received the primary OPV immunization should be given a fourth dose if the third primary dose was administered before the fourth birthday.

B. Contraindications to use of OPV. As a live attenuated vaccine, OPV should not be used for immunizing immunodeficient patients **and** their household contacts (IPV is recommended in these cases).

C. IPV. The primary series consists of four doses of vaccine, usually integrated with DPT immunization. The three first doses can be given at 4- to 8-week intervals, and the fourth should follow 6–12 months after the third. A fifth dose should be given if the fourth dose was given before the fourth birthday. Children who receive primary immunization with the older IPV should obtain a booster dose every 5 years until they reach the age of 18. The need for booster doses for individuals who receive primary immunization with the new enhanced potency IPV is not known at this time. The indications for IPV include: (1) primary immunization of unvaccinated adults at increased risk of poliomyelitis (such as travelers to endemic or epidemic areas; health care or laboratory workers exposed to polioviruses); (2) immunodeficient patients and their household contacts; and, (3) anyone strongly wishing to avoid any risk of OPV-associated paralysis.

D. Past history of clinical poliomyelitis does not preclude the administration of IPV or OPV when otherwise indicated, since infection with one serotype does not provide cross-immunity to the other two.

References

1. Poliomyelitis—United States, 1975–1984. *M.M.W.R.* 35(11):180, 1986. *Current epidemiology of poliomyelitis in the United States.*
2. Advisory Committee on Immunization Practices (ACIP). Poliomyelitis prevention. *M.M.W.R.* 31(3):22, 1982. *Review and recommendations by the CDC.*
3. Hortsmann, D. M., Quinn, T. C., and Robbins, F. C. International symposium on poliomyelitis control. *Rev. Infect. Dis.* 6(Suppl. 2):s301, 1984. *Reports from countries throughout the world on the results of poliomyelitis prevention programs; review of current poliovirus vaccines, research, and prospect for worldwide control.*
4. Update: Poliomyelitis outbreak—Finland, 1984–1985. *M.M.W.R.* 35(6):82, 1986. *Report on a polio outbreak where IPV had been used.*
5. Advisory Committee on Immunization Practices (ACIP). Poliomyelitis prevention: Enhanced potency inactivated poliomyelitis vaccine—supplementary statement. *M. M. W. R.* 36(48):795, 1987. *CDC recommendation for use of new IPV vaccine.*
6. Kim-Farley, R. J., et al. Outbreak of paralytic poliomyelitis, Taiwan. *Lancet* 2(8415):1322, 1984. *Description of an outbreak occurring in a community in which 80% of the infants had received at least 2 doses of OPV.*

58 Measles

Chinh Le

I. The problem

A. Description. Measles (rubeola) is an acute, highly contagious viral infection characterized by fever, cough, coryza, conjunctivitis, a characteristic enanthem (Koplik spots), and a confluent maculopapular (morbilliform) rash. Complications include pneumonia (4%), otitis (2.5%), encephalitis (0.1–0.4%), and others. The illness is spread largely by infectious nasopharyngeal secretions. Measles is usually a self-limited infection, but complications are common. Encephalitis occurs in about 1 in 1000 cases. Measles virus is also associated with subacute sclerosing panencephalitis (SSPE). The case to fatality ratio is reported as 0.1:2.3%.

B. Epidemiology. Efforts are being made to eradicate measles in the United States by extensive use of the live measles vaccine, immunization requirements for school entry, good surveillance systems, and effective public health response to the occurrence of disease. Thus the incidence of measles is rapidly decreasing in the United States, with only approximately 2050–6000 cases reported to the Center for Disease Control yearly. Ninety percent of all counties are free of measles [1,2].

Two epidemiologic trends are of current concern: the emerging importance of imported measles in this country and the persistence of susceptible populations of preschoolers and young adults. Present emphasis is therefore placed on vaccinating not only children at 15 months of age but also susceptible adolescents and young adults (5–10% of persons born between 1950 and 1965 are currently believed to be susceptible).

In the early 1980s, 35% of reported measles cases were classified as preventable. (Among children 16 months to 4 years of age, and adults 20–24 years, this figure was 75%.) Currently, though 15 months is the recommended measles immunization age, less than 80% of United States children are immunized by the age of 2 years, which suggests continuing immunization gaps in susceptible populations. Furthermore, 2–10% of cases were associated with international or out-of-state importations. Therefore, the final eradication of measles in the United States must depend on a universal immunity level achievable only by continuing immunization efforts.

II. Primary prevention

A. Method. The live measles virus vaccine presently used in the United States is prepared in chick embryo cell culture and further attenuated beyond the level of the original Edmonston B strain. It is available in monovalent form and in combinations: measles/rubella (MR) and measles/mumps/rubella (MMR) vaccines.

It is administered subcutaneously. An aerolized form is currently under investigation.

Improperly stored vaccine may result in lack of protection against measles. Directions for proper handling of the vaccine are given in the vaccine package insert and in Table 52-8.

B. Justification

1. **Benefits.** There is no specific treatment for measles. The current vaccine produces an antibody response in 95–98% of the recipients, which has remained detectable in a 15-year follow-up.

   As a result of intensive efforts to vaccinate children in the United States, measles and its complications, including SSPE, have declined more than 99% from the prevaccine era. The benefit/cost ratio of the measles immunization program has been recently estimated to be 14.6 : 1, with a net health care savings of over $5 billion for the 20-year period of 1963–1982. Where outbreaks have occurred, such as in colleges or medical settings, control measures have proved very costly.

2. **Risks and side effects.** Vaccine side effects are summarized in Table 52-2. Children with a personal or first-degree (parent or sibling) history of convulsions have a slightly increased risk of convulsions 5–14 days after vaccination. However, this is not a contraindication to measles vaccination [3]. **Atypical measles** is a severe

hypersensitivity syndrome that occurs after exposure to natural measles virus in some individuals who received killed measles vaccine in the past and rarely in unvaccinated individuals.

III. Recommendations

A. General recommendations

1. Measles vaccine is routinely administered at 15 months of age in healthy infants in combination with rubella and mumps vaccines.
2. Tuberculosis skin testing is recommended before or at the time of measles vaccination, but there is no clinical data that measles vaccine exacerbates tuberculosis.

B. Specific recommendations

1. **Exposure of susceptible persons to wild virus.** Measles vaccination after exposure to natural measles is safe, can usually prevent measles (even when administered up to 14 days after exposure), and can usually control an epidemic in progress. Small children at risk include the following:
   a. **Infants 6–12 months old** at immediate high risk of measles exposure may be immunized and then reimmunized at 15 months; however, 25–50% of infants so vaccinated are unable to sustain an antibody response after the booster doses. An alternative approach for these infants is to administer 0.25 ml/kg of immune globulin (Ig) immediately, and subsequently to administer measles vaccine at or after 15 months of age (at least 3 months should elapse between Ig and measle vaccine administrations).
   b. **Infants 12–15 months old** immunized under the foregoing circumstances do not need to be reimmunized at 15 months of age (except in special circumstances, e.g., school outbreaks). However, if the parents of a child vaccinated at 12–14 months old request revaccination for the child, there is no immunologic or safety reason to deny the request. Since antibody titers following immunization are usually lower than those following natural infection, some infants born since 1963 may become susceptible to measles before 12–15 months of age. Recommendations for selective early vaccination of these children await further studies.
2. **Older individuals** in the following situations should be immunized with live measles vaccine.
   a. Those who have not had medically documented natural measles infection or immunization with live vaccine at, or after, 12 months of age.
   b. Those whose primary immunization regimen included the inactivated, killed vaccine (available in the United States from 1963–1967; in Canada, up to 1970); or the further attenuated vaccine (Swartz strain) with immune serum globulin, or measles vaccine of unknown type, before 1968.
3. Patients with leukemia in remission whose chemotherapy has been terminated for at least 3 months and asymptomatic patients infected with human immunodeficiency virus (HIV) may receive measles or MMR vaccine [3].

C. Precautions and contraindications. See Table 52-8 and Fig. 52-1 for precautions and contraindications when administering viral live vaccine.

References

1. Bloch, A. B. et al. Health impact of measles vaccination in the United States. *Pediatrics* 76(4):524, 1985. *Review on public health impact of measles and measles vaccination programs.*
2. Advisory Committee on Immunization Practices (ACIP). Measles prevention. *M.M.W.R.* 36(17):409, 1987. *Standard review and recommendations by the Centers for Disease Control.*
3. Advisory Committee on Immunization Practices (ACIP). Measles prevention. *M. M. W. R.* 36(29):409, 1987. *CDC updates on measles prevention.*

59 Mumps

Chinh Le

I. The problem

A. Description. Mumps, an acute, generally mild, contagious infection caused by a paramyxovirus, is characterized by painful enlargement of parotid and salivary glands. Thirty percent of the cases are subclinical.

Complications of mumps include meningoencephalitis (severe in 5–10%), oophoritis (5% of cases in postpubertal females), orchitis (20% of postpubertal male patients), neurosensory deafness (1 in 5000 cases), and various inflammations (arthritic and visceral). Infection in the first trimester of pregnancy carries an increased risk of fetal wastage.

B. Epidemiology [1]. Mumps virus is spread by the respiratory route. Vertical transmission has also been described. Although mumps is primarily a disease of young, school-age children, 41.7% of cases in 1984 occurred in 10- to 19-year-olds, and 11.5% occurred in persons older than 20 [1], when complications of the disease are more common. In recent years, about 3000 cases or less of mumps are reported yearly, a 98% decrease since 1968, the year after the live mumps vaccine licensure.

II. Primary prevention

A. Method. Mumps vaccine is a live-attenuated virus vaccine available as a monovalent vaccine, or in combination with rubella or measles, or both, vaccines (MR or MMR). Vaccine side effects are listed in Table 52-2. There is no proved association between mumps vaccination and pancreatic damage or subsequent development of diabetes mellitus.

Vaccination with MMR of persons who were previously immune to one or more of its components is not associated with increased adverse effects. For appropriate vaccine storage, see Table 52-8.

B. Justification. There is no specific treatment for mumps infection. Mumps immune globulin (Ig) is not effective and is no longer available. Mumps vaccine induces protective antibody response in more than 90% of recipients, and immunity may be lifelong. Reported clinical vaccine efficacy ranges from 75–90%.

A benefit/cost analysis based on national data for 1983 determined that an immunization program would have a benefit/cost ratio of 6.7 : 1 and 14.4 : 1, using single-antigen mumps vaccine and combined MMR vaccine, respectively.

III. Recommendations [2]

A. General recommendations. MMR is the vaccine of choice for routine childhood immunization; it is given as a single subcutaneous dose to healthy infants at 15 months of age.

B. Specific recommendations

1. Mumps vaccine is indicated for all young adults (those born after 1957), particularly males believed to be susceptible (i.e., no physician-diagnosed mumps or no records of adequate immunization with live mumps vaccine when 12 or more months of age).
2. Testing for susceptibility before vaccination may be unreliable, not readily available, and not cost-effective.
3. Persons who received killed-mumps vaccine (available from 1950–1978) might benefit from vaccination with live-mumps vaccine.

C. Vaccine precautions and contraindications. See Table 52-8 and Fig. 52-1.

References

1. Mumps—United States, 1984–1985. *M.M.W.R.* 35(13):216, 1986. *Update on epidemiology of mumps in the United States.*
2. Advisory Committee on Immunization Practices (ACIP). Mumps vaccine. *M.M.W.R.* 31(46):617, 25, 1982. *Centers for Disease Control recommendations for use of mumps vaccine.*

60 Rubella

Chinh Le

I. The problem

A. Description. Postnatal rubella (German measles, three-day measles) is an airborne viral infection characterized by a mild systemic illness associated with a generalized exanthema and lymphadenopathy. It can result in abortion, stillbirth, and congenital defects in infants born to mothers infected during the early months of pregnancy [1] (See Chap. 20).

Infection during the first 8 weeks of pregnancy results in a fetal infection rate of about 50%; this rate decreases to less than 10% by the sixteenth week. During the past epidemic years in the United States, congenital rubella had been found in as many as 2% of newborns [2].

B. Epidemiology. Since 1969, the year of the rubella vaccine licensure, the incidence rate of rubella has decreased by 99%, with approximately less than 1000 reported cases a year in the United States [3].

As with measles, the current concerns about rubella are the continuing susceptible population of preschoolers and unvaccinated teenagers and adults, and the importation of rubella from other countries. An estimated 10–15% of young adults remain susceptible to rubella. Although the practice of vaccinating young children has prevented large-scale rubella epidemics, limited outbreaks continue to occur among nonimmunized young adults, including those in colleges and in places of employment—most notably hospitals.

II. Primary prevention

A. Methods. Only the vaccine prepared from attenuated live virus grown in human diploid cell cultures (RA 27/3 vaccine) is currently available in the United States. It is more immunogenic and has the same or lesser side effects than previous rubella vaccines. The vaccine is available in monovalent form and in combinations: measles/rubella (MR), rubella/mumps, and measles/mumps/rubella (MMR).

The rubella vaccine is 95% protective when given to persons 12 months of age and older. Based on available follow-up studies, vaccine-induced protection is expected to be lifelong. Very rarely, viremic reinfection after exposure may occur in vaccinated persons who have low levels of detectable antibody. Conversely, immunity may be present despite the absence of detectable hemagglutination-inhibition (HI) antibodies when more sensitive tests are done.

Routine rubella reimmunization of all children at the time of school entry or just before puberty has been suggested by some authorities. The basis for this recommendation is: (1) gaps in primary immunization; (2) presumed loss of immunity conferred by the previous or present rubella vaccines; (3) insurance against adult susceptibility; and (4) safety of multiple doses. Recent data, however, suggest that secondary vaccine failures appear to be illusory and rare. The patients are actually immune despite seronegativity. Priority should be given to immunizing all preschool and susceptible adoloscents and young adults. For these reasons, universal reimmunization is not recommended at the present time [1, 4].

Some vaccinees intermittently shed small amounts of virus from the pharynx 7–28 days after vaccination, but there is no evidence that vaccine virus is transmissible to contacts.

For **vaccine side effects,** see Table 52-2. Improperly stored vaccine may result in lack of protection against rubella. See package insert and Table 52-8 for proper handling of the vaccine.

B. Justification. The purpose of rubella immunization is to prevent congenital rubella.

There is no treatment for maternal or congenital rubella infection. Administration of immune globulin for postexposure prophylaxis of rubella in early pregnancy does not always prevent congenital infection. Therefore, universal protection by active immunization of young children (with the goal of preventing epidemics) and susceptible young adults is of paramount importance.

The present United States rubella immunization program has reduced the incidence of congenital rubella syndrome (CRS) by 99.2%. Only 5–10 cases of CRS are now reported a year. Because an estimated 10–15% of young adults remain susceptible to rubella and imported cases can start rubella outbreaks if the immunity level in the community is low, the control of rubella can only be achieved by maintaining high immunization levels [1, 3, 5,].

III. Recommendations

A. General recommendations

1. Live rubella virus vaccine is recommended for all children 12 months of age or older. It is routinely given at 15 months of age in combination with measles and mumps vaccine (MMR) as a single, subcutaneous dose.
2. Emphasis is also placed on vaccination of older, susceptible individuals who lack laboratory evidence of rubella immunity or written proof of adequate immunization with rubella vaccine on or after the first birthday. The clinical diagnosis of rubella is unreliable and should not be considered in assessing immune status.
3. When in doubt about rubella immunity and there are no contraindications to receipt of the vaccine, it is justifiable and preferable to administer the vaccine without prior serologic testing, particularly when costs of serology are high and follow-up of identified susceptible persons for vaccination is not assured. Alternatively, potential vaccinees of childbearing age can be screened for rubella susceptibility during premarital and prenatal tests, or during preemployment examination of individuals (both male and female). Susceptible persons should be vaccinated as soon as possible unless there are contraindications.

   Mandatory programs for both sexes for school entry, the military services, medical settings, colleges, or workplaces where women of childbearing age congregate (such as day-care centers, business companies, offices, industrial sites) are effective in maintaining a high level of immunity and are strongly recommended.

B. Specific recommendations

1. **Perinatal immunization of susceptible females**
   a. **Breast-feeding is not a contraindication to postpartum vaccination,** even though the virus may be excreted in breast milk and infants may be infected.
   b. **Administration of Rh immune globulin or blood products is not a contraindication to vaccination.** However, serologic testing should be done at 6–8 weeks to ascertain seroconversion. Vaccination should be extended to include all susceptible women postabortion.
   c. **Vaccination of women of childbearing age.** Accumulating evidence indicates that rubella vaccine is not harmful to the fetus; to avoid the theoretic risk, however, females of childbearing age should be immunized only if they state that they are not pregnant and that they understand that they should avoid pregnancy for 3 months after immunization. Inadvertent rubella vaccination during pregnancy should not be a reason to routinely recommend interruption of the pregnancy, but a final decision must rest with the individual patient and her physician.
   d. **Children of susceptible pregnant women or close contacts** should receive rubella vaccine because: (1) there is no evidence that the vaccine virus is transmissible; and (2) an immunized child is less likely to acquire natural rubella and introduce the virus into the household or into the classroom.
2. **Postexposure immunization of susceptible persons.** As far as use of vaccine or immune globulin after rubella exposure is concerned, there is no evidence that either or both of these measures will prevent rubella infection or congenital rubella syndrome. On the other hand, however, vaccinating a person incubating rubella is not harmful. Ig might be used when a pregnant woman who has been exposed to rubella would not consider termination of pregnancy under any circumstances.

C. Contraindications.

See Table 52-8 and Fig. 52-1 for precautions and contraindications when administering viral live vaccines.

References

1. Advisory Committee on Immunization Practices (ACIP). Rubella prevention. *M.M.W.R* 33(22):301, 1984. *Review and recommendations by the Centers for Disease Control.*

2. Rubella and congenital rubella syndrome—United States, 1984–1986. *M.M.W.R.* 36(40):664, 1987. *Review of current rubella statistics in the United States.*
3. Orenstein, W. A., et al. The opportunity and obligation to eliminate rubella from the United States. *J.A.M.A.* 251(15):1988, 1984. *Review of the success of current rubella prevention programs.*
4. Preblud, S. R. Some current issues relating to rubella vaccine. *J.A.M.A.* 254(2):253, 1985. *Risk/benefit analysis of immunization programs with current rubella vaccine.*
5. International symposium on prevention of congenital rubella infection. Washington, D.C., March 13–15, 1984. *Rev. Infect. Dis.* 7(Suppl. 1):1, 1985. *Review of rubella disease and control programs throughout the world.*

61

Haemophilus Influenzae Type B

Chinh Le

I. The problem

A. Definition. *Haemophilus influenzae* Type B (Hib) is a pleomorphic gram-negative coccobacillus that causes meningitis and other serious, invasive infections such as epiglottitis, septic arthritis, cellulitis, bacteremia, and pneumonia in children and adults. Approximately 3–5% of children with Hib meningitis die and 10–40% of survivors suffer various long-term neurologic sequelae, ranging from severe functional and mental handicaps to hearing loss [1, 2].

B. Epidemiology. It is estimated that invasive Hib disease affects approximately 1 in 1000 children in the United States before their fifth birthday. Hib is the major cause of childhood bacterial meningitis, nearly all cases of epiglottitis, and a substantial number of other bacteremic diseases. It is estimated that 20,000 cases of severe, invasive Hib infections occur a year in children less than 5 years of age, and that the incidence in older children and adults may be increasing as well. The peak incidence of the disease is between 6 and 12 months of age, except for epiglottitis for which the mean incidence of occurrence is 44 months of age [3].

Risk factors for Hib susceptibility, besides young age, include the following [1, 2, 4]:

1. Household contact with a patient with invasive Hib infection.
2. Attendance of a child 2 years of age or less at a large day-care center.
3. Functional or anatomic asplenia, including sickle cell anemia.
4. Immunosuppression and agammaglobulinemia.
5. Ethnicity (Native Americans, Eskimos, and blacks), and other genetic or host characteristics yet to be defined.

II. Prevention

A. Methods. Immunity to Hib disease is associated with the presence of antibodies in the Type B capsular polysaccharide (often referred to as PRP or polyribose-ribitol phosphate), and perhaps other somatic antigens of the Hib. Vaccines consisting of purified PRP and a PRP diphtheria toxoid conjugate vaccine have been licensed in the United States. Based on studies of antibody responses and large clinical trials in Finland, the vaccine's efficacy was estimated to be 90% for children 24 months or older. However, recent post-licensing studies of the PRP vaccine in the United States indicate efficacy rates around 40–80% (range 0–90%). The conjugate vaccine is more immunogenic, but antibody levels indicative of long-term protection were found only in 60% of children vaccinated at 15–24 months of age [2]. The vaccine is not effective for children less than 18 months old. Current studies are underway to develop and license other protein conjugate Hib vaccine(s), which would be more immunogenic and protective for younger children. Since the antibody production is very type-specific, the present PRP vaccine will not protect against *Haemophilus influenzae* diseases caused by other serotypes, nor by nontypable strains (which cause otitis media).

The present Hib vaccines are very safe. High fever (> 38.5 °C) has been reported in less than 1.5% of vaccinees, and mild local reactions in 10–12%. Physicians should be aware that Hib infection may occur in the week after vaccination, prior to appearance of protective antibodies.

B. Justification. Rifampin prophylaxis may prevent disease in household and day-care center contacts, but its use is expensive and often logistically difficult and erratic in large day-care centers. Development of antimicrobial resistance is a constant threat to the efficacy of disease treatment and chemoprophylaxis. These facts underscore the importance of Hib prevention by effective immunization programs.

The present Hib vaccines are not expected to have a significant impact on the overall incidence of Hib diseases since they are suboptimal in children younger than 24 months of age, who comprise 60–75% of all Hib cases in childhood. However, they should have a substantial impact on the disease incidence in children older than 24 months, and on cases of epiglottitis. The present Hib vaccines are an interim measure likely to be replaced by more immunogenic PRP–protein conjugate vaccine(s) in the near future [4].

III. General recommendations

A. The Hib-diphtheria toxoid conjugate vaccine should be given to all children at 18 months of age.

B. Immunization of individuals between 24 and 60 months of age who have not received Hib vaccine is recommended, but priorities should be based on risk of disease. Children 2–3 years of age who attend day-care center facilities should be given a higher priority than older children.

C. The vaccine is not recommended for children under 18 months of age.

D. The vaccine is not recommended for routine use in children older than 60 months of age. However, the AAP recommends its use for children who have chronic illnesses known to be associated with increased risk for Hib disease. The immunogenicity of the Hib vaccine has not been well studied in this group of patients.

E. The Hib vaccine can be given simultaneously with other vaccines but at different anatomic sites. No change in the schedule for the DTP or DT vaccines should be made secondary to the use of the Hib conjugate vaccine.

F. Children immunized at 18–23 months of age with the PRP vaccine (but not with the conjugate vaccine) should receive a booster dose after 24 months of age, preferably 2–6 months after the first.

G. Children who have had invasive Hib disease when they were under 24 months of age most likely failed to mount an immune response to clinical infection. They should therefore still receive the vaccine according to the above recommendations.

H. Vaccination is not a substitute for rifampin prophylaxis in individuals exposed to or carriers of Hib.

References

1. American Academy of Pediatrics, Committee on Infectious Diseases. Hemophilus type b polysaccharide vaccine. *Pediatrics* 76(2):322, 1985. *Recommendations by the AAP.*
2. Advisory Committee on Immunization Practices (ACIP). Update: Prevention of *Haemophilus influenzae* Type b disease. *M.M.W.R.* 37(2):13, 1988. *Recommendations by the Centers for Disease Control.*
3. Cochi, S. L., and Broome, C. V. Vaccine prevention of *Haemophilus influenzae* type b disease: Past, present and future. *Pediatr. Infect. Dis.* 5(1):12, 1986. *Review of epidemiology and prevention of Hib disease.*
4. Granoff, D. M., and Munson, R. S., Jr. Prospects for prevention of *Haemophilus influenzae* type b disease by immunization. *J. Infect. Dis.* 153(3): 448, 1986. *Review of pathogenesis and host factors of Hib, with excellent discussion on present and future Hib vaccines.*

Adult Care

62 Risk Assessment

Norman Kahn

I. Description

A. Definition. Risk assessment is a means of identifying elements in an individual's family history, personal health, present physical and mental condition, and life-style that will shorten that individual's life.

Data have been accumulated in mortality tables that are used to predict for a population group defined by age, sex, and race the most likely causes of death in the succeeding 10 years [1, 2]. Variables influencing mortality that are present in an individual member of the group (risk indicators) are combined with quantitative "weights" (risk factors) to estimate the risk of dying from both specific conditions and their composites [3].

B. Goal. The goal of risk assessment is to provide information to an individual in order to stimulate life-style (behavior) change that will decrease the risk of dying prematurely. This goal is realized through the following steps:

1. Individual becomes **aware** of his or her risk factors.
2. Individual becomes **knowledgeable** that modification of risk factors can alter the risk of dying prematurely.
3. Individual develops the **attitude** that the risk of dying is partially under his or her control.
4. Individual alters **behavior** in ways that are reflected in decreased risk factors.
5. Individual's **risk of dying prematurely** decreases.

C. Relationship to health promotion and disease prevention. In addition to enhancing survival, risk assessment can promote health by facilitating behavior change that leads to improved health status. There is a potential decrease in both mortality and morbidity.

For example, not wearing seatbelts is a risk indicator for dying from a motor vehicle accident. The behavior change to wearing seatbelts not only decreases the risk of mortality, but may decrease the risk of disabling injury for the individual who survives the accident.

D. Assessable conditions. The leading causes of death for a group defined by age, sex, and race may be found in published tables, based on actuarial data [4].

For example, for a white male age 25–29, the 10 leading causes of mortality are: (1) motor vehicle accident, (2) suicide, (3) homicide, (4) arteriosclerotic heart disease, (5) poisoning, (6) drowning, (7) machine accidents, (8) cirrhosis, (9) aircraft accidents, and (10) central nervous system vascular lesions.

The assessment of an individual's risk of developing one of these conditions involves identification of factors in family history, health history, present health, or life-style, for which data exist revealing a correlation between the factor and the development of the condition (e.g., cigarette smoking and lung cancer).

Assessable conditions in the United States include [1]:

1. **Accidents:** aircraft, drowning, falls, fire and explosion, firearms, machinery, motor vehicles, water transport, poisoning.
2. **Alcoholism:** cirrhosis, accidents.
3. **Cancer:** breast, cervix, colon/rectum, lung, uterus.
4. **Cardiovascular disease:** cerebrovascular disease, coronary artery disease, other vascular disease, rheumatic heart disease.
5. **Complications of pregnancy and abortion.**
6. **Diabetes.**
7. **Homicide.**
8. **Pneumonia, bronchitis, and emphysema.**
9. **Suicide.**

E. **Risk factors** for development of and mortality from the above conditions include, in addition to age, sex, and race:
   1. **Accidents:** alcohol habits, drugs and medications, mileage per year, seatbelt use.
   2. **Alcoholism:** alcohol habits.
   3. **Cancer**
      a. **Breast:** family history, history of benign breast disease, breast examination habits, menstrual status, pregnancies.
      b. **Cervix:** socioeconomic status, religion, sexual habits, cervical cytology.
      c. **Colon/rectum:** polyp, rectal bleeding, ulcerative colitis.
      d. **Lung:** smoking habits.
      e. **Uterus:** vaginal bleeding.
   4. **Cardiovascular and other vascular disease**
      a. **Cerebrovascular disease:** blood pressure, cholesterol level, diabetes, smoking habits.
      b. **Coronary artery disease:** blood pressure, cholesterol level, diabetes, smoking habits, exercise habits, family history, weight.
      c. **Rheumatic heart disease:** history of rheumatic fever, presence of signs and symptoms.
   5. **Complications of pregnancy and abortion:** socioeconomic status, religion, sexual habits.
   6. **Diabetes:** family history, weight.
   7. **Homicide:** arrest record, proximity to weapons.
   8. **Pneumonia, bronchitis, and emphysema:** smoking habits, alcohol habits.
   9. **Suicide:** depression, family history, alcohol habits.

II. Techniques

A. **Methods.** Risk assessment tools are used to gather information from an individual to identify risk factors, correlate risk factors with mortality data, and provide that information to the individual.

The health risk assessment (also called health risk profile or health hazard appraisal) is a primary tool for individual risk assessment. It provides a statistical estimate of an individual's risk of dying in the next decade from the assessable conditions of the population. It then provides a comparison of the individual's risk to that of the average for the same age, race, and sex population.

The individual's risk is based on the answers to a questionnaire assessing use of tobacco, alcohol, drugs and medications; automobile mileage and seatbelt use; exercise; family medical history of heart disease, diabetes, breast cancer; personal history of diabetes, pap smears, breast problems, rectal problems, bronchitis, and emphysema; life satisfaction; sleep; personal loss; proximity to violence; marital status; education; employment; and residence. Added to these responses are current physical examination and laboratory data: height, weight, blood pressure, and serum cholesterol [5, 6].

The individual's responses are then computed into an "appraised age" for the individual [1]. The individual with increased risks will have an appraised age older than his or her chronological age. For example, a 28-year-old with an appraised age of 37 has statistically the same risk of dying in the next decade as an individual of the same race and sex who is 37. The tool further reports to the individual the decrease in appraised age to an "achievable age" that can be reached with life-style changes that decrease the relative weight of specific risk factors [1].

The result is an individual profile of current health risks that informs the individual about which risk factors can be reduced by life-style change (e.g., risk of death from accidents is decreased by decreased alcohol consumption). Furthermore, the magnitude of reduction of risk is translated to the patient as a new "achievable age," younger than the current "appraised age," and in some cases, younger than the chronological age.

The weighted "appraised age," while a quantitative measure, is an "odds" statement rather than a prediction for an individual. Its real benefits lie in the objectivity and statistical validity of the data on which the "appraised age" is based, and in the potential for showing the individual not only the necessary changes to make to improve one's health, but a measure of improvement in the individual's "odds," should such life-style changes be made.

There are many variations of the health risk appraisal [6]. Some are designed for women, adolescents, geriatric patients, or workers. An inventory can be obtained from the National Health Information Clearing House [6]. Most utilize statistically predictive tables and thus have the weight of objectivity. Others are based on known associations but cannot be quantitated in the same manner as the health risk appraisal [7]. In a similar sense, a screening protocol based on incidence and prevalence data, average tumor rates of growth, and other objective data, has a statistical predictability to assist in disease prevention decision making.

B. Justification

1. **Effectiveness.** Whereas traditional medical practice intervenes after symptoms of disease have become manifest, health screening attempts to detect signs of disease before they become symptomatic, or at an early, potentially curable state to prevent subsequent disability and death. Risk assessment is designed to provide an intervention in health status before any pathologic condition exists in the individual. In this way, risk assessment, along with health education, can be considered to be the earliest intervention in health promotion and disease prevention [8].

   The effectiveness of the health risk appraisal, as any patient education tool, is only as good as the intervention measures that follow. Such a tool can be said to be effective if it stimulates the patient to progress from awareness, through knowledge and attitude change, to behavior change. Such health behavior change has been shown to be facilitated by health risk appraisal in some populations [9]. Further research is needed to validate sensitivity, specificity, and predictive value of the health risk appraisal.

2. **Risks.** Concern exists regarding the potential for undesirable responses. Many people respond to scare tactics with denial, procrastination, fatalism, or other "change-avoiding" tactics. Similarly, the potential exists for people to react against the health risk appraisal with similar defenses. There is always a risk in interpreting statistics based on group norms as literally predictive for the individual rather than as identification of risky behaviors [10].

   Nonetheless, risk assessment tools have a number of attractions for the health care consumer: There is the "ring of truth" derived from its statistical base; printouts add to the aura of validity; and it is relatively noninvasive, requiring only height, weight, and blood pressure measurements from the physical exam, with measurement of serum cholesterol as the most invasive input.

3. **Costs.** The cost of risk assessment tools varies from free to approximately $50, but most fall in the $10–20 range per individual. This is considerably less than the cost of the annual physical exam and less than a battery of lab tests performed in a "multiphasic screening." As such, the financial barrier to patient acceptance is reduced, although not eliminated entirely for those living on fixed incomes. At any price, preventive medicine frequently is not a priority for people whose financial status permits only basic necessities.

4. **Acceptability.** Perhaps the greatest barrier to risk assessment is what is common to all patient education tools and disease prevention measures: the threat of intervention. It is common to read into objective feedback a perceived expectation from the provider or from the patient that the patient will act on the information, and thus change, which is in itself one of the most threatening of human risks.

III. Recommendations

A. Just as screening is performed more effectively through the use of printed protocols, health promotion is effectively practiced through the use of a health risk assessment instrument.

B. Health risk appraisals vary by target population, inclusion of nutrition or other assessment, and method of scoring (computerized or self-scored); the health care provider should match the instrument to his or her practice [6].

C. When health educators, physician assistants, and nurse practitioners are used in risk assessment and follow-up, it is important for the physician to maintain an active, knowledgeable presence in the process; this underscores for the patient the validity and importance of health promotion.

D. Risk assessment can be performed as part of a periodic health examination, where the focus is on health. However, an equally effective opportunity is at the follow-up visit for previously diagnosed and treated conditions that are now stable. At such time, patients may feel positive and motivated to further promote their health, and the physician will have a few minutes to introduce the process.

As industry is beginning to invest in health promotion for employees, health maintenance organizations and prepaid delivery systems are natural areas for integration of health promotion into health care. Likewise, health insurers are encouraged to invest in potential long-term cost savings through coverage for current risk assessment and health education interventions.

More research is needed, especially in the following areas: behavior modification, health promotion in groups with ethnic and socioeconomic barriers, provider role and impact, risk-benefit of health risk appraisal, sensitivity, specificity, and predictive value of risk appraisal methods, and efficacy in promoting health and containing health care costs [11, 12].

References

1. Hall, J. H., and Zwemer, J. D. *Prospective Medicine* (2nd ed.). Indianapolis: Methodist Hospital of Indiana, 1979. *A practical primer that explains and instructs on the use of the health hazard appraisal.*
2. Robbins, L. C., and Hall, J. H. *How to Practice Prospective Medicine.* Indianapolis: Methodist Hospital of Indiana, 1970. *A classic in the field of health promotion.*
3. Goetz, A. A., Duff, J. F., and Bernstein, J. F. Health risk appraisal: The estimation of risk. *Public Health Rep.* 95(2):119, 1980. *A review of the background and use of health risk appraisal.*
4. U.S. Department of Health and Human Services. Centers for Disease Control. *Mortality Tables.* Atlanta, GA: U.S. Department of Health and Human Services, circa 1980. *Tabulated raw data.*
5. Amler, R. W., Moriarty, D. G., and Hutchins, E. B. (eds.). *Healthier People: The Carter Center of Emory University Health Risk Appraisal Program Guides and Documentation.* Atlanta: The Carter Center of Emory University, January 1988. *Latest update of the Centers for Disease Control HRA, field-tested and based on sound epidemiology.*
6. U.S. Department of Health and Human Services. *Healthfinder.* Washington, DC: Public Health Services, 1985. *An annually updated roster of currently available health risk appraisals (52 in 1985).*
7. Rosser, W. W. Screening in family medicine: The current situation. *J. Fam. Pract.* 6(3):503, 1978. *Describes the "coronary risk assessment sheet," a nonstatistically based, useful office health promotion tool.*
8. Hess, J. W., Liepman, M. R., and Ruane, T. J. (eds.). *Family Practice and Preventive Medicine: Health Promotion in Primary Care.* New York: Human Sciences Press, 1983. *An overview text covering issues from pediatrics to geriatrics in primary care.*
9. Rodnick, J. E. and Bubb, K. Patient education and multiphasic screening: It can change behavior. *J. Fam. Pract.* 6(3):599, 1978. *A one-year follow-up of adults exposed to health hazard appraisal, multiphasic screening, and patient education.*
10. Taylor, R. B. (ed.). *Health Promotion: Principles and Clinical Applications.* Norwalk, Conn: Appleton-Century-Crofts, 1982. *A text/primer with discussions of ethics, the future, and other issues.*
11. Schneiderman, L. J. (ed.). *The Practice of Preventive Health Care.* Menlo Park, CA: Addison-Wesley, 1981. *Broad social and professional coverage of the issues.*
12. Wagner, E. H. et al. An assessment of health hazard/health risk appraisal. *Am. J. Public Health* 72(4): 347, 1982. *A state-of-the-art review.*

63 Accidents

John Robbins

I. Definition. Accidents are unintentional events that result in injury or death.

II. Description. Accidents can be viewed as the outcome of a specific interaction between an individual and the environment. For the purposes of analysis, the actual injury that results from this interaction may be analyzed in three separate time phases: (1) the **preinteraction phase**—the situation that exists prior to the interaction and makes the accident possible; (2) the **interaction phase**—the actual injury phase, in which there is a transfer of energy causing injury; and (3) the **postinteraction phase**—the phase where the injury is attented to.

It is possible for society and the health care provider to intercede in all three phases of the accident. It is important to recognize that one may intervene at any step in the accident process. There is no logical reason why countermeasures must parallel the events leading up to the accident. For example, an individual might be at risk of drowning if he or she cannot swim. Logically, we should teach everyone to swim, but the provision of life jackets may be a simpler approach.

A. In the **preinteraction phase,** a setting is established in which an individual is more or less likely to have an accident. An accident occurs when the task that is demanded is too difficult for the individual to perform. This can happen in three different ways:

1. The task can remain stable, but the individual's ability to perform it may deteriorate—for example, road accidents caused by impaired driver ability from excess fatigue, decreased vision, or alcohol ingestion.
2. The task that is required may become more difficult. The individual's ability does not change, but the conditions become less satisfactory; for example, adverse weather conditions such as ice, snow, or rain increase the likelihood of an automobile accident.
3. The normal variations in the task required and the abilities of the individual become unbalanced; the average task is too difficult for the average individual—for example, the average driver faced with driving over a turning, twisting, narrow roadway.

In each of these cases, one can modify the outcome by adjusting either the individual's performance or the requirements of the task at hand.

B. In the second phase of the accident, the **interaction phase,** in which the actual transfer of energy is taking place, modifications can be made to decrease the injury that results. Modifications in the environment in which the accident occurs may serve to decrease the energy transfer—for example, the use of seatbelts in automobiles, or the use of fireproof bedclothing, which limits the spread of the fire.

C. One may also intervene in the third phase, the **postinteraction phase,** of an accident and attempt to modify the outcome after the actual event has occurred. Examples of intervention are seen in the construction of fire exits or the use of smoke detectors, as well as in the teaching of cardiopulmonary resuscitation (CPR). If we have failed to prevent an automobile accident (phase 1), and the occupant is not wearing his or her seatbelt (phase 2), we may still attempt to decrease the severity of the outcome by having the bystanders perform CPR while awaiting the arrival of the rapidly deployed ambulance (phase 3).

III. Epidemiology. Approximately 4% of the deaths in the United States in 1980 resulted from "accidents." Accidents were classified as the leading cause of death for young adults (ages 15–44) [1]. Annually, over 50 million Americans suffer significant accidental injuries. Ten million of these are classified as disabling injuries (injuries that result in disability continuing for more than the actual day of injury), and more than 100,000 individuals die annually as a result of accidents.

A few major types of accidents are responsible for most morbidity and mortality. Approximately half of these accidental deaths result from motor vehicle accidents, with the peak death rate occurring in individuals between the ages of 15 and 24. The second largest accidental cause of death is falls. Falls become a singularly important factor as age increases. In individuals over 75 years of age, falls account for 75 deaths/100,000 individuals/year. The death rate from falls in the elderly population is greater than the death rate from all causes for individuals ages 1–44. Other major accidental causes of death include drowning, with a peak death rate of 5.4/100,000 in the 15- to 24-year-old age group, and fires, which have a peak death rate in the elderly population of 8.2/100,000.

Specific Causes of Injury: Motor Vehicle Accidents

I. The problem

A. Description

1. Preinteraction phase

a. Deterioration of individual's ability. The most common cause of impaired driver ability is alcohol ingestion. Contrary to the frequently held belief that accidents are caused by mild social drinking, the individuals most commonly involved in a fatal accident have a history of drinking problems and a significantly elevated blood alcohol level [2]. In order for the blood alcohol level to reach what is usually considered a legally intoxicated level (for the purpose of prosecution, 80–100 mg/100 ml), an average individual must consume approximately 6 oz of hard liquor, or 1 quart of beer, or 4 glasses of wine [3]. Individuals with baseline marginal ability, for example, elderly or new drivers, may be more affected by small quantities of alcohol. Problem-drinking individuals should be identifiable to primary care providers.

The increased likelihood of motor vehicle accidents caused by impaired ability also results from coexistent medical conditions. The medical conditions may not actually impair the driver's or pedestrian's ability under normal conditions. However, when the environmental factors become more stressful, the threshold at which accidents occur becomes lower. The individual who may be perfectly safe walking and driving in the daytime with mildly decreased hearing or vision is at much greater risk during the evening hours. The actual limitations of driving by individuals with seizure disorders or similar impairments is a statutory matter in most states. This is of limited importance when compared to more common disabilities such as impaired vision and balance.

b. Increased environmental hazard. Motor vehicle accident death rates are higher at night than during the daytime and are higher in rural areas than in urban areas.

c. Threshold of abilities too low. In many cases, we are requesting unacceptable levels of ability from our drivers or pedestrians. Some roads or intersections are simply too dangerous for some individuals to negotiate, and some vehicles, such as motorcycles, are inherently dangerous.

2. Transfer of energy phase. If an accident cannot be prevented, it is obvious that one should attempt to decrease the damage that is done. The use of seatbelts ranks highest on the list of energy-transfer reduction measures. Seatbelt wearing ranks first, side by side with smoking cessation, as the most important life-style changes that individuals can make to prolong their lives.

B. Epidemiology. In 1980, there were 53,200 Americans killed in automobile accidents. The peak death rates were in the ages 15–24 (44.8/100,000 population), and in the over-75-year-old group (28.0/100,000) [1]. Alcohol is reported to be involved in at least half of all fatal motor vehicle accidents [1]. One study shows that abnormal medical conditions play a role in initiating 15–25% of all crashes (excluding alcohol) [4]. Three times as many pedestrian fatalities occur midblock as at intersections [1], and the death rate for miles traveled is over three times greater at night than during daylight hours (6.93 deaths/10^8 miles traveled at night versus 2.03) [1].

Surprisingly, even though the injury rate is significantly higher in urban areas, the actual fatality rate is greater in rural locations. Not so surprisingly, the death rate per miles traveled is 11 times greater for motorcycles than for other motor vehicles [1].

II. General health promotion

A. Methods. Medical professionals should accept their roles as responsible citizens and should work in their practice settings and communities, and through the media, hospitals, and legislation in at least the following areas, to help implement prophylactic measures for accident prevention, just as they work to prevent the spread of infectious diseases.

1. **Substance abuse.** A history of alcohol ingestion should always be elicited during patient evaluations. One should consider including the Michigan Alcoholism Screening Test in a patient's initial evaluation [5].
2. **Medical disabilities**
   a. **Visual impairment.** After routine vision screening, physicians should consider how decreased vision will affect driving ability.
   b. **Loss of consciousness** (seizures, cardiac arrhythmias, hypoglycemia, or hyperglycemia). In any patient with a recent history of loss of consciousness, physicians should consider the need to restrict driving. Many states require the physician to report such occurrences.
   c. **Physical impairment.** When seeing any patient with weakness, sensory loss, or skeletal abnormality, we must consider his or her fitness to continue driving. As the clinical condition changes with time, the patient may lack the perspective to make his or her own decisions. This is especially important with advancing age.
3. **Lap/shoulder belts.** It is appropriate for health care providers to convince their patients that the use of seatbelts is among the most beneficial of all medical and nonmedical interventions in preventing the loss of life.
4. **Airbags.** Health care providers should encourage their patients to buy cars with airbags. They should also lobby for the general use of these systems.
5. **Roadway improvement.** Health care providers can lobby for controlled access roads, pedestrian overpasses, and crash barriers; changes in road characteristics have been shown to save lives.
6. **Motorcycle helmets.** Health care providers can lobby for laws requiring motorcyclists to wear helmets and can also individually influence their patients. Unfortunately, the price of the individual's right to freedom of choice in not wearing a helmet, and the consequent disability or loss of life is currently borne by society.

B. Justification

1. **Substance abuse.** Treatment for alcoholism has been shown to be effective. The best results are achieved with individuals who have good social support systems and continued employment [6].
2. **Medical disabilities.** Even though it is of unproven efficacy, health care providers can also work with their patients to minimize some of their risks. Individuals should choose vehicles and routes appropriate for their abilities.
3. **Lap/shoulder belts.** Use of lap and shoulder belts combined reduces fatalities by approximately 50%. Injuries are also significantly reduced [7]. If all automobile occupants wore safety belts, it is estimated that 12 000 lives would be saved annually [1]. Driver fatalities have dropped significantly in areas where seatbelts have been required by law [8]. However, no one has clearly shown counseling to be effective in this area [8a].
4. **Airbags.** Passive restraint systems, specifically airbags, which inflate automatically at the time of an accident, appear to be slightly less efffective than combined use of shoulder and lap seatbelts. However, because these passive restraints are not operator-dependent, they function at all times. The overall decreased fatality rate for occupants of cars with airbag-passive restraints, compared to individuals in comparable automobiles, is reported to range from 35–50% [7].
5. **Roadway improvement.** Expenditures on what are considered preventive measures should be viewed as investments for the future. Protective guard rails, traffic lights, pedestrian overpasses, and other highway modifications pay for themselves in decreased injuries and deaths.
6. **Motorcycle helmets.** The fatality rate for individuals not wearing helmets is reported to be 3–9 times greater than for those wearing helmets [9]. The repeal of motorcycle helmet laws has had a significant effect on medical expense and mortality. It is estimated that $61 million could be saved annually if all motorcyclists used helmets [10].

Falls

I. The problem

A. Description and epidemiology. Falls are a significant cause of mortality, especially in the elderly population. Falls are responsible for approximately 50% of the accidental deaths to individuals over 75 years of age [1].

1. **Preinteraction phase**
   a. **Deteriorating individual ability.** High alcohol consumption, neurologic impairment, advanced age, previous history of fractures, and general debility have been shown to correlate with impaired function and therefore with increased frequency of falls.
   b. **Impaired environmental conditions.** It is possible to identify certain situations that predispose the elderly population to falling [11]. The greatest majority of falls in one study population occurred **inside** the home.
   c. **Tasks that are too great for average ability.** Certain tasks are beyond the ability of the average individual. Stairways represent a hazard that may surpass the ability of certain individuals with deteriorated mental or physical conditions.
2. **Interaction phase.** As mentioned above, elderly individuals tend to fall within their own homes, frequently from a recumbent or sitting position and often while going or coming from the bathroom in the middle of the night. Falls going and coming from the bathroom may be aggravated by the hard tile floors that are frequently used in bathrooms.
3. **Postinteraction phase.** A large percentage of elderly individuals live by themselves. It is important that they be able to get help if they fall.

B. Epidemiology. The risk of fractures in women has been shown to rise from less than 1%/year in women under the age of 50 to more than 4%/year in women over the age of 85 [12].

As with motor vehicle fatalities, **alcohol** plays a major role in other injuries. Waller [13], in his study from Sacramento, California, found 70% of individuals over the age of 15 who died within 6 hours of falls had alcohol in their blood. He stated, "Alcohol and problem drinking play a major role in deaths and unintentional injuries off the highway." Physicians should always consider alcohol use or abuse as a predisposing factor for accidents and injuries.

Other **medical impairments** also play significant roles in causing falls. Waller found that, "among persons age 15 or older, 10% died as a result of injuries incurred during an episode of altered consciousness, and 7% died of injuries attributable to other forms of medical impairment."

Brocklehurst, et al. [14], studied predictors of falls in the elderly. The most reliable predictor of falls that resulted in fractured femurs in the elderly population was a previous history of fractures after the age of 60. Patients who had fallen and fractured a bone in the past were at the highest risk for recurrent injury. Neurologic disease was also found to be useful in predicting patients who would fracture their femur: 12% of patients had previous strokes, 12% chronic brain syndrome, 6% parkinsonism, and 13% other neurologic diagnoses. These percentages were significantly greater than a matched control population without fractures. A history of blindness, interestingly, did not correlate with increased falls and fractures. Actual physical state as measured by grip-strength and skin-fold thickness was highly correlated with femur fractures.

The most **common activities** associated with falling were going to or returning from the bathroom. Interestingly, more than one-third of the falls were associated with sitting or lying (i.e., individuals who fell from chairs or out of bed). A highly significant percentage of falls occur when individuals arise at night and in the semidarkness make their way urgently to the bathroom in a semi-awake state.

II. Health promotion

A. Methods

1. **Focus efforts on high-risk individuals.** It is possible for physicians to select individuals who are at high risk for falls and fractures. Physicians should concentrate their efforts at prevention of falls in patients who exhibit one or more of the following risk factors: high alcohol consumption, advanced age, neurologic impairment, previous history of fractures, and general debility.
2. Armed with this information, health care providers should discuss the **home environment** with their at-risk patients. If patients have nocturia, which is not

amenable to therapy, arrangements should be made to facilitate trips to and from the bathroom with proper illumination and handrails, or possible use of a bedside commode.

3. The health care system cannot be considered the gatekeeper for every hazardous activity, yet it would still be prudent for health care providers to **discuss with patients the relative risk of different forms of vocation and avocation,** putting these in perspective vis-a-vis the merits of other medical intervention.
4. If we accept the fact that individuals are going to fall, an effort should be made to **lessen the impact of these falls.** This possibility should be discussed with patients and/or their families. Special arrangements may forestall serious injuries.
5. **Modifications of the environment** may be useful. Proper padding of the floor is a useful intervention. Use of armchairs and beds with siderails that are located close to the floor may also serve to lessen injuries. Obviously, slippery floors and unsafe footwear should be avoided. All of these topics should be discussed with elderly or infirm patients.
6. Efforts can also be directed at **improved bone strength** (see Chap. 75). If falls occur, this may help to prevent fractures. The use of calcium and estrogens in elderly women has been shown to reduce the incidence of fractures. The estrogen use should be weighed against other risk factors: possible uterine malignancy, cholelithiasis, and arteriosclerotic disease [15].
7. **Once an injury has resulted from a fall, it is important that individuals be able to obtain help.** Individuals living by themselves should make arrangements for obtaining help in case of an emergency. Patients who are prone to falls should consider what action they will take should they fall to the ground and be unable to ambulate. Health care providers can discuss with their patients the ways to obtain help. Are telephones accessible? Is it practical to use intercoms to contact a relative, friend, or neighbor? Can burglar alarms be wired with switches that can be easily activated from different rooms in the house, including the bathroom?

B. Justification. The ability to generate a cost-benefit ratio to use with suggested methodologies for the prevention of injury secondary to fall is hampered by the lack of clinical studies. We are unable to define the actual benefits of most of these interventions. Luckily, the cost of the interventions is minimal. Therefore, it is possible to rely on common sense as a justification for many of these interventions.

The major invasive intervention that has been suggested is the treatment of possible osteoporosis. Indications for this therapy are outlined in Chap. 75. To put this problem into perspective, one simply needs to note that 1 in 20 women who live to the age of 80 will suffer a hip fracture.

Recommendations

The following should be incorporated into the ongoing care of all adults by primary care providers.

I. General accidents

A. If a health care provider is going to intervene to prevent an accident, we must be able to predict the predisposing factors that are amenable to this intervention. Individual impairment is probably the most easily observed detectable factor. When the health care provider makes a diagnosis of some form of impairment, he or she should assess the impact that this impairment will have on the individual's life and what intervention can be undertaken to minimize the individual's risks.

B. In every accident situation previously discussed, alcohol consumption has played an important role. The diagnosis of increased alcohol consumption should trigger a major intervening effort on the part of the physician. Treatment programs are registering reasonable success rates. Only if we recognize the condition will we be able to prevent the "accidents" that are precipitated by alcohol consumption.

II. Motor vehicle accidents

A. All patients should be evaluated for excessive alcohol consumption and counseled when appropriate.

B. Seatbelt-wearing or the use of passive restraints is the simplest intervention that will have the most major effect on patient survival.

C. Physicians should assess the competence of their patients to drive safely under various conditions. Patients should be advised about when they may safely operate a motor vehicle.

D. It is especially important that handicapped and elderly individuals be evaluated and counseled as to their abilities and risks as pedestrians. Hearing and visual impairment may significantly raise the risk for pedestrians.

E. Motorcycle helmets should be absolute requirements for anyone who is going to drive or ride as a passenger on a motorcycle.

III. Falls

A. Patients should be screened for alcohol abuse and counseled as to its risk for precipitating falls.

B. It is especially important in elderly individuals to evaluate the environment in which the patients live. An attempt should be made to decrease any obvious hazards. Where indicated, physicians should advocate the use of appropriate equipment, such as bedrails, nightlights, and bathtub grip bars.

C. A mechanism of obtaining help in case of an emergency should be considered for all elderly patients. The morbidity associated with falls is frequently significantly increased by delays in obtaining assistance.

References

1. *Accident Facts 1984.* Chicago: National Safety Council, 1984. *Published annually; see also earlier years. This is the best readily available single source for data on accidents.*
2. Waller, J. A. Injury as a Public Health Problem. In J. M. Last (ed.), *Maxcy-Rosenau Public Health and Preventive Medicine* (11th ed.). New York: Appleton-Century-Crofts, 1980. Pp. 1549–92. *Waller is one of the best-known authors in the field. This chapter summarized well his theories on accidents.*
3. Drinking and driving accidents—does education help? *Br. Med. J.* 2(6148):1352, 1978. *This is one of a number of periodic reviews that appear in the* British Medical Journal *covering the interface between social behavior and medicine.*
4. Waller, J. A. Hunting the evasive solution to medical impairment and highway crashes (editorial). *J. Chronic Dis.* 30(7):393, 1977. *A good reference to non-alcohol-related disability and automobile accidents.*
5. Pokorny, A. D., Miller, B. A., and Kaplan, H. B. The brief MAST: A shortened version of the Michigan Alcoholism Screening Test. *Am. J. Psychiatry* 129(3):342, 1972. *This is one reference source for a relatively useful test for evaluating alcoholism.*
6. Baekeland, F. Evaluation of Treatment Methods in Chronic Alcoholism. In B. Kissin and H. Begleiter (eds.), *The Biology of Alcoholism. Vol. 5: Treatment and Rehabilitation of the Chronic Alcoholic.* New York: Plenum, 1977. Pp. 385–440. *This five-volume treatise on alcoholism represents a very useful reference source.*
7. Department of Transportation. National Highway Traffic Safety Administration. *Occupant Protection Program. Progress Report #2.* Washington, DC: National Highway Traffic Safety Administration, 1979. *An original source for data on the use of restraints and improved highway safety.*
8. McDermott, F. Control of road trauma epidemic in Australia. *Ann. R. Coll. Surg. Engl.* 60(6):437, 1978. *An epidemiologic study showing significant decrease in mortality with legislative-mandated increased seatbelt use.*

8a. U.S. Preventive Services Task Force. Recommendations for automobile occupant protection counseling. *J. A. M. A.* 259:76, 1988. *Summary taken from task force background report.*

9. Department of Transportation. National Highway Safety Administration. *The Effects of Motorcycle Helmet Usage on Head Injuries, and the Effects of Usage Laws on Helmet Wearing Rates—A Preliminary Report.* Washington, DC: National Highway Safety Administration, 1979. *Represents government data supporting the need for motorcycle helmet usage.*
10. Muller, A. Evaluation of the costs and benefits of motorcycle helmet laws. *Am. J. Public Health* 70(6):586, 1980. *A well-presented article demonstrating the economic folly in the repeal of motorcycle helmet laws.*
11. Ashley, M. J., Gryfe, J. I., and Amies, A. A longitudinal study of falls in elderly population. II. Some circumstances of falling. *Age Ageing* 6(4):211, 1977. *Very impressive longitudinal study looking at a large elderly population to see the circumstances surrounding falls.*
12. Garraway, W. M. et al. Limb fractures in a defined population. I. Frequency and distribution. *Mayo Clin. Proc.* 54(11):701, 1979.

13. Waller, J. A. Nonhighway injury fatalities. I. The roles of alcohol and problem drinking, drugs, and medical impairment. *J. Chronic Dis.* 25:33, 1972. *One of the few reviews of the role of alcohol and other impairments in nonhighway fatalities.*
14. Brocklehurst, J. C., et al. Fracture of the femur in old age: A two-centre study of associated clinical fractures and the cause of the fall. *Age Ageing* 7(1):7, 1978. *A retrospective epidemiologic study attempting to ferret out the predisposing factors for fractures of the femur in the elderly.*
15. Riggs, B. L., et al. Effect of the fluoride/calcium regimen on vertebral fracture occurrence in postmenopausal osteoporosis. Comparison with conventional therapy. *N. Engl. J. Med.* 306(8):446, 1982. *Prospective study that illustrates the utility of different regimens of combinations of calcium, fluoride, vitamin D, and estrogens in preventing fractures in postmenopausal women. It is clearly not the last work on the subject but is one step in arriving at a reasonable prophylactic regimen.*

64 Obesity

Faith T. Fitzgerald

I. The problem

A. Definition. There are multiple definitions of obesity. Anthropometric measurements rely on skin-fold thickness, ponderal indices, and height-weight ratios. The latter is most frequent in daily clinical use and originated in the height and weight criteria for each age and sex compiled by the Metropolitan Life Insurance Company in a 1959 report. These analyses, the basis of the frequently referenced charts in professional offices and nutrition literature, were of a life-insured population in the United States between 1935 and 1953 and showed a linear relationship between excess weight and mortality. The "ideal weights" were defined as those in each height/age/sex category at which mortality was lowest. These data have been justly criticized: most insured people in those years were white and of the upper-middle or upper classes. Lower socioeconomic groups and a variety of ethnic peoples other than whites were not included, and leanness in the United States does vary by class and race. The health of people who bought life insurance in those years may have been different from that of the population as a whole. Finally, raw weight, not adiposity, was the criterion used; and, by these same data, football linemen are in a category of morbidity equal to that of some obese individuals. Most startling, recent studies have contradicted this earlier report, and suggest that leanness may be a greater predictor of mortality than fatness in some age categories.

More recent scientific work has used the "body mass index" (weight in kilograms divided by height in meters squared). In the National Center for Health Statistics Survey of 1976–1980, "overweight" was a body mass index equal to or greater than the eighty-fifth percentile of 20–29-year-old men and women. In the survey population, men are "overweight" when the body mass index equals or exceeds 27.8, women at 27.3. By these criteria, about 26% of adults in the United States, or 34 million people age 20–75 years, were overweight.

As a practical matter, most physicians, like most lay people, diagnose obesity by "eyeball analysis," i.e., does the patient appear too fat? We must, in using this diagnostic technique, recognize the influence of our cultural biases (e.g., what is "fat" to an American physician may be normal to a German physician).

B. Description

1. **Etiology.** Given that certain individuals are fatter than others, why is this so? Hypotheses are many and it is probably the case that more than one hypothesis is correct. Genetic influences are clearly operative, and fat parents have fat children. Recent data suggest that this may be the major determinant of adult body weight. In utero and infant feeding patterns have been found to influence ultimate adult weights. Enzymatic, hormonal, and basic bioenergetic systems may differ between the fat and the lean (though whether these are causal or an effect of obesity is subject to heated debate among experts in the field). Differences in the number, size, and metabolic capacity of fat cells are intensely and repeatedly studied, with variable results. Investigators assiduously pursue the influence of exercise and psychologic factors on body weight. All, of course, seek to discover those factors that, once understood, could be manipulated to prevent or reverse the deposition of large amounts of body fat. So far, however, consistent or predictable success in such prevention or reversal has eluded investigators and most obese patients.
2. **The risks of being overweight.** The complications of obesity are many and include the following:
   a. **Mechanical.** The mechanical burden of obesity leads to accelerated degenerative joint disease, especially in the weightbearing joints of the spine, hips, knees, and ankles. Great weight may also, however, increase bony density and so retard the development of osteoporosis.
   b. **Respiratory.** Respiratory compromise in the fat population, among whom

dyspnea is common, may result from increased oxygen demand, increased intraabdominal pressure from a massive pannus, increased work of breathing to lift a thorax burdened with mammae, and fatty obstruction of the upper airway. Sleep apnea in the obese (the Pickwick syndrome) has features in common with that same disorder in the lean, and its direct relationship to obesity needs further study.

c. **Cardiac.** Cardiomegaly is common in fat people and is generally proportionate to body mass; weight reduction decreases left ventricular mass. There is a correlation between obesity and coronary artery disease, but the mechanisms remain poorly understood.

d. **Cancer.** Data suggest that the mortality rates for certain cancers (colorectal and prostatic in men; genital, gallbladder, and breast in women) are higher in the obese.

e. **Iatrogenic.** The body size of the extremely obese patient makes physical, roentgenographic, and nuclear diagnosis more difficult, and surgery and anesthesia are riskier, rendering the fat patient more likely to experience medical misadventure than their leaner agemates.

f. **Dieting.** The ingestion of unbalanced diets has been cited as a risk to the obese. Most fat people undertake multiple schemes to lose weight. The morbidity of the therapy of obesity should be examined: Lipids in the serum of the stable obese are not markedly different from those of the lean cohort but rise during the refeeding following a fast. It is possible that recurrent diets set the stage for periodic hyperlipidemia as patients "fall off the diet wagon." The lithogenicity of bile is greater in the obese than in a matched lean population, but increases most dramatically, with the attendant risk of precipitation of gallstones, during fasting. However, the relationship of periodic diet to the greater prevalence of gallstones in the fat population is not known.

g. **Hypertension.** Hypertension, one of the major complications of obesity, is also a complex issue. The exact relationship of hypertension to obesity remains conjectural, especially when one considers that none of the epidemiologic studies confirming the coincidence of hypertension in the obese controlled for the therapeutic use among the obese of the hypertensive drugs of the amphetamine class. A number of studies show diminution of blood pressure in patients when they lose weight, though the degree is variable and the mechanism controversial. Given the degree, also, of "relapse" to former weight, the long-term effect of weight reduction on hypertension is as yet unknown. The relationship of hypertension to obesity remains an area of intensive inquiry, but two points are clear: (1) the fat patient with hypertension must be carefully questioned about the use of diet pills (amphetamines and phenylpropanolamine), and (2) the fat patient must be treated for his or her hypertension with more than the admonition to "go home and lose weight," since this may be impossible for them.

h. **Diabetes mellitus.** Glucose tolerance is different in the overweight individual, which is no surprise since the normals were established in lean people. There is as yet no good evidence, however, that microvascular diabetes is increased in the obese, nor that angiopathy is improved by weight loss. It may be that obesity is more a complication of diabetes. Whatever the case, glycosuria, infections, cataracts, and neuropathy attributable to diabetes in the fat patient should be treated by attempts at weight loss and by appropriate hypoglycemic agents.

i. **Reproductive.** Obstetric complications of obesity include dystocia (fat women have fat babies). However, the deleterious effects of intrauterine malnutrition are such that an obese woman ought not to be subject to weight loss during pregnancy but should gain weight appropriate to her prepregnancy weight, much as a nonobese woman. Menstrual irregularities in obese women are common and may have to do with fundamental changes in estrogen metabolism or binding, periodic starvation, and stress.

j. **Hyperuricemia.** Hyperuricemia and gout increase with increasing weight and decrease with weight loss. The physician caring for the hyperuricemic fat patient must make careful inquiry about thiazide diuretic use (in some diet pills) and starvation, the ketonemia from which may raise uric acid transiently.

k. **Renal and hepatic risks.** Nephrotic syndrome and fatty liver have been described in some obese patients, though the significance of these limited case reports for the obese population as a whole is uncertain.

l. **Stress.** Psychologic stresses are many in the obese, who are overtly derided in our society. What influence this stress may play on heart disease and hypertension is intriguing but unanswered. Moreover, though we may or may not share it, we should recognize the intense negativity of medical professionals toward the obese, which has been well documented in a number of studies. How these negative attitudes, both within and outside the profession, affect the study and care of the obese has never been rigorously evaluated.

C. Epidemiology. It appears that obesity has a major hereditary component in human beings, compounding the difficulty that individuals encounter in trying to lose weight. Certain data also suggest a far greater prevalence in lower socioeconomic classes in the United States, though whether this is genetically or economically based is unclear.

II. General health promotion

A. Method. The primary prevention of obesity awaits discovery. It is clear that rapid weight loss schemes and subjecting children to diets have significant risks and should be avoided. Overall, regimens involving increased caloric expenditure (exercise) combined with a temperate decrease in caloric intake seem best supported by the literature.

B. Justification. Though studies demonstrate that intrauterine nutrition affects adult weight and that the weight of an infant at 6 months of age may predetermine adult weight, these data cannot be used to justify weight-containment diets for the fetus or infant, which run the risk of intrauterine or perinatal malnutrition. Similarly, though there is no solid evidence to support that the increasing recognition of anorexia nervosa or bulimia (the gorge/purge phenomenon) among young women is a consequence of the national obsession with thinness, this extreme behavior must be of great balancing concern to doctors as they advise the public on the risk of obesity.

III. Specific health promotion

A. Assessment. Overall need for weight reduction should be considered in those patients in whom massive obesity (> 100% over ideal weight) or significant heart disease, diabetes, arthritis, or hypertension are present. No discrete "cut-off" as to ideal weight is scientifically possible.

B. Intervention

1. Methods

a. It is unlikely, given the influence of the media, that physicians will encounter fat patients untouched by the persuasion of the multitudes of weight-loss schemes available. A principal advisory function of the doctor must be to protect the fat patient from the untoward effects of faddism and outright quackery.

b. When weight loss is indicated, individualization of the mode of weight loss is paramount and must be carefully moderated by both patient and physician.

c. As in all good therapy, vigor of the treatment should be matched to the actual deleterious effects of the disorder. Greatest attention should be given to patients with arthritis, symptomatic respiratory disease, heart disease, hypertension, and diabetes. These conditions should be treated as they manifest, **along with** (and not solely by) weight loss.

d. Part of the complete history in the obese includes careful inquiry into the variety of weight-loss nostrums tried in the past, and the education of the patient in the dangers of more radical and expensive schemata of "quick-fix" weight loss.

e. Patients should be encouraged to weigh themselves on the same scale at the same time of day, wearing the same clothing. Women should be specifically reminded about perimenstrual fluid gain and supported in rejecting this as evidence of failure to lose fat.

f. Daily caloric intake for each patient must be individually computed, depending on age, sex, activity, and climate (cold temperatures require more calories). Generally, it should be unnecessary to restrict the diet to fewer than 1000–1400 cal/day, with at least 20% of the caloric content as protein. Small, frequent feedings spread through the day may be more effective than two or three large meals per day. Diets containing 70–80% carbohydrate, 20–25% protein, and 5–10% fat are appropriate.

g. Patients should be reminded that gradual weight loss is preferable to precipitous early drops, and if they lose 1 lb/week they will be 52 lb less 1 year from the initiation of the diet. They should also be warned that early weight loss may be greater than weight loss later on, even with adherence to the same dietary and exercise regimen. This is due to an early diuresis of ketonuria and to the decreased caloric requirements of the body as mass grows less.

h. Exercise, like diet, should be individually tailored to the patient. As with diet, extremes must be avoided. Regular daily exercise for 30–60 minutes is required, rather than sporadic "binge" exercise.

i. Patients should be continually reassured that their failure to lose weight will not cause you to dislike them. Patients are often ashamed to return to their physicians if they have failed to meet their weight-loss goals, and are thereby denied concurrent, necessary therapy for hypertension, diabetes, or other illness.

j. At the extremes of life-threatening obesity, extremes of therapy—including surgical therapies—may be considered. These include jaw-wiring, ileojejunal bypass, and gastric stapling.

2. Justification

a. **Effectiveness.** Data show that 75–95% of all weight-loss regimens fail. Even if the weight is successfully lost, it is most often rapidly regained. No single regimen is uniformly effective, and each should be tailored to the individual. Surgery should be reserved for those with life-threatening obesity that is unresponsive to other therapy.

b. **Risks.** Given the failures of standard therapy, each physician and patient confronted with the problem of simple, uncomplicated obesity must consider the therapeutic ratio of even attempting to lose weight. Cyclic starvation, with returns to previous weight, may be a major factor in some of the morbidity of obesity and eventually may be proved more deleterious than stable obesity. On the other hand, the social sequelae of even uncomplicated obesity are extremely painful for the patient, and this must be taken into account.

Unnecessary "therapy" using unproved methods in the mildly to moderately obese can kill people, as evidenced by the reported deaths and complications of liquid protein diets, starvation, amphetamines, phenylpropanolamine (the agent in most over-the-counter diet pills), thyroid hormone, ipecac, laxatives, diuretics, and bizarre diets.

The large number of complications engendered by ileojejunal bypass make it inappropriate for most, if not all, patients. Gastric stapling and other intestinal interpositionary manipulations are still in the investigational stages, but clearly the risks are such that it must remain largely unwarranted for cosmetic reasons alone.

c. **Costs.** The weight-loss industry is a $13 billion a year enterprise in the United States.

Books, special foods, machines, trusses, camps, exercises, spas, clinics, hypnotism, and magic spells, added to diets and pills, impose a profound financial morbidity on fat patients as well.

IV. Recommendations

A. General health promotion. There is no known effective primary prevention of obesity.

B. Specific health promotion

1. Assessment

a. For those greater than 100% over "ideal weight," weight reduction must be considered.

b. For the others with significant medical conditions that are exacerbated by and in part caused by obesity (e.g., hypertension, arthritis, and diabetes), weight reduction must be considered.

c. In general, no specific cut-off weight is possible for patients.

2. Intervention

a. Advise patients to avoid unproved or dangerous weight-loss methods.

b. Individualize weight-loss programs for each patient.

c. Obese patients with symptomatic respiratory diseases, heart disease, hypertension, and diabetes should be treated with weight loss along with accepted modalities specific to their obesity-associated disorders.

d. Patients should weigh themselves daily as part of their weight-loss monitoring.

e. Calorie counts may be useful.

f. It is generally unnecessary to restrict calories to less than 1000–1400 cal/day.

g. Diets containing 70–80% carbohydrates, 20–25% proteins, and 5–10% fat are appropriate.

h. Expect gradual weight loss.

i. Daily exercise of 30–60 minutes is encouraged.

j. Do not punish patients for failure to lose weight; reward them for success.

k. For those with extreme obesity, surgery may be indicated.

Selected Readings

Alexander, J. K., Ahmad, K., and Cole, V. Observations on some clinical features of extreme obesity, with particular reference to cardiopulmonary respiratory effects. *Am. J. Med.* 35:512, 1962. *Comments on dyspnea, arthritis, cardiomegaly, hypertension, edema, and Pickwick syndrome in the very obese.*
Beller, A. S. *Fat and Thin. A Natural History of Obesity.* New York: Farrar, Straus & Giroux, 1977. *A compendium, extensively referenced, of the data on obesity both medical and cultural. Excellent for lay or professional readers.*
Bray, G. A. (ed.). *Obesity in America.* Bethesda, MD: Department of Health, Education, and Welfare, 1979. *Presents the results of a national conference on obesity covering every aspect of major current knowledge and concerns. Many tables and graphs and 158 references.*
Fitzgerald, F. The problem of obesity. *Annu. Rev. Med.* 32:221, 1981. *A review of the controversies in obesity; extensively referenced.*
Health Implications of Obesity. National Institutes of Health Development Conference. February 11–13, 1985. *Ann. Intern. Med.* 6(pt 2):977, 1985. *A collection of papers and opinions on multiple aspects of obesity.*
Maddox, G. L., and Liederman, V. Overweight as a social disability with medical implications. *J. Med. Educ.* 44(3):214, 1969. *Discusses the social stresses of being fat in America.*
Gwinup, G. Effect of exercise alone on the weight of obese women. *Arch. Intern. Med.* 135(5):676, 1975.
Stunkard, A. J., Foch, T. T., and Hrubec, Z. A twin study of human obesity. *J.A.M.A.* 256(1):51, 1986. *Strongly supports genetic base of obesity.*
Stunkard, A. J., et al. An adoption study of human obesity. *N. Engl. J. Med.* 314(4):193, 1986. *Further data supporting the powerful role of genetics in obesity.*

65

Exercise

T. Warner Hudson

I. The activity

A. Definitions. The following definitions are derived from a number of sources [1, 2, 3, 4]:

1. **Exercise** is planned, structured, and repetitive body, muscle, or muscle-group exertion to enhance physical fitness or its components. Active exercise may be static or kinetic:
   a. **Static** (isometric) exercises produce no joint motion.
   b. **Kinetic** (isotonic) exercises produce joint motion.
2. **Physical fitness** is determined by the individual's ability to perform physical activity, often divided into health-related and skill-related components.
   a. **Health-related components** pertain to health and include but are not limited to the following:
      (1) **Cardiorespiratory endurance:** the ability of the circulatory and respiratory systems to supply fuel and to eliminate fatigue.
      (2) **Muscular endurance:** the ability of a muscle or group of muscles to sustain repeated contractions of a given force.
      (3) **Muscular strength:** the force exerted by a muscle or a group of muscles in a single contraction.
      (4) **Body composition:** the relative amounts of muscle, fat, bone, and other vital parts of the body.
      (5) **Flexibility:** the range of motion available to the body or to a joint.
   b. **Skill-related components** relate more to athletic ability.
      (1) **Power:** the rate at which work can be performed.
      (2) **Speed:** the ability to move the body or any of its parts rapidly.
      (3) **Agility:** the ability to change the direction of movement with speed and accuracy.
      (4) **Coordination:** the ability to use the senses, such as hearing and vision, together with body parts, resulting in smooth, accurate movements.
      (5) **Balance:** The ability to maintain equilibrium.
      (6) **Reaction time:** the time between a stimulus and the beginning of the reaction to it.
3. **Sport:** Any physical activity engaged in for pleasure.

B. Description. The number and types of exercise activities are limitless, and therefore this chapter focuses on a small number of representative activities, mostly of an endurance nature. The emphasis is mainly on the health-related components of physical fitness, although the skill-related components are certainly important. A few important physiologic concepts are described.

1. **Physiology.** Although many of the health benefits and risks of exercise are physiologic and could be included here, only a few principles are explored in this section.
   a. **Maximum oxygen uptake** ($\dot{V}O_2$ max) or **aerobic capacity** is the greatest amount of oxygen that an individual can utilize under the most strenuous conditions of exertion. It is usually expressed as $ml \times kg^{-1} \times min^{-1}$ and is felt to be one of the best measures of cardiorespiratory fitness. At maximal work loads, $\dot{V}O_2$ max plateaus after a brief period in time: 2–5 minutes. The aerobic capacity decreases with advancing age, but it can be increased with training. Aerobic capacity correlates highly with cardiac output. Frequently, aerobic capacity is expressed in METS, which are multiples of resting oxygen consumption, standardized such that $1 \text{ MET} = 3.5 \text{ ml} \times kg^{-1} \times min^{-1}$.
   b. **Cardiac output** is a product of **stroke volume** and **heart rate** ($CO = SV \times HR$). Consequently, there is a direct relationship between heart rate and cardiac output or aerobic capacity [5]. With training, the resting heart rate falls and stroke volume increases. Since maximum heart rate for an individual is fairly constant

Table 65-1. Absolute contraindications to endurance training*

Angina—particularly new or changing patterns
Congestive heart failure symptomatic with ordinary activity
Recent myocardial infarction (less than 3 weeks)—myocardial infarction victims may participate in controlled exercise programs specifically designed for their rehabilitation
Certain arrhythmias—atrial fibrillation, sick sinus syndrome, second and third degree heart block, paroxysmal atrial tachycardia, bundle branch block with coronary artery disease, malignant premature ventricular beats
Severe valvular heart disease (especially aortic stenosis) or outflow obstruction disease (IHSS)
Ventricular or aortic aneurysm
Congenital heart disease—aortic stenosis, coarctation, patent ductus arteriosus (PDA), etc.
Uncontrolled hypertension (greater than 250/115)
Myocarditis or pericarditis
Abnormal exercise test response
Cor pulmonale
Uncontrolled metabolic disorders—hyperthyroidism, diabetes mellitus, adrenal insufficiency
Acute infectious diseases
Active inflammatory arthritis
Recent pulmonary embolism
Medications—coumadin, chemotherapy
Orthopedic problems that prohibit exercise
Transient ischemic attacks

*Some form of very closely supervised exercise may be possible.
Source: American College of Sports Medicine. *Guidelines for Graded Exercise Testing and Prescription* (3rd ed.). Philadelphia: Lea & Febiger, 1986; and B. D. Erb, G. F. Fletcher, and T. L. Sheffield. Standards for exercise treatment programs. American Heart Association Subcommittee on Rehabilitation and Target Activity Group. *Circulation* 59:1084S, 1979.

(but does decline with age), training increases the difference between the resting and maximum heart rates except in pathologic states such as bradycardias. Heart rate is linearly related to exercise intensity unless other stimuli such as environmental conditions, psychologic factors, or disease alter this relationship. It can, therefore, be used to estimate a **target heart rate** for exercising, often expressed as a percentage of maximum heart rate.

2. **Determinants.** A number of factors are important in affecting the performance and results of exercise. These can be grouped into personal, environmental, and activity factors:
   a. **Personal**
      (1) **Genetics.** Certain characteristics, such as height and the ratio of fast-twitch to slow-twitch muscle fibers, are largely genetically determined [4].
      (2) **Underlying conditions.** The presence or absence of a myriad of conditions, diseases, and injuries influences the types, performance, and results of exercise. Some conditions may constitute relative or absolute contraindications to exercise (see sec. **II.A.1.a.** and Tables 65-1 and 65-2).
      (3) **Behavioral factors.** A long list of factors, such as prior participation in sports, perceived health, self-motivation, expected health benefits, perceived spouse support, perceived available time, and behavioral skills, have been shown to be associated with increased likelihood of exercising [5].
      (4) **Demographic variables.** Sex, age, education, occupation, income, and cultural variables influence the choice, type, and performance of exercise. Physical activity typically declines with age, and the higher socioeconomic groups are more active than the lower ones [6].
   b. **Environment.** Important variables include the following: access to facilities; equipment such as shoes, clothing, bicycle, or surface; weather conditions includ-

Table 65-2. Relative contraindications to endurance training that requires supervision

Pregnancy
Stable angina
Congestive heart failure symptomatic with exercise
Asymptomatic coronary or valvular heart disease
Hypertension (greater than 180/110 but less than 250/115)
Peripheral vascular disease—claudication, thrombophlebitis
Respiratory disease—chronic obstructive pulmonary disease, exercise-induced asthma
Recent major surgery
Diabetes mellitus, requiring insulin—exercise decreases insulin requirement
Hepatic, renal, or splenic disorders
Hemorrhagic disease—coagulopathy, history of gastrointestinal or intracranial bleeding
Anemia (hemoglobin less than 10 mg/dl)
Seizure disorders
Marked obesity
Arthritis and disc disease
Recent injuries
Certain medications
Major psychiatric disorders

Source: American College of Sports Medicine. *Guidelines for Graded Exercise Testing and Prescription* (3rd ed.). Philadelphia: Lea & Febiger, 1986; and B. D. Erb, G. F. Fletcher, and T. L. Sheffield. Standards for exercise treatment programs. American Heart Association Subcommittee on Rehabilitation and Target Activity Group. *Circulation* 59:1084s, 1979.

ing temperature, wind, humidity, and air pollution; altitude and hazards such as automobiles or potholes.

c. **Activity**

(1) **Exercise.** The exercise activity itself influences the type of modification and the extent to which the health-related components of physical fitness are modified, as well as the likelihood and types of injuries and other risks that may accrue.

(2) **Training.** The intensity, duration, and frequency of exercise as well as the rate of change in these variables will affect the performance.

C. Epidemiology [7]

Although 80% of Americans are "somewhat or very satisfied" with their condition, 58% do not exercise regularly. The United States Public Health Service goal to have 60% of adult Americans active by 1990 was recently changed to 30%. Currently, one third of Americans do not exercise at all. Americans are, however, quite interested in exercising, as the National Sporting Goods Association 1985 Sports Participation Survey shows [8]. The top 20 sports (rank) engaged in during the past year by all individuals over age 7 were as follows: (1) swimming, (2) bicycle riding, (3) camping, (4) fishing, (5) exercise walking, (6) bowling, (7) exercising with equipment, (8) motor boating, (9) running or jogging, (10) calisthenics, (11) aerobics, (12) billiards or pool, (13) hunting and shooting, (14) softball, (15) hiking, (16) volleyball, (17) basketball, (18) tennis, (19) golf, and (20) roller skating.

II. Specific health promotion

A. Assessment

1. **Methods.** The American College of Sports Medicine (ACSM) states: "Exercise is a safe activity for most individuals. However, it is desirable for adults to have some screening prior to starting an exercise program or taking an exercise test" [9]. There is little consensus about what constitutes a reasonable preexercise medical evaluation, and there are many measurable parameters and tests. The interested reader is encouraged to examine more detailed sources [2, 9, 10, 11]. The following are only guidelines and must be tempered with some consideration of resources available and exercise planned.

   a. **Risk assessment.** A **history, physical examination,** and **cholesterol level** should be obtained to determine if absolute or relative contraindications to an exercise program are present (see Tables 65-1 and 65-2), if major coronary heart disease (CHD) risk factors are present (see Chap. 71), and to contribute to assessment of the current level of physical fitness. A number of useful forms and outlines are available from ACSM [9], from the American Academy of Family Physicians, and from other sources [2]. Review of the personal determinants of exercise, with particular attention to underlying conditions and CHD risk factors, should be appraised at intervals corresponding most effectively to other portions of the periodic health examination.

The ACSM uses the above risk assessment information to make the following broad categorizations of overall health, on which bases they have established the need for further exercise testing [9]:

(1) **Apparently healthy.** No significant risk or injury and no major coronary risk factors. These individuals under age 45 can begin exercise programs without exercise testing (ET). The program should progress gradually and unusual signs or symptoms should be reported. At 45 years of age or older, a maximal ET should be performed prior to beginning an exercise program. ET is also desirable for those already exercising who have reached age 45.

(2) **Individuals at higher risk** have at least one major coronary risk factor (see Chap. 71) and/or symptoms of possible cardiopulmonary or metabolic disease. An ET is recommended in these individuals at any age. In those without symptoms under 35, an ET is not necessary if exercise progresses gradually with some guidance.

(3) **Individuals with disease** have known cardiovascular, pulmonary, or metabolic diseases and should have an ET prior to beginning an exercise program.

b. **Physical fitness assessment.** Although exercise is a safe and healthy activity for most individuals, health care providers should obtain some measure of current physical fitness and exercise habits to further assess risk of exercise for an individual and to safely match new exercise levels with existing levels. The health-related components of fitness can all be measured (Table 65-3); however, cardiorespiratory endurance may be the most helpful category. It is the graded exercise tests in this category that most people refer to as exercise tolerance tests or simply exercise tests, and that provide the best measure of functional capacity.

A number of exercise tests are available and in use [2, 9, 9a].

(1) **Resting heart rate.** In nonpathologic states, heart rate slows with training and is a very gross measure of endurance.

(2) **Heart rate recovery.** The Kasch Pulse Recovery Stress Test may be useful in young (35 years) individuals for determination of training or target heart rate.

(3) **Cycle ergometry.** These tests use a stationary bicycle, but this test favors those with strong quadriceps and is not as easy an activity for many individuals as the treadmill test.

(4) **Treadmill tests.** These are the most widely used and may employ the Balke, Naughton, Ellestad, Bruce, or Åstrand protocols. Cycle ergometry and treadmill tests are supervised, monitored, and interpreted according to criteria that may vary.

The performance, supervision, interpretation, and criteria for abnormal values of these tests are beyond the scope of this book, but the interested reader is referred to recent sources [2, 9, 9a].

2. **Justification**

a. **Test characteristics**

(1) **Risk assessment.** The sensitivity, specificity, and predictive value of these measures have not been adequately studied. However, since they establish prior probability of CHD, by Bayes' theorem they are a determinant of the predictive value for an exercise test in an individual.

(2) **Physical fitness assessment.** More is known about the tests of cardiorespiratory endurance than other fitness parameters. Much has been written about the low predictive value of an exercise treadmill test in asymptomatic young men (4–25%) [12] and the many causes of false-positives and false-negatives [9]. However, the treadmill test's specificity is as high as 100% in one report [13], and its value in high-risk, symptomatic, or diseased patients is well accepted.

b. **Risks** of risk assessment are negligible. Risks of exercise testing can be considerable and depend on the preexisting health of the individual being tested, pay-

Table 65-3. Measuring health-related parameters of physical fitness

Parameter	Test
Cardiorespiratory endurance	Heart rate recovery or graded exercise tests (usually referred to as "exercise tests")
Body composition	Percent body fat
Muscular strength	Bench press
Muscular endurance	Push-ups or sit-ups
Flexibility	Sit and reach

Source: M. L. Pollock, J. H. Wilmore, and S. M. Fox III. *Exercise in Health and Disease. Evaluation and Prescription for Prevention and Rehabilitation.* Philadelphia: Saunders, 1984.

ing attention to contraindications, proper performance and monitoring of testing, stopping the test when appropriate, and having well-trained personnel performing the test who can handle emergencies that may arise [2, 9].

c. **Costs** of risk assessment do not add significantly to the cost of a visit if already occurring for some other reason. Physical fitness assessment in general and exercise testing in particular can be quite expensive, and costs vary widely.

d. **Acceptability** of risk assessment probably could be quite good, although little information is available on how many health care providers actually assess risks of exercise in patients. Acceptability of exercise testing varies widely with provider perceptions of its usefulness and with patient resources.

B. Prescribing exercise

1. **Methods.** With a thorough knowledge of the individual, his or her motivation and other behavioral determinants, risk assessment, level of fitness with exercise testing if indicated, types of exercise(s) currently engaged in or preferred, the environmental condition in which the individual would be exercising, and the time and resources available, it is possible to put together a safe, realistic, and beneficial exercise program for an individual.

There are a number of basic suggestions, some of which are generic to changing any health behavior, that will improve the likelihood of a successful exercise program. These include providing adequate education, assessing motivation, setting realistic short- and long-term goals, advising about equipment and clothing, ongoing reassessment and monitoring, and if possible, choosing an activity that is enjoyable for the individual.

The following recommendations are more specific to the exercise itself, come largely from the ACSM [9], and apply principally to cardiorespiratory fitness. Exercises to promote other measures of fitness such as muscular strength or flexibility are covered in available texts [2, 9].

a. **Types of exercise.** Exercises involving large muscle groups used repetitively, aerobically, rhythmically, and over a long period of time are preferred. Walking, jogging, running, bicycling, swimming, cross-country skiing, rowing, and skating are good examples. Other activities provide interrupted aerobic exercise and are more difficult to monitor: hiking, dancing, and a variety of games and sports. Competition may increase risk of injury.

b. **Intensity of exercise.** Physical activity should be approximately 60–90% of maximal heart rate or 50–85% of aerobic capacity. The rating of perceived exertion (RPE) scale may be a helpful way for individuals to monitor themselves [2]. A good rule of thumb is that the individual should be able to maintain a conversation during the activity.

c. **Duration of exercise.** Fifteen to sixty minutes of continuous exercise is recommended. Lower intensity, longer duration activities result in improvements in cardiorespiratory endurance more readily than high intensity, short duration activities.

d. **Frequency of exercise.** Three to five days per week.

e. **Rate of progression.** Alterations of intensity, duration, and frequency should be gradual as the individual moves from the initial to the improved and then maintenance conditioning stages.

Monitoring of improvements and new symptoms should be part of the program, with reporting to the health care provider of any significant ill effects.

2. **Justification**
   a. **Benefits.** The following partial list is representative:
      (1) **Mortality.** Adequate exercise may add as much as 2 additional years of life for men by age 80 [14] (see sec. **II.B.2.b**).
      (2) **Coronary heart disease.** High-activity groups have less chance of having a myocardial infarction, and, if one occurs, less chance of dying from it, than low-activity groups. This association between high-activity level and lower cardiovascular mortality has been extensively reviewed and is found in the majority of studies [15]. Causality has not been proved, however, and may never be, as studies designed to show whether this association reflects true protection because of activity, or selection because the most fit group inherently exercises more, may be methodologically impossible as well as unethical. Exercise does protect monkeys from morbidity and mortality that is induced by a high-fat diet [16]. As seen below, exercise also exerts a positive effect on several CHD risk factors.
      (3) **Hypertension.** Many uncontrolled studies and a few controlled studies [17] show a moderate reduction in blood pressure with a moderate amount of exercise; many do not [18].
      (4) **Lipids.** Endurance exercise at relatively high levels will increase HDL_2 in men after 7–10 weeks of training [19]. This does not appear to be true in women.
      (5) **Smoking.** Studies show no consistent reduction in smoking [20].
      (6) **Obesity.** Most studies of exercise and weight control show a reduction in weight [20]. Even small amounts of exercise, 30 minutes of walking per day [21], have been shown to be effective in obese, middle-aged women [22].
      (7) **Psychological factors.** There is good evidence that exercise alleviates symptoms reported with mild to moderate depression, reduces some symptoms of anxiety, and may improve mood [22] and sleep patterns.
   b. **Risks.** Lack of controls, unknown denominators, variations with different forms of exercises and intensities, and a number of other variables confound compilation of risk data, but the following are representative:
      (1) **Sudden death.** The risk of cardiac arrest is increased transiently during exercise; however, habitual vigorous exercise is associated with an overall net reduction in cardiac arrest [23]. Individuals with undetected Marfan's syndrome may die suddenly of aortic dissection during vigorous exercise such as basketball, and extreme exertion in individuals with sickle trait appears to increase the risk of sudden death.
      (2) **Injuries** [24]. Overuse injuries are probably the largest category. Thirty-eight percent of runners are injured per year; one third of these injuries are to the knee. Heat-associated illness is a risk on warm, humid days. Bicyclists have a 13% accident rate per year, 62% of whom are injured; one third of these seek medical care. Serious bicycle injuries often involve the head. At least one half of individuals in aerobic classes have been injured doing aerobics. Racquet sports are associated with head, eye, and leg injuries, and tennis elbow. Motor vehicles are a well-known risk to runners and cyclists.
      (3) **Reproductive risks.** Intense exercise associated with weight loss and competition can lead to oligoamenorrhea, hypoestrogenism, infertility, and decreased bone density [25]. (For pregnancy risks, see Chap. 5.) Diminished testosterone levels have been reported in male distance runners ($>$ 65 km/week).
      (4) **Other.** The list of risks is long, but a few other important ones are: increased insulin absorption in diabetics; increased creatine phosphokinase (CPK), lactate dehydrogenase (LDH), and transaminases; hematuria; dermatitis; rhabdomyolysis and myoglobinuria; and gastrointestinal blood loss in distance runners.
   c. **Costs.** The costs are highly variable, usually modest, and certainly affect the choice of participation in sports.
   d. **Acceptability.** Exercise participation in many groups is growing, but the exercise-prevalence gap between different income groups also may be growing.

III. Recommendations

A. Assessment

1. A history, physical examination, and cholesterol level should be performed on adults to determine if contraindications to exercise exist.
2. The behavioral determinants, particularly motivation, of exercise should be analyzed in adults.
3. Current physical fitness should be assessed.
4. Formal exercise testing should be offered to individuals over age 45 or to those who are high-risk or have symptoms of disease.

B. Exercise prescription

1. Exercise is a safe activity for most adults who, after the above assessment, should be encouraged to participate in some form of regular exercise.
2. Type, intensity, duration, frequency, and rate of progression of exercise should be determined for each individual.
3. Environment, costs, and risks should be considered.
4. Monitoring of improvements and signs or symptoms of problems should be included.
5. Safe equipment and conditions should be recommended.

References

1. Caspersen, C. J., Powell, K. E., and Christenson, G. M. Physical activity, exercise, and physical fitness: Definitions and distinctions for health-related research. *Public Health Rep.* 100(2):126, 1985. *Excellent source of definitions.*
2. Pollock, M. L., Wilmore, J. H., and Fox, S. M., III. *Exercise in Health and Disease. Evaluation and Prescription for Prevention and Rehabilitation.* Philadelphia, PA: Saunders, 1984. *An excellent textbook for clinicians and a particularly good source of exercise test protocols.*
3. Scott, W. N., Nisonson, B., and Nicholas, J. A. (eds.). *Principles of Sports Medicine.* Baltimore, MD: Williams & Wilkins, 1984. *Excellent textbook with particular emphasis on injuries.*
4. Committee on Sports Medicine, American Academy of Pediatrics. *Sports Medicine: Health Care for Young Athletes.* American Academy of Pediatrics, 1983. *AAP recommendations, many of which are appropriate to young adults.*
5. Åstrand, P.-O., and Rodahl, K. *Textbook of Work Physiology. Physiological Bases of Exercise.* New York: McGraw-Hill, 1977. *Classic exercise physiology textbook.*
6. Dishman, R. K., Sallis, J. F., and Orenstein, D. R. The determinants of physical activity and exercise. *Public Health Rep.* 100(2):158, 1985. *Good review of factors influencing likelihood of exercising.*
7. Stephens, T., Jacobs, D. R., and White, C. C. A descriptive epidemiology of leisure-time physical activity. *Public Health Rep.* 100(2):147, 1985. *Review of surveys of leisure-time activities.*
8. Clinque, C. Are Americans fit? Survey data conflict. *Physician Sports Med.* 14:24, 1986. *Brief news report.*
9. American College of Sports Medicine. *Guidelines for Graded Exercise Testing and Prescription.* (3rd ed.). Philadelphia: Lea & Febiger, 1986. *Most recent update of a valuable book.*

9a. Guidelines for exercise testing: A report of the joint American College of Cardiology/American Heart Association task force on assessment of cardiovascular procedures (subcommittee on exercise testing). *Circulation* 74:653A, 1986. *Excellent set of exercise testing guidelines.*

10. Erb, B. D., Fletcher, G. F., and Sheffield, T. L. Standards for exercise treatment programs. American Heart Association Subcommittee on Rehabilitation and Target Activity Group. *Circulation* 59:1084s, 1979. *Current American Heart Association recommendations.*
11. Mead, W. F., and Hartwig, R. Fitness evaluation and exercise prescription. *J. Fam. Pract.* 13(7):1039, 1981. *Short, clear review of exercise testing protocols and exercise prescriptions.*
12. Blincoe, W. A., and Lutz, J. F. The prognostic value of exercise testing. *Cardiovasc. Rev. Rep.* 6:347, 1985. *An excellent summary of studies of exercise test characteristics.*
13. Hollenberg, M., et al. Comparison of a quantitative treadmill exercise score with standard electrocardiographic criteria in screening asymptomatic young men for coronary heart disease. *N. Engl. J. Med.* 313(10):600, 1985. *Reports a computer-assisted treadmill scoring system with a specificity of 100%; accompanied by a good editorial.*
14. Paffenbarger, R. S., et al. Physical activity, all-cause mortality, and longevity of college alumni. *N. Engl. J. Med.* 314(10):605, 1986. *Harvard alumni follow-up study demonstrating lower mortality rate with increasing exercise from 500–3500 kcal/week.*

15. Siscovick, D. S., Laporte, R. E., and Newman, J. M. The disease and risks of physical activity and exercise. *Public Health Rep.* 100(2):180, 1985. *An excellent review.*
16. Kramsch, D. M., et al. Reduction of coronary atherosclerosis by moderate exercise in monkeys on an atherogenic diet. *N. Engl. J. Med.* 305(25):1483, 1981. *Shows a protective effect of exercise in monkeys fed an atherogenic diet.*
17. Cade, R., Mars, D., and Wagemaker, H. Effect of aerobic exercise training on patients with systemic arterial hypertension. *Am. J. Med.* 77(5):785, 1984. *A controlled trial showing that moderate exercise (2 miles jogging per day) can reduce mean arterial pressure in hypertensives whether they are taking antihypertension medications or not, in a 3-month period.*
18. Seals, D. R., and Hagberg, J. M. The effect of exercise training on human hypertension: A review. *Med. Sci. Sports Exerc.* 16(3):207, 1984. *Review pointing out the methodologic flaws in most studies of this subject.*
19. Herbert, P. N., et al. High-density lipoprotein metabolism in runners and sedentary men. *J.A.M.A.* 252(8):1034, 1984. *Examines the reasons why* HDL_2 *increases in endurance athletes.*
20. Blair, S. N., Jacobs, D. R., and Powell, K. E. Relationships between exercise or physical activity and other health aerobics. *Public Health Rep.* 100(2):172, 1985. *An excellent review.*
21. Gwinlip, G. Effect of exercise alone on the weight of obese women. *Arch. Intern. Med.* 135:676, 1975. *Study showing 30 min/day walking reduces weight.*
22. Taylor, C. B., Sallis, J. F., and Needle, R. The relation of physical activity and exercise to mental health. *Public Health Rep.* 100(2):195, 1985. *An excellent review.*
23. Siscovick, D. S., et al. Incidence of primary cardiac arrest during vigorous exercise. *N. Engl. J. Med.* 311(14):874, 1984. *Reports a fivefold increase in cardiac arrest during exercise but a net 40% reduction in overall risk of cardiac arrest.*
24. Koplan, J. P., Siscovick, D. S., and Goldbaum, G. M. The risk of exercise: A public health view of injuries and hazards. *Public Health Rep.* 100(2):189, 1985. *A short review.*
25. Drinkwater, B. L., et al. Bone mineral content of amenorrheic and eumenorrheic athletes. *N. Engl. J. Med.* 311(5):277, 1984. *Demonstrates decreased bone density in amenorrheic athletes.*

66 Problems with Alcohol Use

Michael Kan, David Gordon, and Dan Ferrigno

I. The problem

A. Definitions. There are multiple definitions of alcoholism. Three representative definitions follow: DSM-III defines two clinical entities (Table 66-1): alcohol dependence and alcohol abuse. DSM-III-R describes a much broader category of disorders called psychoactive substance use disorders. Alcoholism is a waxing and waning disease, and an affected individual may fulfill the criteria for one, the other, or neither classification at different times of his or her course.

The American Medical Society for the Treatment of Alcoholism and Other Drug Dependencies defines alcoholism as the continued use of alcohol in the face of adverse consequences with compulsion and loss of control.

Finally, though it is elaborated on in detail in the following section, it should be mentioned in the definition of the problem that alcoholism is an affliction that affects not only the individual using alcohol, but that has grave effects on the family and the community of the afflicted.

B. Description. Alcoholism is an illness of multiple etiologies and manifestations. Alcoholism may be more common in individuals with various psychopathologies. Conversely, many mental health professionals believe that alcoholism may mimic almost any psychiatric diagnosis. Multiple attempts have been made to define an alcoholic personality, but to date none have been found reliable. There is evidence of genetic and physiologic predispositions toward alcoholism [1]. Twin studies show 60% concordance for identical twins versus 30% for fraternal twins, and adoption studies also support a genetic predisposition. Family alcoholism, cultural patterns, and peer pressure are strong sociologic factors in the etiology of alcoholism.

1. **Phases of alcohol addiction.** Jellinek [1a] described the natural history of an alcoholic from intensive questionnaire studies of Alcoholics Anonymous (AA) alcoholics. He described a series of phases in alcohol addiction:

   a. **Prealcoholic phase.** Development of a strong association between relief of tension and alcohol use. This develops from occasional episodes to constant use. Tolerance (lessened effect from same quantity of alcohol), in part, can account for this. Tolerance in turn leads to greater quantities of alcohol being used as time progresses.

   b. **Prodromal phase.** This phase is characterized by the onset of blackouts, surreptitious drinking, planning when to get the next drink, gulping drinks, development of guilt feelings about alcohol, and avoiding references to alcohol.

   c. **Crucial phase.** In this phase, the alcoholic loses the control to stop drinking. One drink leads to many more. Social pressures from others to stop drinking develops in response to the alcoholic's increasingly obvious alcohol abuse. The alcoholic responds by rationalizing his or her drinking habits. There are mood shifts from grandiose and aggressive behavior initially, to persistent remorse, marked self-pity, and unreasonable resentments as problems worsen. The alcoholic becomes increasingly isolated, with loss of friends, jobs, and outside interests. Alcohol becomes the alcoholic's best friend. There is family discord, with loss of libido and spouse hostility, which is rationalized into suspicions of infidelity known as alcoholic jealousy. Family members often compensate by either withdrawing from outside social activities or plunging into them. The alcoholic's health deteriorates with nutritional neglect, and eventually he or she is hospitalized for a related problem. Regular morning drinking is a key historic clue characterizing this phase.

   d. **Chronic phase.** This phase is characterized by prolonged intoxications lasting for days and known as "benders." Alcoholic psychoses, impaired thinking, and loss of ethical sense occur in many. Use of rubbing alcohol and other nonbeverage alcohol may occur. Alcohol tolerance disappears and lesser quantities bring on stupor. Indefinable fears and tremors become constant. Psychomotor inhibition results in the inability to perform simple mechanical acts without a drink. Stressors as previous motivations to drink become secondary to the need to control the symptoms of alcohol withdrawal, and obsession with alcohol becomes the primary motivation. Drinking with persons of lower social class, the development of vague religious desires, and a sense of failure (admitting defeat) develops.

Familiarity with this course of decline on the part of the health care provider may lead to earlier intervention. The later the intervention, the more difficult the treatment and the poorer the prognosis (Fig. 66-1) [2].

2. **Family roles.** Alcoholism is known to have profound effects on the family unit as well. Psychological scarring is not uncommon, and groups now exist for both spouses and children of alcoholics. Many "co-alcoholics" go on to become alcoholics themselves or to lead dysfunctional lives. Ashenberg Straussner, et al. [3] described the family system of an alcoholic. The classic work describing the alcoholic family was written by Claudia Black [4]. There is a parallel development in family members of the signs, symptoms, and defense mechanisms of the alcoholic. Isolation, denial, and rationalization develop in parallel. Similarly, irrational behavior, ethical deterioration (often seen in children as crime and other forms of acting-out), guilt, and indefinable fears develop in parallel. Six key roles are also described, termed "survival roles," which family members adopt to maintain homeostasis in the family unit.
   a. **The alcoholic.** Deterioration leads to abdication of roles and responsibilities. Caring for the alcoholic becomes the focal point of the family. The alcoholic's behavior is erratic and unpredictable, and as long as family members are kept busy covering for and second-guessing the alcoholic, they do not notice their own dysfunctions.
   b. **Co-alcoholic (also known as the chief enabler or responsible one).** This person takes over the abdicated roles and responsibilities and is often perversely the butt of the alcoholic's hostility. The co-alcoholic feels virtuous for maintaining the family system and feels hurt and misunderstood when their sacrifice is not fully understood or appreciated by treating professionals, or when attacked by other family members for maintaining the family while allowing the alcoholic to persist.
   c. **Family hero.** The hero's function is to provide worth to the family through successful achievements. Insightful and sensitive, this individual is keenly aware of the distress in other family members and tries to be the "family healer" and make things better for everyone. Often, though professionally successful, this individual feels a sense of personal inadequacy and often goes into a physical or mental health profession.

      The "placator" is another version of this role described by Black [4]. As seen in the family hero, this child is very sensitive to others' feelings and is the nice, apologizing fixer at home and school. The adult often continues to follow the pattern of taking care of others, on both a personal and a professional level. Thus, they will tend to pair with alcoholics and other dysfunctional adults, becoming someone who "loves too much."
   d. **Scapegoat (also known as the "acting-out child").** The scapegoat protects the family from further disintegration by becoming the family "problem" and displacing the focus from the alcoholic to him- or herself. Problem children should be a clinician's clue to look for family alcoholism. The price for the scapegoat is a high risk for alcoholism. Their sensitivity and willingness to take risks often reflect great potential for leadership if attitudes and behavior can be refocused.
   e. **Isolate (also known as the "lost child" or "adjuster").** This role is almost always assumed by a child whose contribution to the family system is to not be a burden. Problems with developing intimate relationships often follow later in life.
   f. **Mascot.** Humor is said to be one of the highest level and most adaptive of all defense mechanisms. The mascot's function is to provide comic relief from the potentially explosive tension ever present in the alcoholic home. They may be the clown who "laughs on the outside while crying on the inside." They are cute, witty, and fun to be around. A mascot may be so good that they go on to succeed on stage or screen.

Recognition of these roles in family members is important to successful treatment so that the family can be guided from mere survival and maladaption to growth and freedom of choice. Recognition of the alcoholic family history may also help the rehabilitation of maladaptive individuals seeking help many years later.

Youth is a particular risk period for the development of alcoholism. The developmental dynamics are experimentation, development of self-identity, rules-testing, and peer pressure. Also, developing judgment, alcohol, and first automobile use are a dangerous combination. Remission may occur as a maturing process, as has been described for narcotic addicts [5]. Cahalan [6] followed a group that was self-identified by surveys and reported one in five people after 3 years no longer had alcohol-related problems; this evidence of spontaneous remission or gradual disappearance of problems shows that the natural history of alcoholism is not an invariable decline.

C. **Epidemiology.** Ten percent of males and 3–5% of females in the United States will become alcoholic at some time in their lives. Approximately 25% of families are affected by serious alcohol abuse. Prevalence of alcoholism is about 10% of all adults and 20% of adults seen in a family practice setting (to as high as 87.5% in some emergency rooms), and accounts for 25% of all hospital expenditures. The costs are staggering [7]. Industrial loss is estimated at $60 billion annually, the criminal justice system spends over $500 million annually, and medical expenses are estimated at $13 billion annually [5]. The total annual cost to United States society exceeds $120 billion.

In 1981, a Kaiser-Permanente study of mortality [8] found the results shown in Table 66-2.

Individuals with cirrhosis and signs of portal hypertension have less than a 5–10% survival at 5 years. Table 66-3 lists other morbidity and mortality statistics associated with alcoholism.

One person dies every 20 minutes from drunk drivers. That equals 80 325-passenger airplanes crashing per year. On an average weekend night, one in ten drivers on the road is drunk, and after 2 A.M., one in four. One of two United States citizens will be in an alcohol-related collision in their life. If Table 66-3 does not affect the reader's sense of safety, think about these facts next Saturday night, when you buckle up.

II. Primary prevention

A. Methods

1. **Public health.** As discussed in Chap. 32, anticipatory guidance by health care providers and parents and school, work, and community programs can be effective in lowering rates of substance abuse, including ethanol.

   An educational model for clinicians should incorporate the following points: (1) information on alcohol and drugs, (2) behavior modification of drinking styles, and (3) establishment of alternative coping resources. This form of educational approach, emphasizing social variables, communicates to the patient the psychosocial dimensions of drinking behavior. Using this model, techniques to minimize stress, such as relaxation training, meditation, and assertiveness training, can be taught either by the physician or an outside source, such as a mental health professional.

   Table 66-4 lists characteristics associated with moderate drinking from the sociocultural norms of low alcoholism groups.

2. **Legislation.** Government has long struggled with controlling alcohol use through legislation. For the most part, efforts from "sin taxes" to constitutional amendments (prohibition) have been ineffective. One area of significant activity is drunk-driving legislation, which may serve as primary prevention of alcohol-related traffic morbidity and mortality (M & M). An extensive review of this subject was done in 1981 by the Insurance Institute for Highway Safety [9]. Tough punishment has been ineffective. M & M tend to decrease for a period of increased public awareness and adjustment, but rates gradually creep back to equal or higher than prelegislation levels.

   The major obstacle encountered is that law enforcement authorities find enforcing such tough laws unpopular and frustrating. A major reason for this frustration is that judges have also been reluctant to impose harsh penalties. Experience has shown that tough legislation is usually undermined by weak enforcement and seldom-applied penalties. Two new approaches have been suggested and are currently under trial in light of this experience. One involved increasing **and** maintaining public perception of widespread enforcement. Some of these plans involve increasing arrest and conviction rates with highly visible publicity of this effort and more obtrusive efforts, such as roadblock testing. Other suggestions include swift, sure, civil penalties: for example, illegal levels of alcohol resulting in automatic roadside confiscation of the license and/or impoundment of the vehicle for a short period of time. Such efforts must include an awareness of the effects of perceived, overly harsh penalties in undermining this effort through increased police

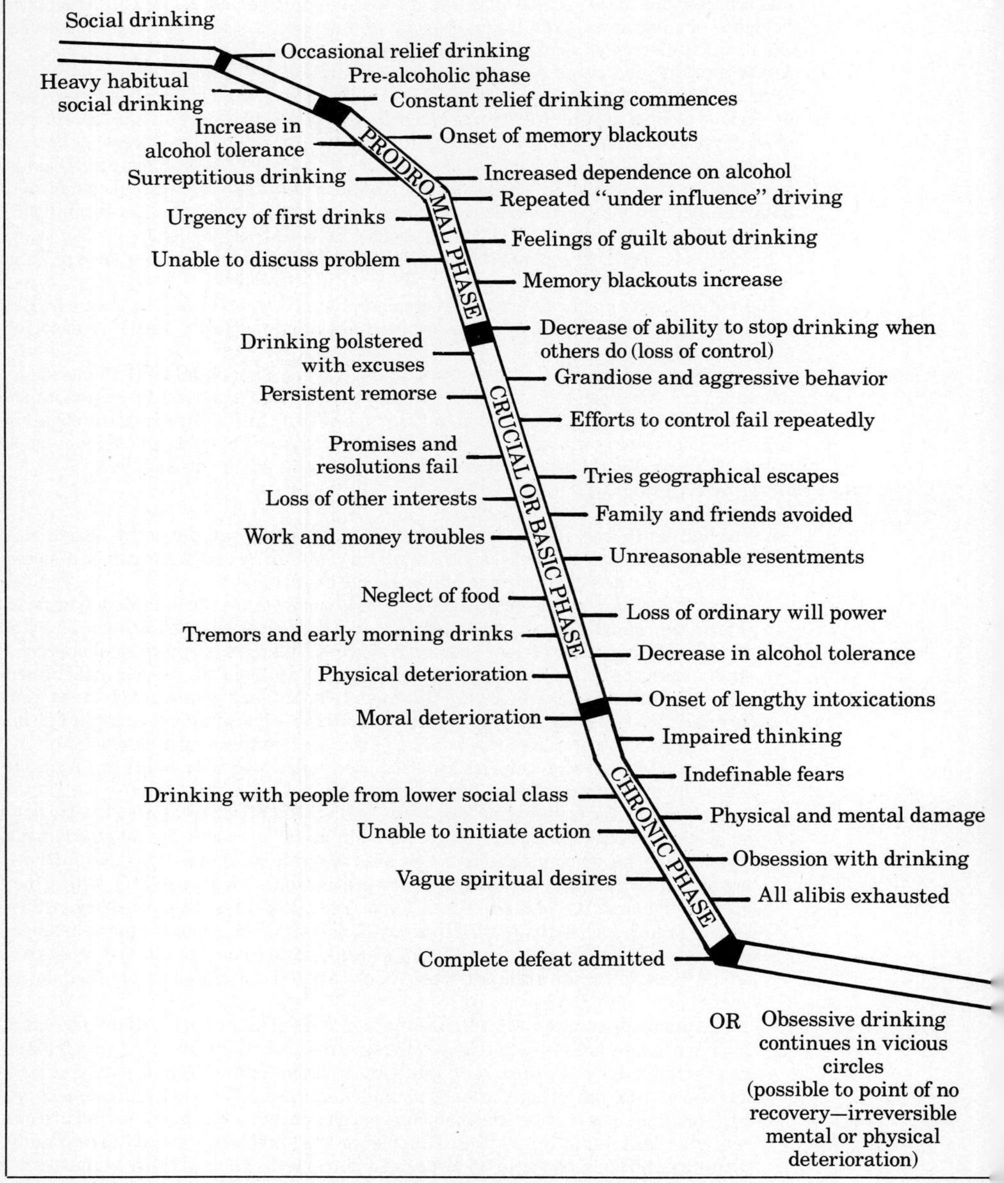

Fig. 66-1. Course of alcohol addiction and recovery. Recovery from the drinking problem may be arrested at any point noted on the chart. The "rock bottom" level is an individual experience and may take place at any point in the developmental process of the individual's alcoholism. (From M. M. Glatt. *The Alcoholic and the Help He Needs* (2nd ed.). London: Priory Press, 1972.)

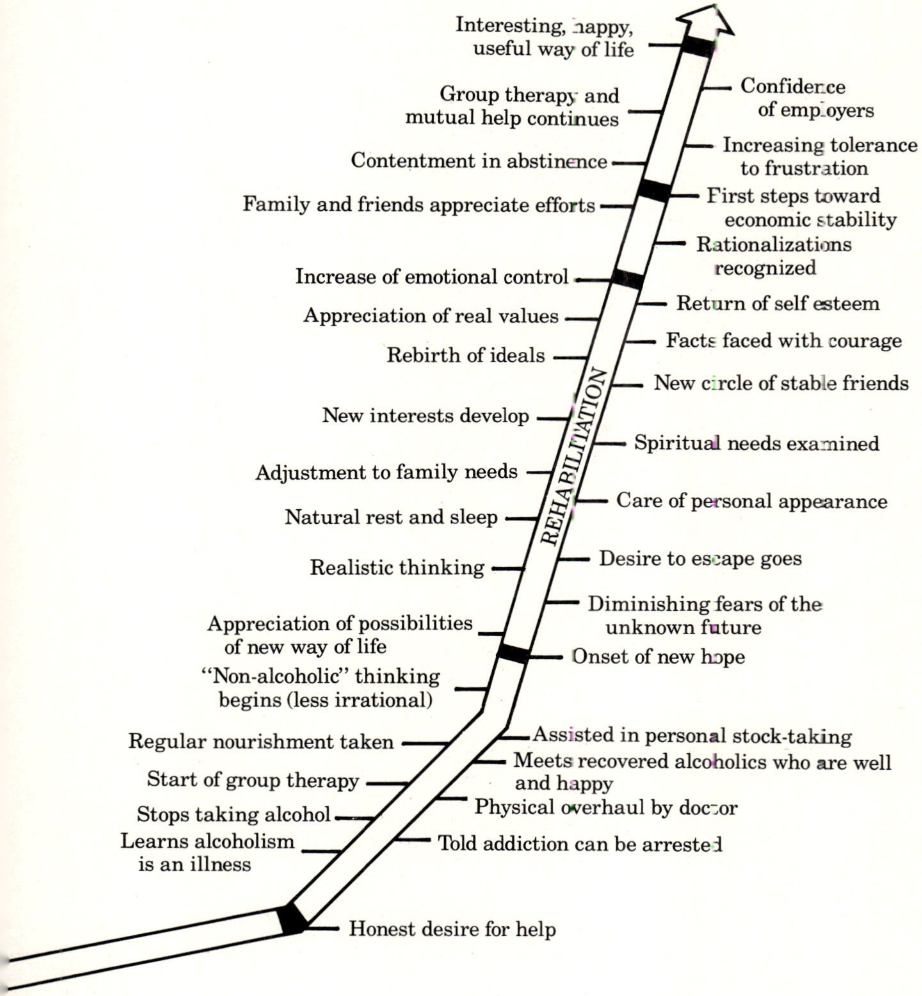
Interesting, happy, useful way of life
Confidence of employers
Group therapy and mutual help continues
Increasing tolerance to frustration
Contentment in abstinence
First steps toward economic stability
Family and friends appreciate efforts
Rationalizations recognized
Increase of emotional control
Return of self esteem
Appreciation of real values
Facts faced with courage
Rebirth of ideals
New circle of stable friends
New interests develop
REHABILITATION
Spiritual needs examined
Adjustment to family needs
Care of personal appearance
Natural rest and sleep
Desire to escape goes
Realistic thinking
Diminishing fears of the unknown future
Appreciation of possibilities of new way of life
Onset of new hope
"Non-alcoholic" thinking begins (less irrational)
Assisted in personal stock-taking
Regular nourishment taken
Meets recovered alcoholics who are well and happy
Start of group therapy
Physical overhaul by doctor
Stops taking alcohol
Told addiction can be arrested
Learns alcoholism is an illness
Honest desire for help

Table 66-1. DSM-III criteria for alcohol abuse and dependence

Diagnostic criteria for alcohol abuse

A. Pattern of pathologic alcohol use: need for daily use of alcohol for adequate functioning; inability to cut down or stop drinking; repeated efforts to control or reduce excess drinking by "going on the wagon" (periods of temporary abstinence) or restricting drinking to certain times of the day; binges (remaining intoxicated throughout the day for at least 2 days); occasional consumption of a fifth of spirits (or its equivalent in wine or beer); amnesic periods for events occurring while intoxicated (blackouts); continuation of drinking despite a serious physical disorder that the individual knows is exacerbated by alcohol use; drinking of nonbeverage alcohol.

B. Impairment of social or occupational functioning due to alcohol use: violence while intoxicated, absence from work, loss of job, legal difficulties (e.g., arrest for intoxicating behavior, traffic accidents while intoxicated), arguments or difficulties with family or friends because of excessive alcohol use.

C. Duration of disturbance of at least 1 month.

Diagnostic criteria for alcohol dependence

A. Either a pattern of pathologic alcohol use or impairment of social or occupational functioning due to alcohol use (see above).

B. Either tolerance or withdrawal:

Tolerance: need for markedly increased amounts of alcohol to achieve the desired effect, or markedly diminished effect with regular use of the same amount.

Withdrawal: development of morning "shakes" and malaise relieved by drinking after cessation of or reduction in drinking.

Source: Reprinted with permission from the American Psychiatric Association. *Quick Reference to the Diagnostic Criteria from the Diagnostic and Statistical Manual of Mental Disorders, Third Edition.* Copyright 1986. American Psychiatric Association.

Table 66-2. Alcoholic death rates

Years alcoholic	Risk of death over general population
0–2	Same
3–5	50% higher
6+	100% higher

Source: Reproduced, with permission, from: A. L. Klatsky, G. R. Friedman, and A. B. Siegelaub. Alcohol and mortality. A ten-year Kaiser-Permanente experience. *Ann. Intern. Med.* 1981; 95(2):139.

leniency, plea bargaining, and decreased convictions. Decriminalizing first offenses except in cases involving injury is suggested to mitigate the confounding effect of leniency.

The experience in Sweden [10] and the work by Grossman et al. [11] suggest that excise "sin taxes" can be effective and can have the same effect as raising the drinking age by 1 year [11]. Excise taxes have been shown to be effective [10], but in the United States taxes have always been considered with ambivalence, and excise taxes have been far outstripped by inflation (adjusted-for-inflation excise taxes in 1985 were at a 51-year low). Excise taxation fails in the United States due to a lack of commitment in the legislative bodies to maintain taxation at discouraging levels [10]. (This should be tempered by the historical perspective that excise taxes have been primarily revenue devices that are **not** part of public health policy or temperance.)

Finally, another area for effective legislation is the "dram shop" reforms. Put simply, bars, party hosts, and others serving alcohol are held financially liable for the actions of persons served alcohol. Financial liability has tremendous impact on today's society, and a number of states have adopted these reforms to varying degrees.

3. **Pregnancy counseling.** Fetal alcohol syndrome risks should always be counseled to pregnant women and **ideally to all women of childbearing age**, since the majority of organogenesis occurs before most women first seek obstetric care (see Chap. 4).

Table 66-3. Alcoholism morbidity and mortality statistics

Entity	Comment
Accidental deaths	One half of road, drowning, fall, and fire deaths related to alcohol use.
Accidents seen in emergency room	22% of home accidents; 15% of work accidents.
Cirrhosis	Ninth leading cause of death in U.S. in 1983.
Brain dysfunction	50–70% alcoholics entering therapy.
Suicide	Over 33.3% of suicides involve alcohol.
Vitamin deficiency	Alcoholism is probably leading cause of this in the United States. Number of cases unknown.
Cardiac problems	Cardiomyopathy caused by alcoholism, as well as exacerbation of other disease entities.
Hematologic problems	Problems with all marrow elements; described neutropenia, anemia, and thrombocytopenia.
Head and neck cancer	10 times the risk in 1983.

Table 66-4. Cultural characteristics associated with alcohol moderation

Traditions and rituals

The use of mind-altering substances is common in history since prehistoric times. Cultural norms have been effective means of moderating use, as in the following examples:

1. Early exposure to use in strong family or religious settings.
2. Parents as an example of moderate use.
3. Viewing alcohol as an accompaniment to a meal or ceremony.
4. Divorcing moral connotations and special attributes from alcohol; it neither proves adulthood or virility nor is especially virtuous or sinful to use.

Social customs

Just as traditions and rituals set a context for moderate and "proper" use of alcohol, socially acceptable behavior associated with its use sets boundaries for defining moderate use:

1. Abstinence accepted as socially proper.
2. Condemnation of excessive drinking and drunkeness.
3. Condemnation of inappropriate behavior (e.g., violence or overt sexuality) secondary to alcohol.
4. No social gatherings primarily for the consumption of alcohol.

4. **Risk index.** Clinicians may improve their ability to do primary and secondary prevention by assessing every patient for alcohol use and risk factors with their routine database. Table 66-5 lists clinically useful clues for risk assessment.

B. Justification

1. **Public health**

   a. **Effectiveness.** Studies show that general public health measures have been of limited effectiveness [9, 10]. Provider impact on alcohol cessation, if inferences can be drawn from provider effectiveness on smoking cessation, may be immensely effective.

   b. **Risks.** Introduction of ideas about alcohol and reaction-formation may increase the likelihood of experimentation (see Chap. 32).

   c. **Costs and acceptability.** Variable costs and acceptability depend on the extent of efforts and family resources. Extensive one-on-one counseling is often expensive. Larger groups, which reduce cost, may dilute the effect of the powerful provider-patient relationship.

Table 66-5. Alcoholism screening

The provider should screen for alcoholism when any of the following are found in the patient's history or physical exam:

History
- Family history of alcoholism
- Depression
- Multiple job changes/absences/injuries
- History of repeated accidents
- History inconsistent with examination
- Family problems
- Requests for tranquilizers
- Complaints of headaches
- Insomnia
- Sexual problems

Examination
- Hypertension (as many as 25% of hypertensives lower their blood pressure with abstension)
- Repeated injuries (or evidence of)
- Agitation with probing of alcohol use (social drinker accepts; alcoholic is hotly defensive)
- Alcohol on breath
- Hepatomegaly/alteration of liver enzymes

2. **Legislation**
   a. **Effectiveness.** "Tough" laws are not effective. Insufficient data exist on new efforts (roadside checks, publicizing of arrests). Only delaying the legal drinking age has been shown to be effective and to reduce accidents from all causes. Sweden considers excise taxes to be a key element in public health policy on alcohol use. If other liability issues, such as medical malpractice, can be considered similar, "dram shop" reform will have significant impact. Health care providers have traditionally taken the lead in pioneering safety legislation, as in the institution of mandatory automobile child restraint devices, and can be equally effective in promoting effective legislation.
   b. **Risks.** Frustration, wasted money, and disillusionment with legal solutions are associated with the failure of legislation to date. Freedom of choice and public health policy have and will always be difficult political issues.
   c. **Costs.** A 1979 General Accounting Office (GAO) report stated that various Alcohol Safety Action Projects (ASAP) are spending millions of dollars, ". . .yet, statistics continue to indicate that, overall, one-half of highway fatalities in the United States are related to alcohol." It concluded that ASAPs did "not show any overall national results." Estimated costs for 1971–1976 were $88 million, for no effect [9].
   d. **Acceptability.** See the discussion of methods in sec. **II.A.**
3. **Risk index**
   a. **Effectiveness** is untried; there are no data.
   b. **Risks.** Broaching the subject of a predisposition to alcoholism based on risk factors may alienate patients, especially alcoholic patients in whom defensiveness and denial are to be expected.
   c. **Costs** include the time used to assess and follow up patients.
   d. **Acceptability** depends on the provider's skill and relationship with the patient.
4. **Pregnancy counseling**
   a. **Effectiveness.** Rosett, et al. [12], in 1983, reported that in a systematic counseling program geared to the severity of alcohol abuse, 67% of women attending three or more sessions reduced their drinking.
   b. **Risks. Not** counseling leaves the health care provider at substantial liability risk and the fetus at substantial morbidity risk.
   c. **Cost** is the time used to counsel the patient.
   d. **Acceptability.** Working with pregnant women to curtail drinking is now a standard of care.

Have you ever felt the need to CUT DOWN on drinking?
Have you ever felt ANNOYED by criticism of drinking?
Have you ever had GUILTY feelings about drinking?
Have you ever taken a morning EYE-OPENER?

Fig. 66-2. The CAGE test. A score of two or more is a positive test. (From J. A. Ewing. Recognizing, confronting and helping the alcoholic. *Am. Fam. Physician* 18:107, 1978.)

1. Do you feel you are a normal drinker? (By normal, we mean you drink less than or as much as most other people.) (No)
2. Does your wife, husband, a parent, or other near relative ever worry or complain about your drinking? (Yes)
3. Do you ever feel guilty about your drinking? (Yes)
4. Do friends or relatives think you are a normal drinker? (No)
5. Are you able to stop drinking when you want to? (No)
6. Have you ever attended a meeting of Alcoholics Anonymous? (Yes)
7. Has drinking ever created problems between you and your wife, husband, a parent, or other near relative? (Yes)
8. Have you ever gotten into trouble at work because of drinking? (Yes)
9. Have you ever neglected your obligations, your family, or your work for 2 or more days in a row because you were drinking? (Yes)
10. Have you ever gone to anyone for help about your drinking? (Yes)
11. Have you ever been in a hospital because of drinking? (Yes)
12. Have you ever been arrested for drunken driving, driving while intoxicated, or driving under the influence of alcoholic beverages? (Yes)
13. Have you ever been arrested, even for a few hours, because of other drunken behavior? (Yes)

Fig. 66-3. The Short Michigan Alcoholism Screening Test (SMAST). The alcoholism-indicating responses are in parentheses. (Reprinted by permission, from M. L. Selzer, A. Vinokur, and L. van Rooijen. A self-administered short version of the Michigan Alcoholism Screening Test [SMAST]. *J. Stud. Alcohol* 36:117, 1975. Copyright by Journal of Studies on Alcohol, Inc., Rutgers Center of Alcohol Studies, New Brunswick, NJ 08903.)

III. Secondary prevention

A. Early detection

1. **Methods.** Every patient contact is an opportunity to update the general database, and continued evaluation and reevaluation for associated problems with alcohol should be part of the health care provider's continuity of care.
   a. **Questionnaires** that may be used include:
      (1) **CAGE questionnaire** [13]: only four questions, and a score of 2 or more is positive (Fig. 66-2).
      (2) **SMAST (Short Michigan Alcoholic Screening Test)** [14]: has 13 questions, 3 or more scored is positive (Fig. 66-3).
   b. **Laboratory measurements**
      (1) **Blood alcohol level (BAL)** measures blood value.
      (2) **Mean corpuscular volume (MCV)** measures red blood cell size on the Coulter counter.
      (3) **Gamma glutamyl transpeptidase (GGT)** is the liver enzyme most sensitive to alcohol metabolism [15].
   c. **Symptoms and signs**
      (1) Question upon suspicion of a problem (see Table 66-5) [16].
      (2) High-risk patients with significant unexplained health problems, social deterioration, or change in mental health should be assessed.
      (3) Consider alcoholism in low-risk patients with the changes discussed in sec. **III.A.1.c.(2)** above.

Table 66-6. Detection of alcoholics with questionnaire or laboratory tests

Tests	Sensitivity %	N_1	Specificity %	N_2	Predictive + %	Predictive − %	Efficiency %
MCV	41	54	87	70	74	62	65
GGT	26	46	85	54	61	57	57
BAL	13	45	97	61	78	56	58
CAGE	72	50	79	57	75	76	76
MAST	86	50	81	57	80	87	83
SMAST	80	50	77	57	76	81	79

Key: N_1=number of patients on which sensitivity is based; N_2=number of patients on which specificity is based; N_1+N_2=number of patients for which test results were obtained; MCV=mean corpuscular volume; GGT=gamma glutamyl transpeptidase; BAL=blood alcohol level.
Source: D. G. Mayfield and R. G. Johnston. Screening Techniques and Prevalence Estimation in Alcoholism. In W. E. Fann et al. (eds.), *Phenomenology and Treatment of Alcoholism.* New York: Spectrum Medical and Scientific Books, 1980.

Table 66-7. Detection of alcoholics with questionnaire and laboratory tests in combination

Test combinations		Sensitivity %	N_1	Specificity %	N_2	Predictive + %	Predictive − %	Efficiency %
	CAGE	86	50	65	55	69	84	75
MCV	MAST	96	50	69	55	73	95	82
	SMAST	90	50	65	55	70	88	77
	CAGE	76	46	66	51	67	76	71
GGT	MAST	89	46	66	51	70	87	77
	SMAST	84	46	66	51	69	83	75
	CAGE	79	44	75	53	74	81	77
BAL	MAST	90	44	81	53	81	91	86
	SMAST	84	44	77	53	77	85	81

Key: N_1=of patients on which sensitivity is based; N_2=number of patients on which specificity is based; N_1+N_2=number of patients for which test results were obtained; MCV=mean corpuscular volume; GGT=gamma glutamyl transpeptidase; BAL=blood alcohol level.
Source: D. G. Mayfield and R. G. Johnston. Screening Techniques and Prevalence Estimation in Alcoholism. In W. E. Fann et al. (eds.), *Phenomenology and Treatment of Alcoholism.* New York: Spectrum Medical and Scientific Books, 1980.

d. **Interval.** All of the above early detection methods would not be unreasonable baseline data to have on all patients, except perhaps BAL. Questionnaires can be done quickly and cheaply in the waiting room, so giving them annually would not be unreasonable. Laboratory measurements should probably be done with the above indications only, or at infrequent intervals that the provider should establish.
e. **Population.** At risk are all ages from early puberty to death. Men are at greater risk. Alcoholic families and certain ethnic groups are more affected: American Indians are more affected than whites or Asians. Less effective acetaldehyde dehydrogenase in Asians leads to "built in" Antabuse effect. **All** socioeconomic groups are at risk. Cultures with the longest history of alcohol use do best at limiting consumption.

2. **Justification**
   a. **Test characteristics** [17] (Tables 66-6 and 66-7).
   b. **Risks.** False-negatives and false-positives may be significant.
   c. **Costs** include the time to administer, plus laboratory fees.
   d. **Acceptability.** Early detection methods should be well accepted. Many are routine. Health care providers may balk at adding additional screening, but the time investment could be minimized by administering questionnaires while waiting to see the provider, or after the examination.

Table 66-8. Estimated treatment utilization

Treatment source	Population served*
NIAAA-funded projects	197,000
Other than NIAAA-funded projects	
Short-stay hospitals	476,000
State and county mental hospitals	111,000
Private mental hospitals	11,000
Drug abuse facilities	17,000
Mental health facilities	286,000
Private physicians' offices	423,000
Community mental health centers	113,000
Outpatient psychiatric clinics	53,000
Halfway houses	36,000
Veterans Administration	133,000
Department of Defense	52,000
Department of Transportation (DWI)	28,000
Indian Health Service	27,000
Alcoholics Anonymous	671,000
TOTAL	2,634,000

Key: NIAAA=National Institute for Alcohol Abuse and Alcoholism.
*The NIAAA data are for 1980; the other data are for 1977.
Source: *The Alcohol, Drug Abuse, and Mental Health National Data Book.* Rockville MD: Alcohol, Drug Abuse, and Mental Health Administration, 1980.

B. Early intervention

1. **Methods.** Once the diagnosis has been made, intervention must require that the individual and/or family enter some form of therapy. Unfortunately, despite the great damage and cost of alcoholism, only 15% of alcoholics receive any treatment.

Methods of intervention have one thing in common. The alcoholic is confronted with the problem, the system of denial is broken down, and personal crisis follows [18]. Alcoholics Anonymous terms spontaneous crisis "bottoming out." Crisis is an element that is instrumental in getting the alcoholic into treatment. Earlier intervention using family, friends, and coworkers to confront the alcoholic is used widely and is well described in the literature. The technique is known as "confrontation." Employee-assistance programs and impaired-professionals programs bring about a state of crisis through the threat of loss of job or license to practice.

Treatment modalities are multiple and diverse, and most programs integrate several methods. Reasonable modalities include (1) medical, utilizing detoxification and sensitizing agents (i.e., disulfiram [Antabuse]), and (2) psychological. The experience with medical management without supportive psychological intervention is poor and dangerous. Some alcoholics will drink with disulfiram or diazepam (Valium) in their system, which can lead to medical emergencies such as coma, Mallory-Weiss tears, or electrolyte imbalances. Medical management must be viewed as a temporizing adjunct to the care of an alcoholic, though when properly used, it can be a valuable component of care.

Psychological treatments include variants of behavior modification (aversion therapy, stress management, assertiveness training, relaxation therapy), psychotherapy, group therapy, family system therapy, and sociocultural modifications such as joining AA. Extended stay, inpatient programs of approximately 30 days offer intensive rehabilitation approaches. Table 66-8 gives some idea of the variety and distribution of treatment modes [19]. It is highly recommended that health care providers attend one AA meeting to learn about that referral source (Table 66-9).

2. **Justification**

   a. **Effectiveness.** Success will depend on the underlying pathology and how success is defined. If complete wellness, abstinence, and mental harmony are the goals, success will be limited, and this in part explains some of the frustration of health care providers in managing alcoholism. If success is defined as altering dysfunction in a family member, returning the alcoholic to a productive life, and reducing alcohol use, success will be greater. We caution the reader to recall

Table 66-9. Characteristics of treatment settings

Setting	Treatment modalities	Patients*
Inpatient		
General hospitals Short-term detoxification units Rehabilitation stay (3–4 weeks)	Medical: frequently pharmacotherapy	Socially stable, fewer years of heavy drinking
State and private psychiatric hospitals	Individual and group psychotherapy, alcoholism education, AA, disulfiram (Antabuse)	Lower middle class, relatively socially and vocationally disabled Severe psychiatric condition or opportunity to interrupt drinking pattern or motivate a resistant patient
Freestanding alcoholism rehabilitation facilities	Nonmedical: lectures, nonpsychodynamic group counseling, AA, family sessions	Socially competent, middle class, working
Aversion-conditioning hospital	Strong medical orientation: detoxification, emetine or faradic conditioning, counseling, group therapy, education, hospital follow-up programs	Socially competent, upper class
Outpatient		
Private physicians' offices	Medical: disulfiram maintenance, symptom management, involvement of spouse and family	Usually alcoholism is not primary complaint
Community mental health centers	Medical, psychological, social services	Broad spectrum of patients
Freestanding outpatient clinics	Medical, psychological, social services	Broad spectrum of patients
Day care	Varied	Broad spectrum of patients
Mental health professionals	Varied	Broad spectrum of patients
Intermediate		
Halfway houses, quarterway houses, recovery homes	Peer-group orientation; food, shelter, supportive services in nondrinking atmosphere	Recovering alcoholics, ambulatory and mentally competent, who usually have no spouse or immediate family

Key: AA=Alcoholics Anonymous.
*Patient descriptors are only rough characterizations.
Source: L. Saxe. *The Effectiveness and Costs of Alcoholism Treatment.* Washington, D.C.: U.S. Government Printing Office, 1983.

that when alcoholism is controlled, the prognosis becomes that of the underlying pathology: marital dysfunction, mental illness, or developmental or coping maladaptation.

The 1983 Congressional Office of Technology Assessment publication on effectiveness and costs of alcoholism treatment provides an excellent compendium of reviews of treatment programs [20]. Prolonged sobriety rates were reported from 30–68% of the programs.

Definition remains a controversy, "normal" drinking versus total abstinence being required to meet criteria for being sober. The Rand studies were long-term studies of patients from eight National Institute on Alcohol Abuse and Alcoholism treatment centers. Remission was defined as abstinence or drinking in moderation. In 4 years, 1976–1980, 7% remained totally abstinent and 54% were drinking with serious problems—down 90% from the initial group. Fifteen percent had died. Many patients required repeat applications of therapy. Comparisons failed to single out any one method or duration of therapy as more effective than others.

Table 66-10. Estimated health care expenditures for alcohol abuse in 1977, by setting (millions of dollars)

Setting	Total expenditures	Expenditures on alcohol abuse-specific illnesses
Alcohol specialty facilities		
Hospital-based facilities		
State and county psychiatric hospitals	$200	$200
Private psychiatric hospitals	34	34
Veterans Administration neuropsychiatric hospitals	29	29
General hospitals with separate psychiatric facilities	43	43
Subtotal	$306	$306
Other facilities and services		
Federally funded community mental health centers	129	129
Residential treatment centers for children	—	—
Halfway houses	37	37
Multiservice mental health facilities	8	8
Other freestanding facilities	198	198
Alcohol specialty units in correctional facilities	3	3
Private practice psychiatrists	18	18
Private practice psychologists	8	8
Subtotal	$401	$401
TOTAL	$707	$707
General health facilities		
Hospital-based facilities		
Community hospitals	$2274	$880
Veterans Administration general hospitals and other facilities	425	321
Other federal facilities	149	84
Subtotal	$2848	$1285
Other facilities and services		
Nursing homes	108	98
Private practice physicians	548	16
Dentists	443	195
Other health professionals	133	62
Drugs and drug sundries	525	232
Other health services	222	90
Volunteer services	103	45
Subtotal	$2082	$738
TOTAL	$4930	$2023

Source: A. M. Cruze, et al. *Economic Costs to Society of Alcohol and Drug Abuse and Mental Illness 1977.* Washington, D.C.: Research Triangle Institute for the Alcohol, Drug Abuse, and Mental Health Administration, Department of Health and Human Services, October 1981.

b. Risks. Intervention may precipitate a crisis resulting in family changes, personal changes, possible depression, and suicide, or steeper decline into alcoholism.

c. Costs. Between 1980 and 1983, the medical costs for 2934 patients from the Federal Employees Health Benefit Program with Aetna Insurance Company were followed after filing claims for alcohol treatment. The majority of patients received inpatient treatment followed by outpatient treatment. For alcoholics less than 45 years old, costs returned to baseline (nonalcoholics). Over 45 years of age, subjects showed some increased costs, which may be explained by a combination of normal aging processes and loss of body resilience as it ages and

Table 66-11. Estimated economic costs of alcoholism in 1977 (millions of dollars)

	Millions of dollars
Core costs	
Direct	
Treatment (for alcoholism and causally related illness	$ 5,637
Support (research, education and training, construction, insurance administration	735
Indirect	
Lost productivity due to	
Premature mortality	$10,715
Morbidity resulting in	
Reduced productivity and lost work time	23,593
Lost employment	2,481
	$36,789
Total core costs	$43,161
Other related costs	
Direct	
Motor vehicle crashes (funeral, legal/court, insurance administration, accident investigation, vehicle damage)	1,782
Criminal justice system	1,685
Social welfare program administration	142
Other (fire losses, fire protection, highway safety)	832
Indirect	
Lost productivity due to	
Alcoholics' incarceration	1,418
Others' lost work time because of motor vehicle crashes	354
Total other related costs	$ 6,213
Total economic costs	$49,374

Source: A. M. Cruze, et al. *Economic Costs to Society of Alcohol and Drug Abuse and Mental Illness 1977.* Washington, D.C.: Research Triangle Institute for the Alcohol, Drug Abuse, and Mental Health Administration, Department of Health and Human Services, October 1981.

endures a severe stress, which leads to accelerated deterioration [21] (Tables 66-10 and 66-11).

d. Acceptability. Multiple modalities exist and therapy must be tailored to the individual. Many object to AA's religious nature and belonging to an "AA community." The key to therapeutic success depends on the practitioner's ability to match the patient and the mode of therapy.

e. Follow-up. Alcoholics commonly see alcohol as their "best friend." It has always been there, numbed the traumas of life's stresses, and provided pleasure and comfort. During treatment, health care providers may need to address issues of grief and loss, emptiness, and the loss of the patient's major coping resource at the time of reemergence into a world made chaotic by their previous alcoholism. Patients may need support and facilitation in the development of new coping resources and friends in order to make a full recovery and begin a new life.

IV. Recommendations. Clinicians should review their practices. Few practitioners approach the prevalence of 10% in the general population in their identified alcoholics population, much less the data showing 20–85+% of patients in medical settings. Alcoholism is prevalent, easily diagnosed when a high index of suspicion exists, and treatable.

A. Primary prevention

1. **Public health.** Health care providers should embody concepts from Table 66-5 into patient education and community service projects. Community physicians, nurse practitioners, physician associates, and so forth often are welcome speakers in public schools and work programs.
2. **Legislation.** For more information contact: National Alcohol Tax Coalition, 1501

Family members

Al Anon: ____________________

Alateen: ____________________

Children of Alcoholics: ____________________

Alcoholics and alcoholism

Alcoholics Anonymous: ____________________

Operation Cork: 8939 Villa La Jolla Dr
San Diego, CA 92037

Films and publications: Free Films (813) 541-7571

Community services*
directory/agency: ____________________

Alcohol Council (local): ____________________

National Institute for Alcohol Abuse and Alcoholism
William Mayer, Director
200 Independence Ave, SW
Washington, DC 20201
(301) 433-3885
(202) 245-6343 (public inquiries)

National Clearinghouse on Mental Health
5600 Fishers Lane
Rockville, MD 20857
(202) 443-4531

National Clearinghouse on Drug Abuse: (Hours: 8:30–4:45)
5600 Fishers Lane
Rockville, MD 20857
(202) 443-6500

Local United Way: ____________________

(usually has lists for alcohol abuse services)

Superintendent of documents
U.S. Government Printing Office
Washington, DC 20402

(for lists of available U.S. agencies' publications)

Miscellaneous (city or county social services):

____

(many locals have publicly funded programs)

*Describes local human service planning. Maintained in California and a few other states by the local community services agency.

Fig. 66-4. Master intervention resource list. Blank spaces are provided for local phone numbers.

16th Street N.W., Washington, DC 20036 (202/332-9110). Join the Council on Alcohol Policy by writing: The Trauma Foundation, Building 1, Room 400, San Francisco General Hospital, San Francisco, California 94110.

3. **Pregnancy counseling.** Consider all women of childbearing age to be at risk, and counsel appropriately.
4. **Risk index.** Incorporate some estimation of risk into the basic health care maintenance workup and periodic physical.

B. Early detection

1. Add the CAGE and SMAST questionnaires to the health care maintenance database.
2. Include MCV and GGT in basic screening labs.
3. Develop a plan for subsequent screenings based on risk profiles and suspicious new problems, especially those affecting social or mental status.

C. Early interventions. Multiple modalities exist and practitioners need to familiarize themselves with local resources. Remember to identify and evaluate alcoholic family members. A basic resource list for use in developing a master resource list appears in Fig. 66-4.

References

1. Schuckit, M. A. Twin Studies on Substance Abuse: An overview. In *Twin Research 3: Epidemiological and Clinical Studies.* New York: Alan Liss, 1981. Pp. 61–70. *Excellent overview on twin studies including classic works by Kaji (1960) and Partanen (1966).*

1a. Jellinek, B. M. *Expert Committee on Mental Health, Alcoholism Sub-Committee, Second Report: Annex 2, The Phases of Alcohol Addiction.* World Health Organization, Technical Report Series, 48, August 1952. *Classic description of phases of alcoholism.*

2. Glatt, N. M. Today's enjoyment—tomorrow's dependency. The road towards the "rock bottom" and the way back. *Br. J. Addict.* 70(Suppl. 1):25, 1975.
3. Ashenberg Straussner, S. L., Weinstein, D. L., and Hernandez, R. Effects of alcoholism on the family system. *Health Soc. Work* 4(4):111, 1979. *Excellent work on alcoholic families.*
4. Black, C. *It Will Never Happen to Me.* Denver: MAC Printing and Publication Division, 1982. *Classic work and workbook for children of alcoholics.*
5. Winick, C. Maturing out of narcotic addiction. *Bull. Narc.* 14(1):1, 1962. *Is experimentation with drugs part of rules-testing in development?*
6. Cahalan, D. *Problem Drinkers.* San Francisco: Jossey-Bass, 1970. *Data on spontaneous remission rates.*
7. Cruze, A. M., et al. *Economic Costs to Society of Alcohol and Drug Abuse and Mental Illness 1977.* Washington, DC: Research Triangle Institute for the Alcohol, Drug Abuse, and Mental Health Administration, Department of Health and Human Services, October 1981. *Review of cost of alcohol, drug abuse, and mental illness in the United States.*
8. Klatsky, A. L., Friedman, G. R., and Siegelaub, A. B. Alcohol and mortality. A ten-year Kaiser-Permanente experience. *Ann. Intern. Med.* 95(2):139, 1981. *Risk quantification of death related to alcohol. Ten-year follow-up study of Kaiser-Permanente.*
9. Insurance Institute for Highway Safety. Drinking-driving laws: What works? *Insur. Inst. Highway Safety, Status Report* 16(5):4116, 1981. *Review of effectiveness of drunk-driving legislation.*
10. Fact Sheets on Sweden. *Facts and Figures about Youth in Sweden.* FS88 Ohfb. Stockholm: The Swedish Institute, December 1983. *Alcohol control program in Sweden and its successes.*
11. Grossman, M., Coate, D., and Arluck, G. M. Price Sensitivity of Alcoholic Beverages in the United States. *Conference on Control Issues in Alcohol Abuse Prevention II: Impacting Communities.* Charleston, SC, September 1984. *Data and theories on excise taxes in the United States.*
12. Rosett, H. L., Weiner, L., and Edelin, K. C. Treatment experience with pregnant problem drinkers. *J.A.M.A.* 249(15):2029, 1983. *Success with prevention of fetal alcohol syndrome.*
13. Ewing, J. A. Recognizing, confronting and helping the alcoholic. *Am. Fam. Physician* 18:107, 1978. *Source of the CAGE questions.*
14. Selzer, M. L., Vinokur, A., and van Rooijen, L. A self-administered short version of the Michigan Alcoholism Screening Test (SMAST). *J. Stud. Alcohol* 36:117, 1975. *Source of the SMAST.*
15. Rosalki, S. B., and Rau, D. Serum-glutamyl transpeptidase activity in alcoholism. *Clin. Chim. Acta* 39:41, 1972. *GGT is a good screen for alcoholic liver disease.*
16. Berry, R. E. Jr., and Boland, J. P. *The Economic Cost of Alcohol Abuse.* New York: Free Press, 1977. *Economics of alcoholism.*
17. Mayfield, D. G., and Johnston, R. G. Screening Techniques and Prevalence Estimation in Alcoholism. In W. E. Fann, et al. (eds.), *Phenomenology and Treatment of Alcoholism.* New York: Spectrum Medical and Scientific Books, 1980. Pp. 33–44. *One of the best references to psychological issues, family issues, and well-researched, well-documented schemes for screening.*

18. Diesenhaus, H. Current Trends in Treatment Programming for Problem Drinkers and Alcoholics. In *Prevention, Intervention, and Treatment: Concerns and Models.* Alcohol and Health Monograph No. 3. Rockville, MD: National Institute on Alcohol Abuse and Alcoholism, Alcohol, Drug Abuse, and Mental Health Administration, 1982. *Review of approaches to the problem.*
19. *The Alcohol, Drug Abuse, and Mental Health National Data Book.* Rockville, MD: Alcohol, Drug Abuse, and Mental Health Administration, 1980. *Good data source on alcohol and drug abuse in the United States.*
20. Saxe, L. *The Effectiveness and Costs of Alcoholism Treatment.* Washington, DC: United States Government Printing Office, 1983. *Deserves special note as the reference describing alcohol programs, costs, and research.*
21. Holder, N. D. and Blose, J. O. Alcoholism treatment and total health care utilization and costs. *J.A.M.A.* 256(11):1456, 1986. *Medical costs analysis of a successful employee assistance program (EAP).*

Selected Reading

American Psychiatric Association. *Diagnostic and Statistical Manual of Mental Disorders, Third Edition, Revised.* Washington, DC: American Psychiatric Association, 1987. *Excellent chapter on psychoactive substance use disorders.*

67 Tobacco Use

Lee Vogel and William A. Norcross

I. The problem

A. Definition. Tobacco use is not limited to cigarette, pipe, and cigar smoking, but includes the increasing use of smokeless tobacco in the forms of chewing tobacco or snuff. On the surface, it might seem that this is an adequate definition of the simple term "tobacco use." However, any definition of tobacco use is incomplete without identifying addiction as the major contributor to continued use. Smoking, chewing, or sniffing tobacco is a learned behavior, usually started in youth as a result of direct and indirect social pressures. Continued use shows a typical substance-abuse pattern by every criteria of addiction, including psychoactive effects, habitual use leading to dependence and compulsive abuse, physiologic and psychological discomfort upon cessation, and a high rate of recidivism among former users. There is no longer any doubt that continued use of tobacco is an addiction.

Finally, the term "passive smoking" must be considered in the complete definition of tobacco use. Passive smoking is the involuntary breathing of exhaled mainstream smoke (which is drawn through the tobacco), and sidestream smoke (which arises from the burning core).

B. Description

1. Physiologic and pathophysiologic effects

a. Ingredients. Cigarette smoke contains about 4000 compounds including carbon monoxide, tar, nicotine, the radioactive alpha-emitter polonium, and two classes of powerful chemical carcinogens—the polycyclic aromatic hydrocarbons and the nitrosamines. These carcinogens are also contained in smokeless tobacco products.

b. Immediate physiologic effects. The immediate physiologic effects of all forms of tobacco use include tachycardia, arrhythmias, bronchial constriction, and elevated blood pressure, cardiac output, and stroke volume, with resultant increased myocardial oxygen consumption. These effects are attributable to nicotine-induced catecholamine release. Use of smokeless tobacco produces blood levels of nicotine comparable to those produced by smoking tobacco. Studies show that nonsmokers exposed to the smoke in a typical work environment have salivary and urinary concentrations of nicotine similar to those found in light smokers. Thus, these nicotine-mediated physiologic effects can be found in smokers, smokeless tobacco users, and nonsmokers in a smoking environment.

c. Blood effects. Chronic smoking increases carboxyhemoglobin, resulting in elevated red cell mass (secondary polycythemia). Nonsmokers may be subject to this effect also, as studies indicate that nonsmokers in smoking environments have carboxyhemoglobin levels equal to those who smoke five cigarettes in 8 hours. This may result from the fact that carbon monoxide concentration in sidestream smoke is 2–3 times that found in mainstream smoke. Evidence suggests that smoking augments platelet aggregation and decreases blood coagulation time, which may account for the relationship between smoking and estrogen-related thromboembolic disease.

d. Drug metabolism. Smoking affects the metabolism of many drugs primarily by induction of the hepatic microsomal enzyme systems. This results in higher dose requirements to achieve the pharmacologic effects of theophylline, pentazocine, imipramine, propoxyphene, diazepam, and chlorpromazine. Smokers have decreased levels of vitamin C, as well as impaired metabolism of vitamin B_{12}.

e. Respiratory pathophysiology. Cigarette smoke impairs ciliary movement and macrophage function in the respiratory system, which contributes to infection and alveolar occlusion. In addition, it induces basal cell hyperplasia and nuclear changes in the bronchial epithelium, probable precursors to respiratory malignancy.

f. Addiction. Over the past 20 years, laboratory and clinical studies indicate that tobacco use shows a typical substance abuse pattern: experimentation leading to regular use and physical dependence, resulting in development of tolerance to the nicotine effect, and requiring increased dosage. Tobacco produces the psychological effects of relaxation and arousal, which have been found to be mediated by nicotine and blocked by mecamylamine by competitive inhibition at brain nicotine receptor sites. Laboratory animals and human studies demonstrate that self-administration patterns are comparable to those of other central nervous system stimulant drugs. The continued use of tobacco products by persons who have suffered serious adverse health effects demonstrates the addicting properties of nicotine. The physical dependence associated with nicotine results in withdrawal symptoms with the abrupt cessation of chronic use. Former users may experience craving for years after cessation and are prone to recidivism. The accumulated evidence unequivocally identifies nicotine in tobacco products as a highly addictive substance.

2. Adverse health consequences

a. Significance. Tobacco use is the leading single preventable cause of premature death in the United States, making it the nation's most important health problem. Serious illness occurs as the result of tobacco use (and possibly as a result of involuntary or passive use), and assumes many diverse forms.

b. Cardiovascular disease. Cigarette smoking is a strong independent risk factor for coronary artery disease and sudden death. Epidemiologic studies indicate that cigarette smokers of any age or sex have a higher incidence of myocardial infarction and sudden death from coronary heart disease, compared with nonsmokers. The risk is dose-dependent, related to the age of onset of smoking, number of cigarettes smoked, number of years of smoking, and depth of inhalation. In addition to being an independent risk factor for coronary artery disease, cigarette smoking acts synergistically with the other major factors—elevated cholesterol levels and hypertension.

Pipe and cigar smokers have a risk of myocardial infarction and sudden death that is intermediate between the risks for nonsmokers and for cigarette smokers. No epidemiologic data are available on cardiovascular risk in association with smokeless tobacco use, although elevation of blood pressure, heart rate, lipid levels, catecholamines, and nicotine levels have been documented in smokeless tobacco users. Women who smoke and use oral contraceptives have a 10-fold higher risk of heart attack than women who neither smoke nor use oral contraceptives.

c. Other vascular diseases. Data from numerous prospective studies have shown an association between cigarette smoking and cerebrovascular disease. Smokers have a higher incidence of stroke mortality than nonsmokers, with a greater risk occurring in the 40–49 year age group, and with little or no effect noted after 65 years of age. Women smokers who use oral contraceptives have been reported to be at increased risk for stroke, especially subarachnoid hemorrhage and thromboembolic events.

Cigarette smoking is a major risk factor for other forms of peripheral vascular disease. Smokers have a two- to threefold increase in mortality from abdominal aortic aneurysm as compared with nonsmokers. The prevalence of aortoiliac and femoropopliteal disease is greater among smokers. An elevated risk for peripheral vascular disease has not been adequately demonstrated for cigar or pipe smokers.

d. Nonmalignant pulmonary disease. Epidemiologic and laboratory data have established a causative relationship between cigarette smoking and chronic obstructive pulmonary disease (chronic bronchitis and emphysema). In addition to the cough accompanied by the excess mucous secretion and phlegm production experienced by many smokers, impairments in pulmonary function have been demonstrated in young, relatively asymptomatic smokers. Cigarette smokers also have an increased risk of mortality from chronic obstructive lung disease compared with nonsmokers, with a dose-response relationship to risk. Development of pulmonary disease (including lung cancer) caused by environmental and occupational agents such as coal dust and asbestos, may be enhanced by smoking. Mortality risks for pipe and cigar smokers are intermediate between those for cigarette smokers and nonsmokers, with risk approaching that of cigarette smokers for those persons who inhale. Passive exposure to tobacco smoke also appears to be related to respiratory illness in both children and adults. Infants and children of parents who smoke have an increased incidence of sudden infant death syndrome (the leading cause of death in the first year of childhood), middle ear effusions, bronchitis, pneumonia, and hospital admissions for respiratory problems in the first year of life. Reactive airway disease appears to be more common among the children of smoking parents. Exposure to tobacco smoke precipitates or aggravates allergic symptoms in both children and adults with respiratory allergies. Studies have not yet evaluated whether passive smoking increases the risk of chronic pulmonary disease such as emphysema. However, persons without a history of respiratory illness who are chronically exposed to environmental tobacco smoke have been found to have diminished small airways function.

e. **Cancer.** The association of cigarette smoking and many types of cancer is well established, and cigarette smoking is recognized as the leading cause of cancer mortality in the United States. Epidemiologic and laboratory studies consistently implicate cigarette smoking as the major causative factor in lung cancer, with an estimate that 85% of cases of lung cancer in men are attributable to cigarette smoking. Lung cancer now accounts for 22% of all cancers in men and 11% of all cancers in women, causing 35% and 19% of all cancer mortality in men and women, respectively. Prevalence rates and mortality risks are directly proportional to the number of cigarettes smoked per day, duration of smoking, levels of tar and nicotine, and absence of filters. Pipe and cigar smokers are also at increased risk for development of lung cancer, although the risk is less than that for cigarette smokers. Although subject to methodologic problems, recent studies suggest an etiologic role for passive smoking in the development of lung cancer in nonsmokers.

Tobacco use is the major causative agent for laryngeal, esophageal, and oral cancer, with studies showing a strong dose-response relation. Alcohol is known to act synergistically with tobacco use to increase the risk of cancer development. Increased risk for these neoplasms is equivalent for smokers of cigarettes, pipes, and cigars. Smokeless tobacco, especially snuff, has also been shown to play a causal role in cancer of the mouth and throat.

Epidemiologic data show an association between cigarette smoking and cancer of the bladder, kidney, and pancreas, while evidence suggesting a relationship between smoking and cervical carcinoma is inconclusive because of methodologic problems. Pipe and cigar smokers have a slightly increased risk of bladder cancer, but a lower risk than cigarette smokers.

f. **Nonmalignant oral and gastrointestinal disease.** It is well known that cigarette, cigar, and pipe smokers have more periodontal disease than nonsmokers, in addition to the unpleasant consequences of smoking such as dental staining and halitosis. Smokeless tobacco is associated with gingival recession and oral leukoplakia, but there is insufficient evidence of an association with periodontitis or tooth decay. Tobacco smoking is implicated in a dose-related manner to the development of duodenal and gastric ulcers. Mortality risk of peptic ulcer disease is 2.5 times greater in cigarette smokers than nonsmokers. Furthermore, adequate therapy of peptic ulcer disease in cigarette smokers appears to be compromised. Studies demonstrate that cigarette smoking significantly diminishes and occasionally abolishes the acid antisecretory effects of cimetidine, which may explain why smokers have a lower rate of healing and a higher incidence of recurrence of duodenal ulcers even while on acid inhibitory drugs.

g. **Fetal effects.** Fetal exposure to maternal smoking adversely affects fetal and neonatal health. Infants born to women who smoke during pregnancy average about 200 gm less in weight than those born to nonsmoking mothers. Smoking mothers have twice the incidence of low birth weight (under 2500 gm) in their infants than nonsmoking mothers, with the risk being dose-related and independent of other factors known to cause low birth weight. Pregnant women who smoke have increased rates of placental abruption, placenta previa, early and late trimester bleeding, premature or prolonged rupture of membranes, and preterm delivery, and consequently have a higher risk of fetal demise. The risks of spontaneous abortion, fetal death, and neonatal death are all dose-dependent.

h. **Passive smoking.** Exposure to tobacco-consumption products in the indoor environment increases one's risk for several health problems, some of which have been described above. To review, most available data indicate a correlation between parental smoking and an increased incidence of respiratory illness (bronchitis, pneumonia, and serous otitis) during the first years of life and possibly later. The most common symptoms associated with involuntary exposure to tobacco smoke are eye and throat irritation, nasal symptoms, and cough. Persons with allergies, asthma, or other underlying pulmonary disease may experience increased symptomatology or even frank respiratory compromise when exposed to ambient tobacco smoke. In persons with coronary heart disease, exposure to environmental tobacco smoke accelerates the development of exercise-induced angina. Finally, while there are conflicting data regarding passive smoking and lung cancer, evidence from human epidemiologic studies and laboratory animal studies suggests that involuntary smoking contributes to the development of lung cancer.

C. Epidemiology

1. **Prevalence patterns.** Despite the widespread public recognition of the harmful effects of tobacco use, smoking remains popular in the United States and is gaining in popularity worldwide. There are now more than 55 million Americans who, on the average, smoke more than 30 cigarettes/day. This includes 1 million new smokers each year, many of whom are teenagers. During the period from 1968–1975, the prevalence of smoking in 15- and 16-year-old girls increased from 10% to 20%, while the prevalence rates for boys of the same age remained unchanged at 18%. A 1982 survey reported that the proportion of United States high school seniors who reported smoking daily was 21%. Among adults, the prevalence of cigarette smoking is declining. In 1983, 35% of American men were smokers, compared with 38% in 1980 and 52% in 1965. Smoking prevalence for women in the United States in 1983 was 29%, compared with 29.4% in 1980 and 34% in 1965. It is encouraging that the prevalence of tobacco-smoking physicians has dramatically declined from 53% in the early 1950s to about 14% currently.

   Various surveys estimate the number of Americans using smokeless tobacco to be from 10–22 million, with at least 3 million of these users being less than 21 years of age. Although detailed national data are not available on smokeless tobacco use, numerous local and state surveys indicate that about 10% of all teenagers, 0–5% of adult females, and 7–15% of adult males use smokeless tobacco products, and the prevalence may be increasing.

2. **Mortality and morbidity.** Although there is a decreasing trend in the prevalence of smoking, tobacco use remains the leading cause of preventable mortality in the United States. Overall mortality is notably increased by smoking. Adult smokers of all age groups have a mortality rate that is more than 1½ times that of nonsmokers. The average reduction in life-expectancy for cigarette smokers is 5–8 years.

   The estimated annual preventable excess mortality from cigarette smoking in the United States exceeds 350,000 each year; that is, approximately 1000 deaths/day are attributable to tobacco. About 30%, or 170,000, of the 565,000 annual deaths from coronary heart disease are thought to be attributable to smoking. In addition, it is estimated that 30%, or 125,000, of the 412,000 annual cancer deaths result from tobacco use. Another 32,000 smoking-related deaths occur in persons with chronic obstructive lung disease. Finally, smoking-related fires are responsible for 1500 annual deaths, or 25% of all fire mortality, in addition to causing 4000 major injuries/year. Besides these adult deaths are the numerous prenatal and neonatal mortalities that are attributable to cigarette smoking.

   Morbidity is also much higher among smokers compared with nonsmokers. As a consequence of the numerous smoking-related illnesses previously described, people who smoke one pack/day have a 50% higher rate of hospitalization. A total of 306 million days of restricted activity and 88 million bed-days annually result from tobacco use.

3. **Cost.** Individuals, industry, and society as a whole pay enormous costs for the tobacco habit. Numerous health economists have estimated the cost of smoking-induced illness to be from $39–55 billion annually, or approximately 10% of the national total health care dollar. This breaks down to total tobacco-related, direct health care costs of more than $16 billion annually, and indirect costs (for lost productivity and lost earnings from excess morbidity, disability, and premature mortality) of $37 billion annually in 1985.

4. **Risk factors.** Because tobacco use is so well accepted in our culture at the current time, any youth or adult is at risk for becoming a tobacco user. Studies show that the great majority of tobacco users begin smoking as teenagers. This age group is at especially high risk for experimentation with tobacco for multiple reasons. Home

environment is an important factor: Children are more likely to smoke if one or both parents smoke, or if they come from a single-parent home. School performance also appears to play a role, with academic or athletic failure contributing to higher smoking risk. Peer pressure contributes to a teenager's decision to smoke and is perhaps the most important factor. Both adults and youths are greatly influenced by the massive advertising campaign of the tobacco industry, which spends more than $2 billion annually to promote tobacco products. Youths are especially vulnerable to using a product that is portrayed in association with glamour, wealth, friendship, sophistication, popularity, maturity, and athletic or sexual prowess.

II. Specific health promotion

A. Early assessment

1. **Methods.** Early assessment of tobacco use requires: (1) a high index of suspicion that any patient who is school-age and older is at risk for being a tobacco user, and (2) the willingness on the part of the practitioner to take a complete tobacco history. Simply put, this means asking every patient if he or she smokes or uses other tobacco products. To be complete and to obtain the most useful information, the practitioner should ask how much the patient smokes, when he or she began smoking, whether the patient has ever tried to quit, and, if so, why he or she returned to smoking. (While the term "smoking" will be used from here on for simplicity, all suggestions apply to the use of other tobacco products.) In addition, the patient should be asked about symptoms attributable to smoking. Finally, the practitioner should inquire about current interest in quitting. Taking a complete smoking history allows the practitioner to praise nonsmokers, to encourage current smokers to quit (even those who have unsuccessfully attempted to quit in the past), and to tailor a quit-smoking message to the individual.
2. **Justification**
   a. **History.** Admittedly, any assessment technique that relies on self-reporting is subject to underidentifying the actual number of tobacco users in any practice, because some patients may be reluctant to have their practitioner know that they are tobacco users. However, according to survey data, 92% of adolescents and 85% of adults who smoke express a strong desire to quit or have recently tried to quit but failed. Given this fact, one might assume that the majority of smokers would honestly report to their practitioner, especially if taking the smoking history was conducted with an attitude of nonjudgment, compassion, and understanding of the difficulty of breaking an addicting habit. Indeed, health surveys show that more than 75% of smokers feel that physician advice would be "somewhat" to "very" effective in helping them to reduce or cease smoking; yet, more than 75% of those questioned stated that their physician had never advised them to quit. Clearly, physicians need to respond to the challenge of the nation's number one health problem by accepting their role in assessing and advising their tobacco-using patient population.

   b. **Cost.** The cost of inquiry is nothing more than a few additional minutes at each clinic visit.

B. Early intervention

1. **Methods.** Practitioners can play an important collaborative role in a patient's attempt to stop smoking. Playing this role requires that practitioners develop some skills in advising their patients about smoking cessation. The underlying principle of intervention is that smoking is an addictive behavior and that the intention to quit smoking represents an important life decision that will require a major change in the way an individual copes with his or her environment. Smoking advice should be offered with an attitude of compassion and patience, combined with belief in the benefits of smoking cessation and a conviction that smokers can quit. Patients should be encouraged to continue their efforts even after several failures. The following suggestions to guide the practitioner are derived from an extensive review of the literature on methods for smoking cessation and maintenance of abstinence.
   a. **Role model.** Practitioners should be nonsmoking role models for their patients and should request the same of their employees. The practitioner's office should reflect his or her intention to promote health and prevent tobacco-related illness. A "No Smoking" sign should be displayed and ashtrays should not be available. Magazines available in the waiting room should exclude publications that accept cigarette advertisements. There should be available literature on the health hazards of smoking and on how to quit smoking, including information on local organized smoking-cessation programs. While the message portrayed by the office atmosphere and staff should be one of firm conviction that tobacco

use is unhealthy, it must also be a message presented without hostility toward the smoker.

b. Deliver a firm "quit smoking" message. Present each tobacco-using patient with an assessment of the health hazards of tobacco use, as well as the healthful consequences of quitting tobacco use. In doing so, practitioners should discuss the short- and long-term consequences of cigarette smoking (as previously outlined). In particular, the message should be tailored to the individual, summarizing the physiologic, social, and economic costs that the patient is already experiencing. Likewise, in discussing the benefits of quitting, the practitioner should emphasize the immediate and short-term health improvements (decreased cough and phlegm production, improved exercise tolerance, better ability to enjoy flavors, decreased halitosis), as well as the improvement in expected longevity and the decreased risk of cancer, heart, and lung diseases. For the user who already has the diagnosis of tobacco-related illness such as obstructive pulmonary disease, coronary artery disease, or peripheral vascular disease, extra effort should be made to help the user understand the direct relationship between his or her smoking behavior and the illness, in addition to the improvement in these conditions afforded by quitting.

c. Suggestions on how to quit. After informing a patient of the hazards of smoking and the benefits of quitting, the practitioner should request the patient to choose a quit date and then write it in the chart. This encourages the patient to put the decision to quit smoking into action. The practitioner should inform the patient that he or she will follow up on the patient's progress by phone or at the next visit, thus giving the patient added incentive for compliance.

There are a number of approaches to smoking cessation. Some initial suggestions that can be offered by the practitioner are as follows:

(1) Have the patient list his or her reasons for wanting to stop and suggest reviewing those reasons daily to provide motivation.

(2) Instruct the patient to keep a log of each cigarette smoked, the activity associated with each cigarette, and a "need rating." Keeping the log wrapped around the package of cigarettes with rubber bands requires its removal, thereby reminding the smoker to use the log. The log is intended to provide the patient with insight into the behavioral forces influencing his or her smoking pattern, and to cause the smoker to reflect on the environmental and emotional factors that precipitate the behavior.

(3) Encourage the smoker to seek the goal of total cessation within 1 week or less of the quitting date, deleting the least-wanted cigarettes or stopping "cold turkey." Progressive reduction of cigarette smoking is easier for some, but this should be used as a prelude to complete cessation within 1 week, as studies show that smokers are rarely able to continue tapering of below 10 cigarettes/day.

(4) Advise the patient and family members to expect irritability within the week after cessation, and that physical discomforts are transient.

(5) Warn the ex-smoker that, as lungs recuperate from smoking, there may be a period of increased cough and sputum production lasting weeks to months.

(6) Encourage new habits to replace smoking, such as relaxation exercise or active exercise to minimize the craving and weight gain associated with smoking cessation.

(7) Provide pamphlets and written hints on smoking-cessation techniques.

(8) Emphasize that patients are learning a new habit of nonsmoking, rather than quitting an old habit.

While a few smokers quit without much effort, most find it a difficult task requiring preparation and perseverance. It should be remembered by practitioners and patients alike that it is not uncommon for a quitter to temporarily go back to an old habit, but that quitting is possible in spite of occasional regressions. A number of helpful suggestions are outlined in "Calling it Quits" [1]. Additional tips for the patient are offered in Fig. 67-1.

d. Follow-up. Ex-smokers are most vulnerable to relapse during the first few months following cessation. During this time, a practitioner will be the most effective in helping a patient to continue with permanent cessation. Follow-up visits or phone contacts can be used to address possible relapse problems. During these contacts, the practitioner can: (1) review the smoking record and help the patient to identify smoking situations to avoid, (2) inquire about success of new healthful habits, (3) encourage patients who did not quit to try again and

1. Make a firm decision to quit, founded on an understanding of the reasons why you want to quit and why you should quit.
2. Make a list of reasons why you want to quit, and review it daily.
3. Consider your decision to quit as developing a positive new habit of nonsmoking, as opposed to quitting an old habit.
4. Make a contract with someone for quitting and plan rewards for yourself with the money saved when you succeed.
5. Make a broader public commitment to family, friends, and co-workers and encourage them to help remind you of your commitment not to smoke.
6. Set a date to quit.
7. Keep a log of smoking behavior (wrapped around a cigarette pack) prior to the quit date.
8. Make a list of places and circumstances associated with smoking (based on the log).
9. Avoid situations in which you usually smoke or would be encouraged to smoke.
10. Begin associating with nonsmokers and former smokers.
11. Discard all tobacco products and smoking paraphernalia (ashtrays, lighters, pipes, matches, etc.).
12. Continually redefine yourself as a nonsmoker or former smoker.
13. Substitute healthy behavior for smoking, including an exercise program, proper eating habits, recreation, and learning new coping behaviors.
14. Remember that there may be some initial physical discomfort, but these withdrawal symptoms will be transient (usually < 1 week).
15. Seek additional help in a smoking cessation program, if necessary.

Fig. 67-1. Hints for the tobacco quitter.

support them in setting a new quit date, and (4) praise patients who have successfully quit smoking.

For those who continue to smoke, the practitioner should review cigarette safety precautions, including use of car ashtrays and avoidance of smoking in bed. Parents should be instructed to smoke out-of-doors and away from the house and enclosed spaces. They should be reminded of the role that they model for their children.

e. Additional methods and therapies. In addition to private practitioner counseling, numerous methods have been developed to help smokers quit, including drugs, aversion therapy, hypnosis, acupuncture, rapid smoking, contingency contracting, and the more publicized use of nicotine chewing gum.

Nicotine chewing gum has become a popular method of smoking cessation and is based on the finding that nicotine substitution can partially relieve the unpleasant withdrawal symptoms of smoking cessation (craving, irritability, anxiety). More recently, transdermal nicotine has been shown to decrease nicotine craving, although no studies have shown efficacy in clinical trials.

At least two studies demonstrate an increased smoking abstinence rate in nicotine gum users compared with controls. Critical review of these studies, however, reveals some methodologic problems (doubtful randomization) with preselection of volunteers and a limited follow-up period of less than a year. In fact, the only double-blind, randomized, controlled trial failed to find a difference in cessation rate between nicotine gum users and control groups that received a doctor's advice with or without literature. Nevertheless, nicotine gum may prove useful when combined with physician advice and supportive counseling in highly motivated individuals with moderate nicotine dependence. Practitioners should bear in mind that while cessation of smoking may result in improved pulmonary health, tobacco-related cardiovascular disease may be mediated by nicotine. For this reason, nicotine substitutes should be used cautiously in patients with cardiovascular disease.

Many drugs, in addition to nicotine, have been tried as substitutes for tobacco. Lobeline, a substance made from dried herbs and the chief ingredient in Nikoban and Bantron, has been promoted as an effective nicotine substitute. However, well-controlled studies demonstrate no better efficacy than placebo. Antianxiety agents such as the benzodiazepines and other sedatives have no proved efficacy in the treatment of tobacco use. Various methods of aversive conditioning have been used, including electric shock and rapid smoking, a form of aversive conditioning in which, over several sessions, smokers inhale smoke every 6 seconds until they are dizzy or nauseated. While studies indicate a long-term abstinence rate of 20–30%, patients must be carefully selected for this technique, excluding those with cardiac or pulmonary disease. During rapid smoking, carbon monoxide levels may reach 10–15% saturation, and some smokers have developed tachycardia, electrocardiogram abnormalities, and respiratory alkalosis. Schick Laboratories has developed a commercial smoking cessation program utilizing shock and rapid smoking techniques.

There are many commercial and voluntary organizations that conduct regular smoking cessation clinics and seminars utilizing combinations of the above therapies. The local chapters of the American Cancer Society and the American Lung Association can provide patient education materials, self-help packets, and smoking cessation clinics based on behavioral modification techniques and group peer support. The Seventh Day Adventists sponsor a Five-Day Plan, a formal smoking cessation clinic offered nationwide that utilizes lectures by physicians and clergymen, explanations of smoking cessation techniques, and group meetings. The Schick Laboratories program mentioned above also offers 8 weeks of reinforcement with weekly group sessions. Smoke-Enders, available nationwide, is a structured smoking-cessation program combining self-awareness, behavior modification, positive conditioning, and periodic group meetings over the course of a year.

Acupuncture and hypnotherapy have not been demonstrated to be more effective than placebo for the treatment of tobacco use, and they are relatively expensive. Nonetheless, any patient strongly motivated to use either of these modalities to effect smoking cessation should be encouraged to do so.

All of the above programs seem to have a similar pattern of efficacy, although well-controlled studies have not been conducted to date. Each method initially helps 40–80% of smokers quit, and 15–25% remain abstinent for 1 year. No single treatment has proved consistently superior to others, although programs with a multifactorial approach achieve slightly higher success rates. Finally, there are some data that suggest that industry-based smoking cessation clinics are more successful than commercial programs (Table 67-1).

f. **Low-tar, low-nicotine "safer" cigarettes.** Finally, for those who are unable to quit entirely, low-tar, low-nicotine cigarettes are available, theoretically with less harmful consequences. The health implications of changes in the tar and nicotine content of cigarettes are unclear. In the past decade, cigarette tar content has declined 32%, and more smokers are using low-tar, low-nicotine brands (92% in 1979 compared with 1% in the 1950s). Recent data, however, indicate that the tar and nicotine content of cigarettes as measured by automatic machine-burning of cigarettes inaccurately underestimates amounts of tar and nicotine. Furthermore, studies indicate that smokers may compensate for lower tar and nicotine by inhaling more. Nevertheless, long-term users of filtered and low-tar, low-nicotine cigarettes have a 10–40% lower risk of lung cancer compared with regular cigarette smokers. Evidence regarding the reduction of risk of coronary heart disease is conflicting, and there is no evidence that filtered low-tar and low-nicotine cigarettes reduce the risk of respiratory disease, peptic ulcer disease, or risk during pregnancy. Practitioners should make it known to patients that only smoking cessation offers clear-cut reductions in health hazards, although low-tar, low-nicotine cigarettes are advisable for those who are unable to quit.

2. **Justification**

   a. **Efficacy.** Perhaps the most important fact for the practitioner to keep in mind is that advice and guidance **can** assist many patients in their smoking cessation efforts. National health surveys indicate that while only 20–30% of smokers express an interest in an organized cessation program, 70% state that they would quit if given unequivocal advice to do so by their physician. Indeed, studies do show that physician advice is effective. When practitioners advise asymptomatic smokers to quit, 5–20% will have quit by 1 year. Russell and colleagues [2] demonstrated that physicians who used simple measures, such as a 2-minute firm explanation of the risks of smoking, distribution of pamphlets on how to quit, and warning of a follow-up on the patient's progress, have 17 times as many patients cease smoking for an entire year as did the control group of physicians. The degree of success of physicians' advice improves with symptomatic patients,

Table 67-1. Information sources

American Cancer Society* 777 Third Avenue New York, NY 10017 (212) 371-2900
American Heart Association* 7320 Greenville Avenue Dallas, Texas 75231 (214) 750-5300
American Lung Association* 1740 Broadway New York, NY 10019 (212) 245-8000
Office on Smoking and Health U.S. Dept. of Health and Human Services 5600 Fishers Lane Park Bldg, Rm. 110 Rockville, MD 20857
Office of Cancer Communications National Cancer Institute National Institutes of Health Bethesda, MD 20205 (800) 638-6694
General Headquarters Five-Day Plan to Stop Smoking Seventh Day Adventist Church* Narcotics Education Division 6840 Eastern Avenue, NW Washington, DC 20012
Schick Laboratories 1901 Avenue of the Stars Suite 1530 Los Angeles, CA 90067
Smoke-Enders* Memorial Parkway Phillipsburg, NJ 08864

*Use your local telephone directory for a listing of local chapters.

especially those who have developed tobacco-related diseases. In one study, after myocardial infarction, 63% of smokers who received an anti-smoking message, literature, and follow-up from their physician quit smoking for at least 1 year, compared with only 27% of those who received routine care. A similar study with chest clinic patients demonstrated a quit rate of 39% in patients advised by their physician to quit, compared with a 19% quit rate in nonintervention controls. With those studies, it becomes clear that practitioners should not underestimate the value of their advice. Based on Russell's study [2], it has been calculated that each practitioner could realistically induce 25 smokers/year to quit. The efficacy of other methods and therapies has been discussed in the previous section.

b. Benefits. Extensive research on the benefits of smoking cessation is encouraging; smoking cessation is associated with reduction in tobacco-related morbidity and mortality. In smokers younger than 65 years, the risk of coronary artery disease declines by approximately 50% within 1 year of quitting, and approaches the mortality risk for nonsmokers about 10–15 years after cessation. The degree of risk reduction is determined by the amount of cigarettes smoked and the duration of smoking before cessation, making early intervention more beneficial. The risk of developing tobacco-related cancers gradually returns to that of nonsmokers approximately 15 years after discontinuation of tobacco products. In patients with smoking-related respiratory symptoms, smoking cessation results in a gradual decrease in the excess risk of mortality from chronic obstructive lung disease in addition to diminishing cough and sputum production. Smokers with fixed reductions in expiratory airflow may avert the process of declining lung capacity. Finally, smoking cessation prior to the fourth month of pregnancy reduces the risk of third trimester complications to that of the nonsmoker.

c. **Costs.** With the exception of the more expensive programs, the cost of methods for smoking cessation is minimal. Largely, what is needed is a few minutes of time at each clinic visit devoted to smoking-cessation advice. In an effort to compare costs of smoking cessation programs with savings on health care expenditures for tobacco-related illnesses, Kristein [3], a health economist, estimated a cost-benefit ratio in 1975. Based on a cessation program cost of $125/person and a 25% success rate, he estimated that 22 million heavy smokers could be treated for $2.75 billion, and that 5.5 million would quit smoking for 1 year. After a 5-year period for the lifetime of the 5.5 million ex-smokers, $5.1 billion/year could be saved; thus, a cost-benefit ratio of 1.8:1.0.

Individual program costs vary widely. The cost of nicotine gum is roughly equivalent to the cost of the cigarette habit itself and declines as the use is tapered. While the Schick program is expensive (currently more than $500), the cost is certainly less than the smoking habit and far less than the costs of smoking-related disease.

d. **Acceptability.** As previously emphasized, the vast majority of smokers express a desire to quit and would welcome practitioner advice. This, combined with the knowledge that practitioners can make a difference in a patient's success in smoking cessation, should increase practitioners' willingness to address their patients' tobacco problems. However, there are at least four major impediments to patient acceptability that must be kept in mind. First of all, anticipated weight gain is a realistic fear that prevents many smokers from quitting. Studies indicate that an average of 5–15 lb is gained after smoking cessation, perhaps secondary to metabolic changes. Smaller gains are possible with appropriate increases in exercise and attention to diet. Second, as previously discussed, smoking cessation requires preparation and perseverance. It is a life-style change that requires much effort. Third, nicotine addiction makes smoking cessation difficult despite acceptability of any particular method. In addition, patient acceptance of nicotine gum may be limited by side effects of bad taste, jaw pain, nausea, heartburn, and hiccups. Finally, while individual smokers may be accepting of attitude changes and smoking cessation therapies, our culture currently encourages tobacco use, at times creating a hostile environment for nonsmoking individuals.

III. Recommendations

A. **Early assessment.** All patients should be asked whether they smoke; when they started; how much they smoke; if they have attempted to quit; if they have a desire to quit; and if they have symptoms attributable to smoking.

B. **Early intervention**

1. Health care providers and their employees should provide role models by not smoking and by offering smoke-free offices.
2. Health care providers should deliver a firm quit-smoking message.
3. Health care providers should offer specific suggestions on how to quit.
4. For follow-up and relapse:
   a. Follow-up visits or phone calls may prevent relapse.
   b. Health care providers should review the smoking record and help the patient to avoid situations likely to cause relapse.
   c. Health care providers should encourage patients who have relapsed and help them to set a new quit date.
5. A variety of therapies for tobacco smoking cessation are available to the motivated patient: aversion therapy, acupuncture, hypnosis, and nicotine chewing gum.
6. Patients who will not quit should be encouraged to smoke low-tar and low-nicotine cigarettes, observe "safe smoking" rules, and smoke in spaces where others will not be exposed to secondhand smoke.

C. **Broader issues.** Many of the factors currently contributing to smoking initiation are beyond the purview of practitioners. However, it is possible for practitioners to assist their tobacco-using patients by early assessment and intervention utilizing the skills outlined in this chapter. The hope for a smoke-free society, however, requires efforts at preventing persons from ever smoking. This will necessitate educational programs directed at our youth to teach decision-making skills prior to development of nicotine addiction (see Chap. 32). In addition, it will require the commitment to create environments where tobacco use is prohibited, whether at school, work, or public places. In addition to efforts directed at assessment and intervention, practitioners should make a commitment to get involved in school education programs and in hospital and legislative committees to aid in the prevention of tobacco use.

References

1. *Calling It Quits.* Bethesda, MD: National Cancer Institute, 1980. *May be obtained through the Office of Cancer Communications, National Cancer Institute, Bethesda, MD 20814.*
2. Russell, M. A., et al. Effect of general practitioners' advice against smoking. *Br. Med. J.* 2:(6184):231, 1979. *Demonstrates that physicians' advice plus literature can increase patients' 12-month rates of smoking cessation by 1–5%.*
3. Kristein, M. M. Economic issues in prevention. *Prev. Med.* 6(2):252, 1977. *Demonstrates beneficial cost-benefit ratio of smoking cessation programs.*

Selected Reading

Cummings, S. R. Kicking the habit: Benefits and methods of quitting cigarette smoking. *West. J. Med.* 137(5):443, 1982. *A brief review of current treatment modalities for tobacco use.*

Doyle, J. T., et al. The relationship of cigarette smoking to coronary heart disease: The second report of the combined experience of the Albany, NY and Framingham, Mass. studies. *J.A.M.A.* 190:886, 1964. *A description of the large epidemiologic data that define the relationship between cigarette smoking and coronary artery disease.*

Fielding, J. E. Smoking: Health effects and control (Part 1). *N. Engl. J. Med.* 313(8):491, 1985. *Part 1 reviews the health risks of smoking, including smoking in pregnancy and passive smoking.*

Fielding, J. E. Smoking: Health effects and controls (Part 2). *N. Engl. J. Med.* 313(9):555, 1985. *Part 2 addresses the treatment of tobacco smoking, including governmental and private-sector measures, and an international perspective on smoking.*

Hammond, E. C. Smoking in relation to the death rates of one million men and women. In W. Haenszel (ed.), *Epidemiological Approaches to the Study of Cancer and Other Chronic Disease.* Bethesda, MD: National Cancer Institute, 1966. Pp. 127–204. *A sample of epidemiologic studies contributing to our knowledge about smoking and chronic diseases.*

Harlap, S., and Davies, A. M. Infant admissions to hospital and maternal smoking. *Lancet* 1:529, 1974. *The children of mothers who smoke are more likely to develop bronchitis and pneumonia during the first year of life.*

Health effects of smokeless tobacco. Council of Scientific Affairs. *J.A.M.A.* 255(8):1038, 1986. *A current review of the data relating smokeless tobacco to multiple chronic diseases, most notably cancer.*

Meyer, M. B., and Tonascia, J. A. Maternal smoking, pregnancy complications, and perinatal mortality. *Am. J. Obstet. Gynecol.* 128(5):494, 1977. *Retrospective study showing that maternal smoking is correlated with perinatal mortality in addition to other complications of pregnancy.*

Schachter, S. Pharmacological and psychological determinants of smoking. *Ann. Intern. Med.* 88(1):104, 1978. *In this review of the data that explores the etiology of chronic smoking behavior, the author demonstrates that smoking is best understood as an addictive behavior.*

Wynder, E. L., and Hoffman, D. Tobacco and health: A societal challenge. *N. Engl. J. Med.* 300(16):894, 1979. *Comprehensive review of the therapy of smoking.*

68 Stress

Jean Ranc and Eric W. Jensen

I. The problem

A. Definition. No single definition of stress is uniformly accepted for scientific purposes; however, common experience and good research suggest that certain events and conditions are stressful and that these are associated with changes in health in some people.

At present, stress is perhaps best defined in terms of the complex and dynamic interaction of the person with his or her environment. This interaction involves three elements, as depicted in Fig. 68-1.

1. **Stressors** are those external and internal events or demands that produce a physical and psychological reaction in a person.
2. **Stress reactions** are the biological and psychosocial changes that can occur in response to stressors. They may vary among individuals and within the same individual over time.
3. **Consequences** are changes in health that may be transient or the result of prolonged and cumulative effects of certain stressors. They may be positive or negative changes in health status, and may be biological, psychological, or social in character.
4. **Mediators** are the factors that modify this three-part sequence to produce individual variations. These mediators help to explain why one person may experience several potential stressors without having any health consequences, while another may have many consequences when confronted with the same stressors. Personality, social supports, and coping style, along with intrinsic biological factors, serve to mediate the stress reaction.

B. Description [1–4]. Stressors may be positive (termed "eustress" by Selye) [5] with creative and motivating aspects, or negative, with debilitating and aversive dimensions that lead to distress. In general, as the arousal in response to stressors increases, a person's performance is enhanced until he or she functions at an optimal level. With excessive arousal, however, performance deteriorates and functioning becomes disrupted. The body reacts to all stressors with a predictable "fight/flight" response, as though preparing for physical attack. This instinctive response was highly functional for our primitive ancestors but often proves inappropriate under the present-day stressful situations that preclude direct action. The chronic and excessive stimulation of the stress response without adequate discharge is associated with physiologic, psychological, cognitive, and behavioral effects that may lead to the onset and maintenance of illness.

The general adaptation syndrome (GAS) of Selye [5] is the model most frequently cited as explanatory of the chain of events set in motion by a stressor. Changes initiated by an environmental stressor are mediated by the central and autonomic nervous system and endocrine system. The cardiovascular, digestive, and muscular systems are directly affected, although every system in the body is involved to a greater or lesser extent. Recent investigations have demonstrated significant changes in the immune system following the common stressor of loss and grief.

The presence of prolonged stress reactions may affect an individual at four levels:

1. **Physiologic**—Increased heart rate and blood pressure; alterations in digestive system; increased muscle tension; release of catecholamines.
2. **Psychological**—Changes in affective state, usually depression, anxiety, emotional lability, and tension; feeling "keyed up;" lowered self-esteem.
3. **Cognitive**—Difficulty concentrating and making decisions; memory lapses; distorted thinking; decrease in mental functioning.
4. **Behavioral**—Decreased performance; avoidance of stressful situations; nervous habits (tics, bruxism); altered eating patterns; somatic symptoms and preoccupation.

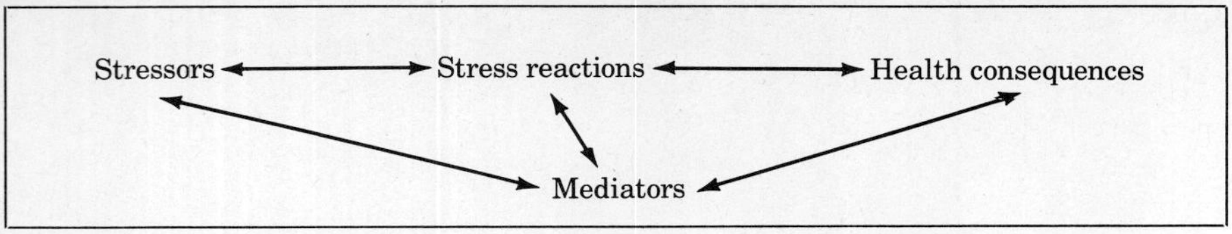

Fig. 68-1. Dynamics of stress.

Stressors do not **cause** illness, but numerous studies have demonstrated a correlation between various stressors and the subsequent onset of disease. Most diseases are multidetermined and no single factor can be said to be causative. However, stress has emerged as a significant component in the onset and progression of many chronic diseases. Table 68-1 lists a number of these "stress-related" disorders.

Mediators, including personality, support systems, and coping strategies, modulate the stress-related factors affecting the impact of stressors. Much recent work has demonstrated a link between the hard-driving, time-urgent, impatient type A personality who represses anger and the onset of coronary artery disease. In a similar fashion, a characteristic "hardiness" is found in those individuals who are relatively stress resistant. This personality trait includes a sense of personal control over external events, deep involvement and commitment in daily activities, and flexibility in adapting to unexpected change and new challenges. These and other dimensions of personality appear to influence disease onset as well as adjustment to chronic illness and response to treatment.

The role of social supports as a buffer to life stress and a modifying factor in stress-illness relationships is well documented. Support from a variety of "significant others," including spouse, family, friends, neighbors, supervisors and co-workers, clergy, and health care professionals can modify the effects of stress, and no single class of supportive individual is crucial to this effect. The individual's sense of being a loved and valued member of a network of people is important.

Coping strategies are those things that people do to avoid or to deal with stressors as they arise. Numerous studies have shown that the ways an individual copes can alter the extent of physiologic arousal that a stressor will induce. Typically, an avoidance coping style tends to increase the impact of stressors, while an active cognitive and behavioral style diminishes this impact.

In most instances, combining the positive mediating factors will result in less illness in persons under stress.

C. Epidemiology. Reliable estimates of the societal burden of stress are difficult to obtain. The pressures of today's life-style both on and off the job are seen as major contributors to decreased productivity, disease, and early mortality. It has been estimated that the direct cost alone (i.e., days lost from work, hospital and outpatient treatment, or death) of executive stress runs to $20 billion/year in the United States. If the direct and indirect costs of blue-collar stress are included (i.e., absenteeism, job turnover, poor quality of work), this $20 billion estimate is only a small fraction of the overall cost [6].

There is abundant evidence that stressful events are related to adverse changes in health. One study found that people who work in excess of 48 hours/week run twice the risk of death from coronary artery disease as those who work fewer hours. Combinations of stressful life events such as death of a loved one, birth of a first child, loss of a job, job promotion, or divorce, increase the risk of having physical or mental illness within 6–12 months following these events. There appears to be a cumulative effect such that increased risk is associated with a greater number of stressful events in the recent past [7].

II. Specific health promotion

A. Early assessment

1. Methods. All patient contacts present opportunities for early and regular assessment of any individual's response to current stresses.

An up-to-date **history and physical** are necessary to determine whether and to what extent the patient's symptoms are stress-related. The assessment should also include a thorough interview to ascertain the source of stressors, current and recent life events changes, the kind and quality of social supports, the patient's coping style, nutrition, and exercise [8], as well as what therapies have been and are currently being utilized.

Table 68-1. Stress-related diseases and conditions

Cardiovascular system
Coronary artery disease
Cardiac arrhythmias
Hypertension
Neuromuscular system
Tension headaches
Migraine headaches
Back pain—muscle contraction type
Respiratory and allergic disorders
Asthma
Hay fever
Immunologic disorders
Lowered resistance
Autoimmune disease
Gastrointestinal disturbances
Peptic ulcer disease
Irritable bowel syndrome
Diarrhea
Nausea and vomiting
Dermatologic disease
Eczema
Neurodermatitis
Acne
Dental problems
Bruxism
Myofacial pain syndrome
Other problems
Fatigue and lethargy
Anxiety
Alcohol, drug, and tobacco abuse
Traumatic injuries

A number of instruments are available that seek to measure individual stress. They vary widely in length and scope as well as documentation of reliability and validity. Unfortunately, there is no one, short, widely used, all-purpose measure for assessing stress in a clinical population. Some that may prove useful include: (1) The two-page *Health Risk Appraisal,* which is widely used to assess health behaviors that impact on illness; (2) the 14-item *Perceived Stress Scale* (PSS), which is suggested for measuring the degree to which life situations are appraised as stressful and for examining the role that such stress plays in the etiology of disease and behavioral disorders; (3) the 28-item *Type A Self-Rating Inventory* for measuring the coronary-prone behavior pattern; and (4) *Stressmap,* a commercially available 11-page inventory that can be self-administered and scored and includes a workbook.

2. **Justification.** The **history and physical** are essential for the assessment of stress-related illness. The **Health Risk Appraisal** [9] is a health education tool that has been widely used but is not very useful for persons under 25 or over 60 years old or for persons who have had a heart attack or other serious medical problems. The **Perceived Stress Scale** [10] has been shown to be reliable and valid in a college-age population and a middle-age group involved in a smoking cessation program. The **Type A Self-Rating Inventory** has been found to be significantly related to an established type A self-report instrument, the Jenkins Activity Survey (JAS) [11], and to an independent behavioral rating based on a standard structured interview

(SI). The **Stressmap** [12] is a comprehensive instrument that provides a multifaceted stress profile, an interpretation, and a structured program for the individual.

Such an assessment involves no risk to the patient and, if well conducted, can serve as introductory education in stress detection for the patient, helping him or her to realize that motivation and self-regulation are crucial for stress management, whether or not the patient commits to a subsequent treatment or training program.

B. Early intervention

1. **Methods.** There are basically three ways to reduce stress: by altering the environment; by changing the person's attitudes and behaviors; and by controlling the physiologic responses by relaxation and related techniques or by chemical means [13, 14].

   a. **Environmental changes** on the community level and in the workplace can significantly reduce the stress experienced in these settings. Stress in the workplace is increasingly recognized as an important factor in absenteeism, injury, and decreased productivity. Many industries are making coordinated efforts to address these issues and alter the deleterious impact of excessive stress on the job. In addition, the individual may instigate changes such as taking a vacation; reviewing social and community activities; and changing jobs, residence, or relationships (even so radical as divorce) to reduce stress.

      Paradoxically, the family can both cause and relieve stress. Such life-cycle events as marriage, childbirth, aging, and death are sources of stress generated in the context of the family that can also be alleviated therein. Work within or outside the family can also serve this dual role. There may be conflicts between career and family responsibilties as well as role overload, underload, or captivity within the family for different members. In addition, outside work stress generating anger, frustration, and depression can be brought home to contaminate the family, or the family can serve as a haven from work stress. On the other hand, work can serve as a means of social support and stress-buffer, especially for women. Helping family members to become more aware of their stressors and of how to utilize the resources within or outside the family can do much to alleviate stress.

   b. **Cognitive and behavioral approaches.** Cognitive and behavioral approaches to stress management may be likened to camera adjustments to ensure clearer and more accurate pictures (perception). The patient examines thoughts, feelings, and impulses, as well as the meanings he or she has assigned to events, learning to clarify problems, and then recognizing and correcting cognitive distortions.

      At the same time, the health care provider, in the mode of stress management counselor, can serve as a catalyst for behavioral change by helping the patient become aware of stressors and learn more effective ways of coping with them.

      Exercise and nutrition habits are important behaviors to monitor in terms of stress management. Exercise on a regular basis will enhance cardiovascular fitness, improve flexibility, and increase strength. Aerobic exercise has a demonstrable effect on physiologic reactivity with a resultant reduction in heart rate and blood pressure as well as a beneficial alteration in lipoprotein profile. Exercise is also a significant factor in weight control.

      Nutrition assessment can be integrated into the history and physical or included by means of a questionnaire to ascertain not only the kind and quantities of food intake, but eating habits and weight history. Nutrition is, of course, a vital factor in weight control and is also important in the reduction of risk factors related to cardiovascular illness and cancer. Reducing caffeine intake can make a significant difference in reducing anxiety-related symptoms, and awareness of food allergies may serve as a valuable tool in stress management.

      Traditional insight-oriented psychotherapy may also play a significant role in stress management in conjunction with the more behaviorally oriented approaches delineated here.

   c. **Controlling the physiologic responses**

      (1) **Progressive muscle relaxation** has proven beneficial in the reduction of everyday tensions and clinically for the management of tension-related syndromes. It can also serve as an adjunctive therapy for easing a person's discomfort from any malady and can be particularly appropriate before and after surgery. It is a skill learned best through individual or group instruction and requires regular, continued practice by the patient to maintain an effective level of competence.

         Progressive muscle relaxation is contraindicated with patients who suffer from affective or thought-disturbance psychoses, or whose reality-testing is tenuous. Patients on medication need to be monitored because relaxation can decrease the dosage required. Since relaxation can induce panic states in patients with high anxiety levels, or release deeply repressed thoughts and emotions in others, the initial training should be under the direction of a professional. Such complications are quite rare, however, and the benefits of relaxation training far outweigh the minimal risks.

(2) **Autogenic training** as a specialized form of relaxation training focuses primarily on handwarming and has proved effective for Raynaud's phenomenon, certain vascular-type headaches, and some anxiety disorders. Here again, close monitoring of progress in self-regulation and resulting physiologic changes is necessary for patients on medication to make adjustments in dosage as needed. As with other forms of relaxation training, emotion-laden thoughts and images may be discharged and be frightening or overwhelming to the patient, so the training needs to be carefully supervised.

(3) **Hypnosis** can be effective in producing deep relaxation or active relaxation to enhace a patient's receptivity to subsequent suggestions. It can also be taken a step further to include self-hypnosis, accentuating the fact that the patient can learn self-control and take an active role in his or her treatment.

Hypnosis has been used in treating stress-related disorders such as migraine, tension headache, asthma, insomnia, and hypertension. However, "hypnosuggestive procedures focusing on deep relaxation and active relaxation have not been shown to be generally more effective than other procedures (such as progressive muscle relaxation, autogenic training, meditation, and various kinds of biofeedback) that have similar aims. In fact, it appears that individual differences are very important here; individuals with certain kinds of characteristics may 'fit' into one type of relaxation procedure and be 'misfits' with another" [14].

(4) **Meditation** in modern forms, simplified and stripped of esoteric trappings and religious overtones, can be therapeutic when applied in clinical practice. It is a "mental device that limits stimulus input by directing attention to a single unchanging or repetitive stimulus" [14]. It has proven effective in reduction of tension and anxiety, for improvement in stress-related illnesses, for increasing productivity, for lessening of self-blame, for mood elevation, and for increased sense of identity and lowered irritability. It has also been shown to have antiaddictive effects for abusers of "soft" drugs, alcohol, or tobacco [14].

Meditation can carry the same risks as relaxation training. Therefore, the patient should be closely monitored by the counselor to provide support and guidance and to recognize when medication adjustments may be required.

(5) " **'Yoga,'** meaning union or oneness with life, is part of an ancient Indian culture. It is a personal self-help system of health care and spiritual development" [14]. Used as a form of meditation, yoga can include simple breathing exercises, deep muscle relaxation, and a type of mental relaxation introduced as passive concentration. It may be preferred by certain individuals and prove more effective for stress-related disorders than other forms of meditation or relaxation, but should be utilized with the same precautions.

(6) "**Biofeedback** may be defined as the technique of using equipment (usually electronic) to reveal to human beings some of their internal physiological events, normal and abnormal, in the form of visual and auditory signals in order to teach them to manipulate these otherwise involuntary or unfelt events by manipulating the displayed signals" [15]. Biofeedback has proved to be an effective treatment for many stress-related disorders, especially when used in conjunction with relaxation training. It provides immediate confirmation of an individual's ability to reduce physiologic arousal, which often correlates with symptom reduction.

Biofeedback is not very helpful as crisis intervention. Hysterical and conversion reaction symptoms are not effectively treated by biofeedback unless used in conjunction with psychotherapy to resolve the unconscious conflict. Caution must be exercised in treating insulin-dependent diabetes because sudden relaxation may result in greatly reduced need for insulin [14]. Severely depressed patients are not good candidates for biofeedback training because of loss of ego strength and lack of motivation.

(7) **Pharmacologic.** A variety of medications are effective in reducing the phys-

iologic arousal associated with stress-related illness. Judicious use of these agents (i.e., analgesics, anxiolytics) can provide significant symptom reduction in a relatively short period of time. The chronic nature of many of these symptoms often requires ongoing treatment with the increased risk of medication overuse and dependence. Symptom control achieved with medications is most effective when combined with some of the self-control strategies described above, providing acute relief while helping the patient develop a long-term approach that includes self-management of stress-related symptoms.

2. **Justification.** All of the above treatments (excluding the pharmacologic) are of minimal risk, have few side effects, and are nonaddictive. They involve a large measure of patient motivation and involvement to be successful. They have all proved to be effective in reducing physiologic arousal, giving the patient more control over how he or she responds to stress. It is also important to note the synergistic benefits that may accrue from coordinating all three facets of stress management: environmental changes, cognitive and behavioral changes, and controlling physiologic responses. At the same time, one must also be aware of the varied responses to specific methods and thus of the importance of designing stress management programs and protocols to meet individual needs. For example, progressive muscle relaxation, autogenic training, hypnosis, meditation, and yoga can all serve as means to the desired end of reducing physiologic reactivity, but which one will be most effective for the particular patient may depend on that person's temperament—for instance, whether they are more cognitively or somatically oriented. In the same way, any of the above methods can be enhanced when coupled with biofeedback, except in individuals who may have an aversion to such instrumentation.

III. Recommendations

A. Specific health promotion. Primary care providers are in a unique position to be aware of the impact of stress on themselves, as well as on their patients. They can serve as role models as they help their patients develop healthy life-styles and strategies for coping effectively with stress. These strategies include good nutrition, regular and appropriate exercise, and specific techniques for altering the physiologic response to stress.

B. Early assessment. Routine medical history-taking should include questions designed to identify current stressors and recent life changes that may be stressful. These data should be incorporated into initial and follow-up visits in order to ascertain the relationship between ongoing stressors and illness progression.

C. Early intervention. The techniques outlined above can be learned by most individuals. Effective learning requires professional supervision during the initial phase to ensure proper skills acquisition and to avoid complications.

When treating an individual with stress-related illness, the primary care provider should consider including some of the behavioral approaches described here as a complement to the ongoing medical treatment. For certain individuals, these techniques will become an integral part of a long-term health and stress management program, and thereby help to prevent or ameliorate future illness.

References

1. Cox, T. *Stress.* Baltimore: University Park Press, 1978. *Good review of theories, models, and research on stress and stress management, including in the workplace.*
2. Dohrenwend, B. S., and Dohrenwend, B. P. (eds.). *Stressful Life Events and Their Contexts.* New York: Prodist, 1981. *Volume 2 in Series in Psychosocial Epidemiology; helpful, but more research than clinically oriented.*
3. Elliott, G. R., and Eisdorfer, C. (eds.). *Stress and Human Health: Analysis and Implications of Research.* New York: Springer, 1982. *This study, sponsored by the Institute of Medicine in 1982, takes a constructive and critical look at the status of stress research. Current research findings are analyzed and discussed, and directions for future study are identified in each of nine panel reports on different aspects of stress. A very useful compendium, perhaps more for the researcher than the clinician.*
4. Everly, G. S. Jr., and Rosenfeld, R. *The Nature and Treatment of the Stress Response: A Practical Guide for Clinicians.* New York: Plenum, 1981. *Emphasizes the role that the individual plays in the creation of excessive stress and therefore the potential for the patient or client to assume self-responsibility for stress reduction. Discusses means of treatment*

including diet, exercise, relaxation, biofeedback, pharmacologic intervention, psychotherapy, hypnosis, meditation, and breath control.

5. Selye, H. *The Stress of Life.* New York: McGraw-Hill, 1956. *A classic by "the father of the stress concept," discussing its discovery and development. Latest revised edition is from 1976.*
6. Beech, H. R., Burns, L. E., and Sheffield, B. F. *A Behavioral Approach to the Management of Stress: A Practical Guide to Techniques.* Chichester: Wiley, 1982. *A lean, concise volume that provides clear definitions and descriptions of stress and stress reactions, means of identification, and analysis, plus discussion of relaxation, cognitive therapy, and biofeedback as stress-reduction techniques.*
7. Gentry, W. (ed.). *Handbook of Behavioral Medicine.* New York: Guilford Press, 1984. *The state of behavioral medicine at mid-decade with particularly pertinent chapters on the sociocultural and psychological dimensions of stress.*
8. Paffenbarger, R. S. Jr., et al. Physical activity, all-cause mortality, and longevity of college alumni. *N. Engl. J. Med.* 314(10):605, 1986. *Study of 16,936 Harvard alumni; impact of physical exercise on their health and longevity.*
9. United States Public Health Service. *Health Risk Appraisal.* Atlanta, GA: United States Department of Health and Human Services, Public Health Service, Centers for Disease Control, 1984. *An easy-to-use health risk appraisal instrument based on sound epidemiology covering the major health risk areas, not just stress.*
10. Cohen, S., Kamarck, T., and Mermelstein, R. A global measure of perceived stress [Perceived Stress Scale (PSS)]. *J. Health Soc. Behav.* 24(4):385, 1983. *A tool for measuring an individual's perceived stress.*
11. Blumenthal, J. A., et al. Development of a brief self-report measure of the type A (coronary prone) behavior pattern. Type A self-rating inventory. *J. Psychosom. Res.* 29(3):265, 1985. *Report of a tool for self-assessment of type A behavior.*
12. Orioli, E. M., Jaffe, V. T., and Scott, C.D. *Stressmap.* San Francisco: ESSI Systems, 1987. *A practical nonquantitative tool for pointing out relative stressfulness of different life areas in an individual.*
13. Hartsough, D. M. and Meyers, D. G. *Disaster Work and Mental Health: Prevention and Control of Stress Among Workers.* Rockville, MD: National Institute of Mental Health, 1985. *Valuable little manual for those concerned with general stress management, as well as with disaster workers.*
14. Woolfolk, R. L. and Lehrer, P. M. (eds.). *Principles and Practice of Stress Management.* New York: Guilford Press, 1984. *An invaluable handbook with experts in their fields discussing their methods of stress reduction, including progressive relaxation, yogic therapy, meditation, hypnosis, autogenic training, biofeedback, cognitive therapy, and pharmacologic therapy.*
15. Basmajian, J. V. (ed.). *Biofeedback: Principles and Practice for Clinicians.* (2nd ed.). Baltimore: Williams & Wilkins, 1983. *The "bible" of biofeedback for physical therapists and rehabilitation, as well as for professionals concerned with tension reduction and stress management.*

69 Suicide

Fran Pepitone-Rockwell and
Don Rockwell

I. The problem

A. Definition. Suicide is the human act of taking one's own life—"self-inflicted, self-intentioned cessation" [1, 2].

B. Description. Suicide is the ultimate self-destructive act—the endpoint on a continuum of behaviors that are life-threatening. It is very useful to consider all life-threatening behaviors as "suicidal" in some sense, since doing so encourages the health care provider to initiate therapeutic interventions. Suicide occurs when an individual's "unbearable anguish" intersects with an unresponsive human network. This clash is lethal for the suicide victim and leaves a permanently etched scar in those left behind. The bases for "unbearable anguish" appear to be twofold—depression and/or hopelessness.

Fortunately, depression is usually time-limited or transient by nature [3]. It contributes to the causes of suicide and at the same time is responsive to psychotherapy, antidepressants, and electroconvulsive therapy. The symptoms of depression are **physiologic** (sleep disorders, especially early morning awakening, appetite loss, constipation, dry mouth, headaches, and fatigue); **psychological** (loss of energy, loss of initiative, and loss of interest in usual pleasures such as sex and recreation; sad mood, low esteem, and an overwhelming sense of guilt; and, finally, social withdrawal); and **interpersonal** (multiple physical complaints, dependency, loss of sense of humor, irritability).

Hopelessness "is the key variable linking depression to suicidal behavior" [1]. The patient who feels hopeless has "tunnel vision," is not likely to have much future orientation, and is therefore more at risk for suicide than the patient who is experiencing only depression. The hopelessness aspect of the suicidal patient implies that the patient sees few or no options and is merely a few steps away from self-annihilation. This emotional state helps us to also understand why some people kill themselves who are not depressed.

Suicide is best understood as a progression of events that culminates with some "last straw." It has been described as "unbearable anguish" by the noted suicidologist Shneidman [4].

> The causes of suicide are multiple and terribly complex and remain one of the great enigmas of human nature. Suicide almost always involves a state of unbearable anguish; the causes of suicide attempts lie in the inadequate response on the part of others to previous suicidal behavior. "The cry for help" is a good phrase to recall.

C. Epidemiology. In the United States every year, about 25,000 people kill themselves; 250,000 make suicide attempts; 2,500,000 threaten suicide; and 25,000,000 have suicidal ideation or engage in life-threatening behavior [5]. Suicide is the tenth leading cause of death in the United States and tends to increase in frequency with increasing age in all Western countries. It is the second leading cause of death in college students and the third for adolescents between the ages of 15 and 19.

Of major interest is the fact that in the course of any 1 year, roughly 1 in 100 patients will threaten suicide, and 1 in 10 will have suicidal ideation. One percent of all deaths are reported as suicides, but the true figure is 2–3 times higher [6]. It has been shown that 75% of suicide victims consulted their physician before acting on their impulses [7]. From 60–74% [3] of suicide attempters have been treated recently by their physician. As many as 10% of suicide attempters see their physicians on the day of, or just prior to, their suicide and are provided with the means for their attempt by the unsuspecting physician.

High-risk "markers" include: (1) patients with a history of prior psychiatric hospitalization—especially hospitalization for depression, where the lifetime risk of suicide may be greater than 15%, (2) patients incurring a major loss (death or divorce and bereavement), (3) the elderly, and (4) alcoholics. A prior history of the above, alone or in combination, requires specific inquiry into current suicidal ideation.

There are some populations whose risk is higher than would be expected on the basis of demographic or other factors. These atypical populations are generally composed of individuals who are more intelligent than average and/or are experiencing unusual change and flux in their lives: students, especially women medical students; young black men or women; Native Americans; Eskimos; gifted individuals; physicians, especially women; immigrants; air traffic controllers; police officers; chemists or pharmacists; and psychologists.

II. Secondary prevention

A. Early detection. "The clues to suicide are either behavioral or verbal, and each of these is either direct or indirect" [4]. Behavioral clues include a suicide attempt, any self-injury, alcohol and other drug abuse, giving one's possessions away, refusal of life-extending procedures, and excessive risk-taking Verbal communications or clues include such statements as: "I wish I were dead," "How do you leave your body to a medical center?" and "I'm going to kill myself." More than 80% of people who have killed themselves have communicated their intent verbally or behaviorally. In most cases, verbal communications occurred close to the time of the suicide, were frequently repeated, and were directed to more than one person [9]. These clues are indicative of the ambivalence or uncertainty of the suicidal person. That is, simultaneously, suicidal individuals experience both the wish to die and the wish to be saved or rescued.

> The pattern of suicide is that a person is highly ambivalent; a person can cut their own throat and cry for help at the same time. And you must not say "Make up your mind." The life of the mind is not that way. Each of us is of several minds; there is a whole "congress of the mind" in our heads all the time, so that we are of different persuasions on key issues. A person who says "Why not let an individual who wants to kill himself (herself) do so" is psychologically naive (and brutal) because the answer to that is "Why not let the same individual, who at the time has fantasies of rescue and intervention, be the object of desired help?" [4]

Certain factors increase the chances of suicide. At age 60, the rate for men increases precipitously. A recent marital disruption or job problem also contributes to significantly increased risk [10].

The theme of loss is of paramount importance in the patient's life. The loss may be a loss of fantasy—for example, the promotion that did not happen or the failure to develop an important relationship, as well as the loss of real things (abortion, move away from home) or people. Living alone increases the risk because of the increase in social isolation and the reduction in person-to-person contacts.

Certain diseases are associated with depression. In some cases, depression is a late effect following viral or other infectious disease, or in association with any chronic, painful process. In some cases, depression can be an acute effect, as in endocrine diseases and many metabolic and nutritional deficiencies. In any postoperative period, the "blues" may be transient or more pervasive [11].

There are a number of drugs that produce depression and, hence, increase the risk of suicide in some susceptible individuals. While the most common depressant is alcohol, any "tranquilizer" or drug with depressant effects can provoke or worsen depressive symptoms. Interestingly, drugs with stimulant effects may also be associated with rebound depression. The amphetamines come to mind first, but much more commonly, ephedrine-type drugs are the culprits in clinical practice. A third large group includes steroids—especially progesterone—and, hence, some birth control pills may, in a small but clinically significant group, provoke a biologic depression.

The final group of drugs includes alkaloids, with reserpine being the most well known. There is a large group of less commonly used drugs that are associated with exacerbation of depression [5].

Most suicidal individuals will discuss their self-destructive thoughts if they are asked to do so. Helpers tend to be the ones reluctant to ask about suicidal ideation, believing that the suicidal person will not discuss it or having the ungrounded fear that talking about suicide prompts suicidal action.

General questions might include "How is your life going?" and more specific ones include "How close are you to suicide now?" and "How would you do it?" In addition to factors noted previously, the following are known to be associated with suicide:

1. Male sex. Men are more likely to complete suicide, although women are more likely to make suicide attempts.
   a. Men are less likely to engage in help-seeking behavior.

   b. Women use less immediately lethal methods.
2. Drug and alcohol abuse.
3. A family history of suicide.
4. Previous suicide attempts, which increase the risk that one will eventually die from suicide.
5. A suicide plan. The person with a suicide plan is to be considered an emergency and in a crisis.

B. Early intervention. The prevention of suicide is a multiple-tiered structure. Primary prevention can be fostered by the clinician by awareness of and, as far as possible, elimination of the common means of suicide. In the United States, this implies a reduction of access to handguns (the number one means) and a reduction in the prescription of potentially lethal drugs (the number two means—primarily sedative and antidepressant drugs). Considerable evidence exists [12, 13] to suggest that, deprived of the symbolically relevant means, persons will not often choose an alternative means of suicide. Clinicians should be exquisitely sensitive to their prescription of sedative/hypnotic drugs, since insomnia and sleep disturbance are common in depression and early morning awakening is a strong predictor of suicide [13].

Suicide prevention centers do not reduce suicide rates, probably because highly lethal individuals do not call these centers. This is not to say, however, that the centers do not serve an important function for the community. Their role as a resource for the acutely and clinically upset is invaluable. The highly lethal person is more likely to contact the clinician, who may inadvertently provide the means of suicide.

The primary problem is recognition by the health care provider of potential risk. Denial by caregivers is far and away the major inhibitor of providing services [6]. The identification of the risk is in and of itself the major therapeutic job. Suicidal individuals usually are willing and able to talk about their anguish, but their experience is that few people in their environment are able to listen. The clinician who makes the diagnosis and allows the patient to ventilate has dramatically reduced the risk of the patient progressing along a suicidal trajectory. Since depression and suicidal ideation are transient, what is required are effective crisis intervention skills and an open channel of communication between clinician and patient.

1. **Assessment.** In routine assessment of patients, clinicians need to keep in mind the risk factors noted above. Tipoffs include: (1) complaints of fatigue, low energy, and depression; (2) positive responses to inquiries about recent losses; (3) a positive history of alcohol abuse; (4) a positive response to routine questions about problems in sleeping; (5) a history of prior psychiatric disorder or depression; and (6) a response elicited in the clinician by the patient of either sadness **or** irritation. Depressed people sometimes make **us** feel depressed or annoyed.

   Alerted to the possibility of this person being at risk, the health care provider is obligated to assess the extent of depression and/or hopelessness by direct questioning. Some clinicians may choose to do this routinely, using a mood-rating scale such as the Profile of Mood States, Zung Self-Rating Depression Scale, or similar scale.

   Assessment will include an evaluation of the level of intentionality—how pressured does the patient feel to attempt suicide—and the level of lethality—what is the plan for suicide.

2. **Management.** General management takes into account several aspects of the suicidal patient. The patient identified as being suicidal or crying for help has already opened the major treatment avenue—that of open communication. The clinician's responsibility is thus to maintain a clear channel of communication with the patient throughout the crisis. Most patients' suicidal crises are short-lived, a matter of hours or days. Being available through this period of labor is indeed life-protecting. One expedient use, often forgotten, is the telephone. Telephone therapy is readily available, time-efficient, and effective. Other crisis intervention strategies can also be employed. Involving the family and dealing with the "last straw" or system-disequilibratory event can be done without great expenditures of time. Consultation with a mental health professional may provide the clinician with a workable plan without having to refer the patient. Involving other members of the treatment team is often useful to patient and clinician alike.

   Specific management is aimed at the specific system of dysfunction. The depressed or suicidal person with a biologic etiology can be managed by:

   a. Removal of organic causes (drugs).
   b. Patient and family education as to the etiology and self-limited nature of the illness.

Table 69-1. Risk factors for suicide

Depression	Prior history of psychiatric hospitalization
Hopelessness	Major loss
Unbearable anguish	Elder age group
Cry for help	High intelligence
Drug and alcohol abuse	Unusual changes in life
Impulsiveness	Chronic illness
Certain medications	Social isolation

c. Judicious use of antidepressant medication.
d. Consideration of a urine and blood drug-screen to evaluate use of other drugs (i.e., bromides, decongestants, and over-the-counter drugs).

The patient whose problems lie more in their individual psychological system needs to be permitted expression and often acceptance of negative feelings about self and others. The empathic clinician can in most cases offer brief (20-minute "hours") crisis intervention and assist the patient in reestablishing a satisfactory equilibrium.

Quite often the dysfunctional system is interpersonal (marriage, family) rather than purely individual. Family or marital counseling is then entirely appropriate, especially for suicidal adolescents. Exploration of covert conflict and hidden agendas may lead the patient to seek more extensive help from appropriate social and mental health professionals.

Treatment is inhibited primarily because of clinician hesitation. That hesitation is often related to lack of information. The rewards for recognizing and effectively managing the suicidal individual are immense. There are few other situations in which the opportunity of lifesaving is so clear and so immediate.

III. Recommendations

A. Early detection

1. Maintain a high index of suspicion and the willingness to explore with a patient the depths of his or her depression and the risk of suicide.
2. Be alert for important risk factors (Table 69-1).

B. Early intervention

1. Understand or eliminate the common means of suicide.
2. Prevent or reduce the social isolation of the suicidal patient by involving the family and others in the treatment.
3. Be available to the patient during periods of crisis.
4. Treat any underlying problems.
5. Assess for possible acute suicidal risk by examining the following:
   a. Presence of a plan.
   b. Psychosis.
   c. Intentionality.
   d. Lethality.
6. Consult with mental health professionals as needed.

References

1. Beck, A. T., Kovacs, M., and Weissman, A. Hopelessness and suicidal behavior. An overview. *J.A.M.A.* 234(11):1146, 1975. *Study illustrating the importance of hopelessness and cognitive restriction in potentially suicidal persons.*
2. Shneidman, E. S. *Definition of Suicide.* New York: Wiley, 1985. *Scholarly review by the world's preeminent suicidologist.*
3. Litman, R. E. Acutely suicidal patients. *Calif. Med.* 104(3):168, 1966. *Review of the crisis aspects of suicidal patients' management*
4. Ross, J. S., et al. The management of the presuicidal, suicidal and postsuicidal patient. *Ann. Intern. Med.* 75(3):441, 1971. *Clinicopathological conference illustrating Shneidman's theories of perturbation and postvention.*
5. Rockwell, D. A. and Pepitone-Rockwell, F. Problems in family practice: The suicidal patient. *J. Fam. Pract.* 7(6):1207, 1978. *Review article on the recognition and acute treatment of suicidal patients.*

6. Rockwell, D. A. and O'Brien, W. Physicians' knowledge and attitudes about suicide. *J.A.M.A.* 225(11):1347, 1973. *Study illustrating physicians' level of knowledge about suicide.*
7. Motto, J. A. and Greene, C. Suicide and the medical community. *Arch. Neurol. Psychiatry* 80(6):776, 1958. *Early study illustrating the presuicidal contacts with primary health care providers.*
8. O'Brien, J. P. Increase in suicide attempts by drug ingestion. *Arch. Gen. Psychiatry* 34(10):1165, 1977. *Study documenting the changing patterns of suicide attempts.*
9. Bernstein, M. The communication of suicidal intent by completed suicides. *Omega* 9(2):175, 1978–79. *Study illustrating the fact that most suicidal individuals signal their pain.*
10. Weissman, M. M. and Klerman, G. L. Sex differences and the epidemiology of depression. *Arch. Gen. Psychiatry* 34(1):98, 1977. *A review of the epidemiology of depression.*
11. Donlon, P. T. and Rockwell, D. A. (eds.). *Psychiatric Disorders, Diagnosis and Treatment.* Bowie, MD: Brady, 1982. *Basic text for primary care physicians.*
12. Dublin, L. I. *Suicide: A Sociological and Statistical Study.* New York: Ronald Press, 1963. *Overview of sociologic aspects of suicide.*
13. Rosen, D. H. The serious suicide attempt. Five-year follow-up study of 886 patients. *J.A.M.A.* 235(19):2105, 1976. *A study of the long-term outcomes of serious suicide attempts.*

II Disease Prevention

70 Screening Tests of Uncertain Value

Steven D. Rose

I. Introduction. The periodic health examination, or "annual physical," means different things to different people, be they patients or physicians. To many, it is a "complete history and physical" and a variety of screening laboratory tests. Some argue that such periodic checkups are valuable for finding and treating early disease, thus preventing later illness and mortality—much like periodic maintenance for automobiles will prevent future untimely breakdowns. Others, however, argue that unlike the evaluation of automobiles, our ability to find disease in asymptomatic people is imperfect, leading to not finding disease when it is there (false-negative tests) and finding disease when in actuality disease is not present (false-positives).

This chapter analyzes some common laboratory tests done routinely in many periodic health examinations. Studies on multiphasic screening examinations will also be presented.

II. Studies of multiphasic screening. There have been many studies looking at multiphasic screening in the laboratory. However, many of these studies simply report abnormalities on one screening examination [1]. These studies tell us little, since many of the abnormalities may be inconsequential, nonspecific, or falsely positive, or may detect diseases that do not have available or necessary therapy. Studies on multiphasic screening should have long-term follow-up to determine whether benefits accrue and outweigh the risks.

The largest and most quoted examination of multiphasic screening is from the Kaiser Permanente Program [2]. Here over 10,000 people were divided into two groups. One group was sent letters of encouragement to undergo a special multiphasic screening program. The control group was **not** urged to do so, although the program was available to them. The battery of tests included hearing and vision testing, tonometry, spirometry, chest x ray, mammograms in women over 48 years of age, urinalysis, serum chemistry panel, gynecologic examination and Papanicolaou (Pap) smear of the cervix, electrocardiogram, sphygmomanometry, sigmoidoscopies for all persons over 40 years of age, and follow-up visits with a nurse practitioner or physician. Although many abnormalities were identified in people undergoing multiphasic screening, after 11 years there were no differences between the two groups with respect to number of days of hospitalization, disability as reported by subjects on surveys, or utilization of outpatient services. Decreased self-reported disability was slightly less in the older males of the study group, but the causes of disability were mainly due to diseases not thought to be helped by periodic screening. The screened group had less disk disease of the back, less back sprain or strain, and fewer circulatory diseases. It would be hard to ascribe this decreased disability to the multiphasic testing.

It is important that there was no difference in overall mortality between the two groups. There was, however, a significant difference in cause-specific mortality due to diseases thought by the authors before the study to be potentially postponable. This was due mainly to the decreased mortality from colorectal cancer and hypertensive disease. On the other hand, there was increased mortality in the screened group from lymphohematopoietic cancer and suicide.

The conclusion from the Kaiser program is that such a wide array of screening tests does not give any tangible benefits when applied to the general population. However, measurement of blood pressure and sigmoidoscopies may have been responsible for decreased mortality for hypertensive disease and colonic carcinoma. These two diseases are discussed in Chaps. 72 and 81.

The other major trial of multiphasic screening comes from the South-East London Screening Study Group [3]. In this study, over 7000 people between the ages of 40 and 64 were randomly divided into control and study groups. After 9 years, no differences were found in morbidity, consultation and hospital admission rates, certified sickness absence from work, or mortality. Tests involved in this study included a symptom questionnaire, occupational data, anthropometry, vision and hearing testing, chest x ray, pulmonary function tests, electrocardiogram, sphygmomanometry, blood count, blood chemistry panels, stool for occult blood, and a basic physical examination.

The main difficulty with studies of this sort is that many tests are done and only general endpoints are measured. A benefit derived from one of the tests for a specific disease may be buried by the large number of tests that are not beneficial. It would be better to consider specific diseases, such as hypertensive disease or cervical carcinoma, and study the specific tests that screen for these diseases such as sphygmomanometry or the Pap smear. Furthermore, important benefits in high-risk populations might not be seen in these studies of general populations. There may be a case for certain screening laboratory tests in identifiable high-risk groups.

III. Criteria for effective screening tests. The criteria for effective screening tests are discussed in Chap. 1. The following is a list of criteria by which all laboratory examinations should be judged:

A. The disease screened for must result in significant morbidity or mortality.

B. The disease screened for should have a sufficient prevalence in the population to justify screening and follow-up costs.

C. The disease must have an asymptomatic period.

D. Treatment of a disease in the asymptomatic state must give a better result or prognosis than treatment begun in the symptomatic stage.

E. Follow-up must be available for abnormal test results.

F. The screening test used should be predictive, safe, inexpensive, and acceptable to the population.

It is obvious from these criteria that every laboratory examination must be evaluated in terms of what disease(s) the test is screening for. Once this is determined, the test can be properly evaluated by the above criteria.

IV. Evaluation of specific screening tests

A. Complete blood count. It is common practice to request a complete blood count (CBC) on any patient undergoing periodic examination. However, it has never been shown that in the asymptomatic nonpregnant adult, the CBC picks up any disease that is worth finding.

A CBC will detect anemia. Anemia does have an asymptomatic period and there is usually effective treatment. The screening test is accurate, simple, and acceptable. Using conventional definitions, screening programs have shown a high prevalence of anemia, ranging from 1% in males to 10% in females, with an increasing prevalence in the elderly. Screening of selected high-risk groups increases the efficiency of any screen. A CBC will find a high prevalence of anemia in women with heavy menses and poor iron intake.

There is no reason to believe that treatment in the asymptomatic stage is any better than treatment after symptoms develop [4]. Surprisingly, symptoms commonly associated with anemia have been shown to have no correlation with hemoglobin levels until values get below 7–8 gm % [5]. In one study looking at women with iron-deficiency anemia and hemoglobin values less than 10.5 gm %, no benefit could be demonstrated with oral iron therapy [6].

Anemia may be considered a sign rather than a disease, and the detection of iron-deficiency anemia would lead to the discovery of diseases causing blood loss. More important would be the discovery of colorectal cancer. However, as discussed in Chap. 81, the stool guaiac is a better test to use in the periodic health examination.

Leukemia is another disease detectable by a CBC. Acute leukemia does not have a long enough asymptomatic period to be detected on a periodic examination. The chronic leukemias do have an asymptomatic period; chronic granulocytic leukemia may be asymptomatic for several months, while chronic lymphocytic leukemia may be present for years without symptoms. However, treatment during the asymptomatic state does not produce a better result than after symptoms have developed.

In conclusion, diagnosing anemia or chronic leukemia with the CBC leads to little or no benefit. Other diseases detectable by the CBC are extremely rare, have no treatment that will improve outcome in the asymptomatic stage, or can be detected more efficiently with other tests.

B. Chemistry panels. Chemistry panels are extremely popular, perhaps due to their ability to provide many tests for little cost. However, one must analyze each of these tests for the disease that they are detecting. Before ordering chemistry panels, one should consider what one would do differently if any one of the tests came back abnormal. Lastly, one must realize that most abnormalities will be insignificant, will lead only to the unneeded expense and risks of further evaluation, and will cause anxiety for the patient.

1. **Electrolytes.** Almost all panels include tests for sodium, potassium, chloride, and carbon dioxide. It is hard to imagine a disease that these tests would detect in asymptomatic people. Abnormalities of electrolytes are seen in many diseases but are rarely seen in asymptomatic populations. Hypokalemia may be a sign of diuretic use and/or laxative abuse and is usually watched for in patients taking diuretics.
2. **Liver function tests.** Screening large populations has resulted in the detection of liver disease in about 1% of adults [1, 2]. It is unknown whether this detection of disease leads to any benefit.

   The diseases being screened for are cirrhosis, hepatitis, and alcoholism. Cirrhosis has a high prevalence in the population and a long asymptomatic period. However, the only treatment is cessation of alcohol intake. One could argue that the worry of progressive cirrhosis could be used to motivate the patient and family toward cessation of alcohol intake. Acute viral hepatitis has an asymptomatic period that is too short for screening. Alcoholic hepatitis is usually symptomatic, and the treatment is alcohol cessation. Elevated liver function tests can be a sign of unrecognized alcoholism and may be helpful to the patient and physician in recognizing the problem. Treatment is available; techniques for changing the behavior of problem drinkers and alcoholics have been effective, especially in those who are employed, socially stable, married, and without significant organic disease, as opposed to the homeless and brain-damaged alcoholics [7]. One study has demonstrated that a group of employed, married, nondeteriorated alcoholics did as well with "advice" as with other techniques such as group and family therapy [8].
3. **Creatinine and blood urea nitrogen (BUN).** These tests detect decreased renal function. Although valuable in the assessment of renal damage in the presence of hypertension and other diseases, unsuspected renal insufficiency is a rare finding in asymptomatic populations and does not lead to treatment that will improve the prognosis. Renal insufficiency is usually a result of known disease such as diabetes, myeloma, and hypertension; there is no known asymptomatic chronic renal disease that has a beneficial treatment. Thus these tests are not worthwhile in the periodic health examination.
4. **Uric acid.** Elevated uric acid does not diagnose gout but simply hyperuricemia. Gout is diagnosed by symptomatic arthritis, with demonstration of urate crystals in joint fluid. The treatment of hyperuricemia has no known benefit before the development of symptoms. There is no evidence that hyperuricemia in the absence of gout leads to urate nephropathy or renal failure. Screening for hyperuricemia as a risk factor for coronary artery disease is also not worthwhile in that elevated uric acid is a weak risk factor, and risk assessment for coronary disease is best done by other tests.
5. **Serum calcium.** The introduction of chemistry panels has led to the discovery of many people with hypercalcemia. Although many of these elevated calciums have led to the diagnosis of hyperparathyroidism, it is unclear what the natural history of this disease is. In the past, the diagnosis was made on symptomatic patients, and therapy was quite effective. However, the high prevalence of asymptomatic hyperparathyroidism found by routine assessment of serum calcium leads one to wonder where all these patients have been in the past. Studies of the long-term follow-up of these patients are needed to assess whether we are diagnosing a treatable disease or simply subjecting many people to unnecessary evaluation with multiple assessments of ionized calcium and parathyroid hormone levels, and possibly to unnecessary surgery.
6. **Blood lipids.** Lipids, especially serum cholesterol, are helpful in establishing a risk for coronary heart disease. This subject is discussed extensively in Chap. 73.
7. **Blood sugar.** In the adult, a blood sugar determination is a screen for noninsulin dependent diabetes mellitus. This is a fairly common disease affecting approximately 3% of the population, a percentage that appears to be increasing each year [9]. Furthermore, the prevalence of diabetes increases with age; the disease is rare before the age of 40 and peaks at about 65 years. Mortality is significant, with the risk of death from cardiovascular disease three times higher in diabetics than in nondiabetics. Morbidity includes blindness, renal failure, coronary heart disease, gangrene, and impotence. There is an asymptomatic period in many cases of diabetes, or an insidious onset of symptoms that may be unrecognized by patients.

   The glucose determination on the autoanalyzer is simple, safe, and accurate. The main difficulty is its interpretation, as there is no general agreement as to what degree of hyperglycemia constitutes diabetes or the need for treatment. The 2-hour postprandial and random sugars are nonspecific, although most would interpret the finding of values greater than 200 dl as diabetes. Most abnormalities, however, are in an intermediate range. Most people with mild degrees of hyperglycemia ("chemical diabetes") do not progress to clinical diabetes [10] Fasting values are more reliable. It does not appear that failure to make a diagnosis of diabetes before the development of persistent fasting hyperglycemia will alter therapy or prognosis [11]. Thus, as opposed to many other tests on the chemistry panel, the normal fasting blood sugar can reassure patients that they do not have the disease screened for.

The main reason that one cannot justify blood sugar determinations in the periodic health examination for asymptomatic, nonpregnant adults is that the treatment available today does not alter prognosis. Although there is much evidence in animals that hyperglycemia itself leads to complications and that control to normal improves these complications, this type of control is not yet achievable in humans. Today's therapy with insulin could possibly do more harm than good in asymptomatic adults with hyperglycemia.

There may be a reason to screen for glucose intolerance in pregnant women [12]. Gestational diabetes mellitus occurs in 2–3% of pregnancies in the United States. Although as a rule the blood sugar swings and degree of complications are not as severe in gestational diabetes as in known diabetes, the same types of complications are seen. These include increased birth weight (difficult deliveries, shoulder dystocia), congenital anomalies, hypoglycemia, and probably increased fetal mortality. As good control of blood sugar in known diabetics during pregnancy has considerably reduced these complications, similar measures may also be effective in gestational diabetes.

A blood sugar, of course, would be helpful in adults with symptoms or diseases that may be related to diabetes. These include recurrent vaginitis or balanitis, cataracts before the age of 50, coronary heart disease, peripheral vascular disease in nonsmokers, peripheral neuropathies, nocturia, polyuria and polydipsia.

Screening for diabetes in the obese patient may be justified. Weight reduction is an effective treatment to reverse glucose intolerance. Healthy overweight people may have few or no health reasons to lose weight; the finding of glucose intolerance would be an important incentive to seriously lose weight and possibly reduce the risk of diabetic complications.

8. **Dangers of chemistry panels.** Chemistry panels or multiphasic screening with a variety of nonspecific tests have definite risks and should not be ordered in the hope that "it might pick up something." Each test has a certain percentage of false-positives; combining many tests increases markedly the likelihood of false-positives. The more one tests a person who actually has no disease, the more likely one will find an abnormal result. This false-positive will often lead to patient anxiety and the risks and costs of further evaluation. Mislabeling of the patient can occur, a serious injustice to healthy people.

   The normal chemistry panel also has drawbacks. As there is little disease that it can pick up, it rules out very little, perhaps only diabetes and hypercholesterolemia. However, many patients and physicians have a conscious or subconscious attitude that the normal chemistry profile indicates health. This false reassurance may lead patients to delay bringing serious symptoms to medical attention and may persuade some physicians to evaluate symptoms less completely than they should.

9. **Conclusion.** Chemistry panels are not indicated in the periodic health examination. In fact, they can lead to false reassurance and to many false-positive results. Arguments can be made to screen for glucose intolerance with fasting blood sugars in the overweight patient and for hypercholesterolemia for coronary heart disease risk.

C. **Urinalysis.** The diseases detected and the components of the urinalysis by which they are detected include: (1) urinary tract infection by pyuria and bacteriuria, (2) renal disease by proteinuria and hematuria, (3) urinary tract cancer by hematuria, and (4) diabetes by glycosuria.

1. **Pyuria and bacteriuria.** Pyuria can be an indication of asymptomatic bacteriuria or covert urinary tract infection. Asymptomatic bacteriuria is found in only 0.5% of males but in 5% of females, with an increasing prevalence with age, occurring in 10–15% of women over 60 [13, 14]. Close to 40% spontaneously remit, and new infections occur in 1% of the total female population in the period of 1 year [13, 15].

   Pyuria is a poor screen for bacteriuria, being present in only one third to one half of asymptomatic females with documented bacteriuria [14]. Furthermore, 3% of women have been shown to have pyuria in the absence of bacteriuria. The chance, then, that pyuria represents true bacteriuria is only 50%. Thus, the pyuria is an inefficient tool for picking up asymptomatic bacteriuria, producing many false-positives and false-negatives.

There is very little reason to screen the general population for asymptomatic bacteriuria. There is a higher mortality associated with bacteriuria in older men and women, but the deaths are not due to causes directly attributable to bacteriuria, such as renal failure [16–18]. Bacteriuria probably accompanies other disease (such as dementia, possibly secondary to fecal incontinence) and has no causal effect. There are no controlled trials that demonstrate a better outcome with treatment of asymptomatic bacteriuria in the nonpregnant adult (see Chap. 10). Antibiotics will be effective in about 80%, but it has been found that only one half will continue with sterile urine after 1 year [13]. Without antibiotics, 36% were found to spontaneously develop sterile urine. Thus, for all the work of screening with follow-up cultures, the actual benefits are dubious. Furthermore, risks and costs of treatment must be kept in mind.

The other diseases that pyuria might indicate, such as renal tuberculosis, are quite rare or present with obvious symptoms, during which time effective treatment is available.

2. **Proteinuria.** The dip stick can detect albumin at concentrations as low as 30 mg/100 dl, but the vast majority of proteinuria will be benign essential or orthostatic proteinuria and thus of little consequence. Very rarely, chronic nephritis may be picked up. As this group of diseases is extremely infrequent in asymptomatic people and, furthermore, has no treatment outside dialysis and transplantation in the end stage, screening cannot be justified.
3. **Hematuria.** Hematuria is frequently present with bladder cancer and less often with renal cancer. One study of dye stuff workers using hematuria as a screening test resulted in a sensitivity of 72% and a specificity of 79% [19]. The 23% false-positives in this high-risk group would be increased markedly in a general population where the prevalence of urinary cancer is less than 0.01%. One study found that 98% of people with asymptomatic microscopic hematuria had benign causes, with 44% of the total having no cause discernible [20]. The costs and risks of evaluating these cases would vary according to the type of evaluation performed: urinary cytology, intravenous pyelogram (IVP), or cystoscopy.

   In addition to the above, there is no evidence that early detection of bladder cancer, the least rare of the urinary cancers, improves the prognosis. However, some recommend that screening be carried out in high-risk groups, mostly those working with chemical dyes. The screening proposed is not for hematuria but uses cytologic examination of the urine [21].

D. Chest x ray

1. **Lung cancer.** Lung cancer is the number one cause of cancer mortality in men and is rapidly becoming the leading cause in women. The chest x ray and sputum cytology have been studied as screening tests in the hope of finding early resectable and curable disease. Unfortunately, studies on screening have not found significant improvement with early detection. Chest x rays were taken every 6 months for 3 years in a British study of over 29,000 men, and survival was compared to cases found without screening in the control group of about 25,000. The 5-year survival was 15% in the 101 cases found in the screened group, and 6% in the 76 cases in the control group, an insignificant difference [22]. Only 65 of the 101 cancers in the screened group were found by the routine chest x ray, with the rest presenting at a time between the screening exams. The Philadelphia Pulmonary Neoplasm Project screened over 6000 males every 6 months for 10 years and found 121 cancers. The 5-year survival was a disappointingly low 8%, the same as the national statistics for unscreened patients [23, 24]. The Kaiser trial randomized over 5000 people to the multiphasic screening program, finding after 11 years 25 lung cancer deaths, compared to 26 in the control group [2].

   The problem with lung cancer is its rapidly fatal and progressive course. By the time it is noticeable on the chest x ray, it is usually not curable. In fact, 90% of new cancers in the Philadelphia study were symptomatic prior to the detection on chest x ray. The smallest detectable size of 0.6 cm represents already over 26 doublings of the original cancer cell [25]. This means that 60% of the tumor's total growth has already been achieved. Small increase in the 5-year survival for screened cases may be due not to early resection but to earlier diagnosis, and thus a longer survival time despite an inexorable progression of disease (lead-time bias). Screening may also select our slow-growing tumors that are curable even with late diagnosis (length-time bias).

In any event, the routine chest x ray in the periodic health examination cannot be justified for finding lung cancer, as no benefit has been found. Routine screening of older men who smoke also cannot be recommended, as the grim results of the above studies were from such a high-risk population.

Dangers of the screening chest x ray, besides its impressive cost, include the generation of false-positives. One study found four false-positives for every true case. Coupled with the insensitivity of the chest x ray, screening will result in exaggerated fear in many patients and their families, and false reassurance to others. Such time, energy, and money would be better spent on smoking cessation.

Combining sputum cytology with the chest x ray does increase detection. The Johns Hopkins Lung Project, the Mayo Lung Project, and the Memorial Sloan-Kettering National Lung Program have looked at dual screening (chest x ray and sputum cytology) in heavy smokers over the age of 45 [26]. In the initial prevalence screen, 160 cancers were found in 21,127 men (prevalence of 0.58%) who had the dual screen. This compares to 0.62% in 10,233 men having a chest x ray only. Of the cancers detected by the dual screen, 123 (77%) were detected by the chest x ray (including 30 by cytology also) and 37 (23%) were detected by cytology alone. One half of these tumors were in stage I and of those, 47% were detected by the chest x ray, 31% by cytology alone, and 7% by both. The 5-year survival for stage I tumors was almost 80%. Taking all cancers discovered, the 5-year survival was much lower. Interestingly, if a cancer was discovered radiographically, the 5-year survival rate was 33%, which compares to 85% for cancers found by cytology alone.

Despite these encouraging results, it is still unclear if this increased early detection leads to improved survival. As the investigators of these programs note, screening asymptomatic people results in the discovery of a disproportionate number of tumors with long latent periods, while faster, more malignant cancers are underrepresented. It is very likely that some of these tumors are so indolent that they would not have progressed to clinical importance before the patient dies of other causes. Nobody knows the natural history of cancers that cannot be seen radiographically at the time of diagnosis. Additionally, lead-time bias is still a problem with the above studies.

An analysis of incidence cases (cancers found over time in the population with negative screens at the initial exam) with an unscreened control, would reduce the above biases of the prevalence studies. None of the studies have an unscreened control group, but dual screening was compared to the chest x ray alone. In the Mayo Lung Project [27], 109 incidence cancers were found in the dual screened group during follow-up, compared to 78 in the chest x ray group (2.4% versus 1.7%). Of the 109 cancers, 70 were found by screening, the rest coming to attention between the 4-month screens. Unfortunately, 28 were small-cell cancers (unresectable) and of the 81 non-small cell cancers, 32 were resectable. The Memorial Sloan-Kettering Cancer Center had similar results with 97 incident cases found by the dual screen, and 107 by chest x ray screening alone. In both studies, sputum cytology was not very productive, finding relatively few cancers not seen on the chest x ray.

The above studies are evaluating a very intensive screen. There is a considerable expense to frequent cytology, which requires an accomplished cytotechnologist. False-positives will be more frequent too. A follow-up evaluation of an abnormal chest x ray can cost from less than $100 to over $1000, depending on the amount of workup. False-positive cytologies are less frequent but do occur. In one study of over 6000 subjects, 34 had positive sputum cytologies with negative chest x rays. After evaluation, six of these were eventually found to have cancer of the lung, and two to have cancer of the larynx. Evaluation of the cytologies for occult cancer can be extensive with repeated bronchoscopies and biopsies. The American Cancer Society notes that the financial costs of such a workup can be well over $1000, and the psychological costs extremely high. If all smokers over the age of 45 were screened every 4 months with a false-positive rate of 0.5% to 2.0%, over 500,000 people/year would undergo a difficult and unnecessary evaluation to find one lung cancer. This is a main reason why the American Cancer Society does not recommend routine screening for lung cancer with the chest x ray or sputum cytology [23].

2. **Tuberculosis.** The other major disease picked up by a chest x ray is tuberculosis. This is a disease of considerable consequence, and it can be treated in the asymptomatic stage to give a better prognosis, if not for the patient, then for the people

who come in contact with the patient. However, as reviewed in detail in Chap. 96, the skin test is a more efficient screening test. Screening mini chest x rays has been successful in high-risk populations, such as in alcohol detoxification centers, where compliance for skin-test reading is poor.

E. Electrocardiogram

1. **Coronary heart disease.** As noted in Chap. 71, the resting electrocardiogram (ECG) is quite inaccurate for detecting coronary heart disease (CHD), with poor sensitivity, specificity, and predictive value. Seventy-three percent of people in Framingham, Massachusetts, who developed a myocardial infarction had previously normal ECGs. False-positives would lead healthy people to unnecessary concern for their hearts. Furthermore, there is no treatment yet for asymptomatic CHD outside of risk-factor reduction, which is advocated regardless of the cardiogram. Many ECGs are ordered as a "baseline" to be compared with cardiograms taken later when the patient develops symptoms. However, it has been shown that such baseline cardiograms have little if any effect on the management of patients with new cardiac symptoms [28].
2. **Ventricular arrhythmias.** Arrhythmias are frequently found in screening cardiograms. Premature ventricular contractions (PVCs) have been found in 1% of Air Force recruits, 4% of life insurance applicants, and 7% of male factory workers, increasing from 2–15% with age [29-31]. Ventricular arrhythmias on Holter monitoring are even more frequent, with one half of male medical students without heart disease and with normal echocardiograms having PVCs.

   As opposed to the patient with heart disease, especially with a prior myocardial infarction, patients with PVCs but with no history of hypertension, heart disease, or left ventricular hypertrophy are at no higher risk for infarction or sudden death than those without arrhythmias [29-31].

   The routine ECG does not find disease that requires any treatment or change in management in asymptomatic people. It is relatively expensive for screening and carries the usual psychological costs of false-positives. It furthermore gives false reassurance to people who should reduce risk factors and report new symptoms.

F. Thyroid function tests (TFTs)

1. **Hyperthyroidism.** The common causes of hyperthyroidism are Graves' disease, toxic multinodular goiter, and toxic adenoma. Hyperthyroidism is not rare; Graves' disease was found in 0.97% of a private practice in Connecticut, and in 1.58% in a British community study conducted in Whickham [32, 33]. Most of these cases were previously diagnosed, but a significant number of unexpected cases were found. In the Whickham survey, seven women were found out of 2745 people (0.26%) who had no history of thyroid disease. The Connecticut study found six new cases (0.39%). Hyperthyroidism was found unexpectedly in eight women (five with Graves' disease and three with toxic nodular goiter) out of 2606 adults (0.31%) in a Kaiser multiphasic screening program.

   Thyroid function tests include an assay for serum thyroxine (T_4) and triiodothyronine uptake (a measure of thyroxine-binding globulin) from which a free thyroxine index (FTI) can be calculated. The tests are quite accurate. In the Kaiser screening program, the FTI identified all cases of hyperthyroidism and gave only three false-positives [34]. The predictive value of an elevated FTI was then 73%. The additional risk, expense, and psychological burden of the evaluation of false-positives are not significant.

   Once found, there is effective treatment with drugs, radioactive iodine, or surgery. However, there is no reason to believe that treating hyperthyroidism in the asymptomatic state offers any benefit over treatment once symptoms or signs have developed. Screening during a periodic health exam may result in finding 1–2 cases/1000 people screened. Although there are no studies, the nature of the disease suggests that most if not all of the cases found would be found a few months or perhaps a year later when symptoms develop and become more prominent. Death from undiscovered hyperthyroidism is exceedingly rare and represents an unusual lack of clinical suspicion in the face of signs and symptoms of the disease.

   Hyperthyroidism often presents in the elderly where signs and symptoms can be quite nonspecific. Patients over the age of 60 with tachyarrhythmias or nonspecific fatigue and weakness should be evaluated. However, routine thyroid function tests for hyperthyroidism in healthy adults should not be one of our health priorities.
2. **Hypothyroidism.** The prevalence of hypothyroidism varies with the manner in which the disease is defined. A low FTI is found in approximately 0.5% to 1.0% in screened patients. Overt hypothyroidism was found in 1% of the Whickham sur-

vey. Subclinical hypothyroidism with an elevated thyroid stimulating thyroid hormone (TSH), a low serum thyroxine but normal serum triiodothyronine (T_3), was much more common, occurring in 10% of postmenopausal women. In a British study screening 2000 patients admitted to the hospital, 46 (2.3%) were found to have hypothyroidism, 42 of these cases being newly diagnosed [35].

The asymptomatic period, or more correctly the period of clinically unsuspected hypothyroidism, is probably longer than that for hyperthyroidism. Cases are often diagnosed after years of nonspecific mild symptoms that improve with therapy. Again, high clinical suspicion, especially in postmenopausal women, should prompt one to order TFTs. Cases found in screening programs have either suggestive signs and symptoms or some nonspecific symptoms to prompt one to order TFTs. Completely asymptomatic people have been found with subclinical hypothyroidism: a high TSH, a low T_4, and a normal T_3. It is not yet established what the natural history of this abnormality is and whether treatment improved morbidity and mortality.

TFTs are quite accurate and safe as described above. In the Kaiser study, the FTI was 100% sensitive, and the predictive value of a low FTI for hypothyroidism was 67%. Follow-up risks and costs for false-positives are not significant.

Although screening TFTs for finding undiagnosed hypothyroidism will find treatable disease, the test should not be routinely applied for the general population. However, TFTs may be ordered often in high-risk groups such as postmenopausal women and in clinical situations where hypothyroidism is not uncommon (e.g., depression, psychiatric disorders, fatigue, apathy, and general deterioration of health).

V. Recommendations

A. A common battery of tests available today are not as helpful as they appear. The chemistry panels are often appropriate for following hospitalized patients who have abnormal electrolytes or changing hepatic and renal function but are not appropriate for outpatient screening. Furthermore, the inclusion of many of the tests on panels appears to be based more on the technical ability to perform the test inexpensively than the test's ability to screen for disease.

B. One should evaluate each test for the disease that it is to detect. The disease must fulfill the above-described screening criteria to be useful.

C. Extremely few tests will qualify for the general population as a whole, and few will qualify even for high-risk groups. Arguments may be made to order a serum cholesterol, a fasting blood sugar in the obese, and thyroid function tests in postmenopausal women. Other tests should be ordered not for screening but in evaluation of symptoms or physical findings.

D. One must always keep in mind the often irreparable harm that can result from the inaccuracy present in all tests. False-positives can lead to expensive and risky evaluation, and unnecessary patient concern and worry. Normal batteries, false or not, reassure patients who should be working to alter unhealthy life-styles, or who have disease that is undetectable by the panels, resulting in the patient ignoring important symptoms and delaying their presentation to the physician.

References

1. Rowe, I. L., and Larsen, L. H. Evaluation of automated multiphasic health testing of referred patients by genetal practitioners. *Med. J. Aust.* 2(7):214, 1977. *Multiphasic tests in 752 patients referred from general practitioners, finding much disease, little of any consequence.*
2. Dales, L. G., Friedman, G. D., and Collen, M. F. Evaluating periodic multiphasic health checkups: A controlled trial. *J. Chronic Dis.* 32(5):385, 1979. *The Kaiser prospective randomized trial on multiphasic screening, showing no significant beneficial effect of a large battery of tests.*
3. The South-East London Screening Study Group. A controlled trial of multiphasic screening in middle-age: Results of the South-East London Screening Study. *Int. J. Epidemiol.* 6(4):357, 1977. *A prospective randomized trial finding no difference in mortality and general endpoints with multiphasic screening.*
4. Elwood, P. C. Anemia. *Lancet* 2(7893):1364, 1974. *A review by a prominent investigator on anemia.*
5. Elwood, P. C., et al. Symptoms and circulating haemoglobin level. *J. Chronic Dis.* 21(9):615, 1969. *Study shows symptoms thought to be associated with anemia do not correlate with level of hemoglobin until levels are below 7–8 dl.*

6. Elwood, P. C., and Hughes, D. Clinical trial of iron therapy on psychomotor function in anaemic women. *Br. Med. J.* 1(717):254, 1970. *Iron replacement did not improve symptoms in 47 women with iron-deficiency anemia.*
7. Baekeland, F., Lundwall, L., and Kissin, B. Methods for the Treatment of Chronic Alcoholism: A Critical Appraisal in Research Advances in Alcohol and Drug Problems. In R. Gibbins, et al. (eds.), *Research Advances in Alcohol and Drug Problems.* New York: Wiley, 1975. Vol. 2, Pp. 247–327. *A review.*
8. Edwards, G., et al. Alcoholism: A controlled trial of "treatment" and "advice." *J. Stud. Alcohol* 38(5):1004, 1977. *Both methods had the same effectiveness.*
9. *Report of the National Commission on Diabetes to the Congress of the United States.* Bethesda, MD: National Institutes of Health, 1975. *Five-year follow-up report on the Birmingham Diabetes Survey of 1962.*
10. Birmingham Diabetes Survey Working Party. *Br. Med. J.* 3(718):301, 1970. *Five-year follow-up of people with glucose intolerance, with 82.5% not progressing to diabetes.*
11. Siperstein, M. D. The glucose tolerance tests: A pitfall in the diagnosis of diabetes mellitus. *Adv. Intern. Med.* 20:297, 1975. *Review of the nonspecificity of the glucose tolerance test, arguing that the fasting blood sugar is more useful.*
12. Centers for Disease Control. Public health guidelines for enhancing diabetes control through maternal- and child-health programs. *M.M.W.R.* 35:201, 1986. *A summary of screening for gestational diabetes.*
13. Asscher, A. W., et al. The clinical significance of asymptomatic bacteriuria in the nonpregnant woman. *J. Infect. Dis.* 120(1):17, 1969. *Original study of asymptomatic bacteriuria and its treatment.*
14. Kass, E. H. Asymptomatic infections of the urinary tract. *Trans. Assoc. Am. Physicians* 69:56, 1956. *A frequency of positive Gram stains, urine cultures, and pyuria in asymptomatic female outpatients.*
15. Asscher, A. W. *The Challenge of Urinary Tract Infections.* New York: Grune & Stratton, 1980. *A review.*
16. Evans, D. A., et al. Bacteriuria and subsequent mortality in women. *Lancet* 1(8264):156, 1982. *This study (and those in references 17 and 18) find increasing mortality in the elderly with bacteriuria, but due to causes such as "senile cachexia" and cerebrovascular disease and not to causes related to bacteriuria.*
17. Dontas, A. S., et al. Bacteriuria and survival in old age. *N. Engl. J. Med.* 304(16):939, 1981. *See reference 16.*
18. Sourander, L. B., and Kasanen, A. A 5-year follow-up of bacteriuria in the aged. *Gerontol. Clin.* 14(5):274, 1972. *See reference 16.*
19. Crabbe, J. G., et al. The cytological diagnosis of bladder tumors among dye stuff workers. *Br. J. Indust. Med.* 13:270, 1956. *Cytologic methods used in screening 1800 men for bladder cancer.*
20. Greene, L. F., O'Shaughnessy, E. J. Jr., and Hendricks, E. D. Study of five hundred patients with asymptomatic microhematuria. *J.A.M.A.* 161(7):610, 1956. *Two percent of those with microhematuria had neoplasms.*
21. Trott, P. A. Cytological screening for cancer of the bladder. *Proc. R. Soc. Med.* 69(7):496, 1976. *A review arguing for screening for bladder cancer in people with high risk due to occupational exposure.*
22. Brett, G. Z. The value of lung cancer detection by six-monthly chest radiographs. *Thorax* 23(4):414, 1968. *Found screening with chest x rays did not result in better survival.*
23. Eddy, D. Cancer of the lung. *CA* 30(4):199, 1980. *An excellent review of the current status of lung cancer screening.*
24. Boucot, K. R., and Weiss, W. Is curable lung cancer detected by semiannual screening? *J.A.M.A.* 224(10):1361, 1973. *The answer was no for chest x rays every 6 months.*
25. Spratt, J. S. Jr., Ter-Pogossian, M., and Long, R. T. The detection and growth of intrathoracic neoplasms. The lower limits of radiographic distinction, the antemortem size, the duration, and the pattern of growth as determined by direct mensuration of tumor diameters from random thoracic roentgenograms. *Arch. Surg.* 86:283, 1963. *Found that tumors are not generally discernable on chest x rays until they reach a diameter of 6 mm.*
26. The National Cancer Institute. Early Lung Cancer Cooperative Study: Early lung cancer detection program: Summary and conclusions. *Am. Rev. Respir. Dis.* 130(4):565, 1984. *Summary of three major prevalence studies on lung cancer screening.*
27. Woolner, L. B., et al. Mayo Lung Project: Evaluation of lung cancer screening through December 1979. *Mayo Clin. Proc.* 56(9):544, 1981. *Ongoing study of intensive cytologic screening for lung cancer.*
28. Rubenstein, L. Z., and Greenfield, S. The baseline ECG in the evaluation of acute cardiac

complaints. *J.A.M.A.* 244(22):2536, 1980. *Found that baseline ECGs rarely affected decision to hospitalize or manage differently patients with acute cardiac symptoms.*

29. Rodstein, M., Wolloch, L., and Gubner, R. A mortality study of the significance of extra systoles in an insured population. *Trans. Assoc. Life Insur. Med. Dir. Am.* 54:91, 1971. Article also appears in *Circulation* 44:617, 1971. *Articles in references 29–31 report ventricular arrhythmias on routine ECGs as being common but not a risk factor for sudden death in the absence of heart disease and left ventricular hypertrophy (LVH).*
30. Fisher, F. D., and Tyroler, H. A. Relationship between ventricular premature contractions on routine electrocardiography and subsequent sudden death from coronary heart disease. *Circulation* 47(4):712, 1973. *See reference 29.*
31. Weis, A. N., et al. Relationship of premature ventricular contractions and left ventricular hypertrophy to sudden cardiac death. *Circulation* 40(Suppl. 3):III-213, 1969. *See reference 29.*
32. Tunbridge ,W. M., et al. The spectrum of thyroid disease in a community: The Whickham Survey. *Clin. Endocrinol.* 7(6):481, 1977. *A community screening study for thyroid dysfunction.*
33. Baldwin, D. B., and Rowett, D. Incidence of thyroid disorders in Connecticut. *J.A.M.A.* 239(8):742, 1978. *Over 1500 people screened during an annual physical examination for thyroid disorders.*
34. dos Remedios, L. V., et al. Detecting unsuspected thyroid dysfunction by the free thyroxine index. *Arch. Intern. Med.* 140(8):1045, 1980. *A study from Kaiser Permanente of the free thyroxine index as a screen for thyroid dysfunction.*
35. Bahemuka, M., and Hodkinson, H. M. Screening for hypothyroidism in elderly inpatients. *Br. Med. J.* 2(5971):601, 1975. *Found screening worthwhile in 2000 geriatric inpatients.*

Suggested Reading

Sox, H. C., Jr. (ed.). *Common Diagnostic Tests. Use and Interpretation.* Philadelphia: American College of Physicians, 1987. *A collection of detailed discussions of common diagnostic tests; includes the Blue Cross and Blue Shield guidelines.*

71 Coronary Heart Disease

Steven D. Rose

I. The problem

A. Description. The natural and treated history of coronary heart disease (CHD) is quite variable. There is a long asymptomatic phase of developing atherosclerosis in the coronary arteries, a process that appears to begin in young life and progresses at varying rates with age. Arteriography and autopsy studies in people without symptoms of CHD estimate that the prevalence of CHD in adults over 40 is 4%. However, this rate increases with age and in males, as shown in Table 71-1 [1]. These prevalence rates also increase with the presence of the risk factors listed in Table 71-2.

Asymptomatic atherosclerosis progresses to symptomatic CHD at various rates and in different ways. Initial manifestations in men are myocardial infarction (MI) (45%), angina pectoris (23%), and sudden death (11%). Thus, irreversible damage that may include death occurs in the majority by the time symptoms appear. Furthermore, people with established CHD have coronary artery atherosclerosis at a stage so advanced that regression is difficult to induce. No treatment other than risk-factor reduction is currently available for asymptomatic CHD.

The course of CHD is quite different in women. Premenopausal women have an extraordinarily low rate of CHD. In the Framingham study, no case of CHD death of MI occurred in 8500 person-years of observation [2]. The reason for this protection is not known and can only be explained in part by the lower prevalence of CHD risk factors in premenopausal women. When CHD does occur, it presents most often as angina [3]. With natural or surgical menopause, there is an abrupt increase in both risk factors and CHD. Hypertension, less common in young women than in young men, is most common in postmenopausal women. The same is true of elevated total cholesterol and diabetes. Mortality from CHD is still less for women than men, although CHD remains a major source of illness and death for women. The risk factors are as important for women and even more so for diabetic women. In fact, diabetic women have as much CHD as diabetic men. Also, women who do develop CHD have the same poor prognosis as men. CHD in the postmenopausal woman presents as angina somewhat more than half of the time. When presenting as an MI, the prognosis is actually worse in women, with 50% of patients in the Framingham study being dead in 5 years.

B. Epidemiology. In the United States, CHD has been the number one cause of death for more than 30 years. However, mortality rates over time have been far from stable. Deaths due to diseases of the heart were relatively stable in the beginning of the century. In 1920, mortality from CHD began to rise, and this rise continued unabated for over 30 years. The peak occurred in the mid 1960s, and for largely unknown reasons CHD mortality has been declining ever since. Furthermore, this decline appears to have accelerated in 1973 such that the absolute reduction is well over 25%.

The reasons for this decline are not at all clear. This country has had a reduction in the levels of CHD risk factors during this time, but the decline in CHD mortality has exceeded what would be expected from the observed lowering of risk factors. The same is true for improved treatment of CHD. The decline began well before the rise of coronary bypass surgery. This decline is not worldwide; some countries have had an increase in CHD. Of further interest is that if one divides CHD mortality into acute myocardial infarction and chronic ischemic heart disease, one sees that the decline is limited to the former, while mortality from the latter has been relatively stable [4].

Despite the declining CHD mortality, CHD is still by far the major cause of death in the United States. In 1978, 434 deaths/100,000 population between the ages of 35 and 74 were due to CHD, more than twice the mortality rate for all cancers. The periodic health exam should address CHD if only for its high prevalence in our society. Moreover, CHD attacks people in their prime, depriving them, their families, and society of many productive years of life.

Table 71-1. Prevalence of coronary heart disease (CHD)

Age	Prevalence of CHD: Men (%)	Prevalence of CHD: Women (%)
30–39	1.9	0.3
40–49	5.5	1.0
50–59	9.7	3.2
60–69	12.3	7.5

Source: Modified from G. A. Diamond and J. S. Forrester. Analysis of probability as an aid in the clinical diagnosis of coronary-artery disease. *N. Engl. J. Med.* 300(24):1350, 1979.

Table 71-2. Risk factors for coronary heart disease

1. Definite
   - Reversible
     - Smoking
     - High blood pressure
     - Low HDL
     - High cholesterol
     - Oral contraceptives (in smokers)
   - Fixed
     - Older age
     - Male sex
     - Family history
     - Diabetes
2. Probable
   - Inactivity
   - Type A personality
   - Obesity
3. Not independent
   - High triglycerides
   - Gout
4. Not risk factors
   - Coffee
   - Refined sugars
   - Alcohol

Key: HDL=high density lipoprotein.

II. Primary prevention

A. Methods. Primary prevention of coronary heart disease (CHD) focuses on altering known reversible risk factors. The three major factors are smoking, hypertension, and hypercholesterolemia. Less important factors include exercise, obesity, stress, and personality type. The methods for identifying and altering each of these risk factors are discussed in other chapters. Screening recommendations from the American Heart Association were published [14].

Age and family history cannot be treated but are assessed because they multiply the significance of treatable risk factors. Diabetes, though treatable, is a risk factor even when blood sugar is well controlled.

A cardiovascular risk profile can be developed easily by history (age, family history of CHD, smoking, inactivity), measurement of blood pressure, and determination of total and high density lipoprotein (HDL) cholesterol. All risk factors should be reversed, but if one wants to quantify the risk, values can be plugged into tables [5], and an approximate numerical risk of developing CHD in the next 6 years can be calculated.

Risk reduction requires many life-style changes, and one should start with reasonable goals that will produce the greatest reduction in risk. Efforts should focus first on the big three reversible factors: smoking, hypertension, and hypercholesterolemia. Birth control pills should be discouraged in women over the age of 35, especially in those who smoke. An exercise program has many benefits and may reduce other risk factors. Weight reduction should be encouraged, although it is often a difficult and painful process, frustrating for both the physician and patient. One should first concentrate on the more significant factors, especially smoking. Weight reduction often occurs when one is pursuing a low-fat diet for hyperlipidemia and an exercise program.

A risk profile may be assessed arbitrarily every 5 years in low-risk patients. In high-risk patients, assessments should be more frequent, perhaps at each visit. Risk-factor reduction is mostly a struggle involving patient compliance with life-style changes, so frequent feedback and encouragement are important.

B. Justification. Although it is recommended to reduce CHD risk factors in everyone, one should keep in mind that there is little if any evidence to show that risk-factor reduction is effective in the general population. Trials using the general population have not shown any reduction in coronary mortality with risk-factor reduction. The World Health Organization (WHO) studied multiple risk factor reduction in a randomized trial in the general population [6]. The intervention included dietary modification, smoking cessation, weight reduction, exercise, and drug treatment of hypertension. A reduction in fatal and nonfatal coronary events or total mortality was **not** found.

The main rebuttal to the above is that the trials were not carried on long enough with enough people to show a difference. CHD develops over 30–40 years, attacking people in middle and older ages. Risk-factor reduction over this long a period has never been and probably never will be studied. Furthermore, intervention is less effective in those at low and moderate risk. Inclusion of these people in the above trials makes the benefits of intervention more difficult to find.

A second approach to primary prevention of CHD would be to identify the people at highest risk and apply risk-factor reduction to them. Unfortunately, the evidence is still not strong that this approach is effective. The Oslo Heart Study intervened on smoking and cholesterol reduction under medical supervision and **did** find a reduction in CHD. However, the Multiple Risk Factor Intervention Trial (MRFIT), looking at high-risk men in the United States, did not show any reduction in CHD or total mortality in the intervention group. Again, this trial was short in comparison to the long, asymptomatic development of CHD. Furthermore, a difference may have been missed in part because of the coincidental lowering of risk factors in the control group, which showed a lower CHD event rate than expected. If this is the real reason, then one could conclude that simply identifying men at high risk and reassessing them every year, as was done with the control group here, was as effective in reducing CHD as the elaborate, expensive, and intensive programs applied to the study group.

Because CHD is so widespread, more cases of CHD will be found outside of the high-risk group than in it. Perhaps we should rethink and identify the group at low risk. We would then apply risk-factor modification to the rest of the population. It has been estimated that if we could reverse risk factors in the American population to the level of those of lowest risk (the present lowest quintile or 20%), CHD rates would decrease by two thirds [7]. That is, two thirds of CHD may be prevented if nobody smoked, mean cholesterol were 205 mg/dl, and mean blood pressure through middle age were 120/80 and not 136/86. This, of course, means asking millions of people who will never develop CHD to reduce risk factors. However, the stakes (death) are high, and if risk-factor reduction is without harm and acceptable in this large population, then it can be justified. The case is further strengthened when risk factors are also tied to other diseases (hypertension with stroke, and smoking with emphysema and cancer).

A good randomized trial on risk-factor reduction in CHD over an appropriate period of time will not be done, as it would be prohibitively expensive. One then has to make a decision on the effectiveness of risk-factor reduction based on the large amount of epidemiologic and laboratory evidence (discussed in other chapters) showing strong correlations of the risk factors with CHD. These studies strongly suggest that reduction of hypertension, of tobacco use, and of high serum cholesterol over many years will reduce CHD.

Reducing risk factors other than the "big three" seems to be of much less importance. Inactivity and obesity may not be important independent risk factors by themselves, but weight reduction and exercise are methods to lower blood pressure and improve lipid levels and glucose intolerance. Recent data from the Framingham study has found that obesity does contribute independently to CHD risk [8]. The hard-driving, impatient, often frustrated, time-conscious, anxious personality (type A) may have increased risk, but the efficacy of reversing this behavior is unknown. Gout and hyperuricemia are associated with other risk factors and are not helpful in risk assessment. Birth control pills are probably a negligible risk except in women over the age of 35 (especially smokers), and risk in this group may continue at some degree despite discontinuation of the birth control pills. Factors popularized in the lay press that have not been associated with an independent increased risk of CHD include refined sugar and alcohol [3]. As alcohol may increase blood pressure, moderation or cessation should be addressed in hypertensive patients. Coffee is probably not an important factor. Coffee does increase the heart rate transiently and may lead to a rise in serum cholesterol. Many studies have looked at the contribution of coffee to the development of CHD and have given inconsistent results. It now appears that coffee in moderate amounts (2 cups/day) is not an important risk factor. Larger amounts may result in a small but independently increased risk for CHD. One aspirin taken every other day has been shown to reduce coronary events in people not known to have heart disease [13]. However, there was not even a trend toward reduced mortality. One must consider possible side effects of lifelong aspirin use. Further study is needed before it can be recommended for the general population for CHD reduction.

III. Secondary prevention

A. Early detection methods

1. **The history.** Patients are to be asked not just if they have chest pain but if they have any uncomfortable sensation in the chest, neck, or jaw area that is brought on by exertion. The history will likely yield higher results in those at high risk. However, the history is not sensitive, with most CHD presenting the first time as an MI or as sudden death.
2. **Risk factor identification.** Although used to predict the development of CHD, risk factor identification cannot be used as a screen for CHD because of its lack of sensitivity and specificity. This is true even for those at the highest risk. In the Framingham study, the 10% of people at high risk accounted for only 20% of the CHD found.
3. **The resting ECG.** The resting ECG can identify some people with old infarcts. Almost 25% of the MIs in the Framingham study were identified by routine ECGs rather than through hospitalization at the time of the MI. However, the ECG is very insensitive. In the Framingham study, 73% of people who developed myocardial infarction had normal ECGs before the MI. On the other side, false-positive ECGs—ST depression and T-wave inversions—are quite frequent and will lead many healthy people to worry unnecessarily.
4. **The exercise electrocardiogram.** Exercise treadmill testing (ETT) is more accurate but not to the level that it can be used as a screening test on asymptomatic individuals [9]. The sensitivity is only around 60%, and false-positives run at about 10% depending on the criteria used. If the prevalence of CHD in the screened population is about 5%, ETT will be positive in 128 of 1000 people. Of these positives, only 33 will be shown to have real disease. Seventy-five percent of the positive results will be in people who have no disease at all. Further evaluation means more expensive (thalium scans) and risky (cardiac catheterization) procedures. Furthermore, people with false-positive results undergo the stress and worry of these tests and the concern of having serious heart disease. In groups with a lower prevalence of CHD, the situation is even worse. If women aged 40–49 (CHD prevalence of 1% by Table 71-1) are screened with ETT, 94% of the positive results would be in people without disease.

   ETT screening in asymptomatic people of extremely high risk will find disease somewhat more accurately. Males over the age of 50 with risk factors are often subjected to ETT before embarking on a training program. Still, one must consider that even with a prevalence as high as 10%, more than half of the positive results will be false. To get 80% of the positives as true positives, the prevalence of disease has to be over 25%. This may correspond to the population of older males with multiple risk factors.

   ETT has also been proposed as part of a risk factor profile rather than as a diagnostic test. Studies in asymptomatic men show a 10-fold increase in risk for those with positive tests. The Seattle Heart Watch Study showed that in those with one or more conventional risk factors, CHD risk increased from 1–30 times as exertional risk factors determined by ETT (e.g., 0.1 mV ST depression during recovery, exercise duration <6 minutes) increased from 1 to any 3 exertional risk factors [10]. However, in those without any conventional risk factors, exercise testing did not add anything to risk assessment.

   The difficulty with ETT for risk assessment is that both physicians and patients do not yet view ETT as risk assessment but as diagnosis. People without CHD may develop undue fear knowing that their ST segments depress with exercise. In screening and risk assessment, one should adhere to Hippocrates' adage, "Above all else, do no harm." The potential harm with a positive ETT is considerable and may result in cardiac cripples and fear in healthy people.

   ETT is also quite expensive for a screening test. Routine ETTs cost from $150–250. The use of ETT even in asymptomatic people at high risk would lead to considerable expense. Furthermore, the cost of evaluating the large number of false-positives that would result from such a screening program would be more than the cost of the ETT screening program itself.

B. Early intervention [11].
The main reason that screening for CHD cannot be recommended is that there is no known intervention that can be applied in the asymptomatic individual that will improve outcome. The discovery of asymptomatic CHD should not

lead to any treatment such as coronary bypass surgery or beta-blocker therapy unless the patient is on a research protocol to determine the effect of such therapy compared to controls. This lack of an effective treatment in asymptomatic people with CHD is the main reason that screening for CHD has not been recommended by others analyzing this problem, such as the Canadian Task Force on the Periodic Health Exam and the report on screening by Frame and Carlson [12].

Although finding asymptomatic CHD may give incentive to people to reduce risk factors, the time and expense of screening would be perhaps more appropriately applied to efforts to reduce risk factors in everyone. Smoking should be discontinued for many health reasons, whether CHD is present or not. Likewise, hypertension should be identified and controlled for reasons outlined in Chap. 72. As discussed in Chap. 73, treatment of hyperlipidemia should be extended to all people with unfavorable lipid levels and not just those with known CHD. Lastly, the effectiveness or risk-factor reduction in people with established CHD is less hopeful than in those without CHD, as coronary lesions are often too advanced. Smoking cessation, however, does improve outcome in survivals of an MI, and this will likely benefit those with CHD present.

IV. Recommendations

A. Primary prevention. Primary prevention of CHD is recommended and should focus on risk factor identification and reduction.

1. Discontinue smoking.
2. Control hypertension.
3. Reduce total cholesterol-HDL ratio.
4. Discontinue oral contraceptives in smokers and women over 35.
5. Promote weight reduction in the obese.
6. Encourage regular exercise.

B. Early detection. Screening for CHD is not recommended in the periodic health exam.

1. There is no sufficiently accurate screening test.
2. Treatment in the asymptomatic stage is not known to be beneficial.

References

1. Diamond, G. A., and Forrester, J. S. Analysis of probability as an aid in the clinical diagnosis of coronary-artery disease. *N. Engl. J. Med.* 300(24):1350, 1979. *Uses incidence of CHD by age, sex, and symptoms to determine the predictive value of four tests: ETT, cardioxymography, thallium scintigraphy, and cardiac fluoroscopy.*
2. Gordon, T. Cardiovascular risk factors in women. *Prac. Cardiol.* 5:137, 1979. *Review of Framingham study.*
3. Kannel, W. B. Some lessons in cardiovascular epidemiology from Framingham. *Am. J. Cardiol.* 37(2):269, 1976. *Quantifies the risk of cardiovascular disease with risk factors of varying degrees and combinations.*
4. Stallones, R. A. The rise and fall of ischemic heart disease. *Sci. Am.* 243:53, 1980. *An interesting and well-written analysis of the possible reasons for the decline in CHD in the United States.*
5. Brittain, E. Probability of coronary heart disease developing. *West. J. Med.* 136(1):86, 1982. *Tables for calculating CHD risk. Based on the Framingham study.*
6. Multifactorial trial in the prevention of coronary heart disease: 3. Incidence and mortality results. *Eur. Heart J.* 4(3):141, 1983. *A randomized trial of risk-factor prevention groups in the general population. No reduction of CHD was found.*
7. Stamler, J. Primary prevention of coronary heart disease; the last 20 years. *Am. J. Cardiol.* 47(3):772, 1981. *Describes the progress of CHD prevention and what is left to be done.*
8. Hubert, H. B., et al. Obesity as an independent risk factor for cardiovascular disease: A 26 year followup of participants in the Framingham Heart Study. *Circulation* 67:968, 1983. *Obesity found as an independent risk factor for CHD.*
9. Froelicher, V. F., and Maron, D. Exercise testing and ancillary techniques to screen for coronary heart disease. *Prog. Cardiovasc. Dis.* 24(3):261, 1981. *Excellent review of screening tests for CHD, concentrating on exercise testing.*
10. Bruce, R. A., De Rouen, T. A., and Hossack, K. F. Value of maximal exercise tests in risk assessment of primary coronary heart disease events in healthy men. Five years' experience of the Seattle Heart Watch Study. *Am. J. Cardiol.* 46(3):371, 1980. *Study of symptom-limited exercise testing as a part of CHD risk factor profiling.*
11. Olson, R. E. Mass intervention vs. screening and selection intervention for the prevention of coronary heart disease. *J.A.M.A.* 255(16):2204, 1986. *A well-written commentary sum-*

marizing the problems in the prevention of CHD and arguing for screening and intervention in those at high risk.

12. Frame, P. S. A critical review of adult health maintenance. Part 1: Prevention of atherosclerotic diseases. *J. Fam. Pract.* 22(4):341, 1986. *An update of the original Frame and Carlson report on screening. Screening for CHD is not recommended, but screening for and treatment of risk factors are.*
13. Steering Committee of the Physicians' Health Study Research Group. Preliminary report: Findings from the aspirin component of the ongoing Physicians' Health Study. *N. Engl. J. Med.* 318:262, 1988. *A placebo-controlled trial that shows that aspirin reduced the incidence of coronary events.*
14. Grundy, S. M., et al. Cardiovascular and risk factor evaluation of healthy American adults. A statement for physicians by an ad hoc committee appointed by the Steering Committee, American Heart Association. *Circulation,* 75:1340A, 1987. *An in-depth discussion of risk factor screening from the AHA. The recommendations are more extensive than those of this chapter (e.g., ECG, chest x ray).*

72 Hypertension

Steven D. Rose

I. The problem

A. Definition. Hypertension, or high blood pressure, is conceptually defined as blood pressure high enough to lead to morbidity and mortality not seen as frequently with lower levels of blood pressure.

Despite consensus on the significant health risks attending elevation of blood pressure, controversy exists concerning the specific "cut off" blood pressure measurement that defines hypertension. Not only has the blood pressure value defining hypertension not been clearly established, but the time and place that blood pressure measurements should be taken has not been agreed on. This chapter defines hypertension from the therapeutic point of view—that is, the level of diastolic blood pressure measured at a given time and place during the day at which one should initiate treatment to improve survival and decrease morbidity. Thus, our working definition of hypertension will be a diastolic blood pressure (DBP) measured above 90 mm Hg on three separate occasions at the physician's office.

This working definition is based on the results of recent studies demonstrating benefit with treatment [1–3]. The Hypertension Detection and Follow-up Program (HDFP) found that treatment reduced significantly the 5-year mortality from all causes (i.e., total mortality) in patients with average diastolic blood pressures above 90 mm Hg at entry into the study [1, 2]. A similar trial in Australia found benefit from treatment at DBPs above 95 mm Hg; people in the 90–95 mm Hg range were not studied [3]. There have been no studies that examine the effect of therapy on DBPs below 90 mm Hg. Systolic blood pressure (SBP) has unfortunately not yet been studied in a therapeutic trial, despite a strong correlation of increased SBP with mortality and morbidity. However, most authorities would define a significantly elevated SBP as one above 160 mm Hg. The Systolic Hypertension in the Elderly Project (SHEP) is currently studying this problem.

Numerically, then, hypertension is a blood pressure over 160/95. Pressures under 140/90 may be considered normal. Defining hypertension based on the decision to treat with levels of 140–160/90–95 varies for each individual, as the prognosis of elevated blood pressures at any levels varies with cardiovascular risk factors that may occur with hypertension, such as age, male sex, high serum cholesterol, diabetes, smoking, and family history of heart disease.

B. Description. Hypertension is simply high blood pressure. Its importance, however, is as a part of diseases to which it appears to contribute. Hypertension is a major risk factor for the development of the major killers in Western countries: coronary heart disease and stroke. Hypertension can also lead to renal failure and congestive heart failure. Uncontrolled hypertension lowers life expectancy significantly; the severity of the effects of elevated blood pressure are related directly to the blood pressure level [4].

The vast majority of hypertension is essential hypertension, where the cause is unknown. Although this large group may be heterogeneous with many different but as yet undiscovered causes, it was in this group that mortality was decreased with treatment. The other forms of hypertension are fairly rare.

Secondary hypertension due to renal causes (parenchymal and renovascular), endocrine causes (Cushing's syndrome, primary aldosteronism, pheochromocytoma), and other causes (oral contraceptives, coarctation of the aorta) occur in 10–15% of hypertensives in referral centers. With the exception of oral contraceptives, secondary hypertension is much rarer in the primary care setting. Surgically reversible hypertension is even rarer, forming less than 1% of hypertensives in one large referral center [5].

C. Epidemiology and risk factors. Elevated blood pressure is one of the most common life-threatening chronic diseases in the United States. About 15% of the American population has blood pressure above 160/95 mm Hg, and approximately twice that many have blood pressure greater than 140/90 mm Hg, thus increasing the risk of serious hypertensive complications [4, 6]. The prevalence is similar for males and females but is twice as prevalent in the black population as in the white. The majority of hypertension is mild hypertension where the DBP is between 90 mm Hg and 104 mm Hg. In the HDFP, 70% of hypertensive patients were in this range. One half of these mild hypertensives were in the 90 mm Hg–95 mm Hg category, and 15% were in the 100 mm Hg–104 mm Hg group [2].

The most important risk factor known for the development of hypertension is inheritance [6]. From the study on monozygotic and dizygotic twins [7], it has been estimated that the genetic contribution to the variance of blood pressure is 64% for DBP and 82% for SPB, a finding that emphasizes the importance of the family history in the periodic health examination and the need to aggressively screen first-degree relatives and siblings of known patients with hypertension.

Excessive salt intake and obesity appear to be the most important environmental determinants of hypertension and are discussed below.

II. Primary prevention

A. Methods. The primary preventive measures examined are salt restriction and, for those 15% or more overweight, weight reduction.

1. **Salt restriction.** When one reads articles on salt restriction, one can be easily confused when salt is alternately measured in terms of grams of salt, grams of sodium, and milliequivalents (mEq) of sodium. Sodium chloride, or salt, is made up of 23 parts sodium to 35.5 parts of chloride (the respective atomic weights of each element). That is, sodium makes up somewhat less than 40% of salt. Thus, when one orders a 4-gm sodium diet, one gets a 10-gm salt diet. One mEq of sodium equals 23 mg of sodium, or 58.5 mg of salt.

   The normal American diet averages about 10–12 gm of salt/day, with a wide range from under 3 gm to over 20 gm. This average 10–12 gm of salt corresponds to 4–5 gm of sodium, and 170–200 mEq of sodium. It is estimated that one third of this is due to salt added to food, so a no-added salt diet may reduce the normal intake to 6.5–8.0 gm of salt. About 3 gm of this salt is present naturally in food, and 46 gm occur with processing of foods. Thus, by restricting the salt shaker and avoiding high-salt foods, one can achieve considerable salt restriction without specially prepared "diet" foods or a cardboard diet. The degree of salt restriction will vary for each person, depending on the risk (family history of hypertension), the presence of other cardiovascular risk factors (hypercholesterolemia, smoking, glucose intolerance, family history of heart disease), and the presence of coronary disease.

   People should be encouraged to change their dietary habits gradually to better ensure compliance with measures to limit salt intake and reduce weight. People who salt their food before tasting it should be encouraged to try tasting first; eventually, the salt shaker will be used less and less. People can be made aware of foods extremely high in salt, both the obvious (potato chips, pretzels, peanuts) and the not-so-obvious (dill pickles, processed foods, frozen dinners, and many restaurant foods, especially fast food and Chinese). Label reading and cooking with spices other than salt should be encouraged. Diet techniques and lists of sodium content in common foods are readily available [3].

2. **Weight reduction.** The technique of weight reduction is beyond the scope of this chapter. Generally, calorie restriction should be combined with an exercise program. Diets should be permanent changes in life-style instead of short-term, rapid weight-loss diets. Success is seen when diet is combined with behavior modification or peer reinforcement, as in organizations such as Weight Watchers or Overeaters Anonymous.

B. Justification

1. **Effectiveness**

   a. **Salt restriction.** There is some suggestive but inconclusive evidence that salt restriction will prevent the development of hypertension [9, 10]. Epidemiologic studies show that cultural groups with diets low in salt do not show an elevation of blood pressure with advancing age as do cultures that consume a large amount of salt. This observation is also true for nonindustrialized societies with high-sodium diets, indicating that the Western life-style and other factors that are absent in these primitive high-salt cultures are not primarily responsible. In addition, populations with low-sodium diets show an elevation of blood pressure when switched to high-sodium diets, indicating that genetic differences are also not completely responsible. Many people in our culture can lower their blood pressure with salt restriction [11]. On the other hand, many people cannot lower their blood pressure, and some individuals' blood pressures increase with salt restriction. Cross-cultural studies are criticized for not defining hypertension, not measuring sodium excretion or intake, and not taking into account many cultural differences other than sodium intake. Futhermore, some cultural differences in salt intake appear to occur at extremes not seen in American society (ranging from < 1 gm to over 18 gm/day). Most studies within cultures have not found salt intake to correlate with blood pressure. Those that do find a correlation find it to be extremely slight [10]. Thus, the salt theory is not yet proved or disproved. Considering the evidence on the development of hypertension in cultures with high-sodium diets, the fact that at least some people (over 50%) respond to moderate salt restriction and the benign nature of such restriction in those who comply, physicians may recommend salt restriction with the caveat to patients that there is no guarantee of benefit.

b. **Weight reduction.** Obesity is proposed as a predisposing factor for hypertension. A correlation between body weight and blood pressure has been shown, although it is slight and the individual variations are great. Unfortunately, no studies have yet taken into account the use of diet pills, which may elevate blood pressure. There has been no study of normotensive obese people to show that weight reduction prevents the development of hypertension. However, studies have shown that hypertensives who are 15% overweight can lower their blood pressure with weight loss alone, even if ideal weight is not obtained [12, 13].

2. **Risks or side effects.** The major concern of salt and calorie restriction is the lowering of the quality of life by denying life's pleasures. No doubt some lives can be made miserable by strict dietary changes, and thus one has to be moderate. Many people can happily adapt to restricted diets. Salt restriction is particularly easy to adapt to when other spices are substituted and new ways of cooking are found. As of now, there are no known medical risks of sodium restriction down to the recommended 70–80 mEq/day. Cultures presently exist living on less than 70 mEq of sodium/day, and normal active people have been shown to tolerate extreme restriction to less than 10 mEq/day without apparent untoward consequences.

3. **Costs.** Cost of sodium restriction itself is nothing. The major cost is in counseling and educating people. Weight reduction costs vary considerably, from negligible to considerable, if behavior modification and extensive counseling are needed.

4. **Acceptability.** Some people will adapt to these measures easily, and some will never adapt. As a large fraction will find them acceptable, one should offer these measures and give everyone who is at risk a chance, being more aggressive only with those with the highest risk, such as offspring of hypertensive patients.

III. Secondary prevention

A. Early detection

1. Methods

a. **Performance.** The measurement of blood pressure by sphygmomanometry is simple, but many mistakes are made. All practitioners should be familiar with the American Heart Association (AHA) Committee Report on the recommendations for blood pressure measurements [14]. Important points of this report and common mistakes are described here.

The patient should be seated comfortably with the forearm supported at heart level. Although blood pressure may not differ much in the standing, sitting, or supine positions, it does differ somewhat; the sitting position is usually the most convenient position and is the position used in the studies showing benefit from treatment. More important, one should assure that the arm is at heart level (approximately at the fourth intercostal space at the sternum). Raising the arm will falsely lower the reading, while lowering the arm will falsely raise it. Errors due to arm position may result in measurement errors as high as 10 mm Hg.

A very common error is made by using a cuff that is too small for the subject's arm. The length of the bladder of the blood pressure cuff should ideally be 80% of the circumference of the arm. To allow standard sizes of cuffs to fit the many differently sized arms one sees in practice, the AHA report recommends that the bladder length be at least 75% of the circumference of the arm. This should allow for a measurement error of no more than 5%. Table 72–1 gives the length and appropriate arm circumference for a variety of standard cuffs. Note that the standard adult cuff will not fit many adult arms, and its use may result in an overestimation of blood pressure by as much as 30–40 mm Hg. Note also that many cuffs have a range marked on them by a line that is inaccurate, and thus the cuff should be re-marked [15]. Ideally, one should avoid cuffs that overlap

Table 72-1. Standard cuff measurements

Arm circumference (cm)	Cuff name	Bladder length (cm)	Bladder width (cm)
5–7.5	Newborn	5	3
7.5–13	Infant	8	5
13–20	Child	13	8
17–26	Small adult	17	11
24–32	Adult	24	13
32–42	Large adult	32	17
42–50	Thigh	42	20

Source: Adapted from W. M. Kirkendall, et al. Recommendations for human blood pressure determination by sphygmomanometers. *Circulation* 62(5):1146A, 1980.

or encircle more than 100% of the arm circumference. However, it has not been shown that oversized cuffs give falsely low blood pressures. As for the width of the bladder, it should be one half of the length.

To measure blood pressure, the radial pulse is palpated and the cuff is inflated to about 30 mm Hg above the disappearance of the pulse. Not palpating the pulse disappearance may occasionally result in an underestimation of the systolic blood pressure by as much as 40 mm Hg. This error results from the auscultatory gap, a temporary diappearance of sounds in the pressure ranges between the SBP and DBP. One should be sure that the stethoscope is over the brachial artery, the location of which was found previously by palpation. The pressure is then released at about 2–3 mm Hg/second. SBP is noted when initial tapping sounds are heard. The DBP is measured in adults by the disappearance of the sounds, a point called phase V. Recommendations have swung back and forth as to whether to use phase IV, the muffling of sounds, or phase V. Again referring to the HDFP and other studies, phase V was used to determine the DBP. Thus, the practitioner should use the same (in children, however, phase IV is recommended). One should also be careful not to exert too much pressure with the stethoscope on the artery as this will produce sounds below the true DBP.

The muffling of sounds usually occurs at a cuff pressure 5–10 mm Hg higher than the directly measured intra-arterial DBP. The disappearance of sounds occurs at cuff pressures very near the true DBP. Important exceptions include measurements in infants, children, and adults with hyperkinetic states, such as hyperthyroidism, aortic insufficiency, and after exercise. In these cases, the sounds may well disappear well below the DBP and muffling may be the more accurate reading. In these situations then, all three pressures should be recorded (e.g., 160/90/40) with the pressure at the muffling used as the DBP.

There is also a tendency for examiners to not write down accurately the pressures they see on the manometer. Rounding off to even numbers leads to insignificant errors, but rounding off to 0's or 5's (e.g., to 160/90 when the reading is 163/92) is to be avoided. Furthermore, there is a tendency for physicians to round consistently downward, perhaps motivated by a wish for the patient to be well or to avoid dealing with abnormal results. DBPs of 90–95 often become 85–90 by this systematic error.

To get representative readings, it is helpful to note factors that may affect blood pressure, such as extreme anxiety, emotional turmoil, and especially pain. Although blood pressures may be elevated by the mere presence of a physician, these measurements are still representative because this blood pressure probably accompanies the many everyday stresses that people experience.

Serial readings on either different days or on the same visit help to establish a representative mean blood pressure reading. The HDFP identified their subjects by finding an initial DBP above 95 mm Hg and then an average greater than 90 mm Hg of two subsequent readings.

Home blood pressure recordings are interesting but of limited use. Home blood pressures are usually lower than office blood pressures, but again it is the office blood pressure that has been used in the studies. If home blood pressures were

Table 72-2. Common mistakes in the measurement of blood pressure

Cuff size too small
Arm position not at heart level
Muffling of sounds used instead of disappearance
Equipment not serviced annually
Tendency to read abnormal readings as normal

used in these studies, one may have found that the level of DBP to treat was as low as 80 mm Hg.

Manometers should be serviced annually. The air vent and filter at the top of the mercury manometer tube needs service, as dirt will cause the mercury to respond slowly to decreasing cuff pressures during measurement. Aneroid manometers need calibration annually, and this can be done against a functional mercury manometer.

Attention to the common errors listed in Table 72-2 will result in reliable blood pressure readings. The therapeutic trials are quite careful to avoid these mistakes. For the practitioner to achieve the same benefit (reduction of mortality) with the least amount of harm (overdiagnosis), he or she must also adhere to these easily achievable standards.

b. **Screening interval.** There are no data indicating the optimum screening interval. Since the complications of hypertension are related to the degree and duration of elevated blood pressure, blood pressure should be measured routinely in all adult patients by sphygmomanometry at least every 1–2 years. More frequent measurements would be made in those with high "normal" pressures or with pressures from 140–160/90–95.

c. **Interpretation.** At least three separate blood pressure measurements should be taken to accurately assess the patient for existing hypertension. If the average of the three DBP measurements is greater than 90 mm Hg or the average of the SBP measurements is greater than 160 mm Hg, the patient is considered to have hypertension.

d. **Population.** The population to be screened is all adults. For the office practitioner, it is good policy to take blood pressures on all patients.

2. **Justification.** Hypertension is defined, practically speaking, by sphygmomanometry, and thus the test is 100% sensitive and specific when used correctly as discussed above. There are no medical risks or side effects, the cost is negligible, and acceptability is high.

B. Early intervention

1. Methods

a. **Nonpharmacologic.** The major nondrug interventions are sodium restriction and weight reduction. Other modalities include exercise, biofeedback, and relaxation techniques. Methods of sodium restriction and weight reduction were discussed extensively under primary prevention (see **II.A 1.** and **II.A.2**).

Aerobic exercise can both aid in weight reduction and help bring down blood pressure. A training effect can be seen with 20–30 minutes of aerobic exercise (brisk walking, jogging, swimming, bicycling) 3–4 times a week. The heart rate should achieve 70% of maximum predicted (70% of 220 minus a person's age). One effective trial employed 60-minute workouts of walking and jogging to 70–80% of maximum heart rate. Hypertensive patients should start exercise programs gradually. A treadmill test may be helpful in assessing a person's maximum heart rate and blood pressure response to exercise. Such a test will help the patient judge the degree of exercise that he or she should achieve during workouts.

Behavior modification can range from simply identifying common situations resulting in stress to formal biofeedback programs. Health care providers should be aware of the programs available in the community. Stress management sessions are often carried out in group sessions. Just realizing that one predictably has stress (e.g., automobile driving, family arguments involving power plays) and employing basic stress reduction techniques can reduce a considerable amount of stress.

Alcohol consumption should be kept moderate. Too much daily alcohol may elevate blood pressure. Hypertensive patients should be not only advised against heavy alcohol consumption but also told what specific amounts are worrisome. Daily alcohol should not exceed 2 oz, which corresponds to 4 12-oz beers, 16 oz of wine, and 4 oz of 100-proof liquor.

It should be remembered that patients on nonpharmacologic therapy should be followed as closely as those on drugs for blood pressure response. These therapies should also not be abandoned when drug therapy is initiated.

b. Pharmacologic. Drug therapy for hypertension is usually straightforward. The stepped-care approach is still alive and well in modified form [10, 17]. After all, the best studies showing benefit from treatment used a stepped-care approach.

The first drug is usually a diuretic, although often a beta blocker is used first. For diuretics, lower doses than used previously are recommended. For example, chlorthalidone is started at 12.5 mg/day and should not exceed 50 mg/day. Hydrochlorthiazide has been used in 50–100-mg or even 200-mg doses. It is best to start with 12.5–25.0 mg and not go much higher than 50 mg, as higher doses do not appear to be more effective and only increase side effects. If the blood pressure cannot be controlled on a low dose of a diuretic, a second drug should be employed.

The second drug can be a beta blocker or a diuretic, if that was not the first drug. Reserpine at 0.1 mg/day was used quite a bit in the HDFP trial. Calcium channel blockers and angiotensin-converting enzyme inhibitors are also now in use. Further guidelines for drug therapy can be found elsewhere, as in the Joint National Committee Report [16] and other references [17].

2. Justification

a. Nonpharmacologic. In a number of trials, salt restriction has been shown to lower blood pressure in hypertensive patients. The effectiveness of salt restriction is variable, and while many will not respond, the majority of patients will benefit. Additionally, it appears that salt restriction will allow antihypertensive drugs to be more effective at lower doses and will also diminish the amount of potassium loss associated with diuretics.

Weight reduction has also been associated with lowering of blood pressure, and this effect is independent from and additive to salt restriction. The major problem is that long-term weight reduction is exceedingly difficult, with many failures. Nevertheless, patients should be advised to lose weight, as some, albeit few, will be able to comply.

Modest but important blood pressure drops have been demonstrated from exercise programs. A randomized trial using 60-minute workouts of walking and jogging to 70–80% of maximum heart rate (as determined on a treadmill exam) for 16 weeks showed a 7 mm drop in DBP, while nonexercising controls had an average 3 mm rise. Systolic blood pressure dropped 12 mm compared to 7 mm in controls.

Behavioral therapy has shown long-term reductions in blood pressure. Although randomized trials have not yet been conducted, these techniques are very likely helpful, impose little risk, and likely have other health benefits as well.

b. Pharmacologic. The HDFP and other trials [1–3] have shown conclusively that pharmacologic treatment of hypertension will reduce morbidity and mortality. As hypertension is an asymptomatic disease until complications such as stroke and heart failure appear, early treatment to prevent these complications is more beneficial than treatment after complications (symptoms) have started.

One should not be misled by the results of the Multiple Risk Factor Intervention Trial (MRFIT) [18] that suggest to some that treatment of hypertensive patients is not that beneficial. This trial randomized men at high risk for CHD into a special intervention group (SI) and a usual care group (UC). The SI group had fairly aggressive treatment and counseling to reduce hypertension, smoking, and serum cholesterol. The results were negative, largely due to the unexpected lowering of CHD risk factors and low mortality in the UC or control group. In looking for an explanation for the negative results, a subgroup was found for which treatment was associated with a poor outcome. Many have cited this group of hypertensive men with ECG changes as evidence that diuretic treatment may be harmful. This is fallacious reasoning as the trial was never designed to look at this group specifically. If one looks at enough subgroups for differences, one will find a "significant" difference by chance eventually. This is a valid method to generate hypotheses, but not to prove them. In fact, this group has been looked at in other trials, and the MRFIT results were not reproduced, indicating that the poor outcome in the MRFIT was a chance finding.

c. **Risks and side effects** [16, 17]. The side effects of the drugs used to treat hypertension are considerable. The thiazide diuretics can lead to hypokalemia, hyperuricemia, hyperlipidemia, glucose intolerance, rashes, and allergic disorders. The beta blockers can lead to drowsiness, lethargy, and bronchospasm.

Many of the agents appear to cause decreased sexual activity and impotence. On the other hand, most patients can find a compatible drug regimen with acceptable or minimal side effects. It is important that enough people tolerated drugs well enough in the drug trials to show an overall decrease in morbidity and mortality.

d. **Costs.** Costs for drugs vary considerably depending on the regimen. A low-dose diuretic may cost $7–15/month. Combined with a beta blocker, prices range from $15–35/month. More expensive regimens can run well over $50/month.

e. **Acceptability.** Although acceptable to many, the biggest problem with drug therapy for hypertension is noncompliance. People may not take the medicine because of lack of motivation or unwanted side effects. Even without any side effects, it is hard to get people to take the medicine for a disease that has no symptoms. Physicians should take this not as an argument to discontinue treatment, but as a way to identify noncompliers (lack of drug effect) and to attempt to increase compliance.

IV. Recommendations

A. Primary prevention

1. For the general public, there are no solid recommendations specifically to reduce the risk of the development of hypertension.
2. For those at risk—family history of hypertension, high normal blood pressures, and risk factors for the development of coronary heart disease—salt restriction and weight reduction are prudent recommendations.

B. Secondary prevention

1. **Early detection.** Blood pressure measurement by sphygmomanometry should be taken every 1–2 years.
2. **Early intervention.** Weight reduction, exercise, salt restriction, and antihypertensive drugs are recommended.

References

1. Hypertension Detection and Follow-up Program Cooperative Group. Five-year findings of the hypertension detection and follow-up program. I. Reduction in mortality of persons with high blood pressure, including mild hypertension. *J.A.M.A.* 242(23):2562, 1979. *An important randomized trial showing a reduction in total mortality by treating hypertension, including mild hypertension.*
2. Hypertension Detection and Follow-up Program Cooperative Group. Five-year findings of the hypertension detection and follow-up program. III. Reduction in stroke incidence among persons with high blood pressure. *J.A.M.A.* 247(5):633, 1982. *Found a reduction of stroke mortality in all race/sex subgroups of the stepped care group.*
3. The Australian therapeutic trial in mild hypertension. Report by the Management Committee. *Lancet* 1(8181):1261, 1980. *A double-blind placebo trial; mortality reduced in those treated for DBP ranging from 95 mm Hg–110 mm Hg.*
4. Kannel, W. B., Schwartz, M. J., and McNamara, P. M. Blood pressure and risk of coronary heart disease: The Framingham Study. *Dis. Chest* 56(1):43, 1969. *Reviews the relationship of the level of blood pressure to the subsequent development in 14 years of coronary heart disease.*
5. Tucker, R. M., and LaBarthe, D. R. Frequency of surgical treatment for hypertension in adults at the Mayo Clinic from 1973 through 1975. *Mayo Clin. Proc.* 52(9):549, 1977. *Review of surgically remediable hypertension at the Mayo Clinic.*
6. Borhani, N. O. Prevention of death and morbidity associated with hypertension in the community: A ten-year appraisal, 1972 to 1982. *Heart Lung* 11(1):48, 1982. *Review of the epidemiology of hypertension and changes occurring in the last 10 years.*
7. Borhani, N. O., et al. Genetic variance in blood pressure. *Acta Genet. Med. Gemellol.* 25:137, 1976. *The National Heart and Lung Institute study of 514 monozygotic and dizygotic twins, showing that blood pressure levels are genetically controlled to a considerable extent.*

8. Salt and high blood pressure. *Consumer Rep.* 44(3):147, 1979. *A discussion written in lay terms on how to avoid salty foods.*
9. Freis, E. D. Salt, volume and the prevention of hypertension. *Circulation* 53(4):589, 1976. *Review of evidence supporting salt restrictions as preventing the development of hypertension.*
10. Langford, H. G. Electrolyte intake, electrolyte excretion, and hypertension. *Heart Lung* 10(2):269, 1981. *A concise review of evidence for and against salt and potassium correlating with blood pressure.*
11. MacGregor, G. A., et al. Double-blind randomized crossover trial of moderate sodium restriction in essential hypertension. *Lancet* 1(8268):351, 1982. *Demonstrates effectiveness of moderate salt restriction in hypertensives.*
12. Sims, E. A., and Berchtold, P. Obesity and hypertension: Mechanisms and implications for management. *J.A.M.A.* 247(1):49, 1982. *A review of the evidence linking obesity and hypertension, focusing on management, not prevention.*
13. Stamler, J., et al. Prevention and control of hypertension by nutritional-hygienic means. Long term experience of the Chicago Coronary Prevention Evaluation Program. *J.A.M.A.* 243(18):1819, 1980. *Weight reduction in coronary-prone men resulted in blood pressure reduction.*
14. Kirkendall, W. M., et al. Recommendations for human blood pressure determination by sphygmomanometers. *Circulation* 62(5):1146A, 1980. *The AHA recommendations for correct technique of blood pressure measurement.*
15. Manning, D. M. Avoiding sphygmomanometer-cuff "hypertension" [letter]. *N. Engl. J. Med.* 306(2):108, 1982. *Points out that manufacturers' labeled range of cuff for arm size is often inaccurate in that the bladder may not surround at least 75% of the arm.*
16. The 1984 report of the Joint National Committee on Detection, Evaluation, and Treatment of High Blood Pressure. *Arch. Intern. Med.* 144:1045, 1984. *Well-written summary on the various methods used to control hypertension.*
17. Kaplan, N. M. Treatment of Hypertension: Drug Therapy. In *Clinical Hypertension* (4th ed.). Baltimore: Williams & Wilkins, 1986. Pp. 180–272. *An excellent review of the drugs and discussion of a modified stepped care/substitution approach.*
18. Multiple Risk Factor Intervention Trial Research Group. Multiple risk factor intervention trial: Risk factor changes and mortality results. *J.A.M.A.* 248(12):1465, 1982. *The well-known MRFIT trial.*

73 Hyperlipidemia

Steven D. Rose

I. Description. Hyperlipidemia represents a variety of disorders with multiple causes. This chapter focuses on the most common hyperlipidemias that relate to the development of coronary heart disease (CHD).

A. Hypercholesterolemia. Hypercholesterolemia is a very common finding in the United States. How common it is depends on the definition. Severe familial hypercholesterolemia with xanthomas is quite rare; the Framingham study found 6 cases in 5127 men. They all had serum cholesterol levels greater than 400 mg/dl and a strong family history of premature CHD, and all 6 died before the age of 50 [1]. The more common acquired mild hypercholesterolemia is asymptomatic and important because of its strong association with premature CHD. Based on the bell-shaped distribution of serum cholesterols in the United States, hypercholesterolemia is commonly defined as a serum cholesterol above 265 mg/dl. The prevalence by this definition is about 1 in 20 people, or 5%. More recently, opinion has settled on >240 mg/dl, which includes 25% of the U.S. population [27].

However, if one looks at the world distribution of serum cholesterols, one would find most of the United States population at the high end, making the majority of adult Americans hypercholesterolemic. A more functional definition of this disease is a serum cholesterol above a level where there is an increased risk for premature CHD. Like blood pressure, there is no cut-off level; the risk of CHD drops as the serum cholesterol drops [2]. It appears, however, that an acceptable minimal risk is seen somewhere between 180–200 mg/dl [1, 3]. This would make most adults in the United States hypercholesterolemic, making this disease, like CHD, a major public health problem.

Like hypertension, mild hypercholesterolemia has a long asymptomatic period and is not dangerous by itself but because of what it leads to—premature CHD. Identification and treatment of hypercholesterolemia is an attempt to prevent CHD, the most common cause of death in this country. The risk of CHD increases with the level of total cholesterol and with the number and extent of associated CHD risk factors. It is to be noted that the majority of people with mild hypercholesterolemia do not develop CHD but are only at increased risk. This is analogous to many known risk factors of disease, such as smoking with lung cancer.

Hypercholesterolemia is also secondary to a number of diseases, which are listed in Table 73-1.

B. High density lipoprotein (HDL). This fraction of cholesterol is important because the level correlates more strongly with CHD than total serum cholesterol [4]. In Norway, with 6595 young males, NDL levels made a threefold greater contribution to CHD risk than low density lipoprotein (LDL), a measure of cholesterol [5]. However, the association is inverse, with the CHD risk increasing as the HDL decreases. Currently, there are no clear definitions of high, normal, or low HDL levels, yet a utilitarian approach could be as described above for hypercholesterolemia. American values commonly vary between 30 mg/dl and 80 mg/dl. CHD risk appears to be high at levels below 45 mg/dl, intermediate at 45–65 mg/dl, and low at greater than 65 mg/dl [6, 7].

As with other lipids, CHD risk varies at each level depending on other CHD risk factors. A table of multipliers for CHD risk with HDL levels is given in Table 73-2 from the Framingham study [7]. This table is based on men and women 50 years and older but is probably applicable at all ages. Noteworthy is that the total serum cholesterol had no relationship with CHD risk in the older group at Framingham, whereas LDL did weakly and HDL did quite markedly.

The lipid parameter that may correlate the most with CHD risk is the ratio of either total cholesterol or LDL to HDL. In screening 572 asymptomatic men in the Air Force, 132 men had a positive exercise treadmill test. Of these, 14 of 16 men (89%) found to have significant CHD by angiography had a cholesterol-HDL ratio greater than 6 [8].

Table 73-1. Conditions associated with secondary hypercholesterolemia

Hyperthyroidism
Nephrotic syndrome
Acute intermittent porphyria
Dysglobulinemia
Obstructive liver disease
Antihypertensive medicines (e.g., thiazides, propranolol)
Androgenic steroids
Uncontrolled diabetes mellitus

Table 73-2. Cardiovascular risk multipliers for high density lipoprotein (HDL)

HDL (mg/dl)	Men	Women
30	1.82	
35	1.49	
40	1.22	1.94
45	1.00	1.55
50	0.82	1.25
55	0.67	1.00
60	0.55	0.80
65	0.45	0.64
70		0.52

Source: Reproduced, with permission, from: W. Kannel, W. Castelli, and T. Gordon. Cholesterol in the prediction of atherosclerotic disease: New perspectives based on the Framingham study. *Ann. Intern. Med.* 1979; 90(1):85.

Only 4 of the other 102 (4%) with angiographically normal coronary arteries had a ratio greater than 6. Of 14 men with CHD but less than 50% stenosis, 4 had a ratio greater than 6. In this group of young asymptomatic men with positive stress tests and a prevalence of disease of 12%, the sensitivity of the ratio for significant CHD was 89%, and the predictive value of a positive test was 64%. The predictive value for any CHD was 82%, and the predictive value of a ratio less than 6 for no disease was greater than 98%.

C. Hypertriglyceridemia. Hypertriglyceridemia is common. Levels greater than 200 mg/dl are found in 10% of adults, and twice as frequently in males as in females. Although hypertriglyceridemia is associated with CHD, the relationship appears unimportant in the absence of hypercholesterolemia [1]. Elevated triglyceride levels and elevated very low density lipoproteins (VLDL, the major lipoprotein fraction that contains triglycerides) are not established as important risk factors for CHD.

Hypertriglyceridemia is typically asymptomatic. Besides CHD, this disease is associated with peripheral vascular disease, hyperuricemia, diabetes, alcoholism, and gout. Very high levels of triglycerides lead to eruptive xanthomas. The rare patient with levels greater than 1000 mg/dl may have lipemia retinalis and the complications of type V hyperlipoproteinemia (raised VLDL and chylomicrons), which are chiefly abdominal pain and pancreatitis. Treatment of this rare group with diet after symptoms have developed is quite effective. Diet and drug treatments of mild hypertriglyceridemia have no known effect except that they may simultaneously lower serum cholesterol.

II. Secondary prevention

A. Early assessment

1. Methods. The important screening tests are the serum total cholesterol and the HDL. These tests require a blood sample with the following precautions [9]:

a. Procedure

(1) The patient should be sitting. A recumbent position may decrease lipid levels as much as 12%. This effect is seen after only 5 minutes of recumbency.

(2) Do not draw samples after a myocardial infarction (MI). Cholesterol levels drop to a nadir 7–20 days after an MI. Samples should be delayed 2–3 months after infarction.

(3) Avoid prolonged venous occlusion, which may increase lipid levels as much as 22% after 5 minutes.

(4) Avoid hemolysis that falsely elevates cholesterol levels with widely used colorimetric methods for cholesterol determination.

(5) Check with the laboratory for collection requirements, as some lipid analyses require immediate storage of blood samples at 4 °C (ice water bath).
(6) Drawing blood directly into evacuated blood tubes is preferred to drawing into a syringe because the shorter procedure reduces the changes of hemolysis, and evaporation is prevented as the blood is not exposed to the air.
(7) The patient should be fasting. Actually, fasting has little effect on cholesterol levels as opposed to triglyceride levels, the determination of which requires a 12–14 hour fast. High levels of cholesterol on nonfasting casual specimens are probably accurate, but they may be inaccurate with grossly lipemic serum.
(8) Hyperbilirubinemia interferes with the widely used colorimetric methods.

It is best for physicians to check with their laboratories, as the method of analysis determines the accuracy in the face of interference by hyperbilirubinemia, hemolysis, and lipemic serum.

Serum cholesterol measurements can now be fairly accurately recorded with a fingerstick method. This method is advantageous in terms of both cost and quick feedback for patients.

b. Population. Given that a relatively high cholesterol is widely prevalent in the United States, a serum cholesterol should be obtained in all adults. As age increases, the relationship of serum cholesterol weakens and the effects of intervention lessen. It might be appropriate to not screen people over the ages of 65–70.

c. Interval. No solid recommendation for a screening interval can be given. As a general guideline, people at low risk for CHD and with previous low serum cholesterol levels would not need repeat measurements as often as those with other CHD risk factors or previously borderline or high cholesterol levels. Every 5 years may be reasonable for those at low risk, while those with borderline high levels may be screened annually. For those attempting to lower their cholesterol through diet or medicines, frequent determinations are needed not only for the assessment of treatment and risk, but also for feedback to the patient as a means to increase compliance.

2. Justification

a. Test characteristics. The screening tests recommended are a total cholesterol and an HDL level. Screening for hypertriglyceridemia is not justified in that it is not an independent risk factor for CHD. Actually, most hypertriglyceridemia is accompanied by low levels of HDL, a much more powerful CHD risk factor. Extreme hypertriglyceridemia leading to pancreatitis is too rare to screen for, and early detection in the asymptomatic period is not known to improve prognosis. There is no real debate that the level of total serum cholesterol is related to the development of CHD. This relationship has been consistently found in studies both within populations and across populations. The International Atherosclerosis Project, with over 23,000 autopsies in 14 countries, and Keyes' Five Year Study of 12,000 men in seven countries, showed a high correlation of the average serum cholesterol of each population with the occurrence of CHD. This same relationship is found when examining individuals in the United States. Population studies from Framingham, New York, Minnesota, and others show that the serum cholesterol is a strong independent risk factor for the development of CHD.

It is not clear that below a certain level of serum cholesterol the risk of CHD continues to diminish. In several studies in the United States, the incidence of CHD was actually higher in the group with the lowest 20% of serum cholesterols (roughly lower than 180 mg/dl) than in the next highest group (about 180–200 mg/dl). Furthermore, the association is not so strong in women as in men.

The association is less dramatic with increasing age but still holds, even in advanced ages. Because the Framingham study showed no relationship of serum cholesterol with the risk of CHD in people over the age of 60, many physicians mistakenly believe that lipid levels are unimportant in this age group.

More recent studies of the Framingham cohort have shown that lipoprotein fractions of the serum cholesterol, LDL, and HDL, correlate well with the development of CHD in all age groups, including people in their eighties [6, 7]. In fact, HDL appears to be the most powerful, single lipid measurement for the risk of CHD for all ages, male and female [4, 5]. Table 73-2 gives the relative risks, with levels of HDL less than 45 mg/dl being particularly risky.

The cholesterol-HDL ratio is relatively new, and unlike total cholesterol, has not been studied in many epidemiologic, animal, and human dietary studies. However, it has proved to be more predictive than total cholesterol, especially in the older age groups. With further research, tables of values with associated risk will be developed. For now, values over 6 carry an enormous risk of developing CHD.

b. **Costs.** Laboratories offer many different lipid tests, and the health care provider should check for the least costly way to get an HDL and a total cholesterol (or LDL). Chemistry panels such as the SMAC-20 cost from $10–20 and are the cheapest if they have been ordered for other reasons. However, as discussed in Chap. 70, these panels are not indicated in routine health care and are only occasionally ordered for other problems in patients under the age of 50. They should not be ordered for lipid determination alone. Many labs offer lipid panels that include a total cholesterol and HDL, but often include unnecessary tests such as a lipoprotein electrophoresis. These panels can be expensive if the electrophoresis is included ($15–30). An HDL and total cholesterol combination is offered by some labs for around $8–15. Fingerstick cholesterols are quite inexpensive. The reagent cost of the test should be about $1 with additional cost for the fingerstick and collection, all of which can be handled by the physician and the office personnel.

B. Early intervention

1. Methods

a. **Diet.** The serum cholesterol and HDL levels are interpreted here as CHD risk factors and not in the diagnosis of CHD. High levels of serum cholesterol (risk increases as levels increase over 200 mg/dl) and low levels of HDL (see Table 73-2) are indications for aggressive counseling for the reduction of reversible CHD risk factors. Smoking is extremely risky for anybody with a high cholesterol level. Likewise, high blood pressure should be well controlled with a goal of 140/90 or below (Chap. 72). Regular exercise as outlined in Chap. 65 will raise HDL levels and thus may decrease CHD risk. Moderate (2 oz/day) alcohol intake can also raise HDL levels, but note that the fraction of HDL raised with alcohol is not the one that correlates with CHD risk. Furthermore, it is not wise to recommend alcohol to people who do not drink. Total abstainers may have very good reasons not to drink, such as an inability to keep from drinking less than 2 oz/day. The health risks of excess alcohol far outweigh the dubious benefits of moderate alcohol intake.

For physicians accepting the validity of the diet-heart hypothesis, diet modification can be successful in many people. Although many recommend the low-fat diet for all Americans, we should perhaps be more aggressive with people with increasingly high levels of cholesterol and low levels of HDL. A 1% increase in serum cholesterol is associated with a 2.66% increase in the risk of CHD. Thus, at increasing levels of cholesterol, the absolute risk of CHD rises considerably.

For details on the diet, the reader should refer to the references [10, 11, 27]. Generally, people are to reduce fat, preferably to 20–25% of total calories. Since much fat is found in certain common animal food, the diet will reduce considerably the intake of beef, pork, and dairy products (other than nonfat dairy products). Complex carbohydrates such as starch, vegetables, and beans will become a larger percentage of the diet. Frying will give way to broiling and other methods where fat is reduced. For the fat that is consumed, vegetable fats (oils and margarines) are preferred over lard and butter.

Physicians are able to give these general guidelines, but to obtain optimum compliance other resources will be necessary. Although many motivated people can adapt for themselves with recommended reading and cookbooks, others will need (along with their family) comprehensive diet counseling by nutritionists, dietitians, or other nonphysician personnel. Resources in many communities can aid people in the techniques of the low-fat diet. However, physicians should avoid sending people to organizations that employ fad diets, drastic weight loss programs, and vegetarian or "health food" diets high in cheese, butter, other dairy products, and expensive but unnecessary vitamins. Fat restriction should be gradual and should emphasize new, tasty food rather than concentrate on what one cannot eat. Although this discussion has particularly emphasized fat reduction, it is usually recommended that dietary cholesterol be reduced to 300 mg/day

(1 egg has about 250 mg of cholesterol). Some advocate a reduction to 100 mg/day. Again, the degree of modification can be individualized, watching the response of the serum cholesterol and HDL levels, and the reduction of other risk factors. Note that the degree of response of cholesterol levels to diet is quite variable, with some people having to make fairly drastic changes to achieve the same degree of cholesterol-lowering as others who modify their diet less.

The goal cholesterol level has to be individualized based on other risk factors. Remember that populations with the lowest rates of CHD have average values of 140–180 mg/dl. It appears that in the United States, average cholesterol levels of 180–200 mg/dl are associated with a low risk of CHD. At levels above 200 mg/dl, the risk increases. Not everyone can achieve this level, but the present average U.S. cholesterol value of 220 mg/dl can be lowered to the 200 value.

b. Drugs. For those with quite high cholesterol values, drugs may be indicated if diet therapy fails to bring the serum cholesterol below 265 mg/dl or an LDL below 190 mg/dl [28]. In the Lipid Research Clinics-Coronary Primary Prevention Trial, the successful drug was a cholestyramine resin that was given as 6 packets or 24 gms/day in 2–4 equal doses. Gastrointestinal side effects are the most common, especially constipation and heartburn. Patient compliance in pratice is never as good as in clinical trials and may present a real problem. Cost is also a problem. Although prices may come down, the drug can cost up to $150/month. Niacin is considerably cheaper. Its efficacy was seen in the Coronary Drug Project with postmyocardial infarction patients, but only after 10 years when an 11% lower mortality was seen. It can be given in 500-mg tablets, 3–12/day. The main side effect is cutaneous flushing, which led to compliance problems in the above study. Gastrointestinal side effects also occur along with some increase in glucose and uric acid levels. A recent trial in Finland has shown a 34% reduction in coronary endpoints over 5 years in men taking gemfibrozil at a dose of 600 mg twice a day [29].

There are many other agents, such as clofibrate, probucol, and lovastatin, but trials looking at the benefits of lowering lipids with these agents have not been done. One should not prescribe an agent just because it can lower serum cholesterol. Lovastatin is a promising new drug that effectively lowers cholesterol with few side effects. Unlike the bile acid sequestrants, niacin and gemfibrozil, the effect of lovastatin on CHD is not yet known. The Coronary Drug Project showed that one agent, clofibrate, did lower serum cholesterol and reduce the risk of CHD, but the drug was also associated with a significantly higher total mortality.

2. Justification

a. Effectiveness. The usefulness of screening for hypercholesterolemia depends partly on the validity of the lipid or diet-heart hypothesis. This hypothesis claims that the dietary consumption of fat and cholesterol is directly related to the risk of CHD and that this risk is reflected through the serum cholesterol or its component lipoprotein fractions. If this hypothesis is valid, then physicians should screen their patients for hyperlipidemia and should recommend diet modification for those people with the disease. The evidence for and against the diet-heart hypothesis will be reviewed briefly, and the reader may find more thorough discussions in recent excellent reviews [12–18].

The idea that dietary changes will alter the serum cholesterol and the risk of CHD is controversial. The reason for the controversy is that this hypothesis is nearly impossible to test in a prospective, randomized trial, considering the large number of subjects required and the difficulty of diet alteration and monitoring. Ongoing surveys in free-living subjects are likewise difficult due to present-day crude measures of diet, such as the 24-hour diet recall.

Nevertheless, animal and epidemiologic studies quite consistently give results supporting the hypothesis. Animals given high-fat and high-cholesterol diets develop atherosclerotic lesions that regress when the diet is changed to contain low fat and low cholesterol. These changes correspond to the rise and fall of serum cholesterol. Metabolic studies in humans show that the serum cholesterol rises and falls in accordance with changes in the dietary content of saturated fat and cholesterol. Epidemiologic studies support the belief that changes in diet reduce CHD in humans. International studies of different populations consistently show low rates of CHD in countries consuming high carbohydrates and low-fat diets, while countries such as Finland and the United States with high-fat diets have high rates of CHD. Other diet variables such as sugar consumption and hardness of the water are not found to be related to CHD. Studies of migrant populations also support the hypothesis. Japanese people living in Japan, Hawaii, and California show a consistent relationship between dietary fat, serum cholesterol, and the rate of CHD; the lowest of all three is found in the native Japanese men and the highest in the California migrants, with the Hawaiian group being intermediate [19]. Within the United States, vegetarian groups have considerably lower cholesterol levels. Seventh Day Adventists have lower mortality rates than the general population. Although this may be due in part to life-style (which includes abstinence from smoking), nonvegetarian Adventists have mortality rates 34% lower than the United States population, while those rates are 57% lower for the lactovegetarian Adventists and 77% lower for the pure vegetarian Adventists [20].

Although the above evidence is highly incriminating for the belief that dietary fat leads to CHD, it is not as conclusive as randomized diet trials. Most of the trials to date have been seriously flawed and do not test the hypothesis adequately. Experimental diets have usually been fairly high in total fat (35–40%), not so much reducing the amount of fat as substituting much of the saturated fat with polyunsaturated fat. With this diet, which does not correlate with any diet of the epidemiologic studies in living societies, mean serum cholesterol levels do not decrease appreciably and in no trial were they less than 210 mg/dl, well above the desired 150 mg/dl to 200 mg/dl range. Secondly, many trials use people with established CHD that is possibly too far advanced for significant short-term improvement with modest diet modification to occur.

The Multiple Risk Factor Intervention Trial (MRFIT) unfortunately did not give evidence for or against the lipid hypothesis [21]. In the trial, high-risk men were randomized to two groups, one of which was referred back to community physicians (Usual Care Group—UC), while the other group was given a program designed to reverse the risk factors of smoking, hypertension, and hyperlipidemia. There was no significant difference in mortality between the groups at the end of 7 years. However, serum cholesterol dropped in both groups, and cardiovascular mortality was unexpectedly low in the UC group. An annual cardiovascular mortality rate of 2.8/1000 was found as opposed to an expected 4.8/1000 for these men at high risk. The lack of a difference in mortality between the two groups would be very difficult to show. Thus, this trial was not able to adequately test the hypothesis of a reduction of mortality resulting from risk-factor intervention.

Positive results were seen, however, in a similar trial done in Norway on high-risk normotensive men [22]. Risk reduction concentrated on smoking cessation and lowering of serum cholesterol. By diet modification, serum cholesterol fell 13% lower than the control group. Smoking cessation occurred in 25% of the test group as compared with 17% of the control group. At the end of 5 years, the incidence of myocardial infarction and sudden death was significantly lower (by 47%) in the intervention group.

The Lipid Research Clinics-Coronary Primary Prevention Trial (LRC-CPPT) did show that lowering serum cholesterol by a drug (cholestyramine) reduces mortality and morbidity from CHD [23]. This study is often quoted as proof of the lipid hypothesis. Indeed, men with serum cholesterol levels above 265 mg/dl taking cholestyramine for 7 years were able to lower the average serum cholesterol by 8.5% more than controls. This was associated with a 19% lower incidence of CHD.

As exciting as this study is in showing that lowering serum cholesterol can lead to a lower CHD incidence, one must note that the results may not be applied to the practice of preventive medicine as extensively as is now being seen [15, 24, 25]. First of all, the trial did not prove or even examine the diet-heart hypothesis. This was a drug trial; the study group and the controls had the same diet. Secondly, the study was done with people in the upper 5% of serum cholesterol. The average serum cholesterol initially was over 290 mg/dl. It is not known if lowering serum cholesterol from levels lower than those studied to even lower levels will result in any benefit. Furthermore, the benefits in this high-risk group were less than overwhelming. Deaths from CHD may have been 19% less in the treated group, but this represented a reduction of CHD deaths from 8.6% to only 7.0%. This means that a physician would treat 200 patients over 7 years to prevent 3 deaths from CHD. More important, total mortality did not differ between the treated subjects taking the drug and the controls. This important point is often overlooked. Finally, to achieve these modest benefits, people had to take the drug six times a day and endure its side effects. The cost of the drug is considerable, with treatment running in the neighborhood of $150/month.

Because of the immense cost, it is doubted that there will ever be a well-designed, randomized, controlled trial to test the diet-heart hypothesis. Therefore, physicians will have to decide for themselves from the available evidence what to recommend to patients. If diet does prevent CHD, the benefits would be considerable and obvious.

b. Risks. The risks of recommending diet therapy are nebulous, but one must be aware of the possibilities. The most serious possibility proposed so far is an increase in cancer, especially large bowel cancer. Two studies have shown an increase in cancer with diets high in polyunsaturated fats. Although other studies have not confirmed this, one should be quite cautious [26]. More established harmful effects of polyunsaturated diets (where total fat is near 40%) include increased formation of gallstones but a decrease in bowel cancer. There is no known population presently on a high-polyunsaturated-fat diet, and thus we do not know all of the long-term benefits and risks. Thus, any diet recommendation should not include adding polyunsaturated fat or merely substituting polyunsaturated fats for saturated fats, but should stress reducing total fat intake as much as possible, preferably to less than 30% of calories. Reducing total fat and cholesterol in the diet has no known risks, and people switching to such diets in vegetarian societies have not developed the possible complications of the high-polyunsaturated-fat diets.

There are also ethical risks in recommending fairly drastic life-style changes without being able to guarantee benefits. In fact, physicians do this all of the time by recommending that people lose weight, exercise, reduce salt, get adequate sleep, reduce stress, and quit smoking. Except for smoking, the evidence for the benefits of all the above recommendations is much weaker than for a change to a low-fat diet. Even critics of the diet-heart hypothesis often recommend many life-style changes, the benefits of which are much less well known [17]. Although many authorities support the diet-heart hypothesis, there are some prominent critics [13, 15, 16, 28]. Health care providers must weigh the arguments and decide as they would for any clinical problem. Furthermore, physicians making no recommendations in regard to diet are, in fact, then recommending the present American diet. People often ask their physicians for diet recommendations, so one has to have some form of answer. There are millions of diets that are presently being recommended throughout the country, and some of these diets have some significant risks. The low-fat diet is an attractive alternative.

c. Acceptability. The main problems posed by the low-fat diet are social and psychological. Physicians hesitate to deny people one of life's enjoyments for undetermined benefits. Low-fat, low-cholesterol diets, however, can be quite enjoyable and even exciting as one learns how to cook or to seek out foods conforming with the diet. The diet can make use of a large variety of spices and recipes from cuisines of other countries. Asian, Mexican, Mediterranean, African, and Middle Eastern cultures have developed delicious meals that are low in fat and cholesterol. However, people able to make such a change, like people able to quite smoking and maintain an exercise program for themselves, may well find life not devoid of pleasure, but actually more enjoyable after taking control of their lives and doing something to improve their health.

In summary, testing for hypercholesterolemia meets most of the criteria for inclusion in the periodic health exam. The disease is a major common problem, there is a long asymptomatic period, and the screening test is simple, safe, and fairly accurate. Treatment with diet before symptoms (CHD) may well lead to improved outcome as discussed above. The treatment itself is safe, although its major limitation is its acceptability.

III. Recommendations

A. Early detection

1. Serum cholesterol and HDL should be obtained in all adults with the objective of identifying the risk of developing CHD.
2. Repeat lipid measurements should be obtained every 3–5 years (arbitrary). Those with unfavorable levels may have more frequent measurements taken to give both the physician and the patient feedback on the patient's efforts to reduce risk.

3. Those with total serum cholesterol greater than 200 mg/dl, or HDL less than 45 mg/dl, have unfavorable lipid values with an increased risk for CHD.
4. The physician should also note whether diseases causing hypercholesterolemia are present (see Table 73-1).

B. Early intervention. Risk increases with increasingly unfavorable values; recommendations and treatment should be likewise increasingly aggressive.

1. Other CHD risk factors should be reduced (smoking, hypertension, obesity).
2. Dietary fat should be reduced to 25–30% of total calories, and cholesterol to no greater than 300 mg/day.
3. Drugs should be prescribed for those with extremely high values of cholesterol (>265) who do not respond to diet.

References

1. Kannel, W. B., et al. Serum cholesterol, lipoproteins, and the risk of coronary heart disease: The Framingham study. *Ann. Intern. Med.* 74(4):1, 1971. *Total serum cholesterol proves to be the most useful lipid measurement for CHD risk.*
2. Stamler, J., Wentworth, D., and Neaton, J. D. Is the relationship between serum cholesterol from risk of premature death from coronary heart disease continuous and graded? Findings in 356,222 primary screenees of the Multiple Risk Factor Intervention Trial (MRFIT). *J.A.M.A.* 256(20):2823, 1986. *Examination of over 350,000 men showing the risk of CHD with serum cholesterol is continuous and that there is no cut-off for hypercholesterolemia, for the MRFIT Research Group.*
3. Relationship of blood pressure, serum cholesterol, smoking habit, relative weight and ECG abnormalities to incidence of major coronary events: Final report of the pooling project. *J. Chronic Dis.* 31(4):201, 1978. *Pooling project report on risk factors and major coronary events.*
4. Castelli, W. P., et al. HDL cholesterol and other lipids in coronary heart disease: The Cooperative Lipoprotein Phenotyping study. *Circulation* 55(5):767, 1977. *Found decreased HDL as independent risk factor in five populations.*
5. Miller, N. E., et al. The Tromso heart-study: High-density lipoprotein and coronary heart disease: A prospective case-control study. *Lancet* 1(8019):965, 1977. *Inverse relation of HDL and CHD in a 2-year study.*
6. Gordon, T., et al. High density lipoprotein as a protective factor against coronary heart disease. *Am. J. Med.* 62(5):707, 1977. *The Framingham study results showing the strong correlation of HDL and CHD in men and women over the age of 50. In this age group, both total cholesterol and triglycerides were not found to correlate independently with CHD.*
7. Kannel, W. B., Castelli, W. P., and Gordon, T. Cholesterol in the prediction of atherosclerotic disease: New perspectives based on the Framingham study. *Ann. Intern. Med.* 90(1):85, 1979. *A review of the Framingham study that focuses on the relation of serum cholesterol, LDL, HDL, and VLDL as CHD risk factors. Noteworthy are the risks in older age groups and in people with other risk factors.*
8. Uhl, G. S., et al. Relation between high density lipoprotein cholesterol and coronary artery disease in asymptomatic men. *Am. J. Cardiol.* 48(5):903, 1981. *A study showing utility of cholesterol-HDL ratio in asymptomatic Air Force aviators with positive screening treadmill tests.*
9. Bachorik, P. S., and Wood, P. D. S. Laboratory Considerations in the Diagnosis and Management of Hyperlipoproteinemia. In B. M. Rifkind and R. I. Levy (eds.), *Hyperlipidemia: Diagnosis and Therapy.* New York: Grune & Stratton, 1977. *Review of a technique of lipid measurement.*
10. Connor, W., and Connor, S. Dietary Treatment of Hyperlipidemia. In B. M. Rifkind and R. I. Levy (eds.), *Hyperlipidemia: Diagnosis and Therapy.* New York: Grune & Stratton, 1977. *An excellent, detailed discussion on the low-fat diet, or the "alternative diet." Includes food lists and recipes.*
11. American Heart Association. *Cookbook* (3rd ed.). New York: Ballantine, 1979. *Recipes for low-fat (30%), low-cholesterol diets.*
12. Inkeles, S., and Eisenberg, D. Hyperlipidemia and coronary atherosclerosis: A review. *Medicine* 60(2):110, 1981. *A well-written, concise review of the evidence for and against the diet-heart hypothesis.*
13. McMichael, J. Fats and atheroma: An inquest. *Br. Med. J.* 1(6157):173, 1979. *Cites evidence*

against the diet-heart hypothesis and warns of the hazards of polyunsaturated diets. Balance this article with the rebuttal by J. Mann [14].

14. Mann, J. I. Fats and atheroma: A retrial. *Br. Med. J.* 1(6165):732, 1979. *Rebuttal to article by McMichael. The two articles illustrate the problems of the present state of dietary trials. Both agree that diets high in polyunsaturated fats are not yet warranted.*
15. Ahrens, E. H. Dietary fats and coronary heart disease: Unfinished business. *Lancet* 2(8156-8157):1345, 1979. *One of the better-written arguments against the current diet recommendations for preventing CHD. Written by a well-known lipid investigator.*
16. Hulley, S. B., et al. Epidemiology as a guide to clinical decisions—II. Diet and coronary heart disease. *West. J. Med.* 135(1):25, 1981. *A logical interpretation of the diet-heart hypothesis, arguing for an individual approach to diet recommendations.*
17. Mann, G. V. Diet-Heart: End of an era. *N. Engl. J. Med.* 297(12):644, 1977. *A famous and often-quoted argument refuting the diet-heart hypothesis. One should also read the rebuttals in the letters to the editor in the* N. Engl. J. Med. *298:106, 1978.*
18. Borhani, N. O. Primary prevention of coronary heart disease: A critique. *Am. J. Cardiol.* 40(2):251, 1977. *Reviews diet trials and finds the diet-heart hypothesis not proved or disproved.*
19. Keys, A., et al. Lessons from serum cholesterol studies in Japan, Hawaii, and Los Angeles. *Ann. Intern. Med.* 48(1):83, 1958. *Found dietary fat, total cholesterol, and CHD correlating among three Japanese populations.*
20. Phillips, R. L., et al. Coronary heart disease mortality among Seventh-Day Adventists with differing dietary habits: A preliminary report. *Am. J. Clin. Nutr.* 31(10 Suppl):S191, 1978. *Found CHD correlates with different diets and life-styles.*
21. Multiple risk factor intervention trial: Risk factor changes and mortality results. Multiple risk factor intervention trial research group. *J.A.M.A.* 248(12):1465, 1982. *A national multicenter trial of risk-factor reduction in high-risk men.*
22. Hjermann, I., et al. Effect of diet and smoking intervention on the incidence of coronary heart disese. Report from the Oslo study group of a randomized trial in healthy men. *Lancet* 2(8259):1303, 1981. *Randomized trial showing reduction of CHD with smoking cessation and diet modification. Often referred to as "Oslo II."*
23. The Lipid Research Clinics Coronary Primary Prevention Trial results. I. Reduction of incidence of coronary heart disease. *J.A.M.A.* 251(3):351, 1984. *This is the LRC-CPPT that showed that men with a very high serum cholesterol can lower their CHD mortality with cholestyramine.*
24. Borhani, N. O. Prevention of coronary heart disease in practice. Implications of the results of recent clinical trials. *J.A.M.A.* 254(2):257, 1985. *An excellent, even-handed update to reference 14, with recent clinical trials discussed, including the LRC-CPPT.*
25. Consensus Conference. Lowering blood cholesterol to prevent heart disease. *J.A.M.A.* 253(14):2080, 1985. *A recent NIH consensus-panel report recommending fairly aggressive lowering of serum cholesterol. The recommendations are reasonable, but the case is overstated.*
26. Ederer, F., et al. Cancer among men on cholesterol-lowering diets: Experience from five clinical trials. *Lancet* 2(7717):203, 1971. *Review and analysis of previous diet trials; found no evidence of cancer with these diets.*
27. Report of the National Cholesterol Education Program expert panel on detection, evaluation, and treatment of high blood cholesterol in adults. *Arch. Intern. Med.* 148:36, 1988. *An elaboration of reference 25 with a good review of the "expert" national recommendations and details of dietary management.*
28. Palumbo, P. J. National Cholesterol Education Program: Does the emperor have any clothes? *Mayo Clin. Proc.* 63:88, 1988. *A rebuttal to the fairly strict recommendations of reference 27.*
29. Frick, M. H., et al. Helsinki Heart Study: Primary-prevention trial with gemfibrozil in middle-aged men with dyslipidproteinemia. *N. Engl. J. Med.* 317:1237, 1987. *Randomized double-blind trial showing gemfibrozil reducing coronary heart disease over 5 years.*

74 Glaucoma

Doug Campos-Outcalt

I. The problem

A. Definition. There are three criteria used to characterize glaucoma: (1) an increase in ocular pressure, usually defined as greater than 20–21 mm Hg, (2) cupping and pallor of the optic disk, and (3) typical visual field defects that are characteristic of glaucoma, as described by Armaly [1], which early in the disease are asymptomatic. Elevated intraocular pressure without associated visual field defects is referred to as **ocular hypertension**.

Glaucomas are classified into two main categories: primary and secondary. Primary glaucomas are further subdivided into three categories: open angle, closed angle, and congenital. In open-angle glaucoma, the angle between the cornea and iris is normal, while in closed-angle glaucoma, this angle is narrowed. The most common type of glaucoma is primary open-angle, followed in frequency by secondary and primary closed-angle glaucomas. Primary open-angle and the asymptomatic closed-angle and secondary glaucomas are those types for which the discussion of screening applies since they can exist in an asymptomatic state. Low pressure glaucoma is characterized by visual field defects and cupping, yet intraocular pressure is less than 21 mm Hg. Low pressure glaucoma can constitute up to 18% of all glaucoma cases and 37% of previously undiagnosed glaucoma discovered by screening [2].

According to the National Society for the Prevention of Blindness, 1 out of 7 new cases of blindness is due to glaucoma, accounting for 6600 new cases each year in the United States. It is thought that blindness results more frequently from secondary glaucoma than from primary glaucoma because it is more severe and more difficult to control, even though it is less common [3, 4]. It is unclear, therefore, how much blindness is due to the asymptomatic glaucomas for which screening is advocated.

B. Description. Aqueous humor is produced by the ciliary body and moves from the posterior chamber through the pupil into the anterior chamber. It then leaves the eye through the trabecular meshwork and canal of Schlemm. In glaucoma, the sequence of events is believed to be as follows: the outflow of aqueous humor is decreased; aqueous humor continues to be produced and the intraocular pressure elevates; elevated pressure causes ocular nerve damage and cupping; ocular nerve damage leads to visual field defects that can progress to blindness. The level of pressure that ocular nerves can tolerate varies from individual to individual.

C. Epidemiology. The prevalence of elevated intraocular pressure (> 21 mm Hg) varies by study from 3–12.7% in those over the age of 40 years [5–7]. The prevalence of elevated intraocular pressure increases with age from an average of 5% of the population at 40–44 years to 10% at 55–59 years, and 15% at 70–75 years [8].

The prevalence of chronic open-angle glaucoma in these same studies varies between 0.35% and 0.93%. The prevalence of all types of glaucoma varies from 0.84–1.30%. Therefore, only about 10% of those with elevated intraocular pressures have some form of glaucoma.

The prevalence of glaucoma increases with age. In the Ferndale study, there was a 0% prevalence at age 40–44 years, 0.9% at age 55–59 years, and 1.3% at age 70–74 years [8]. The prevalence of glaucoma also increases with the level of intraocular pressure. Even so, at 30 mm Hg, only 30% will have visual field defects, and at 35 mm Hg, 50%.

There are other subgroups of the population that seem to have a higher risk of glaucoma. There is an association between diabetes and open-angle glaucoma [9]. Family history of the disease is probably an added risk factor, and blacks may be at increased risk [10].

Studies that have examined the incidence of glaucoma among those having ocular hypertension have shown a low incidence of glaucoma in this group over a 5- to 10-year period [1, 11–16, 22]. Even at the higher levels of intraocular pressures (24–30 mm Hg), most people having ocular hypertension do not develop visual field defects within 5–10 years [1]. The studies from glaucoma referral centers show incidences of 0, 6.0, 9.3, and 16.0% [11, 13, 15, 16]. The studies involving general population surveys resulted in incidences of 0.5, 1.0, and 3.2% [1, 12, 14, 22].

At first glance, these combined data seem somewhat contradictory; 10% of those with elevated intraocular pressures have glaucoma, yet a much smaller percentage of ocular hypertension patients will develop glaucoma over 5–10 years. These data have been analyzed by Anderson and explained by his concept of variable sensitivity [17]. It appears that each individual has his or her own threshold of intraocular pressure, beyond which ocular nerve damage and visual field defects develop. For some, this threshold is 21 mm Hg, for others it is 18 mm Hg (explaining low pressure glaucoma), and for others it is 35 mm Hg (explaining high intraocular pressures with no visual field loss). Approximately 10% of the population is susceptible to ocular nerve damage at pressures above 21 mm Hg. At higher pressures, a greater percentage is susceptible.

A number of unsuccessful attempts have been made to find ways to predict which patients who have ocular hypertension are at increased risk of glaucoma [13, 15].

II. Secondary prevention

A. Early detection

1. Methods

a. Tonometry

(1) Description. There are three methods currently used to measure intraocular pressure: Schiotz, applanation, and noncontact tonometry.

(2) Performance. Schiotz tonometry is the most widely used office modality. It is less acccurate than applanation tonometry, but errors can be decreased markedly if it is performed by someone experienced in the use of a Schiotz tonometer [18].

When using the Schiotz tonometer, the patient is recumbent and the eyes are anesthetized by a topical anesthetic. The lids are held open without placing pressure on the eyeball. While the patient focuses on a fixed object, the tonometer is brought toward the cornea from the temporal side and held above the cornea without touching it for several seconds. Once the patient is relaxed, the tonometer is gently lowered until it rests on the cornea. The amount of corneal indentation is indicated on a scale that can be converted to ocular pressure using a calibration table.

Applanation tonometry is used mostly by ophthalmologists, since the device is part of the standard slit-lamp.

Noncontact tonometry uses puffs of air to indent the cornea and is more practical for screening large numbers of patients. The noncontact tonometer is reliable except at high levels of intraocular pressures.

(3) Interpretation. All tonometry measures the amount of corneal indentation that is converted to ocular pressure, using tables in the case of a Schiotz tonometer. The cut-off for normal pressure is usually 21 mm Hg.

b. Ophthalmoscopy. The use of routine ophthalmoscopy by primary care providers (looking for a cup-disk ratio of 0.5 or greater) has been compared to tonometry in only one small study [19], and largely remains an unproved screening method.

c. Visual field screening. One of the newer, more promising developments in the area of glaucoma screening has been the automated perimeter for visual field screening. There are now a variety of automated perimeters available. As more experience is gained and cheaper versions of automated perimeters become available, this modality might replace all others. It is not, however, currently available to most primary care providers.

2. Justification

a. Test characteristics (Table 74-1).

b. Risk and side effects. Frequent mistakes using tonometry include measuring the pressure before the patient is fully relaxed and placing pressure on the eye while retracting the eyelids. Contact tonometry, Schiotz or applanation, can infrequently result in complications including corneal abrasions, local reactions to the anesthetic, and transmission of infections. Noncontact tonometry requires neither topical anesthesia nor florescein, and therefore does not have these risks.

c. Costs (Table 74-2).

d. Acceptability. Tonometry can cause some minor discomfort, but it is usually well tolerated. Perimetry is well accepted by most patients.

B. Early intervention

1. Methods. Once an individual has been found to have a pressure of $\geq$ 21 mm Hg,

Table 74-1. Screening tests

	Sensitivity (%)	Specificity (%)	+ Predictive value (%)	− Predictive value (%)	Total predictive value (%)
Tonometry [3][a]	66	91	10	99.0	90
Fundoscopy [4, 20][b]	85	83	7	99.7	83
Automated perimetry [3, 4, 21]	85–100	81–96	82	100.0	99

[a]Tonometry will not detect low tension glaucoma, which represents up to one third of previously undiagnosed cases of glaucoma.
[b]The problem with these numbers is that they are obtained in studies using disk photography to study the optic disk.

he or she should be referred to an ophthalmologist for further evaluation. If medication is indicated, it will generally include one or more of the following medications:

a. Beta blockers (timolol)
b. Cholinergics (pilocarpine, carbachol)
c. Adrenergics (epinephrine)
d. Carbonic anhydrase inhibitors (acetazolamide)
e. Anticholinesterases (echothiophate)

2. **Justification**

a. **Effectiveness.** Glaucoma meets most of the criteria for justifying screening. It has a significant effect on quality of life, there is an asymptomatic period, an acceptable method of treatment is available, and there are tests that can detect the disease in the asymptomatic stage. However, efficacy of treatment has to be accepted on faith rather than evidence. Glaucomatous visual field defects are generally considered irreversible. Therefore, if treatment is efficacious, early intervention should improve the outcome. Considering how widely held is the belief that visual field loss can be prevented or minimized by treating elevated intraocular pressure, this lack of supporting clinical evidence is surprising. Most authorities would agree, however, that patients with documented visual field defects secondary to ocular pressure (those who have crossed their thresholds) should be treated.

More controversy exists concerning whether to treat those having ocular hypertension. In spite of no evidence of efficacy, some suggest treating ocular hypertensives who have a strong risk factor for developing glaucoma such as extremely high pressures, family history, advanced age, and disks suggestive of early damage.

b. **Risks and side effects.** Medical therapy for glaucoma is usually safe although each drug can produce local and systemic side effects. Cholinergics can cause miosis, decreased night vision, and local irritation. Anticholinesterases have been implicated in cataract formation, retinal detachment, and the precipitation of closed-angle glaucoma. Epinephrine can also cause the onset of angle-closure glaucoma as well as tachycardia and increased blood pressure. Timolol can produce bradycardia, bronchospasm, and local irritation. Carbonic anhydrase inhibitors frequently cause nausea, vomiting, diarrhea, metabolic acidosis, and, less frequently, facial paresthesias, renal calculi, blood dyscrasias, and cutaneous reactions.

c. **Acceptability.** Anti-glaucoma medications are usually well accepted although they can be associated with the compliance problems involved with the treatment of asymptomatic disease.

III. Recommendations

A. Screening should start with tonometry for those over the age of 40 years. Those with pressures of 20 mm Hg or less can be rescreened every 5 years up to age 60, and every 2 or 3 years thereafter.

B. Those with confirmed pressures of 21 mm Hg or greater should be referred to an ophthalmologist for two reasons: to determine if visual field defects are present, and if so, to diagnose what type of glaucoma the patient has.

C. The management of those with ocular hypertension will need to be discussed with the consulting ophthalmologist. Those who are at higher risk for the onset of glaucoma (those with pressures $\geq$ 30 mm Hg, suspicious disks, or a family history of glaucoma) are often started on therapy before the onset of visual field defects. Many opthalmologists would suggest being aggressive in following up on ocular hypertension by doing visual field screening frequently or looking for any changes in optic disks with serial photography. It should be remembered that up to 10% of the population can have ocular hypertension, and the potential cost of such recommendations needs to be kept in mind.

D. The screening approach described will detect 66–80% of the glaucoma cases, missing only those with low pressure glaucoma. The population in the pressure range of 17–20 mm Hg presents a special problem. It cannot be recommended that they be referred for visual field testing. Thirty percent of the population falls within the 17–20 mm Hg pressure range [6]. While one out of ten individuals with ocular pressures greater than or equal to 21 mm Hg will be found to have glaucoma, 1 out of 200–300 with pressures of 17–20 mm Hg will have the disease.

E. In the setting where automated perimetry is available, it is recommended that this method replace tonometry as a primary screening tool, with referral of those with visual defects characteristic of glaucoma.

References

1. Armaly, M. F. Ocular pressure and visual fields. A ten-year follow-up study. *Arch. Ophthalmol.* 81(1):25, 1969. *Community-based glaucoma detection program in Iowa. Includes 10-year follow-up.*
2. Hollows, F. C., and Graham, P. A. Intra-ocular pressure, glaucoma, and glaucoma suspects in a defined population. *Br. J. Ophthalmol.* 50(10):570, 1966. *Community-based glaucoma detection program in Wales; 0.84% prevalence of glaucoma.*
3. Anderson, D. R. *The Detection of Glaucoma as Part of a Periodic Health Examination. A Report to the Task Force on the Periodic Health Examination.* Canada: Health Standards Directorate of Health and Welfare, 1978. *Comprehensive summary of evidence for and against various glaucoma screening maneuvers.*
4. Bengtsson, B. Aspects of the epidemiology of chronic glaucoma. *Acta Ophthalmol.* (Suppl 146):1, 1981. *Community-based glaucoma detection program in Sweden, including a 10-year follow-up.*
5. Bankes, J. L., et al. Bedford glaucoma survey. *Br. Med. J.* 1(595):791, 1968. *Community-based study in England; 3% prevalence of ocular hypertension; 0.93% prevalence of glaucoma.*
6. Stromberg, U. Ocular hypertension. Frequency, course and relation to other disorders occurring in glaucoma, as seen from mass survey of all inhabitants over 40 years of age in a Swedish town. *Acta Ophthalmol.* (Suppl 69):1, 1962. *Community-based study in Sweden; 3.3% prevalence of ocular hypertension; 0.35% prevalence of chronic open-angle glaucoma.*
7. Armaly, M. F. On the Distribution of Applanation Pressure and Arcuate Scotoma. In G. Paterson, S. J. Miller, and G. D. Paterson (eds.), *Drug Mechanisms in Glaucoma.* Boston: Little, Brown, 1966. Pp. 167–189. *Same population as reference 1; 12.7% with ocular hypertension; 1.3% with glaucoma.*
8. Graham, P. A. and Hollows, F. C. A Critical Review of Methods of Detecting Glaucoma. In L. B. Hunt (ed.), *Glaucoma: Epidemiology, Early Diagnosis and Some Aspects of Treatment.* Edinburgh: Livingstone, 1966. *Early review of glaucoma.*
9. Becker, B. Diabetes mellitus and primary open-angle glaucoma. *Am. J. Ophthalmol.* 71(1):1, 1971. *Review of the literature on diabetes and glaucoma.*
10. Sasovetz, D. Open-angle glaucoma in blacks: A review. *J. Natl. Med. Assoc.* 69(10):705, 1977. *Superficial review of the literature.*
11. Norskov, K. Routine tonometry in ophthalmic practice. II. Five-year follow-up. *Acta Ophthalmol.* 48(5):873, 1970. *Zero of 72 eyes with ocular hypertension developed glaucoma over 5 years.*
12. Perkins, E. S. The Bedford glaucoma survey. I: Long-term follow-up of borderline cases. *Br. J. Ophthalmol.* 57(3):179, 1973. *Four of 124 patients with ocular hypertension developed glaucoma over 5–7 years (see reference 22).*
13. Wilensky, J. T., Podos, S. M., and Becker, B. Prognostic indicators in ocular hypertension. *Arch. Ophthalmol.* 91(3):200, 1974. *Three of 50 patients with ocular hypertension developed glaucoma over an average of 6 years.*
14. Graham, P. A. The definition of pre-glaucoma. A prospective study. *Trans. Ophthalmol. Soc. UK* 88:153, 1969. *One of 232 patients with ocular hypertension developed glaucoma in 3.5 years.*
15. Kitazawa, Y., et al. Untreated ocular hypertension. A long-term prospective study. *Arch.*

Ophthalmol. 95(7):1180, 1977. *Seven of 75 patients with ocular hypertension developed glaucoma over 10 years.*

16. David, R., Livingston, D. G., and Luntz, M. H. Ocular hypertension—a long-term follow-up of treated and untreated patients. *Br. J. Ophthalmol.* 61(11):668, 1977. *Twelve of 117 eyes with ocular hypertension developed glaucoma over 3.5 years.*
17. Anderson, D. R. The management of elevated intraocular pressure with normal optic discs and visual fields. I. Therapeutic approach based on high risk factors. *Surv. Ophthalmol.* 21(6):479, 1977. *Excellent summary of glaucoma data and presentation of threshold theory.*
18. Spector, R., et al. Should tonometry screening be done by technicians instead of physicians? *Arch. Intern. Med.* 135(9):1260, 1975. *Clinic-based screening project. False-positives decreased by over 60% in the second half of the study.*
19. Hammond, E. A., and Begley, P. K. Screening for glaucoma: A comparison of ophthalmoscopy and tonometry. *Nurs. Res.* 28(6):371, 1979. *Lack of randomization between ophthalmoscopy and tonometry and frequency of patients being screened with both methods casts doubt on results. Both methods showed similar sensitivities and specificities.*
20. Douglas, G. R., Drance, S. M., and Schulzer, M. A correlation of fields and discs in open-angle glaucoma. *Can. J. Ophthalmol.* 9(4):391, 1974. *Examination of the correlation between optic disks and visual fields in open angle glaucoma.*
21. Heijl, A., and Drance, S. M. A clinical comparison of three computerized automatic perimeters in the detection of glaucoma defects. *Arch. Ophthalmol.* 99(5):832, 1981. *Three automated perimeters compared.*
22. Perkins, E. S. The Bedford glaucoma survey. II: Rescreening normal population. *Br. J. Ophthalmol.* 57(3):186, 1973. *See reference 12.*

75 Osteoporosis

Felicia Stewart

I. The problem

A. Definition. Clinicians, radiologists, and pathologists usually can agree on the clinical diagnosis of osteoporosis in its advanced form. Unfortunately, there is no single accepted set of diagnostic criteria for this problem at earlier states of severity. A good clinical description of osteoporosis is that of Stillman [1].

> Osteoporosis exists when bone strength reaches a state where there is a risk of fracture under conditions of ordinary skeletal stress. . . . In osteoporosis, the bone cells, bone matrix, and bone crystals are normal. Also normal are serum concentrations of calcium, phosphorus and alkaline phosphatase. Since the external dimensions of osteoporotic bone are also normal, the reduced size of trabeculae and cortex—the hallmark of the disease—causes structural weakness and increases the risk of fracture.

B. Description. The etiology of osteoporosis is not fully understood. Gradual loss of bone mass has been documented for both men and women beginning in the fourth decade and continuing thereafter as an almost universal "normal" aging phenomenon. Loss is usually cumulative, so an individual's bone mass at any point in time depends on his or her initial bone mass and on the subsequent rates of loss over time. Many factors appear to influence maximum bone mass and rates of loss, including genetic predisposition, endocrine milieu, diet, exercise, and renal function. Age is often associated with decreased physical activity and with reduced dietary calcium intake. Diminished intestinal absorption of calcium, increased renal calcium loss, and reduced renal production of 1,25-dihydroxy-vitamin D have also been documented in association with aging. Any decrease in serum calcium resulting from negative calcium balance leads to a physiologic increase in parathyroid hormone activity, and thus to loss of bone mineral content.

Women experience an interval of accelerated bone loss beginning at the time of natural or surgical menopause and continuing for several years. The precise role of ovarian steroids in bone metabolism is not yet understood, although the importance of ovarian hormone loss has been well documented. Estrogen may mediate bone sensitivity to parathyroid hormone, or may influence bone metabolism through its effects on growth hormone levels, calcitonin, collagen, lysis, vitamin D metabolism, intestinal absorption of calcium, or in other ways not yet elucidated. Progestogens, too, may influence bone [2]. Within a few years after loss of ovarian hormones, a new equilibrium is established, and the woman's rate of bone loss decreases to approximate that of her male contemporaries. Because women begin with a smaller skeletal mass, experience a period of more rapid loss with menopause, and have a longer lifespan, they are more likely than men to suffer clinically significant osteoporosis. Progressive bone loss of osteoporosis affects trabecular bone more than cortical bone and involves the central skeleton earlier than the pheripheral bones. Demineralization ultimately affects the entire skeleton.

Skeletal fragility caused by osteoporosis leads to fractures that occur "spontaneously" or with trivial skeletal stress. Back pain caused by anterior wedge compression fracture of lower thoracic or lumbar vertebra is a common first symptom of osteoporosis. The severe, midline, lower back pain usually subsides after 4–6 weeks unless additional fractures occur. Pain is increased by bending over but is not usually complicated by nerve root compression pain. Loss of height is a consequence of vertebral compression fractures, as is the exaggerated spinal curvature of "dowager's hump." Other common fracture sites include distal radius (Colles' fracture) and hip (femoral neck, intertrochanteric, or avulsion of the trochanter). Periodontal disease may also be linked to loss of alveolar bone in the mouth.

The diagnosis of osteoporosis requires exclusion of other diseases that cause skeletal fragility and may present similar clinical or radiologic findings. Other diseases to consider include: metastatic cancer (especially breast), myeloma, osteomalacia, osteogenesis imperfecta tarda, lymphoma, leukemia, and Paget's disease.

C. Epidemiology. Osteoporosis is a common problem. Attempts to estimate incidence, however, are confounded by the absence of uniform diagnostic criteria. Most writers in the field conclude that a large majority of hip fractures in the elderly, as well as spontaneous vertebral compression fractures, should be attributed to osteoporosis, with only a small minority attributable to severe trauma or to other disorders. Fracture rates in the elderly therefore provide an index of the prevalence of severe osteoporosis; it is likely that clinically significant but less advanced disease involves a proportional, and large, percentage of the elderly population. As many as 270,000 hip fractures/year occur among the 45 million or so postmenopausal women in the United States. These fractures are responsible for approximately 20,000 deaths annually. Hip fracture incidence and mortality are highest among the very elderly (10 hip fractures/year/1000 white women over 75 years of age, with a mortality as high as 30%), but are nevertheless a significant problem for younger women as well (two hip fractures/1000/year in the age group 50–64) [3]. Spinal compression fractures have been reported in as many as 25% of white women age 60, and 50% of white women over 75. Overall incidence estimates for symptomatic osteoporosis vary widely and probably reflect characteristics of the specific populations under study. A median estimate is that 25% of postmenopausal women are at risk for developing this problem.

Data on morbidity associated with osteoporosis are limited. The 50–70 fractures/1000 women/year that may be expected among untreated women with documented osteoporosis, however, incur substantial morbidity—chronic pain, orthopedic deformity, compromised pulmonary function, disability in ambulation, and, as a consequence of hip fracture complications, death.

D. Risk factors and groups. The most important risk factors for osteoporosis are age, sex (female), and race (nonblack). With the exception of Eskimo men and men with medical problems such as alcoholism, clinically significant osteoporosis is uncommon in men before the seventh or eighth decade. Bone mass varies with ethnic group and race, as well as sex, and is highest among blacks and lowest among white women of Northern European ethnic origin. Osteoporosis is rare among black women, but does occur among brown-skinned women and women of Asian origin.

Some writers believe that there is a subgroup within the population of women at risk for osteoporosis who lose bone mass at an abnormally rapid rate. Other authors disagree and believe instead that deficiencies in initial bone mass, calcium metabolism, diet, and life-style, rather than abnormally rapid loss, result in clinically significant osteoporosis for some women and not for others [1]. The possibility of identifying rapid bone losers would have important implications for prevention but has not yet been demonstrated.

Numerous medical problems are associated with an increased risk of osteoporosis. Problems that cause or reflect an altered endocrine milieu, impaired calcium absorption, physical immobilization, or require use of drugs that can induce iatrogenic osteoporosis can all affect osteoporosis risk. Some of the risk factors listed in Table 75-1 have been documented by epidemiologic studies of fracture rates; other factors have been identified through clinical observation, and some are based on theoretical grounds in relationship to calcium metabolism.

II. Primary prevention

A. Methods. There is no accepted regimen for prevention of osteoporosis. Exercise, calcium supplementation, estrogen treatment at the time of menopause, menopausal progestogen treatment, and fluoride have been shown to reduce bone-density loss measured radiologically in small studies.

Epidemiologic studies of variations in fracture rates among populations that differ in dietary calcium and in average levels of physical activity lend support to the hypothesis that primary prevention of osteoporosis may be possible. Further support for this concept may be provided by the observation that within the elderly population there are individuals who do not appear to lose bone mass: as many as 20–30% of elderly women and a slightly larger percentage of men maintain stable bone density despite aging [4].

Lacking a pathophysiologic understanding of the reasons for individual susceptibility to osteoporosis, most writers in the field stress the importance of optimal physical activity and calcium balance as reasonable approaches to primary prevention.

Reduced fracture rates have been documented for estrogen treatment initiated at the time of menopause [5]. Although benefit in reducing fracture risk has not yet been reported in research, hormone replacement treatment for women who experience premature hypoestrogenism for any reason is also recommended by most experts. Temporary estro-

Table 75-1. Risk factors for osteoporosis

Fair complexion, transparent skin, sparse hair[a]
Northern European ancestry[b]
Slender (low quetelets' index wgt [lb]÷Hgt [in.]<0.030)[b]
Small (Hgt $\leq$ 62 in.)[b]
Skinfold thickness low[a]
Family history of osteoporosis, vertebral or hip fracture[a]
Smoking[a]
High-protein diet
Sunlight exposure $\leq$ 3 hours/week[b]
Outdoor games—low frequency[b]
Low calcium intake
High caffeine intake
Excessive vitamin A intake
Medical problems and treatment
Early menopause ($\leq$ 44)[b]
Premature menopause (surgical or spontaneous)[a]
Amenorrhea—hypothalamic, hyperprolactinemic[a]
Hypogonadism (male)[a]
Turner's syndrome[a]
Klinefelter's syndrome[a]
Immobilization—3 weeks[b]
Hemiplegia[a]
Polio[a]
Multiple sclerosis[a]
Kidney disease
Hyperthyroidism or history of[a]
Diabetes mellitus[b]
Renal calculi or history of[a]
Gastrectomy[a]
Intestinal malabsorption[a]
Lactase deficiency[a]
Inflammatory bowel disease[a]
Alcoholism[a]
Rheumatoid arthritis[a]
Ankylosing spondylitis[a]
Parkinsonism[a]
Medications
Aluminum-containing antacid
Dilantin
Heparin
Furosemide[a]
Thyroid treatment ($\geq$ 3 grains daily or 300 mg levothyroxin)[a]
Corticosteroid[a]

[a]Female
[b]Non-black

gen deficiency, such as that associated with hypothalamic amenorrhea or hyperprolactinemia, can cause significant loss of measured bone mineral content. Similarly, premature menopause that occurs spontaneously or as a result of oophorectomy is associated with an increased risk for subsequent osteoporosis. Aggressive clinical management to ensure an uninterrupted, adequate estrogen level is an appropriate primary prevention measure, whenever possible.

1. **Maintaining adequate calcium balance.** Negative calcium balance results in physiologic bone resorption to maintain normal serum calcium concentration at the expense of bone mass. Many researchers feel that the current recommended daily allowance for calcium of 800 mg is not sufficient for adult and elderly women. In measured calcium balance studies of women age 35–50, researchers concluded that

Table 75-2. Calcium supplement products

Product	Calcium dose/tablet (mg)	Dose for 1 gm elemental calcium (tablets)	Comments
Calcium carbonate			
Caltrate 600	600	2	Least expensive; may cause constipation or flatulence
Os-Cal 500	500	2	
Tums	200	5	
Calcium gluconate	50–60	17–20	More expensive; less constipation
Calcium lactate	80–100	10–13	Not suitable for patients with lactose intolerance
Calcium phosphate	600	2	Inexpensive; additional phosphate may not be desirable
Chelated calcium	50–150	7–20	Intermediate cost
Bone meal	Not recommended		May be contaminated with toxic metals
Dolomite	Not recommended		May be contaminated with toxic metals

premenopausal and hormonally treated postmenopausal women required 990 mg calcium daily to maintain zero calcium balance. Untreated postmenopausal women required 1504 mg daily [6]. Dietary surveys show that the average elderly woman consumes only 400–600 mg of calcium daily. Clearly, increased dietary calcium or calcium supplementation is necessary (although probably not reliably sufficient) for prevention of osteoporosis in such women.

Recommendations regarding dose and timing for calcium supplementation vary. Many authors recommend routine supplementation with 1 gm elemental calcium daily for perimenopausal and postmenopausal patients. Patients with very low dietary calcium intake may require a slightly higher supplementation dose to ensure a total of 1.5-gm daily intake. Calcium is best absorbed in multiple daily doses, and a bedtime dose may help to counteract the increased calcium loss that occurs with fasting and immobilization during sleep. Optimal calcium absorption requires adequate vitamin D. Approximately 15–60 minutes of sunlight daily or supplementation of 400 IU daily should provide an adequate vitamin D level. Because excessive vitamin D can stimulate bone resorption, daily intake in excess of 1000 units should be avoided. Some calcium products are listed in Table 75-2.

Calcium balance is influenced by several factors besides calcium intake. Excessive dietary protein, vitamin A, and common drugs such as caffeine, nicotine, and antacids may adversely affect calcium absorption and urinary calcium excretion.

2. **Maintaining optimal physical activity.** Bone mass and architecture are influenced by the local (intrinsic) response of bone tissue to mechanical stress exerted by gravity and by muscular activity. Numerous studies have documented bone loss in response to immobilization and localized bone increase in response to specific occupations or sports [7].

Physical activity is often quite limited among elderly patients. The sedentary habits of a lifetime may be compounded by common medical problems such as cardiovascular disease or orthopedic problems and result in severely restricted daily levels of physical activity.

Although there are no large-scale studies to document the effectiveness of exercise in preventing osteoporosis, nor to indicate what level of exercise would be sufficient for maintaining bone, the issue of exercise and physical activity nevertheless may be an appropriate concern for clinicians and patients as well.

3. **Avoiding iatrogenic causes of osteoporosis.** Drugs that can cause osteoporosis (see Table 75-1) should be avoided whenever possible, and treatment duration and dose should be evaluated carefully. With the risk of bone loss in mind, periodic evaluation of thyroid replacement may be especially worthwhile since doses of 3 grains dessicated thyroid (150μg levothyroxine) or more may be supraphysiologic, and the dose needed may change with age. When medical recommendations or procedures involve immobilization, the possible impact on bone loss should be considered. Similarly, whenever hypogonadism is diagnosed or one of the other medical problems associated with osteoporosis risk is identified, medical management should include attention to preservation of skeletal integrity.

B. Justification

1. **Maintaining adequate calcium balance**

   a. **Effectiveness.** Small prospective studies of elderly women have shown calcium supplementation to be effective in reducing the rate of bone loss measured radiographically compared to the loss experienced by untreated control subjects. Bone loss observed with 700–1000 mg elemental calcium treatment is, however, greater than that observed with estrogen treatment in studies that compare the two approaches [8].

   There are no research data to show whether dietary modification with regard to caffeine, optimal (moderate) protein intake, nicotine, or antacids is effective in improving calcium balance or preventing bone loss.

   b. **Risks and side effects.** Recommendations to minimize dietary caffeine and to avoid smoking and excessive protein involve negligible risk and are in concert with general health recommendations. The importance of these issues among elderly women, however, deserves emphasis. Many such women choose high-protein diets because of their concerns about weight control.

   Most authors believe that risks of calcium supplementation are minimal when total calcium intake is 1–2 gm. Potential risks of calcium overload include hypercalcemia, hypercalcuria, and renal stones. For this reason, supplementation in excess of 2 gm daily, concomitant treatment with vitamin D, or treatment of a patient who has a history of renal stones, endocrinopathy, or is immobilized require careful monitoring for hypercalcemia. Relative contraindications to calcium supplementation include primary hyperparathyroidism, idiopathic hypercalcuria, sarcoidosis, renal impairment, sodium depletion, metabolic alkalosis, or thiazide diuretic therapy [9]. A patient with one of these problems who also needs calcium supplementation would require frequent assessment of calcium balance status. The Federal Drug Administration (FDA) has warned [10] that lead levels as high as 20 parts/million have been detected in samples of dolomite and in bonemeal preparation intended for use as a calcium supplement. Ingesting these products in large doses (> 10 gm daily) might expose the individual to unacceptable levels of lead intake.

   c. **Costs.** Recommendations regarding protein, caffeine, and nicotine involve no direct cost (possibly a cost saving). Calcium supplementation of 1 gm daily costs from \$2–15/month, depending on the calcium preparation selected.

   d. **Acceptability.** Maintaining adequate calcium intake through diet is difficult or unacceptable for many elderly patients. Approximately 1 qt of milk, or 36 oz of cottage cheese, or 3 cups of yogurt provides 1 gm of elemental calcium. Milk intolerance is common among elderly women, and obtaining adequate calcium from dairy products severely limits the calories available for consumption of other foods. For these reasons, calcium supplements are often preferable.

   Most patients tolerate calcium supplements in the 1-gm range well. Preparations containing magnesium or chloride may cause gastrointestinal irritation for some individuals. Selection of a preparation that requires fewer tablets daily may improve patient compliance.

   Recommendations regarding diet, use of stimulants, and drugs are acceptable (often welcome and expected) to most patients. Because change in life-style is required for their implementation, however, compliance may be a significant issue.

2. **Maintaining optimal physical activity**

   a. **Effectiveness and benefits.** Two widely quoted studies have shown that a modest exercise regimen may be enough to produce measurable improvement in bone status [11, 12].

   However, it seems unlikely that exercise alone will prove to be sufficient in prevention of osteoporosis. Significant bone loss has been documented among women athletes who have hypothalamic amenorrhea and low estrogen levels as a consequence of their athletic activity. Researchers suspect that bone loss occurs in these patients despite high exercise levels because of abnormally low estrogen.

b. **Risks and side effects.** Pursued in a prudent manner, the risks of exercise are minimal. For patients who are not accustomed to exercise, a gradual and gentle regimen is essential to avoid early injury or discouragement. Walking, swimming, weight training, and stationary bicycle riding are recommended for beginners, 3–5 times weekly for 15–60 minutes. A period of slow warm-up before and gradual cooling down after exercise may help prevent muscle injury, but stretching exercises should not be attempted before warm-up and may not be a good idea for elderly athletes. Preexercise cardiac stress testing should be undertaken for patients with hypertension, elevated cholesterol, or family history of myocardial infarction [13].

c. **Costs.** Costs depend on the specific form of exercise chosen and may be as little as $25–50 annually for suitable walking shoes.

d. **Acceptability.** Patients often need very specific recommendations and considerable encouragement to implement an exercise plan. Physicians may find it helpful to become acquainted with community resources that offer organized classes or exercise groups for senior citizens.

3. **Avoiding iatrogenic causes of osteoporosis.** There are no research data available to document the role of iatrogenic factors in osteoporosis or the effectiveness of medical attention to this issue. The risks of possible bone loss must be weighed against the potential risks to the patient of medical treatment curtailed or substituted.

III. Secondary prevention

A. Early detection

1. **Methods.** There is no accepted screening regimen for detection of early osteoporosis. Abnormalities in serum or urine calcium, phosphorus, and alkaline phosphatase usually indicate some other metabolic problem (such as hyperthyroidism); these values remain within the normal range despite clinically significant osteoporosis. Some authors have noted an elevation in the urinary hydroxyproline-creatinine ratio, elevated plasma parathyroid hormone, or lower-than-average serum progesterone among osteoporotic subjects [14]. None of these, however, have been shown to be of value as potential screening tests.

Conventional xray can detect osteoporosis only after loss of 30% or more of bone mass. More sensitive radiologic techniques such as radiogrammetry and radiographic photodensiometry have been used in research on bone loss but are of limited clinical value. They can be used only for assessment of peripheral bone (usually arm and hand), while the earliest and most important bone loss in osteoporosis occurs in the axial skeleton.

Photon absorptiometry involves little radiation exposure, is quite sensitive and precise, and is fairly economical. Single-beam photon absorptiometry can be used to evaluate peripheral bone, typically os calcis or radius. Dual-beam photon absorptiometry permits assessment of vertebral bone but is less widely available and is somewhat more costly.

Quantitative computerized tomography (CT) scan can also be used to assess axial bone. Because of the substantial xray exposure involved, as well as the cost, this technique has not been widely adopted as a screening measure.

CT scan, dual-beam, and single-beam absorptiometry are all being actively investigated as tools for routine screening or screening of selected groups. This approach may be of particular relevance when screening results might affect a decision about hormone replacement treatment. Clear evidence for the value of these screening methods in predicting future fracture risk is lacking [15], although good correlation between low peripheral-bone mineral content and the incidence of both spine and nonspine fracture has been documented in small, short-term research [16].

Patients at risk of osteoporosis because of other medical problems, drug treatment, or premature loss of gonadal hormones, as well as nonblack women in the perimenopausal age group, should be identified for education about maintaining adequate calcium balance and exercise. These issues are discussed in Sec. **II.** In addition, consideration should be given to possible methods of skeletal surveillance, and the advantages and disadvantages of hormone treatment should be assessed and discussed with the patient.

Carefully measured height and arm span are simple clinical parameters that can

Table 75-3. Falls in the elderly

Major causes of falls
Accidents
Orthostatic hypotension
Dizziness or vertigo
Drugs (sedative, antihypertensive, diuretic, hypoglycemic, alcohol)
Syncope (sudden loss of consciousness)
Drug attacks (sudden fall without loss of consciousness)
Neurologic dysfunction
Environmental factors associated with falls at home
Unstable furniture
Throw rugs
Frayed carpet
Low beds and toilets
Objects on floor
Creaky stairs
Poor rails
Poor lighting
Pets

Source: National Institutes of Health. *Osteoporosis. National Institutes of Health Consensus Development Conference Statement.* Bethesda, MD: National Institutes of Health, 1984. Vol. 5, No. 3.

be used to detect loss of height. Height loss from vertebral crush fractures indicates clinically advanced osteoporosis and therefore is not an "early" detection method. When height loss is found, however, further evaluation and clinical intervention are indicated. Similarly, midline, lower-back pain should be recognized as a possible first symptom of significant osteoporosis.

2. **Justification.** When osteoporosis is suspected, or for patients at high risk for osteoporosis, or when a decision about hormone replacement treatment might be affected, absorptiometry or CT scan may be justified. Data are not available, however, to indicate appropriate testing intervals, specific population recommendations, or justification for these modalities in routine osteoporosis screening.

B. Early intervention

1. **Methods**

a. **Minimizing the risk of falls.** Falls account for two-thirds of accidental deaths in people over 65. Accidents are the fifth leading cause of death in this age group, a reflection of the steady increase in the incidence of falls and severity of complications with age. Complications, in turn, reflect in part the skeletal fragility of osteoporosis. Prevention of osteoporosis morbidity, thus, should logically address accident and fall prevention. Obvious correctable environmental hazards and major causes of falls are listed in Table 75-3. Appropriate treatment of medical problems that can contribute to falls, home assessment to reduce environmental hazards, and teaching of adaptive behavior such as slow rising, gait training, and falling techniques may all be appropriate steps in prevention of fall morbidity [17].

b. **Hormone treatment.** Treatment with oral estrogen is effective in preventing loss of bone density. Many experts now recommend estrogen treatment as a routine measure for osteoporosis prevention for all nonblack menopausal women. FDA-approved package labeling for estrogen now includes arrest of osteoporosis progression as an approved treatment indication for which estrogen is "probably" effective, and a national Consensus Conference on Estrogen use sponsored by the National Institutes of Health has recognized osteoporosis prevention as an acceptable indication for long-term use of estrogen [18].

When the use of estrogen is contraindicated, progestin can be given alone for treatment of vasomotor symptoms and also may have a beneficial effect on bone metabolism. Research on benefits and risks of treatment with progestin alone is quite limited.

Progestin used cyclically, in conjunction with estrogen, has been more extensively studied and appears to confer effective protection against hyperstimulation of the uterus. Data on bone mineral content provide some assurance that

Table 75-4. Estrogen relative potency

Estrogen preparation	FSH suppression	Corticosteroid binding globulin increase	Sex binding globulin increase	Angiotensinogen increase
Piperazine estrone sulfate (Ogen)	1.1	1.0	1.0	1.0
Micronized estradiol (Estrace)	1.3	1.9	1.0	0.7
Conjugated estrogen (Premarin)	1.4	2.5	3.2	3.5
Diethylstilbestrol	3.8	70.0	28.0	13.0
Ethinyl estradiol	80–200*	1000.0*	614.0	232.0

Key: FSH=follicle-stimulating hormone.
*Estimate in absence of parallelism.
Source: C. A. Mashchak, et al. Comparison of pharmacodynamic properties of various estrogen formulations. *Am. J. Obstet. Gynecol.* 144(5):511, 1982.

Table 75-5. Estrogen equivalents*

Diethylstilbestrol	1.00 mg
Conjugated estrogens	5.00 mg
Mestranol	0.08 mg
Ethinyl estradiol	0.05 mg

*Estrogens with approximately equal biologic effects.
Source: A. G. Gilman, et al. (eds.). *The Pharmacologic Basis of Therapeutics* (6th ed.). New York: Macmillan, 1980.

protection against bone loss is maintained or possibly improved by the addition of progestin [19].

For these reasons, combination treatment utilizing estrogen alone for 12–15 days, followed by estrogen and progestin together for 10–13 days, followed by 5 or 6 drug-free days each month is rapidly gaining clinical acceptance as the best approach when hormone treatment is used.

A variety of estrogen products and several alternative progestin products are available. Although there is no conclusive evidence that their effects in postmenopausal treatment differ significantly, conjugated estrogens and medroxyprogesterone acetate are by far the most commonly recommended and have been most thoroughly studied. Estrogens and progestins vary widely in potency (Tables 75-4 and 75-5) and also differ in their effects on lipid metabolism. Progestins differ in their relative androgenic, estrogenic, and antiestrogenic potency, as well as their effect on estrogen receptors. Some authors believe that C-21 progestins such as medroxyprogesterone acetate, megestrol acetate, or chlormadinone acetate, are preferable to C-19 derivatives including norgestrel, norethindrone, or ethynodiol diacetate, because of the elevation in low-density lipoprotein that has been reported with C-19 but not with C-21 compounds [20]. Others, however, feel that the differences in reported lipid effects can be attributed primarily to the dose of progestins involved, and that C-21 progestins at comparable dose levels would exhibit similar undesirable characteristics.

Recent histologic and receptor assay studies have addressed the issue of optimal progestin dose and timing. These studies suggest that treatment for at least 13 days in each cycle may provide optimal suppression of the endometrium, and that a lower dose of progestin (1 mg of norethindrone or its equivalent) may be sufficient to provide a maximal effect [21]. In one study, a dose of medroxyprogesterone acetate of 5 mg for 10 days was sufficient to reduce endometrial estrogen receptor levels for women receiving a conjugated estrogen dose of 0.625 mg daily or less, but 10 mg was required for women receiving higher doses [22]. Other researchers, however, have reported less consistent reduction in receptor levels with medroxyprogesterone acetate at all doses as compared to more uniform results with other progestins [23]. Because the effect of progestin on lipid metabolism is dose-related, using the lowest effective dose is desirable.

Large-scale clinical studies of cyclic combined hormone treatment, documenting reduced hyperplasia and carcinoma rates, have involved primarily conjugated estrogen 0.625 mg daily with medroxyprogesterone acetate 10 mg or norethindrone acetate 5 mg given for 10 days in each cycle [24]. Because this is an important basis for confidence in the safety of combined hormone treatment, it may be prudent to utilize these dose levels until alternative approaches are shown to be equally effective or superior clinically. Data to document the relative safety of weekly-administered estrogen and of transdermal estrogen are limited, though they may be reasonable options for patients who experience unacceptable side effects with more traditional treatment. If progestin side effects are a problem, however, a reduction in progestin dose is a reasonable option and would be preferable to omission of progestin or to shorter treatment duration.

For treatment with progestin alone, oral preparations and parenteral medroxyprogesterone acetate have been utilized. Data on the effect on bone of progestin used alone are very limited but suggest that oral medroxyprogesterone acetate, 20 mg daily, significantly decreases urinary calcium-creatinine and hydroxyproline-creatinine ratios. The decrease observed is not as great as that observed with estrogen treatment but is significantly greater than the reduction observed with similar doses of megestrol acetate [2].

Vaginal administration of estrogen can result in significant systemic absorption. Use of 2–4 gm of conjugated estrogen cream daily, the package recommendation, introduces 1.25-2.50 mg of drug, and results in serum levels in the range expected for oral therapy with 0.300–0.625 mg daily [25]. Clearly, this treatment would not be suitable for a patient in whom estrogen is contraindicated. A significantly smaller dose of vaginal cream, 0.5 gm containing 0.3 mg of conjugated estrogen daily, may be sufficient to control vaginal atrophy symptoms with little or no measurable increase in serum estrogen levels [25].

c. **Other methods.** Fluoride, anabolic steroids such as OD 14 and Stanozolol, calcitonin, and pulsatile treatment with vitamin D or parathyroid hormone followed by calcitonin or diphosphonate have all been proposed for treatment of osteoporosis [3] but must be considered investigational approaches at the present time. Sodium fluoride has not been approved by the FDA for use in osteoporosis and is associated with frequent adverse reactions. As many as 40% of women experience serious side effects such as nausea and vomiting, anemia, plantar fascial syndrome, synovitis, or fluorosis with fracture. When vitamin D and calcium are prescribed with fluoride, significant hypercalciuria and hypercalcemia may occur [26]. Although fluoride may prove to be an important treatment approach in the future, its use clearly requires careful supervision.

2. **Justification**

a. **Effectiveness and benefits.** No data are available to assess the effectiveness of early identification and education for patients at risk of osteoporosis, or the effectiveness of fall-prevention measures in reducing osteoporosis morbidity.

Multiple prospective studies have shown that estrogen treatment can arrest bone mineral loss in menopausal women. Several retrospective, case-control studies have documented reduced fracture risks among treated women. Bone preservation is most effective when treatment is initiated within 3 years after menopause, and when the estrogen dose is at least 0.625 mg of conjugated estrogen daily or its equivalent [3]. A randomized comparison of calcium (0.5 gm) plus placebo, versus calcium with combined cyclic estrogen and progestin treatment, found that 51 placebo patients suffered a 5.7% loss of bone mineral content over 36, while 43 hormone-treated patients had a 3.7% increase in bone mineral content (Fig. 75-1). The results of this study indicate that calcium supplementation of 0.5 gm is not sufficient to prevent loss of bone mineral and that combination hormone treatment can prevent bone loss and may actually result in some gain in bone mineral [19]. Effective bone protection with aggressive calcium supplementation and lower-dose estrogen (conjugated estrogen 0.3 mg daily) has been documented in one small study [27]. Women in this study maintained a total daily calcium intake of 1500–2100 mg, and significant bone less occurred in the group using calcium alone.

When estrogen treatment is stopped, bone loss can be expected to resume. Some researchers believe that treatment cessation is followed by a period of exces-

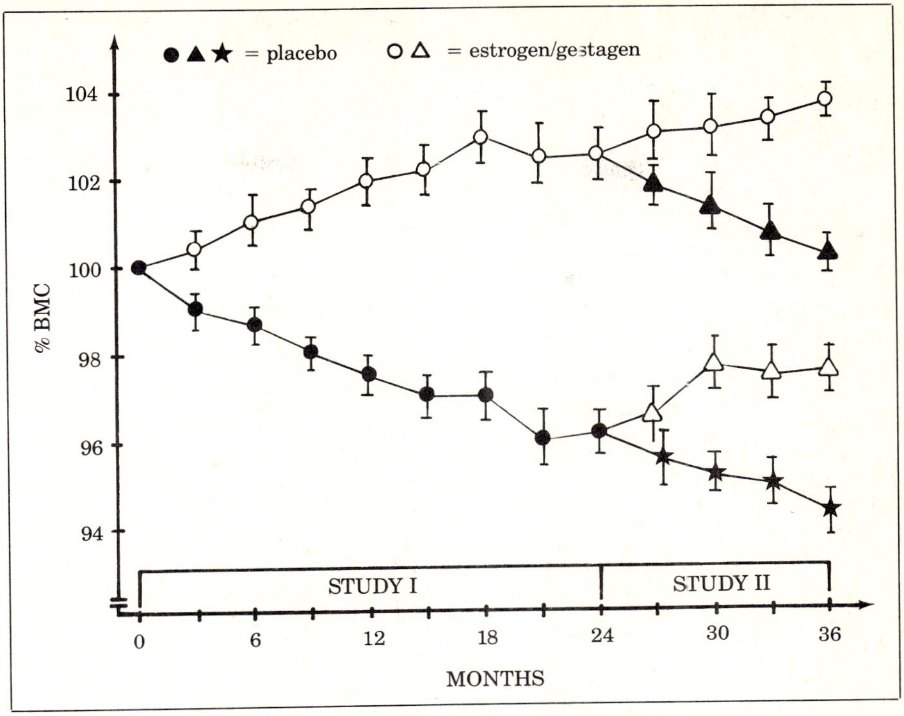

Fig. 75-1. Bone mineral content as a function of time and treatment in 94 (study I) and 77 (study II) women soon after menopause (crossover study of placebo [calcium 0.5 gm alone] versus estrogen and progestin with calcium 0.5 gm). (From C. Christiansen, M. S. Christensen, and I. Transbol. Bone mass in postmenopausal women after withdrawal of oestrogen/gestagen replacement therapy. *Lancet* 1[8218]:459, 1981.)

sively rapid bone loss similar to that observed during the first few years after menopause [3]. If treatment cessation does result in a period of rapid loss, then it is conceivable that a woman who starts and stops treatment several times might experience a greater loss of bone than she would have had with no treatment at all. For this reason, intermittent treatment should be avoided whenever possible until further research is available to clarify this issue.

Hormone treatment confers other benefits, unrelated to osteoporosis prevention. **Vasomotor symptoms** of menopause are usually controlled when an estrogen dose of 0.625 mg conjugated estrogen or its equivalent is used. Progestin treatment also is often effective in eliminating this problem. Hot flashes are not believed to be medically dangerous but may contribute to other menopausal symptoms such as irritability or depression when flushes are severe enough to disturb sleep. **Atrophic vaginitis** with thinning of vaginal epithelium, loss of elasticity, diminished lubrication response to arousal, more alkaline pH, and atrophy of the urethra often associated with dysuria, frequency, and urgency are usually controlled with estrogen administered vaginally or orally in doses smaller than those required for control of vasomotor symptoms.

In older reviews, estrogen effects on **cardiovascular disease** are often discussed as risks of treatment. Although analysis of data from the Framingham study documented increased risks for cardiovascular disease among postmenopausal estrogen users [28], most recent research has suggested that estrogen treatment may reduce cardiovascular diseases risks, possibly because of estrogen effects on lipid metabolism [29]. Several retrospective, case-control studies have found significant protection (relative risk 0.4–0.9) against cardiovascular disease for current and past estrogen use compared with untreated controls. The finding that estrogen treatment reduces low-density lipoprotein

Table 75-6. Endometrial cancer incidence at Wilford Hall, 1975–1979

	Patient-years of observation	Patients with cancer	Incidence (per 100,000)
Estrogen-progestin users	7063	5	70.8
Estrogen users	2302	10	434.4
Estrogen vaginal cream users	1318	1	75.9
Progestin or androgen users	761	0	
Untreated women	2477	6	242.2
Total	13,921	22	158.0

Source: R. D. Gambrell, Jr. Clinical use of progestins in the menopausal patients: Dosage and duration. *J. Reprod. Med.* 27(8 Suppl.):531, 1982.

cholesterol and increases high-density lipoprotein is also consistent with a protective effect against cardiovascular disease. Progestins, on the other hand, have been shown to reverse the beneficial HDL/LDL shift induced by estrogen, and cardiovascular disease risks associated with oral contraceptive use have been shown to be related to progestin dose. Whether or not C-21 progestins given in equipotent doses would have the same undesirable lipid and cardiovascular risk effects is not known [30].

b. Risks and side effects of hormone treatment

(1) Endometrial hyperstimulation. Among women treated with estrogen alone, as many as 18–32% develop endometrial hyperplasia, and 6–10% develop adenomatous hyperplasia. These women also experience an increased risk of endometrial carcinoma, with a relative risk of as much as 4.8% after 5 years, and 8.5% after 10 years of treatment. Thus, an excess of approximately eight cases of endometrial carcinoma/1000 women/year can be expected after 10 treatment years [30]. Despite the increase in incidence, however, the use of estrogen is not associated with an increase in mortality from endometrial cancer among estrogen-treated women [31]. Their low mortality may be due to earlier, more aggressive evaluation and treatment, or to tumor-characteristic differences between spontaneous and "estrogen-induced" malignancies, or to other, unrelated, beneficial effects of estrogen on mortality [32]. Unfortunately, abnormal vaginal bleeding does not always occur early in the course of these problems, so routine endometrial sampling is necessary for detection of hyperplasia and carcinoma when estrogen is used alone.

The cyclic use of progestin along with estrogen protects the endometrium against hyperstimulation. The incidence of hyperplasia is reduced to 2% when progestin is given for 10 days, and to zero with 12-day exposure [30]. Researchers in another small study found that endometrial response to progestin dose could be predicted by the cycle day of bleeding onset. When the progestin dose given was sufficient to delay bleeding onset until 11 days or more of progestin had been completed, the endometrial biopsy samples reliably showed a normal secretory pattern [33]. The incidence of endometrial carcinoma in one study was significantly lower for women receiving combination hormone treatment than for women receiving no hormone treatment (Table 75-6) [24].

Particular caution is justified in management of women who are at risk for endometrial carcinoma because of obesity, diabetes mellitus, infertility, irregular menses and failure of ovulation (especially polycystic ovary disease), or liver disease. These patients face an excess risk because of prolonged exposure to unopposed endogenous estrogen [34]. Excess risk is also documented among patients with estrogen-producing neoplasm. Whenever hormone treatment is considered for such patients, thorough pretreatment evaluation including endometrial sampling is indicated.

(2) Breast disease. The role of exogenous hormones in breast cancer is controversial. Some studies have found a decreased risk, some an unchanged risk, and some a slightly increased risk of breast cancer among women treated with unopposed estrogen compared to untreated patients. Some studies of breast cancer risk with combination estrogen and progestin treatment indicate that progestins may provide some protection against breast cancer [35], and some experts recommend that estrogen treatment be combined with cyclic progestin even for women who have undergone hysterectomy. Others, however, feel that the evidence available regarding breast cancer is not sufficiently persuasive to justify progestin use in this situation, since possible adverse effects on lipid balance may be involved.

(3) **Gallbladder disease.** The incidence of gallbladder disease among estrogen-treated postmenopausal women in the Boston Collaborative Drug Surveillance Program was 218/100,000 compared to 87/100,000 among nonusers (relative risk 2.5). Effects of progestin on this risk, if any, are not known, although cholelithiasis is more common among oral contraceptive (estrogen and progestin) users than among the general population.

(4) **Other serious medical conditions.** Studies of oral contraceptive users and some studies of menopausal estrogen patients, have linked hormone treatment to elevation in blood pressure, abnormal glucose tolerance, thromboembolic disease, stroke, and myocardial infarction. The Boston study as well as more recent studies of cardiovascular disease [29], however, have failed to document any increase in the risks for these problems among menopause-treatment patients. Some authors have identified individual women who appear to have idiosyncratic hypertension associated with menopausal hormone treatment. For this reason, routine monitoring of blood pressure is recommended [20].

(5) **Rare or minor side effects.** When combination hormone treatment is used, uterine withdrawal bleeding occurs in 97% of women 60 or younger; the proportion gradually decreases to about 60% for women 65 or older. Other side effects occur in approximately 10% of women. Nausea, usually transient, is a common estrogen side effect. Mastodynia may be transient or may improve with a decrease in estrogen dose or an increase in progestin. Edema, bloating, and irritability can be aggravated by progestin but may improve with a decrease in estrogen dose. Lower abdominal cramps and dysmenorrhea may improve with a change in progestin or use of a prostaglandin-inhibiting analgesic [24]. Side effects reported for estrogen use, including the use of oral contraceptives, include the following: breast enlargement, galactorrhea, enlargement of uterine fibroids, cholestatic jaundice, hepatic adenoma, chloasma or melasma, erythema multiforme, erythema nodosum, rash, loss of hair, hirsutism, intolerance to contact lenses, headache, migraine, dizziness, depression, chorea, change in weight, reduced carbohydrate tolerance, aggravation of porphyria, change in libido, and adverse effects on a fetus exposed during pregnancy. Edema resulting from estrogen or progestin might aggravate other medical conditions including asthma, epilepsy, migraine, heart disease, or kidney disease.

Contraindications for use of estrogen and progestin are listed in Table 75-7. All patients who receive hormone treatment should be taught to watch for the danger signs of serious medical complications [Table 75-8].

c. **Risk-benefit assessment of intervention options.** Neither the effectiveness of adequate calcium supplementation nor that of exercise have been studied sufficiently to permit risk-benefit assessment in comparison to hormone treatment. Studies of calcium so far have used fairly small doses (in most cases < 1 gm), and this may explain the superior effectiveness seen with hormone treatment in these comparisons.

Considering hormone treatment separately, many authors have estimated mortality and morbidity of prevented osteoporosis versus endometrial carcinoma mortality and morbidity caused by treatment. Because endometrial carcinoma mortality is quite low and osteoporosis so common, many conclude that the risk-benefit ratio justifies hormone treatment even for estrogen used alone. The risk-benefit ratio would favor combined progestin and estrogen treatment even more strongly if future data confirm a protective effect against endometrial cancer or against cardiovascular disease.

Cost/benefit analysis of estrogen treatment was undertaken in 1980 by Weinstein [36]. He assumed that women taking estrogen had a risk of endometrial cancer 8.0 times as great, a risk of breast cancer 1.5 times as great, and a risk of hip or wrist fracture 0.33 times as great as untreated women. He concluded that estrogen treatment of all women 50–65 years of age would prevent 55,000 hip fractures and would cause 27,000 cases of endometrial and breast cancer,

Table 75-7. Contraindications to estrogen treatment

Absolute
Pregnancy
Estrogen-dependent neoplasia, known or suspected
Undiagnosed vaginal bleeding
Acute or severe chronic liver disease
Acute phlebitis
History of severe thrombophlebitis or thromboembolic disease associated with estrogen
Relative
High risk for thrombosis: such as trauma, immobilization, sepsis, myocardial infarction, congestive heart failure, cerebrovascular accident
Severe hypertension or history of estrogen-induced hypertension
Diabetes mellitus (monitor blood sugar)
Gallbladder disease
Endometrial hyperplasia
Migraine headaches
Kidney disease
Liver disease
Epilepsy
Asthma
Uterine leiomyomata
Depression

Table 75-8. Danger signs for patients: Serious estrogen complications

1. Abnormal vaginal bleeding: Any bleeding that occurs during the days you are taking pills
2. Pain in the leg (calf) or chest, shortness of breath, coughing blood
3. Severe headache, dizziness, faintness, or vision problems
4. Breast lump
5. Jaundice (yellow skin)

and 38,000 cholecystectomies. His analytic model for cost versus "quality-adjusted life expectancy" concluded that estrogen treatment is cost-effective in menopausal women with prior hysterectomy or osteoporosis, but not as a prophylactic measure in asymptomatic women with intact uteri. If this analysis is adjusted to reflect a reduced risk for endometrial cancer with combined progestin and estrogen treatment, then prophylactic hormone treatment for asymptomatic and osteoporotic women, with or without prior hysterectomy, would all be cost-effective.

The primary issue, however, that must be clarified before conclusive prevention and treatment recommendations can be made, is whether adequate calcium intake and appropriate exercise can result in bone preservation comparable to that achieved with hormone treatment.

d. Costs. Annual costs are $25–40 for 0.625 mg conjugated estrogen 25 days monthly; and $25–60 for 10 mg medroxyprogesterone acetate 10–13 days monthly. The medication cost for 20 mg medroxyprogesterone acetate daily is $85–185/year. In addition, hormone treatment may require more frequent physician visits and procedures than would otherwise be necessary. Endometrial biopsy (approximately $100) may be recommended on a periodic basis. Biopsy or diagnostic dilation and curettage (approximately $500–1000) may be required for evaluation of bleeding in some cases.

e. Acceptability. Providing hormone treatment is straightfoward and easily accomplished by the health care provider. For patients, however, acceptability is a major issue. The climate of fear regarding uterine cancer risk is widespread and intense. A patient may react with skepticism to reassurances about low cancer mortality rates or the power of progestin to prevent it. For her, medical facts reported in the media have always stressed grave risk and may have undermined her confidence in the medical judgment that would advocate use of a drug known to cause cancer.

The resumption of monthly vaginal bleeding because of treatment is often distinctly unwelcome. Similarly, the occurrence of medical minor side effects such as nausea, mastodynia, or edema can be major obstacles for women embarking on preventive treatment. Also, the necessity to remember daily medication and to cope with frequent medical follow-up visits may seem intrusive for a woman who has no health problems that otherwise require her to do so.

IV. Recommendations

A. Primary prevention

1. Encourage everyone to maintain adequate calcium balance throughout life.
   a. Maintain adequate calcium intake through diet or calcium supplementation. Children and young adults should have an intake of 800–1000 mg elemental calcium daily; pregnant and lactating women, 1300–1500 mg; adults, including treated postmenopausal women, 1000 mg; and untreated postmenopausal women, 1500 mg.
   b. Assure adequate vitamin D through sunlight exposure (15–60 minutes daily) or supplementation (400 units daily).
   c. Avoid excessive dietary protein, as well as excessive vitamins A or D.
   d. Avoid smoking and caffeine.
   e. Whenever possible, avoid drugs, including aluminum antacids, that may adversely affect calcium balance.
2. Encourage everyone to maintain physical activity throughout life.
3. Avoid iatrogenic causes of osteoporosis whenever possible. Consider preservation of skeletal integrity as an important aspect of medical management. Whenever possible, ensure uninterrupted, adequate estrogen replacement for women who experience temporary or permanent premature hypoestrogenism.

B. Early detection

1. Record measured height and weight annually and measured armspan when height loss is suspected.
2. Identify patients at risk of osteoporosis because of medical problems, premature hypogonadism, or drug treatment, and nonblack women of perimenopausal age, for education regarding calcium balance and exercise. Consider dietary survey or other approaches that may reinforce education efforts. Consider diagnostic methods for skeletal surveillance. Assess advantages and disadvantages of hormone treatment and discuss with patient.

C. Early intervention

1. Initiate evaluation and management of medical problems that may contribute to accidental falls; educate patients about assessment and correction of environmental hazards.
2. Reinforce (or institute) calcium supplementation or high dietary calcium intake. Provide educational materials [37].
3. Consider initiation of hormone treatment. Discuss possible benefits, risks, and side effects with patients. Assess contraindications and endometrial carcinoma risk status. Inform patient of possible disadvantages of intermittent treatment. Initiate treatment if patient and clinician agree.
4. Monitor serum calcium and phosphorus annually for 2 years (to identify asymptomatic hyperparathyroidism unmasked by treatment).
5. If hormone treatment is not elected, establish periodic surveillance of calcium balance, exercise status, and symptoms or signs of osteoporosis, and reassess advisability of hormone treatment periodically. Consider bone mineral content evaluation.

References

1. Stillman, T. G. Can osteoporosis be prevented? *Geriatrics* 35(2):95, 1980. *A short and clear review of osteoporosis differential diagnosis, risk factors, and treatment options.*
2. Mandel, F. P., et al. Effects of progestins on bone metabolism in postmenopausal women. *J. Reprod. Med.* 27(8 Suppl):511, 1982. *This supplement includes eight articles summarizing current research on progestins in relationship to the menopausal woman.*
3. Lindsay, R., and Herrington, B. S. Estrogens and osteoporosis. *Semin. Reprod. Endocrinol.* 1(1):55, 1983. *The first issue of this new journal is edited by Leon Speroff, M.D., and is entirely*

devoted to menopause. It includes comprehensive reviews of key controversial topics in management of perimenopausal patients.

4. Sandler, R. B. Etiology of primary osteoporosis: A hypothesis. *J. Am. Geriatr. Soc.* 26(5):209, 1978. *A brief review of epidemiologic and metabolic data on osteoporosis etiology.*
5. Ettinger, B., Genant, H. K., and Cann, C. E. Long-term estrogen replacement therapy prevents bone loss and fractures. *Ann. Intern. Med.* 102(3):319, 1985. *Quantitative assessment of fracture incidence among postmenopausal women using estrogen alone (compared to case-matched controls).*
6. Heaney, R. P., Recker, R. R., and Saville, P. D. Menopausal changes in calcium balance performance. *J. Lab. Clin. Med.* 92(6):953, 1978. *A landmark study of calcium balance among white, Roman Catholic nuns in Nebraska.*
7. Smith, E. L. Exercise for prevention of osteoporosis: A review. *Physician Sports Med.* 10(3):72, 1982. *An interesting review of data concerning bone remodeling and physical stress.*
8. Recker, R. R., Saville, P. D., and Heaney, R. P. Effect of estrogens and calcium carbonate on bone loss in postmenopausal women. *Ann. Intern. Med.* 87(6):649, 1977. *An early landmark study of the efficacy of estrogen and calcium treatment.*
9. Calcium for postmenopausal osteoporosis. *Med. Lett. Drugs Ther.* 24(623):105, 1982. *A brief review of calcium supplementation, including available calcium products, dose ranges, and prices.*
10. Advice on limiting intake of bonemeal. *FDA Drug Bull.* 12(1):5, 1982. *FDA warning on lead contamination of calcium supplement products.*
11. Aloia, J. F., et al. Prevention of involutional bone loss by exercise. *Ann. Intern. Med.* 89(3):356, 1978. *One of the very few prospective studies of exercise in relation to bone loss.*
12. Smith, E. L., Jr., Reddan, W., and Smith, P. E. Physical activity and calcium modalities for bone mineral increase in aged women. *Med. Sci. Sports Exerc.* 13(1):60, 1981. *One of the very few prospective studies of exercise in relation to bone loss.*
13. Shangold, M. M. How exercise benefits older women. *Contemp. Obstet. Gynecol.* 19:81, 1982. *A short and very practical guide for clinicians in recommending an exercise program.*
14. Upton, G. V. The perimenopause: Physiologic correlates and clinical management. *J. Reprod. Med.* 27(1):1, 1982. *An exhaustive review of data on hormone physiology in menopause written by the Associate Director of Clinical Research, Wyeth International Ltd.*
15. Cummings, S. R., and Black, D. Should perimenopausal women be screened for osteoporosis? *Ann. Intern. Med.* 104(6):817, 1986. *An analysis of issues relevant to screening policy for absorptiometry and CT scan.*
16. Wasnich, R. D., et al. Prediction of postmenopausal fracture risk with use of bone mineral measurements. *Am. J. Obstet. Gynecol.* 153(7):745, 1985. *Study of 1098 postmenopausal women showing statistically significant correlation between os calsis density percentile and fracture risk.*
17. Rubenstein, L. Z. Falls in the elderly: A clinical approach. *West. J. Med.* 138(2):273, 1983. *A practical guide to reducing accident risks in the elderly.*
18. United States National Institutes of Health. *Osteoporosis. National Institutes of Health Consensus Development Conference Statement.* Bethesda, MD: National Institutes of Health, 1984. Vol. 5, No. 3. *Expert review of salient issues in osteoporosis prevention as of 1984.*
19. Christiansen, C., Christiansen, M. S., and Transbol, I. Bone mass in postmenopausal women after withdrawal of oestrogen/gestagen replacement therapy. *Lancet* 1(8218):459, 1981. *One of the first studies of bone mass with cyclic combined estrogen and progestin treatment.*
20. Hammond, C. B., and Maxson, W. S. Current status of estrogen therapy for the menopause. *Fertil. Steril.* 37(1):5, 1982. *A comprehensive review of estrogen pharmacology, pathophysiology of estrogen withdrawal, and risks and benefits of estrogen treatment.*
21. Whitehead, M. I., et al. Effects of estrogens and progestins on the biochemistry and morphology of the postmenopausal endometrium. *N. Engl. J. Med.* 305(27):1599, 1981. *One of the few studies to address optimal dose and timing for progestin treatment.*
22. Gibbons, W. E., et al. Biochemical and histologic effects of sequential estrogen/progestin therapy on the endometrium of postmenopausal women. *Am. J. Obstet. Gynecol.* 154(2):456, 1986. *Small study of progestin effects on cytosolic estrogen receptor concentration.*
23. Lane, G., et al. Is Provera the ideal progestogen for addition to postmenopausal estrogen therapy? *Fertil. Steril.* 45(3):345, 1986. *Small study of progestin effects on nuclear estradiol receptor concentration and endometrial ultrastructure.*
24. Gambrell, R. D. Jr. Clinical use of progestins in the menopausal patients: Dosage and duration. *J. Reprod. Med.* 27(8 Suppl):531, 1982. *The first large-scale clinical study to document the effectiveness of progestin in counteracting uterine hyperstimulation with estrogen treatment.*

25. Deutsch, S., Ossowski, R., and Benjamin, I. Comparison between degree of systemic absorption of vaginally and orally administered estrogens at different dose levels in postmenopausal women. *Am. J. Obstet. Gynecol.* 139(8):967, 1981. *A comparison of oral and vaginal absorption of estrogen.*
26. Riggs, B. L., et al. Effect of the fluoride/calcium regimen on vertebral fracture occurrence in postmenopausal osteoporosis. *N. Engl. J. Med.* 306(8):446, 1982. *A comparative study of calcium, fluoride, and estrogen showing reduced fracture rates.*
27. Ettinger, B., Genant, H. K., and Cann, C. E. Postmenopausal bone loss is prevented by treatment with low dosage estrogen with calcium. *Ann. Intern. Med.* 106(1):40, 1987. *A small (N=73) but important study.*
28. Wilson, P. W. F., Garrison, R. J., and Castelli, W. P. Postmenopausal estrogen use, cigarette smoking, and cardiovascular morbidity in women over 50. *N. Engl. J. Med.* 313(17):1038, 1985. *The most important epidemiologic study (Framingham, 1200 women), which has found an adverse effect of estrogen on cardiovascular morbidity.*
29. Stampfer, M. J., et al. A prospective study of postmenopausal estrogen therapy and coronary heart disease. *N. Engl. J. Med.* 313(17):1044, 1985. *A very large epidemiologic study (121,000 nurses) published concurrently with the Wilson study that found a significant protective effect for estrogen use on coronary artery disease.*
30. Whitehead, M., et al. Avoidance of endometrial hyperstimulation in estrogen-treated postmenopausal women. *Semin. Reprod. Endocrinol.* 1(1):41, 1983. *A review of data concerning estrogen and progestin and dose.*
31. Chu, J., Schweid, A. I., and Weiss, N. S. Survival among women with endometrial cancer: A comparison of estrogen users and nonusers. *Am. J. Obstet. Gynecol.* 143(5):569, 1982. *A landmark study documenting significantly better survival among endometrial cancer victims that had used estrogen, compared to victims who did not have a history of estrogen use.*
32. Bush, T. L., et al. Estrogen use and all-cause mortality. Preliminary results from the Lipid Research Clinics Program Follow-up Study. *J.A.M.A.* 249(7):903, 1983. *If confirmed, the findings of this study may have enormous significance: All-cause mortality among 2269 white women age 40–69 using estrogen was 0.37 times that of nonusers (3.4/1000 compared to 9.3/1000).*
33. Padwick, M. L., et al. A simple method for determining the optimal dosage of progestin in postmenopausal women receiving estrogens. *N. Engl. J. Med.* 315(10):930, 1987. *An innovative, clinically useful approach to assessment of adequate progestin dose.*
34. Ziel, H. K. Estrogen's role in endometrial cancer. *Obstet. Gynecol.* 60(4):509, 1982. *A concise summary of data on the relationship between endometrial cancer and estrogen exposure.*
35. Gambrell, R. D. Breast disease in the postmenopausal years. *Semin. Reprod. Endocrinol.* 1(1):27, 1983. *A summary of data on breast cancer risk with hormone treatment.*
36. Weinstein, M. C. Estrogen use in postmenopausal women—costs, risks, and benefits. *N. Engl. J. Med.* 303(6):308, 1980. *One of the few published attempts to quantify costs, risks, and benefits of estrogen treatment.*
37. Notelovitz, M., and Ware, M. *Stand Tall: The Informed Woman's Guide to Preventing Osteoporosis.* Gainesville, FL: Triad, 1982. *This 200-page, softbound book provides clear, comprehensive information and a balanced, practical viewpoint on all aspects of osteoporosis including calcium balance and a levelheaded overview of hormone treatment. An excellent book to recommend to patients.*

76 Breast Cancer

Lois F. O'Grady

I. The problem

A. Description. Early diagnosis of breast cancer is important because survival varies tremendously according to the severity of the disease at diagnosis (Table 76-1). A patient with a small tumor and negative axillary nodes (stage I) has a greater than 85% chance of 5-year survival free of disease after primary therapy (surgery, radiation, or a combination). If a patient has a larger tumor, evidence of extensive local spread, or involvement of the axillary lymph nodes, her chances of survival drop off dramatically. It is important to find ways to diagnose more patients at stage I, when the disease is more curable. Recent studies show that age at diagnosis is also prognostically significant [1].

B. Epidemiology. Carcinoma of the breast is the most common malignancy of nonsmoking women in the United States and is second only to lung cancer in smokers. One of every 12 women (8%) will develop the disease during her lifetime. Over 120,000 new cases are recorded each year, and over 35,000 women die of the disease yearly.

There are certain known **risk factors** for development of breast cancer (Table 76-2). Many are minor associations, but three are major:

1. A woman who has a cancer in one breast has a risk of 0.8%/year of developing cancer in the opposite breast.
2. Family history is very important in assessing risk. Breast cancer in maternal relatives increases the risk for a given patient. If the cancers in the family occur premenopausally or bilaterally, the risk is greater.
3. The fibrocystic condition has long been known to increase the incidence of breast cancer. From the studies of DuPont and Page [2], we now know that it is primarily fibrocystic disease of the proliferative type (about 30% of the fibrocystic population) that increases the risk by a factor of 2. If it is atypical hyperplasia, the risk is 5 times that of the general population. Women who have atypia and a positive family history of breast cancer carry a risk 11 times that of women with nonproliferative breast disease and a negative family history. This study also demonstrates that risks are additive.

II. Secondary prevention

A. Early detection

1. Methods [3,4]

a. Physical examination by medical personnel

(1) Performance. As part of the routine examination, the breasts are inspected while the patient is seated and disrobed. One looks for variation in contour and skin changes such as *peau d'orange.* There is no need to palpate the breasts while the patient is sitting.

After the patient lies down, place one of her arms over her head. This stretches the breast over the chest wall and permits the examiner to compress and roll each segment of the breast between the flat portion of the fingers and the chest wall. The breast is compressed, or "milked," for examination of secretion.

The process is repeated with the other breast.

(2) Interpretation. The examiner searches for areas of breast tissue that stand out as different from the rest of the breast: areas of nodularity that do not spread out when palpated, as normal tissue does, and dominant masses.

Any discoloration of fluid secretion is abnormal.

(3) Age, interval. The breast should be examined as part of every general examination. Special attention should be directed to the breasts after age 30. Examination should occur yearly after age 40, and every 4 months in high-risk patients.

Table 76-1. Breast cancer survival statistics

Stage	Patients (approximate %)	5-year survival free of disease (%)
I: Small, localized tumor	50	80–90
II: Tumor >2 cm, axillary nodes	35	60–65
III: Large tumor, local invasion, multiple nodes	8	40
IV: Metastatic at diagnosis	7	<10

Table 76-2. Risk of developing breast cancer

	Relative risk
Some increase	
Nulliparous	1.5x
Late age of first pregnancy (10–15-year post-menarche)	1.5x
Early menarche; late menopause	1.5x
Postmenopausal estrogens	1.5x
Major increase	
Fibrocystic condition, especially proliferative lesions	1.5–4x
History of previous breast cancer	5x
Bilateral breast cancer in family	5x
Premenopausal breast cancer in family	3–5x
Relative with premenopausal, bilateral cancer	9x
Patient with atypical hyperplasia on biopsy and family history	11x

(4) Follow-up. Abnormalities are evaluated with aspiration of cysts or biopsy of masses.

b. Breast self-examination (BSE)

(1) Performance. Classically, self-examination includes inspection before a mirror, examination while upright, and examination while supine. This author agrees with Mahoney [5] that these techniques are cumbersome and time-consuming, and that there is some lack of compliance. In this author's opinion, the easiest and most effective technique is for the woman to lie comfortably in bed, raise one arm over her head to stretch the breast across the chest wall, and palpate with the fingers of the opposite hand. There is no need for cream, soap, or powder to make the breast "slippery."

(2) Age, interval. BSE can be taught to women at any age, even in high school; it is easily learned and can be reinforced repeatedly through medical or community educational efforts. BSE is learned most effectively when taught by a physician after he or she has examined the breasts. At that time, the patient can be reassured that any irregularity found in the breast is "normal," and she should be encouraged to look for changes in the future. Although instruction by the physician is ideal, other medical care workers and even trained nonmedical personnel can teach BSE.

BSE should be done just after the menstrual period, when the breast is least engorged and tender. In postmenopausal women, a specific date each month can be selected for the examination. Although it is not stressed by most health educators, it is appropriate for the woman's sexual partner to become an aide in the monthly health maintenance ritual.

(3) Follow-up. Abnormalities should be evaluated by a physician within 4–6 weeks.

c. Mammography. There are two points about mammography that must be stressed: (1) It is an adjunct to regular medical care and not a replacement for a good, thorough physical examination, and (2) it is not used to determine the malignancy of a discrete mass in the breast. A new discrete mass must be evaluated by aspiration and/or biopsy, regardless of the mammographic interpretation. In this situation, the mammograph is used to screen the rest of the breast, and the opposite one.

(1) **Performance.** The new techniques of film screen mammography provide excellent images at reduced radiation exposure—less than 0.5 rad per examination. With this technique, the breast is compressed on the x ray plate, and some women note mild discomfort.

(2) **Interpretation.** It is not 100% accurate, and its accuracy is only as good as the skill of the interpreter; know and communicate with your mammographer. Mammography is more accurate in older women, who have more fat in the breast for better contrast.

(3) **Age, interval, population.** In its recent revision of The Cancer Related Health Checkup, the American Cancer Society (ACS) modified its standard recommendations slightly:

(a) BSE for all women over 20.

(b) Physical examination every 3 years between the ages of 20 and 40, and yearly thereafter.

(c) Baseline mammography between the ages of 35 and 40, yearly over the age of 50.

(d) Women between the ages of 40 and 50 should be screened every 1–2 years. This recommendation may assume more importance if recent reports of increased survival for women diagnosed between ages 45 and 50 are true.

The ACS points out that these recommendations emphasize the role of the personal physician in determining the need for mammography. This may be so, but it also places the personal physician right in the middle of a major controversy without guidelines.

Women who are at higher risk of developing breast cancer (see Table 76-2) may need routine mammography starting in their 30s. At the same time, these women may be (theoretically) more susceptible to the effects of radiation. Women who are at low risk may not need mammography as often. At a 1986 conference of oncologists in northern California, there was a general agreement that a good approach for low-risk women might be three yearly mammograms beginning in the mid-40s, and if negative, every 2 years thereafter. The author believes there is merit in such an approach, but it should be emphasized that this is not the recommendation of the ACS.

2. **Justification.** Most breast cancers grow slowly and therefore a malignancy is present in the breast for many years before it is diagnosed [6]. Because of this, breast cancer is a disease for which screening is most important and that fits the usual criteria for effective screening: it is numerically significant; it has very effective primary treatment (surgery or radiotherapy); it has a long asymptomatic but detectable period; early therapy provides cures, whereas delayed therapy leads to death; and, effective screening methods are available.

a. **Physical examination by medical personnel**

(1) **Test characteristics.** Sixty percent of breast cancers are detected by physical examination alone [4]. There is little information about false-negative examination, but we do know that 80% of lesions identified as abnormal are benign in young women, and 20% are benign in older women.

(2) **Risks.** There is no risk to the examination. There is some risk of infection or bleeding from needle aspiration of cysts, or needle biopsies of masses. However, the risk of missing a cancer far outweighs the very low risk of these procedures.

(3) **Costs.** The examination is part of regular examination and does not add to cost. Needle aspirate of cysts is not costly. Needle or excisional biopsy cost varies across the country.

(4) **Acceptability.** A careful and considerate examination of the breasts is quite acceptable. Needle aspirates are uncomfortable but not painful. Most women accept biopsies but are very fearful about potential outcome. They need kind and thoughtful reassurance.

b. **Breast self-examination**

(1) **Test characteristics.** BSE has been shown to be an excellent method of screening the breast for new masses, which, in turn, can be brought to medical attention. It does not increase the number of cancers detected but does increase the percentage of tumors that are detected while they are still stage

I from 50% to over 70%, and the tumors are smaller [7–10]. This, in turn, results in a higher percentage of "cures."

The Cancer Detection Center of the University of Minnesota performed over 50,000 exams in 9000 women [4]. Of the cancers found, 56% were found at the annual exam, and 44% by the women doing monthly self-examinations between their yearly visits. Eighty percent of the cancers were stage I, and the 5-year survivals were close to 90%.

(2) Risks. The only risk is anxiety. There is some suggestion that the earlier in life a woman begins regular BSE, the less anxious she is during her high-risk years.

(3) Costs. BSE is the most cost-effective screening test that this author knows [9]. Once taught, it costs nothing save the follow-up costs of breast lump evaluation.

(4) Acceptability. The more often BSE is taught, the greater the number of women who practice it. The compliance rate is reported to be 50% [11] but is probably less. This author suspects that we will see more of this patient participation in cancer prevention, such as self-examination of the testes.

c. Mammography

(1) Test characteristics. The first study that showed clearly the effectiveness of mammographic screening for breast cancer was that conducted by the Health Insurance Program of New York [7]. In the control group, 46% of the cancers were stage I (small, high percentage of cure); but in the group that had regular examinations and mammography, 70% of the tumors were stage I. However, the only statistically significant decrease in mortality was in women over 50 years of age. This latter fact has been of importance in setting the current screening recommendations by the ACS.

The recent report of the Breast Cancer Detection Demonstration Project showing that screening women in their forties was virtually as effective as screening older women has rekindled interest in screening younger women [12]. However, several European studies have failed to show a benefit for women under 50 [13–16]), and, as yet, there has been no change in the screening recommendations of the American Cancer Society, the National Cancer Institute, or the United States Preventive Services Task Force [17, 18].

The European studies confirm the value of mammography screening, demonstrating a 50–70% reduction in mortality [13–16]. Of note, there is benefit even in women screened only once or twice.

A mammogram is not 100% accurate either in detecting a cancer that is present or identifying a cancer-free breast. Like all radiographs, mammographs depend on contrasts between tissues of different densities. In a menopausal female, when the breast tissue itself has decreased in amount and has been replaced by more fatty tissue, there is good contrast between the breast and a malignant mass. However, in young women, nursing women, and women with extensive fibrocystic disease, there is less contrast and, subsequently, less reliability. In actual fact, in young women the test is only 85% accurate (much less so in nursing women and those with an extensive fibrocystic condition), whereas in older women it is 95% accurate. It is due to consideration of these two problems that the American Cancer Society has recommended routine yearly screening for women only after the age of 50—the test is more accurate, the risks of long-term radiation exposure are minimized, and screening is more effective in older women.

(2) Risks. In earlier years, mammography resulted in a relatively high radiation dose to the breast. It has been known for years that the breast is quite sensitive to the effect of radiation in inducing malignancy.

Many people felt that routine yearly mammography over a 40- or 50-year span would induce more malignancy than it would detect at a curable stage. Recent technical advances have decreased the dose of radiation per test to a more acceptable level, less than 1 rad, the total dose for two films of each breast (four films). Indeed, the newest techniques of film screen radiography give beautifully clear radiographs, deliver under 50 mrad/exposure, and cost $50 to $200 for the films and their interpretation. This means that mammography is safer and can be used as a regular diagnostic test, as long as it reliably detects the cancers at a curable stage.

(3) Costs. The addition of mammography to physical examination or BSE increases the cost by $50–$200, but also the "detectability" of small cancer, from 50% to in excess of 90%.

On a national basis, the costs for yearly mammography are staggering—in the billions of dollars. This fact needs careful consideration in future recommendations. The studies may be cost-effective on a personal level but are unacceptably high on a national level.

(4) **Acceptability.** Film screen mammography requires that the breast be compressed between the machine and the x ray plate. Some women find this uncomfortable.

d. **Thermography** is included only to emphasize that it is **not** a reliable method of screening. Theoretically, it is ideal because it poses no risk to the patient. However, it has a very high false-positive and false-negative rate and cannot be recommended in its present state of technology, despite its relatively low cost ($75).

e. **Ultrasound.** The major advantage of ultrasound is that it does not use ionizing radiation. However, it is not as sensitive or specific as mammography in detecting malignancy and cannot be recommended as a routine detection/screening tool.

Ultrasound does have a role in determining the solid or cystic character of a mass identified on mammography. Cost ranges from $100–$250, depending on mode, equipment, and area of country.

f. **Computerized tomography** [19]. At the present time, computerized tomography (CT) is too time-consuming and cumbersome to be used for screening, and its cost ($400–$700) is prohibitive.

B. Early intervention

1. Methods

a. Once a mass in the breast has been identified, it must be removed or diagnosed as benign. There are three acceptable methods:

(1) **Aspiration** of cystic material with disappearance of the mass; and, most important, no recurrence after 3 months. If it recurs, it must be excised.

(2) **Needle biopsy** (large-bore or core) with definitive diagnosis of benignity.

(3) **Excisional biopsy.**

b. If a lesion is identified on mammography but no mass is palpated, it must still be biopsied. This is accomplished by placing a needle tip into the center of the lesion under mammographic or CT control, injecting dye markers to guide the biopsy, or performing direct dissection along the needle to the tip where the biopsy is performed.

2. Justification

a. If the lesion is benign, it gives reassurance and allays fear. If malignant, proper therapy can be instituted. The earlier a tumor is diagnosed, the greater the chance that it will be stage I with its associated greater disease-free survival. This has been documented in many studies [7, 12].

b. **Risks.** The risks of needle aspiration and biopsy are small and consist of a chance of bleeding or infection. The risk of missing a cancer far outweighs the very small complication rate.

c. **Costs** vary depending on procedure and area of the country. At the University of California, Davis Medical Center, 1986 costs to the patient were as follows:

(1) Aspiration including cytology—$164.

(2) Needle biopsy and pathology—$164.

(3) Excisional biopsy—$465

d. **Acceptability.** Needle aspirates are minimally painful and quite acceptable. Larger needle biopsy or excisional biopsy requires local anesthesia, but the procedures are very acceptable to the patients—especially if they have the fear of cancer allayed by a benign finding.

III. Recommendations

A. Early detection

1. Recommendations are guidelines, to be used with several basic tenets in mind:

a. No diagnostic method is infallible.

b. No diagnostic method is superior to a concerned, careful practitioner.

c. If clinical suspicion of a mass is high, rely on your suspicion, not the test.

d. A discrete mass in the breast requires aspiration or biopsy; use mammography to screen the rest of the breast.

e. When in doubt, biopsy.

2. The recommendations shown in Table 76-3 represent the author's personal guide-

Table 76-3. Recommendations for screening*

Age	Low risk	High risk
30		Baseline mammogram. Begin yearly physical examination. Reinforce BSE.
35	Baseline mammogram. Reinforce BSE.	Increase physical examination to every 4 months.
40	Yearly breast examination.	Periodic mammogram every 2 years.
50	Reinforce BSE. Three yearly mammograms. If negative, mammography every 2 years.	Increase periodic mammogram to once every year.
70		?Decrease periodic mammogram to every 2 years.

*At age 20, a detailed history should be taken and a physical examination performed to assess risk. The patient should be taught BSE with periodic reinforcement.
Key: BSE=breast self-examination.

lines for routine health checks for breast cancer. Some of these follow the ACS guidelines; the reasons for the others have been outlined above.

The recommendations for the frequency of screening for breast cancer, and the method used, depend on the patient and her relative risk of developing the disease (see Table 76-2). For example, a patient who had a malignancy in one breast at age 39 would require yearly mammography thereafter. If a patient has a severe fibrocystic condition, we would rely more heavily on BSE and frequent physician examination, because mammography has a higher false-negative rate in these patients.

B. Early intervention

1. If the mammogram or sonogram shows a cystic lesion, aspiration and observation for recurrence are recommended.
2. If a solid mass is identified, needle or excisioned biopsy is recommended.
3. If a lesion is identified on mammogram but no mass is palpated, needle localization and biopsies should be performed.

References

1. Adami, H. O., et al. The relation between survival and age at diagnosis in breast cancer. *N. Engl. J. Med.* 315(9):559, 1986. *One of two recent studies suggesting that women diagnosed with breast cancer in their late 40s have a 10% survival advantage.*
2. DuPont, W. D., and Page, D. L. Risk factors for breast cancer in women with proliferative breast disease. *N. Engl. J. Med.* 312(3):146, 1985. *Excellent study in which patients who had biopsy were followed for 25 years to determine which pathologic changes were associated with later development of cancer.*
3. Health and Public Policy Committee, American College of Physicians. The use of diagnostic tests for screening and evaluating breast lesions. *Ann. Intern. Med.* 103(1):143, 1985. *Good review of advantage and disadvantage of various tests.*
4. Carlile, T. Breast cancer detection. *Cancer* 47(5 Suppl):1164, 1981. *Good review of detection methods.*
5. Mahoney, L., and Csima, A. Clinical screening for breast cancer (letter). *N. Engl. J. Med.* 306(9):546, 1982. *Brief editorial comment.*
6. Von Fournier, D., et al. Growth rate of 147 mammary carcinomas. *Cancer* 45(8):2198, 1980. *Details the growth rate of cancer, followed mammographically.*
7. Shapiro, S. Evidence on screening for breast cancer from a randomized trial. *Cancer* 39(6 Suppl):2772, 1977. *Report of Health Insurance Plan (HIP).*
8. Gilbertsen, V. A. The earlier detection of breast cancer. *Semin. Oncol.* 1(2):87, 1974. *Review of early studies.*

9. Foster, R. S. Jr., et al. Breast self-examination practices and breast-cancer stage. *N. Engl. J. Med.* 299(6):265, 1978. *Documents the effectiveness of BSE.*
10. Huguley, C. M. Jr., and Brown, R. L. The value of breast self-examination. *Cancer* 47(5):989, 1981. *Extensive statistical data.*
11. Baines, C. J., et al. Changes in breast self-examination behavior in a cohort of 8214 women in the Canadian National Breast Screening Study. *Cancer* 57(6):1209, 1986. *Reports behavior modification toward increased BSE frequency.*
12. Seidman, H., et al. Survival experience in the Breast Cancer Detection Demonstration Project. *CA* 37:259, 1987. *Results of the American trials suggesting a screening benefit for women under 50.*
13. Verbeek, A. L., et al. Reduction of breast cancer mortality through mass screening with modern mammography. First results of the Nijmegen project, 1975–1981. *Lancet* 1(8388):1222, 1984. *Shows that mammographic screening does reduce mortality.*
14. Collette, H. J., et al. Evaluation of screening for breast cancer in a non-randomized study (the DOM project) by means of a case-control study. *Lancet* 1(8388):1224, 1984. *Shows a marked decrease in mortality in women screened for detection of breast cancer.*
15. Tabar, L., et al. Reduction in mortality from breast cancer after mass screening with mammography. *Lancet* 1(8433):829, 1985. *Results of the Swedish trials.*
16. Breast screening: New evidence [editorial]. *Lancet* 1(8388):1217, 1984. *Comments on the study above (DOM project) and other studies showing similar results.*
17. U.S. Preventive Services Task Force. Recommendations for breast cancer screening. *J. A. M. A.* 257(6):2196, 1987. *Recent U.S. Preventive Services Task Force recommendations.*
18. Bailar, J. C. Mammography before age 50? *J. A. M. A.* 259(10):1548, 1988. *Editorial, supporting task force recommendations and accompanied by excellent original article by David Eddy, et al.*
19. Kopans, D. B., Meyer, J. E., and Sadowsky, N. Breast imaging. *N. Engl. J. Med.* 310(15):960, 1984. *Good review of all imaging procedures.*

77 Cervical Carcinoma

Richard H. Oi

I. The problem [1]

A. Description. It is a reasonable assumption that the detection and eradication of the precursor lesions of squamous cell carcinoma of the cervix has resulted in a dramatic decrease in the death rates from this disease. Routine surveillance techniques have proved to be easily applied, economical, and effective.

1. **Natural history of squamous carcinoma of the cervix.** The squamocolumnar junction (SCJ) is embryologically determined and is usually present at the anatomic external os of the cervix (Fig. 77-1A). It may also occur on the portio of the cervix; this condition is designated *ectropion* (Fig. 77-1B). The natural history of columnar epithelium is to undergo "squamous metaplasia" (Fig. 77-2). Squamous metaplasia is most active during adolescence and first pregnancy but continues to occur throughout reproductive life such that the columnar epithelium is replaced by mature squamous epithelium. In an older, postmenopausal woman, therefore, the SCJ is often well within the endocervical canal (Fig. 77-1C). The area of the cervix involved with the metaplastic change is designated the transformation zone (TZ) and is the site that is most often influenced by an oncogenic factor, resulting initially in an atypical precursor that, unattended, has the potential to undergo a further oncogenic alteration resulting in malignant squamous epithelium (Fig. 77-3). The precursor lesion designated "dysplasia" has subsets determined by the degree to which dysplastic cells occupy the thickness of the involved epithelium. Mild, moderate, and severe dysplasia and carcinoma in situ demonstrate one-quarter, one-half and three-quarter to full thickness involvement of the epithelium, respectively. More recently, as the result of newer concepts in the biology of the precursor lesion, an alternative histologic terminology, cervical intraepithelial neoplasia (CIN), has been proposed and is utilized [1]. CIN grades I, II, and III correspond to mild dysplasia, moderate dysplasia, and severe dysplasia/carcinoma in situ, respectively.

   The exact degree or grade of CIN is not as important as recognizing that neoplastic cells capable of malignant transformation are present and that there are minimal or more substantial numbers of these cells available for transformation. Epidemiologic evidence points to an average period of more than 10 years for progression from the serious degrees of the precursor lesion to invasive carcinoma. It is estimated that approximately 30% of patients with CIN III (severe dysplasia/carcinoma in situ) will progress to invasive cancer. It is important, however, to realize that all cervical intraepithelial neoplasia, even CIN I and CIN II, is at risk for developing invasive cancer, although the risk of transformation is less immediate with the lesser lesions.

   Anatomically, CIN borders the squamocolumnar junction and may extend distally, being limited by the native squamous epithelium, and proximally may extend into the endocervical canal. This zone, therefore, must be clearly recognized, as it represents the area at risk for neoplastic proliferation and the area that must be sampled for cytologic screening.

2. **Human papilloma virus (HPV).** Infection of the genital tract is now a very common disease. Certain cytologic and histologic changes occur within the cervical epithelium that are produced by HPV. These have led to subsequent identification of papilloma virions by electron microscopy, of gene-specific antigens by immunohistochemistry, and of HPV DNA sequences by hybridoma technology, in these condylomatous and noncondylomatous wart virus lesions of the cervix, vagina, and vulva [2].

   Some of these lesions have been shown to be associated with aneuploid cells and represent morphologic expression of specific HPV subtypes [3]. HPV subtypes have

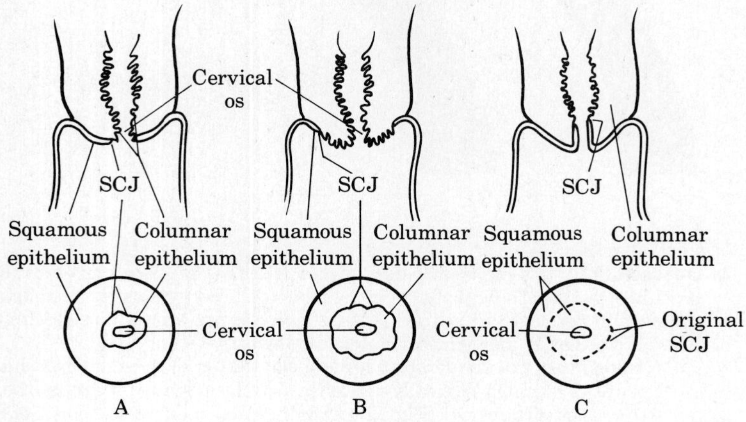

Fig. 77-1. A. The squamocolumnar junction (SCJ) is at the anatomic external os. B. Ectropion. The SCJ is on the portio of the cervix. C. Postmenopausal.

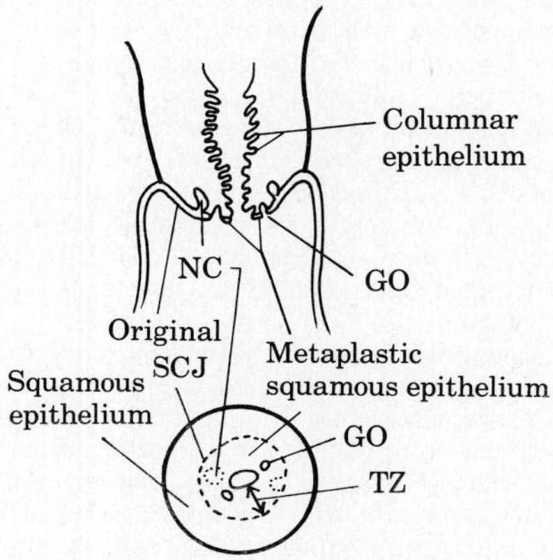

Fig. 77-2. Squamous metaplasia. The columnar epithelium has undergone transformation to squamous epithelium resulting in nabothian cyst (NC) formation and leaving "gland openings" (GO) within the zone of transformation (TZ).

been equated with varying malignant potential: types 6 and 11 are seen in anogenital condylomata and lesser degrees of CIN; types 16 and 18 have a high correlation with aneuploidy and the development of genital tract squamous carcinoma [4]. Though the association may not be causal, there is preliminary information that HPV associated with concurrent or sequential infection with herpes virus (HPV), coupled with immunologic changes, may initiate cervical squamous cancer.

B. **Epidemiology.** For the year 1986, the United States can expect to see 14,000 new cases of invasive cervical cancer, some 41,000 cases of carcinoma in situ (CIN), and 6000 deaths from the disease [5].

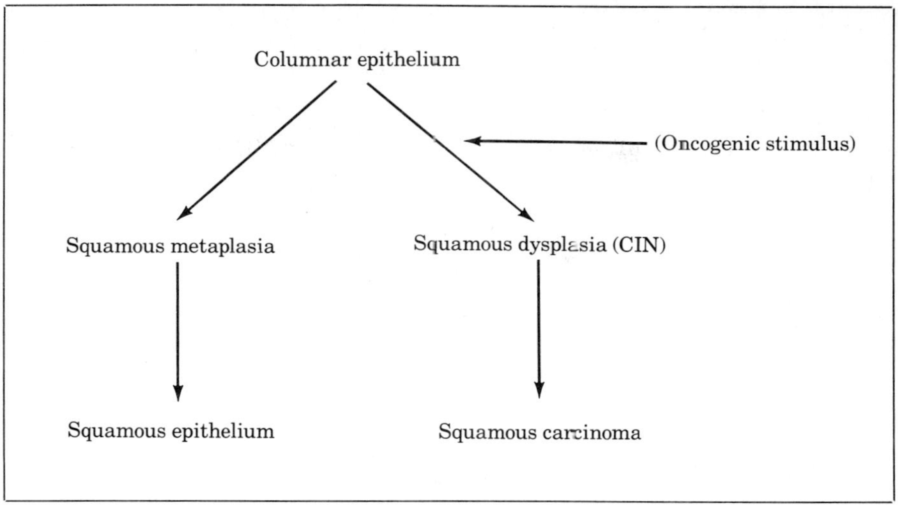

Fig. 77-3. Transformation of cervical epithelium.

C. Risk factors. Cervical neoplasia appears to be confined almost exclusively to women who have had coital activity and may be loosely designated a venereal disease. A compilation of epidemiologic data concludes: (1) early sexual activity, before age 17, and multiple sexual partners are the most important risk factors in the genesis of early cervical cancer, and (2) other factors such as gravidity, circumcision, and coital frequency were either covariable or were not important [6]. The increased risk related to early sexual activity may be correlated with the active metaplastic change that occurs in the cervix during adolescence, and this tissue may be more susceptible to oncogenic stimuli. Multiple sexual partners increases the risk of exposure to a "high-risk male" who may introduce a transmissible agent important in the development of cervical neoplasia.

The concept of a high-risk male contributing to the causation of cervical cancer is suggested by the following reports: (1) The second and third wives of males whose first wives developed cervical cancer show a higher-than-expected incidence of the same [7], (2) Males with penile cancer more often than chance have a spouse who developed cervical cancer [2], and (3) The presence of penile warts is associated in female consorts with warty atypias, intraepithelial neoplasia, and carcinoma.

The role of sexual activity is further noted in the following: (1) cervical carcinoma is most frequent among prostitutes, (2) cervical carcinoma is almost nonexistent in adult virginal women, and (3) cervical cancer is frequently found in patients who have or have had other venereal diseases, including syphilis, gonorrhea, trichomonas, genital herpes, and, especially, HPV infections.

II. Primary prevention methods. The following may be helpful but are of unproved value:

A. Teenage women should be informed of the advantages of delaying sexual relations until after their cervical epithelium has become more mature, less unstable, and, therefore, less likely to be influenced by any exogenous oncogenic factors.

B. These same women who decide to become sexually active should be encouraged to use barrier methods of contraception, to have available condoms, or to advise their consorts to use condoms for contraception as well as for disease control.

C. These women should be encouraged to establish a regular pattern of gynecologic examination to include Papanicolaou (Pap) smear screening.

III. Secondary prevention

A. Early detection methods

1. The Pap smear

a. Description. Neoplastic cells have decreased cell cohesiveness and are readily shed from tumor surfaces. The staining and evaluation of these cells form the basis of exfoliative cytology as developed by Papanicolaou.

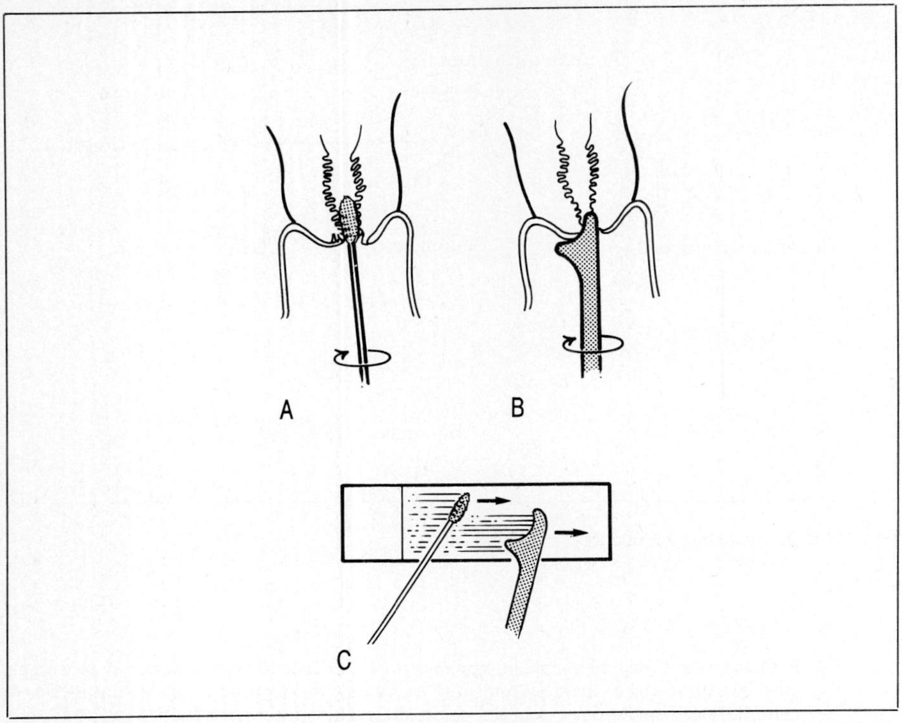

Fig. 77-4. Sampling technique. A. Cotton swab within the cervical canal, especially with a nulliparous or postmenopausal cervix, in which the squamocolumnar junction (SCJ) is in the endocervical canal. B. Spatula to obtain sample from the ectocervix and, when possible, to include the SCJ. C. Both specimens are evenly spread on one slide and may overlap each other.

b. Technique. The transformation zone, including the squamocolumnar junction, is the area at risk for development of CIN and is therefore the area that must be included in the smear sample. If the cervix is patulous and the TZ and SCJ are readily accessible, there should be minimal problems in adequately obtaining a proper cytologic specimen. The cervix in a nulliparous woman will present an os with a reduced diameter and the SCJ may be present within the endocervical canal, requiring a greater effort to sample the tissue at risk. The use of an endocervical cotton swab or endocervical aspiration technique is essential in this circumstance. Similarly, in postmenopausal women, the SCJ and TZ may be well within the cervical canal, making endocervical canal sampling mandatory. Important points to remember in collecting Pap smears include:

(1) Douching should be avoided immediately prior to the examination, and the patient should not be menstruating. Ideally, the sample should be obtained 10 days or more after the onset of any menses.

(2) Lubricants should not be used at any time prior to obtaining cytologic specimens.

(3) Two samples should be obtained: one from the ectocervix with a spatula, and the second from the endocervical canal with a cotton swab or bulb aspirator. Both specimens are uniformly and thinly spread on one slide, perhaps separating the two by placing the endocervical specimen on one half and the ectocervical specimen on the other half of the slide. The endocervical specimen is usually obtained first, as it is the less likely to "dry out" before the ectocervical smear is obtained. The specimens may overlap when being placed onto the slide (Fig. 77-4).

(4) The specimen should then be fixed immediately to avoid drying and distortion of the cytologic material. Ideally, the slide should be immediately immersed in a 95% alcohol solution, but as a satisfactory alternative, a variety of spray fixatives are available to immediately coat the slide. It is permitted to dry and is then sent to the laboratory for staining and evaluation.

(5) Vaginal pool specimens obtained from the posterior fornix are of minimal value in cervical cancer screening and are not part of the usual screening practice.

c. **Equipment**

(1) **Cervical spatula.** A variety of spatulae are available but all are designed such that one component is introduced into the cervical canal as the circumferential "scraping" of the cervical epithelial surface is performed (Fig. 77-4B). Different designs alter the length and shape of the endocervical canal component, place serrations on the "scraping" edge, or utilize plastic instead of wood in the basic construction. It is important to sample within the endocervical canal; but this is probably better accomplished by a cotton swab within the cervical canal or by aspiration of the endocervical canal, and therefore any reasonably designed spatula would suffice, complemented by an endocervical swab or aspirate.

(2) **Endocervical sampling.** Ideally, a tapered and blunted plastic tube with a 30-ml bulb aspirator should be utilized to obtain an endocervical specimen. It has been a general experience, however, that a cotton swab introduced into the canal seems to be a reasonable alternative to the bulb aspirator.

It is important to reemphasize that whatever equipment is used, the TZ should be clearly identified and included in the cytologic sampling.

d. **Interpretation.** Cytology reports usually contain a description of the material obtained and some type of statement as to the nature of the lesion that can be anticipated. Numerical classification (i.e., classes I - V) without a narrative statement is no longer acceptable, nor are simple positive or negative reports. More important, the clinician should clearly understand the implications of the report and establish a comfortable rapport and communication with the cytologist, and both should monitor the sensitivity of the screening test.

e. **Screening intervals.** There have been several recommendations as to when Pap smears should be initiated and how long the screening intervals should be. In 1982, the Canadian Task Force on Cervical Cancer Screening Programs updated their 1976 report [8, 9]. Condensed versions are listed in Table 77-1. The recommendation to increase the interval between Pap screening is primarily an economic one and is also based on the availability of an appropriate registry for surveillance so that smears are not obtained less often than recommended and so that adequate follow-up is ensured. The Canadian report recommends that women have screening annually between the ages of 18 and 35, and thereafter every 5 years. High-risk patients require more frequent screening, and the report recommends that they should not be discouraged from having smears more frequently than every 5 years. The American Cancer Society (ACS) recommendations were similar to those of the Canadian Task Force [10], but these have been revised to agree with those of the American College of Obstetrics and Gynecology [14]. ACS, ACOG [11], and the International Academy of Cytology all now advocate annual screening, and ACOG adds that routine smears are a practical mechanism to encourage women to have periodic gynecologic examinations.

Screening intervals are based on that type of cervical cancer that develops slowly through an intraepithelial stage and responds to therapy. There are, however, reports of patients under the age of 25 who have clinical cancer and who present a type of rapid onset disease that may be less responsive to treatment and, obviously, to prevention. There are other anecdotal reports of cancers being detected in patients after five negative smears. Less-than-yearly screening may be suboptimal for these groups of patients, further supporting the recommendation for annual screening.

f. **Pap smear after hysterectomy.** If the reason for hysterectomy was to eliminate a precursor lesion, and, certainly, the surgery was a radical procedure for the treatment of squamous carcinoma, screening should be initiated at 3- to 6-month intervals and indefinitely on a semiannual basis. In the case of hysterectomy for benign disease, vaginal vault Pap smears would detect vaginal intraepithelial neoplasia or early invasive carcinoma. These are less common lesions, more often seen in postmenopausal women, and screening intervals may be extended to every 5 years until age 60. However, ACOG recommends annual cytologic screening.

Table 77-1. Recommendations on Pap smear screening

Canadian Task Force, 1982

1. Women who have had sexual intercourse should generally be advised to have screening annually between the ages of 18 and 25, and thereafter every 5 years until age 60.
2. Women over 35 who are at high risk should not be discouraged from having smears more frequently than every 5 years if they request them.
3. Women over the age of 60 with repeated satisfactory smears without significant atypia may be dropped from a screening program for squamous cell carcinoma of the cervix.

American Cancer Society [14]

1. Women who are 18 years or older and women who are or have been sexually active should receive an annual Pap test and pelvic examination.
2. Once a woman has had three or more consecutive normal Pap smears, the screening can be performed less frequently at the discretion of the physician.

American College of Obstetrics and Gynecology

1. Cervical/vaginal cytology examinations should be performed in any sexually active women, regardless of age, and should be done in all women at age 18 or if there is any abnormal bleeding or discharge.
2. Patients with initial negative examination should have a repeat Pap smear to rule out false-negative results, preferably at 6 months, but certainly within 1 year.
3. Premenopausal women should have smears taken yearly after one or more negative smears, not only to screen for potential malignancies, but also to encourage women to have periodic gynecologic checkups.
4. Asymptomatic postmenopausal women should have smears taken yearly. Cervicovaginal cytologic examination is not adequate screening for postmenopausal bleeding.

2. Justification

a. Test characteristics. Sensitivity, specificity, and predictive values are difficult to assess since there is no way to identify with certainty who actually has cancer.

b. Risks. The test itself is without risk and the principal risk of the Pap smear is that it may be misread. False-positive tests may lead to unnecessary conization of the cervix requiring anesthesia and the minimal risks of hemorrhage, infection, and, even rarer, reproductive difficulties. The false-negative rate of a single smear may be as low as 5% to as high as 50%, either because of sampling error or misreading, and is the reason that repeat smears on a yearly basis are encouraged.

c. Costs. The direct cost for the Pap test ranges from $5–15, exclusive of the cost of the examination during which the test is performed.

d. Acceptability. Except for the discomfort of the pelvic examination, the Pap smear does not cause any pain and therefore is a very acceptable test. Any need for repeat examinations is equally acceptable to patients.

B. Early intervention

1. Diagnosis and evaluation

a. Colposcopic examination, using a well-illuminated binocular stereoscopic microscope, will permit successful identification and biopsy confirmation of precursor lesions.

b. Eradication is accomplished by several methods:

(1) Cryosurgery is an essentially painless procedure in which the abnormal epithelial presence is destroyed by freezing. Treatment failures approximate 7–10%.

(2) Laser therapy is a very precise method of literally vaporizing the abnormal epithelium. Destruction of the entire transformation zone is recommended. Treatment failures are similar to that of cyrosurgery.

(3) Conization. Circumferential surgical excision of the transformation zone containing the abnormal epithelium is used primarily as a diagnostic tool and secondarily as therapy. Treatment failures of 2–10% may occur.

Table 77-2. Cervical cancer mortality and survival

Year	Estimated cancer deaths	Estimated new cases
1973	8700	
1976	7700	20,000
1982	7100	16,000
1986	6800	14,000

(4) **Hysterectomy.** Hysterectomy, usually vaginally, is definitive therapy for patients who have completed their childbearing and are interested in permanent sterilization.

2. **Justification.** Since the widespread acceptance of cytologic screening for cervical cancer in the 1960s, the incidence and mortality rate for cervical cancer has declined steadily (Table 77-2) [12].

This decline has occurred in part because of earlier diagnosis of invasive lesions but more so because a well-defined asymptomatic precursor lesion with a substantial latent period can be detected, the eradication of which will preclude progression to invasive carcinoma. The identification of the precursor is possible because a convenient, painless, noninvasive, reproducible technique, the Pap smear, has been developed and is being utilized with greater frequency. The early intervention maneuvers described earlier have been combined with the screening tools to produce this steady decline in invasive disease. Early detection of cervical cancer and cancer precursors through screening, along with early intervention for these lesions, are, therefore, effective methods in the prevention of morbidity and mortality due to cervical squamous carcinoma [13].

IV. Additional considerations

A. **Adenocarcinoma of the cervix.** Pap smears, performed properly, can and do detect early adenocarcinomas of the cervix. Adenocarcinoma accounts for up to 8–10%, if not more, of the cancers that occur in the cervix and are also considered to exist in an asymptomatic precursor stage. They originate within the endocervical canal from glandular epithelium. Endocervical aspiration technique or cotton swab samples are especially important in the detection of these lesions.

B. **Vaginal carcinoma** should be considered if cytologic samples demonstrate malignant squamous cells and no cervical lesion is identified after appropriate evaluation.

C. **Endometrial carcinomas** will exfoliate malignant cells that may appear in the specimen obtained from the cervix, especially in the endocervical aspirate or cotton swab sample.

D. **Ovarian and fallopian tube carcinomas** may also be occasionally detected by the Pap smear sample.

It should be emphasized, however, that cytologic specimens obtained from the cervix are unsatisfactory for the detection of any other genital malignancies.

V. Recommendations

A. **Primary prevention.** Epidemiologic data would indicate that the following may be beneficial in primary prevention:

1. Sex education encouraging adolescent women to delay sexual activity until after the cervical epithelium has become more mature and less likely to be influenced by sexually transmitted factors.
2. Use of barrier methods of contraception, especially condoms.
3. Becoming sexually exclusive; avoiding multiple consorts.

B. **Secondary prevention**

1. **Early detection.** Cancer of the cervix is the only cancer for which there has been long-term, widespread, successful screening.
   a. Pap smears should be obtained when a woman has been or is sexually active, or by age 18, and should be repeated within a year to reduce the false-negative rate, and obtained at least yearly thereafter.
   b. The Pap smear is an easily performed, painless, accurate, and very acceptable screening test.
   c. Identification of women with abnormal smears then requires colposcopic evaluation and directed biopsies to establish accurate diagnosis of precursor lesions.

2. Early intervention

a. Eradication of the highly curable precursor lesion by cryotherapy, laser vaporization, or conization has resulted in the reduction in incidence and mortality of cervical squamous carcinoma.

b. Hysterectomy in women who have completed childbearing, with preservation of ovarian function, if appropriate, is definitive therapy.

References

1. Richart, R. M. Cervical intraepithelial neoplasia. *Pathol. Annu.* 8:301, 1973. *Defines pathobiology of precursor lesions and justifies newer terminology based on the pathobiology.*
2. Baird, J. P. The causation of cervical cancer. Part II: The role of human papilloma and other viruses. *Clin. Obstet. Gynecol.* 12(1):19, 1985. *Categorization of viruses in the etiology of cervical squamous cancer, especially with reference to the role of human papilloma virus.*
3. Syrjanen, K. J. Current view on the condylomatous lesions in uterine cervix and their possible relationship to cervical squamous cell carcinoma. *Obstet. Gynecol. Surv.* 35(11):685, 1980. *Review of the relationship between cervical condylomata and cervical squamous cell carcinoma.*
4. Crum, C. P., et al. Human papillomavirus type 16 and early cervical neoplasia. *N. Engl. J. Med.* 310(14):880, 1984. *Report of DNA hybridization techniques correlating the presence of HPV types with histology and concluding that lesions demonstrating the presence of HPV 16 correlate with presence of abnormal mitotic figures in flat warts, and that these lesions are precursors of invasive squamous carcinoma of the cervix.*
5. *Cancer Statistics* 26(1):14, 1976; 32(1):15, 1982; 36(1):9, 1986. *Survey of all cancers as tabulated by the National Cancer Institute.*
6. Rotkin, I. D. A comparison review of key epidemiologic studies in cervical cancer related to current searches for transmissible agents. *Cancer Res.* 33(6):1353, 1973. *Comparison review of epidemiologic studies that provide support for key sexual risk variables to be important in cervical squamous carcinoma.*
7. Kessler, I. I. Human cervical cancer as a venereal disease. *Cancer Res.* 36(2 Part 2):783, 1976. *Discussions of a controlled epidemiologic study on the role of the male coital partner in cervical carcinogenesis.*
8. Walton, R. J. Task force on cervical cancer screening programs. *Can. Med. Assoc. J.* 114(11):981, 1976. *Task Force report that includes a description of the natural history of carcinoma of the cervix, philosophy of the screening process, components of a practical screening program, and considerations and recommendations for cervical cytologic screening.*
9. Cervical cancer screening programs: Summary of 1982 Canadian task force report. *Can. Med. Assoc. J.* 127(7):581, 1982. *A summary of the 1982 task force report, updating the 1976 material, dealing especially with frequency of screening, laboratory quality control, and follow-up mechanisms.*
10. Eddy, D. Cancer of the cervix. *CA* 30(4):215, 1980. *American Cancer Society recommendations for cervical cytologic examination based principally on the Walton report of 1976.*
11. The frequency with which cervico-vaginal cytology examination should be performed in gynecologic practice. *ACOG Technical Bulletin* No. 9, 1975. *The American College of Obstetrics and Gynecology "response" to the American Cancer Society guidelines.*
12. Axtell, L. M., and Meyers, M. H. *Recent Trends in Survival of Cancer Patients, 1960-1971.* Bethesda, MD: National Cancer Institute, 1974. *Stage and treatment distributions and relative survival rates of cancer of the cervix uteri.*
13. Stenkvist, B., et al. Papanicolaou smear screening and cervical cancer. What can you expect? *J. A. M. A.* 252(11):1423, 1984. *Cancer screening experience and lifetime follow-up in three Swedish counties in which more than 90% of the total female population between age 30–59, 53% between 60–69, and 25% older than 70 were screened over a 10-year period, demonstrating a major reduction in the incidence of invasive cervical cancer.*
14. Cancer society revises stance, calls for yearly Pap smears. *Med. World News* Dec. 14, 1987. P. 25. *Summarizes the revisions of the American Cancer Society recommendations, which now agree with the ACOG recommendations.*

78 Endometrial Carcinoma

Richard H. Oi

I. The problem

A. Description. Most cancers of the endometrium are adenocarcinomas and appear to arise in the context of abnormal, unopposed, prolonged estrogenic stimulation. Excessive proliferation of the endometrium occurs, which may then proceed to hyperplastic change with its various subsets, and a subsequent neoplastic transformation into atypical hyperplasias, and finally adenocarcinoma (Fig. 78-1). Consensus is that hyperplastic changes without atypia are probably at minimal risk of undergoing malignant transformation, but atypical hyperplasia is a true precursor lesion and has great risk, unmodified or untreated, of proceeding to adenocarcinoma. As such, there is a precursor lesion that has a latent period of perhaps 2 – 8 years and that can be treated or modified to prevent progression to cancer [1, 2].

B. Epidemiology. There has been a dramatic rise in the incidence of carcinoma of the endometrium, which now ranks as the most common malignancy of the female genital tract. Thirty-six thousand new cases and 2900 deaths are anticipated in the United States from this disease in the year 1986. This represents more than twice the number of invasive cervical carcinoma [3]. Overall, 5-year survivals approximate 70–75%, but early stage I lesions have a good prognosis, with up to 90% 5-year survivals. In more advanced stages, 5-year survival varies from 25–50%. Clearly, then, early detection of endometrial carcinoma will improve the mortality relative to this disease.

C. Risk factors [1, 4, 5]

1. Although endometrial carcinoma may occur in the absence of an altered hormonal milieu, abnormal and prolonged estrogenic stimulation is a primary risk factor for this malignancy [4].
   - **a.** Exogenous estrogen administration has been implicated, and a four-fold increase in risk has been identified in postmenopausal women on estrogen therapy [6]. The risk is related to the dosage of estrogen used and the length of time it has been prescribed. Addition of progestational agents to the estrogen administration has been shown to dramatically reduce the risk of developing endometrial carcinoma [11]. It is of interest that the cancers identified in estrogen users are more often well-differentiated lesions confined to the endometrial cavity and therefore are associated with good prognosis.
   - **b.** Excessive endogenous estrogen production increases the risk and includes conditions such as:
     - **(1)** Hormone-producing tumors of the ovary, especially granulosa cell tumors and theca cell tumors. These are fortunately unusual neoplasms, but should be considered especially in postmenopausal patients.
     - **(2)** Chronic anovulation and unopposed estrogen stimulation such as with sclerocystic ovary syndrome.
2. Obesity has a strong correlation with endometrial carcinoma.
   - **a.** Obesity is associated with high estrogen levels, as adipose tissue is one of the most important compartments in the extragonadal conversion of androgen precursors to estrone [8].
   - **b.** Hypertension and diabetes are risk factors, probably because of their known strong association with obesity, and are only indirectly associated with carcinoma.
3. Nulliparous women account for one half of endometrial carcinomas. Nulliparity and low parity are related to persistent estrogen stimulation uninterrupted by the effects of pregnancy. However, obesity, anovulation, and infertility may represent a more general expression of a total endocrinopathy that predisposes to carcinoma.
4. Women who experience late menopause, after age 50, have a slight excess of endometrial carcinoma.

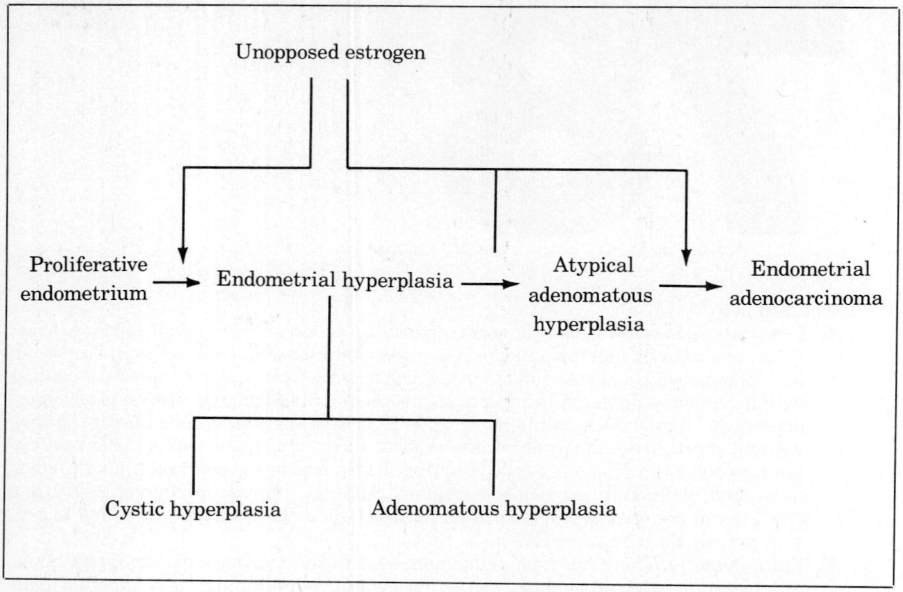

Fig. 78-1. Spectrum of endometrial changes from benign to malignant associated with unopposed stimulation by endogenous or exogenous estrogens.

5. Notably, women at risk of endometrial cancer are also at increased risk of developing breast cancer [9].

II. Primary prevention. The following considerations are worth noting in primary prevention:

A. Combined estrogen/progesterone contraceptive use appears to have a protective effect on the development of endometrial carcinoma [10]. This effect appears to be limited to women who have used them for 1 year or longer, and was especially significant in nulliparous women.

B. Postmenopausal estrogen therapy should be modified to use the lowest possible effective dose to control symptoms and to avoid stimulating the endometrium, and should be used for as limited a time as is clinically feasible. Use of progestational agents for a minimum of 10, or better, 13 days, is also protective if used cyclically with estrogen therapy [11].

C. Patients with chronic anovulation and, therefore, unopposed estrogen stimulation, should be considered for progestational therapy: i.e., patients with polycystic ovary syndrome who are not interested in ovulation induction, and perimenopausal women who, because of anovulation, develop irregular bleeding and endometrial hyperplasias.

D. Prevention and treatment of obesity in perimenopausal and postmenopausal women may also reduce the risk of endometrial carcinoma.

III. Secondary prevention

A. Early detection

1. Low risk. There are not, at present, methods to screen low-risk women for asymptomatic endometrial hyperplasias or cancers that are as simple, acceptable, and productive as the Pap smear is for carcinoma of the cervix.

2. High risk

a. There are individuals whose risk of endometrial cancer is high and who may be considered for histologic screening examination:

(1) A nulliparous or low-parity, obese female over the age of 50 who is still menstruating may be offered endometrial sampling.

(2) Nulliparous, low-parity, asymptomatic postmenopausal women with estrogenic effects on vaginal hormonal evaluation may have a 13-fold increased risk of endometrial carcinoma, especially if they are 5 or more years postmenopausal, and they should be considered for endometrial sampling.

(3) Patients on postmenopausal estrogen replacement therapy, even with added progesterone, may benefit from periodic endometrial surveillance.

b. A second group of women with abnormal symptoms or findings should be thoroughly investigated with histologic sampling:

(1) Postmenopausal women with Pap smear results suspicious for hyperplastic, estrogen-stimulated, or neoplastic endometrial changes.

(2) Women with postmenopausal bleeding.

(3) Perimenopausal women with abnormal, irregular bleeding.

3. **Methods**

a. **Pap smears,** which are so effective in the detection of cervical cancers, have a false-negative rate of up to 60% in patients with known endometrial carcinoma. This detection rate can be improved, especially by obtaining endocervical canal samples, especially by aspiration [12].

(1) The presence of endometrial-type cells in a Pap smear obtained from a postmenopausal woman is significant and should prompt investigation for hyperplastic and neoplastic lesions of the endometrium [13].

(2) Vaginal hormonal cytology demonstrating an estrogenic effect in a woman more than 5 years post-menopause suggests further investigation as to possible estrogen-producing ovarian lesions, and secondarily, endometrial lesions.

b. **Cytologic techniques.** Available tests all require introducing various appliances into the uterine cavity, which causes enough discomfort that it becomes difficult to establish the technique as a routine screening procedure and makes it difficult to encourage patients to return for repeat screening. Furthermore, intrauterine sampling techniques that depend on interpreting exfoliated cells instead of tissue fragments cause less discomfort but have a much lower detection rate. Obtaining more tissue and therefore more accurate diagnoses by endometrial biopsy using a larger caliber, often metallic, currette is quite accurate but has the major disadvantage of causing much more pain and discomfort.

Another disadvantage with the cytologic specimen is that it cannot be simply transferred to a slide, stained, and examined, but instead requires suspension in saline, either filtration or centrifugation, and subsequent staining. Finally, because the endometrial cavity is being invaded, it requires specialized sterile instruments, adding considerably to the expense of the procedure.

Techniques for obtaining cytologic specimens include:

(1) Gravlee jet washer

(2) Isaacs endometrial cell sampler

(3) Mi-Mark Helix Instrument

(4) Endometrial brush

These methods have a significant rate of inaccuracy, and none compares with the accuracy rate of the endometrial biopsy [14, 15].

c. **Endometrial biopsy** techniques utilize mechanical or manual suction applied to a variety of cannulas, both metallic and plastic, that permit tissue diagnosis rather than cytologic screening. The caliber of the cannula used is inversely related to the discomfort of the procedure but directly related to the amount of tissue obtained and, therefore, to the accuracy of diagnosis. These include packaged units such as:

(1) Masterson endometrial biopsy device (Gyneco, Inc., New Jersey)

(2) Vakutage device (Warner Chilcott, New Jersey)

(3) Vabra aspirator (Cooper Laboratories, New York)

Standard endometrial biopsy curettes include: (1) Novak curette, (2) Randall curette, and (3) Milex curette.

d. **Dilatation and curettage** (D & C), keeping the endocervical material separate from the endometrial tissue (fractional curettage), is the definitive procedure in evaluation of endometrial pathology but requires general anesthesia and is obviously not a screening procedure.

e. **Hysteroscopy,** endoscopic visualization of the uterine cavity, permits a more direct method of examining and sampling the endometrium. Though outpatient office hysteroscopy is possible, general anesthesia is usually required for thorough evaluation.

4. **Justification.** There is not yet a simple, acceptable, sensitive, and reproducible screening test for endometrial carcinoma. Techniques for both cytologic and histo-

logic sampling of the endometrium require introducing appliances into the endometrial cavity and, as a result, cause unavoidable pain and discomfort precluding application as acceptable screening tests. The "screening techniques" are also relatively expensive. Screening for endometrial carcinoma or its precursors appears not to be a practical strategem in the reduction of morbidity and mortality due to endometrial carcinoma. Moreover, although there are women with endometrial carcinoma who are asymptomatic [16], the majority of patients present with irregular, abnormal bleeding, as do women with precursor hyperplasias of the endometrium. They, of course, should be evaluated with endometrial sampling techniques. Endometrial sampling of postmenopausal women with an estrogenic effect or endometrial cells on Pap smears may be justified and may also be considered for evaluating the asymptomatic high-risk woman.

B. Early intervention (treatment)

1. Endometrial hyperplasia

a. This is considered a reversible lesion and may be treated medically with cyclic progestational agents and the endometrium resampled after three or four cycles. Progestational therapy then may be continued until there is no longer any cyclic withdrawal bleeding, that is, until there is no longer any significant estrogen-stimulated endometrium.

b. If medical therapy does not correct the hyperplasia, or if there are other indications for surgery such as leiomyomata, hysterectomy is justified.

2. Atypical adenomatous hyperplasia

a. This is a precursor lesion and can be successfully treated by hysterectomy.

b. If the patient is a poor candidate for surgery, high-dose, continuous progestational agents may be used, then endometrial tissues should be resampled.

3. Adenocarcinoma. Early detection should identify early-stage cancers, which have a good prognosis and survival with hysterectomy and bilateral salpingo-oophorectomy.

IV. Recommendations

A. Primary prevention. Although not principally used to prevent endometrial carcinomas, considerations in the management of other health areas that may have impact in the primary prevention of endometrial carcinoma include:

1. Combined estrogen/progestin contraceptives appear to have a protective effect on the development of endometrial carcinoma.
2. Postmenopausal estrogen therapy should use the lowest possible estrogen dose, should be used cyclically, and should be combined with 10–13 days of progestin (see Chap. 75).
3. Patients with chronic anovulation and, therefore, unopposed estrogen stimulation should be considered for progestational therapy.
4. Prevention and treatment of obesity in peri- and postmenopausal women may reduce the risk of endometrial carcinomas.

B. Secondary prevention

1. Early detection

a. Routine screening of low-risk, asymptomatic women is not recommended.

b. Evaluating high-risk, symptomatic individuals with histologic sampling may be worthwhile.

c. Postmenopausal individuals with abnormal Pap results suggesting abnormal endometrial changes should be evaluated using histologic sampling techniques.

d. Women with abnormal, irregular, or postmenopausal bleeding should be evaluated for the possibility of endometrial hyperplasia or carcinoma.

2. Early intervention

a. Early intervention would detect reversible hyperplasias that can be treated medically, or atypical hyperplasias that can be removed surgically and therefore obviate progression to adenocarcinoma.

b. Early intervention should identify adenocarcinomas confined to the endometrium, which can be successfully treated by hysterectomy.

References

1. Gusberg, S. B. An approach to the control of carcinoma of the endometrium. *CA* 30(1):16, 1980. *Discussions on the pathobiology of precursor lesions and risk factors, techniques of early diagnosis, and treatment problems related to endometrial carcinoma.*

2. Gusberg, S. B., and Kaplan, A. L. Precursors of corpus cancer. IV. Adenomatous hyperplasia as stage 0 carcinoma of the endometrium. *Am. J. Obstet. Gynecol.* 87:662, 1963. *Study of patients with adenomatous hyperplasia who subsequently developed endometrial carcinoma.*
3. Silverberg, E., and Lubera, J. Cancer statistics, 1986. *CA* 36(1):9, 1986. *Survey of all cancers as tabulated by the Centers for Disease Control.*
4. Berg, J. W., and Lampe, J. G. High-risk factors in gynecologic cancer. *Cancer* 48(2 suppl):429, 1981. *Epidemiologic survey of risk factors associated with genital cancers.*
5. Glassburn, J. R. Carcinoma of the endometrium. *Cancer* 48(2 suppl):575, 1981. *Prognostic factors in endometrial carcinoma and recommended therapy as determined by stage of disease and associated prognostic factors.*
6. Mack, T. M., et al. Estrogens and endometrial cancer in a retirement community. *N. Engl. J. Med.* 294(23):1262, 1976. *Survey of a retirement community establishing a causal relationship between the use of postmenopausal estrogen replacement therapy and endometrial adenocarcinoma.*
7. Gordon, J., et al. Estrogen and endometrial carcinoma. An independent pathology review supporting original risk estimate. *N. Engl. J. Med.* 297(11):570, 1977. *Pathology review of the endometrial histology in the survey by Ziel and Finkle validating the original estimate and conclusions that estrogen replacement therapy plays a part in the pathogenesis of endometrial carcinoma.*
8. Siiteri, P. K. Steroid hormones and endometrial cancer. *Cancer Res.* 38(11 part 2):4360, 1978. *Reviews factors associated with the risk of developing endometrial carcinoma especially as related to elevated production of estrone in peripheral nonendocrine tissues from androgen precursors.*
9. McMahon, B., and Austin, J. H. Association of carcinomas of the breast and corpus uteri. *Cancer* 23:275, 1969. *Study of the frequency and types of other primary tumors, especially carcinoma of the breast, seen in patients with endometrial adenocarcinoma.*
10. Oral contraceptives and cancer risks. *M. M. W. R.* 31(29):393, 1982. *Analysis of multicenter case study indicating that oral contraceptive users are half as likely to develop ovarian and endometrial cancer.*
11. Gambrell, R.D. Jr., et al. Reduced incidence of endometrial cancer among postmenopausal women treated with progestogens. *J. Am. Geriatr. Soc.* 27(9):389, 1979. *Prospective study demonstrating a reduced incidence of endometrial carcinoma in postmenopausal women using cyclic estrogen-progestogen as compared to estrogen alone.*
12. Ng, A. B. The cellular detection of endometrial carcinoma and its precursors. *Gynecol. Oncol.* 2(2-3):162, 1974. *Assessment of various sampling procedures in the detection of endometrial carcinoma, including posterior vaginal fornix cytology, cervical canal aspiration, and direct endometrial cavity sampling.*
13. Ng, A. B. P., et al. Significance of endometrial cells in the detection of endometrial carcinoma and its precursors. *Acta Cytol.* 18(5):356, 1974. *Report of the association of desquamated endometrial cells seen in smears obtained from postmenopausal patients and the presence of endometrial cancer or its precursors.*
14. Isaacs, J. H., and Wilhoite, R. W. Aspiration cytology of the endometrium: Office and hospital sampling procedures. *Am. J. Obstet. Gynecol.* 118:679, 1974. *Report of a technique utilizing aspiration cytology in the detection of endometrial carcinoma.*
15. Anderson, D. G., et al. The cytologic diagnosis of endometrial adenocarcinoma. *Am. J. Obstet. Gynecol.* 125(3):376, 1976. *A comparison of different techniques in sampling the endometrial cavity and their relative efficacy in accurate diagnosis of endometrial carcinoma.*
16. Hofmeister, F. J. Endometrial biopsy: Another look. *Am. J. Obstet. Gynecol.* 118:773, 1974. *Report of 20,677 endometrial biopsies as a practical and economic method of early detection and diagnosis of endometrial carcinoma, in which 17% were found to be asymptomatic.*

79 Ovarian Carcinoma

Richard H. Oi

I. The problem

A. Description. The ovary can give rise to a variety of tumors derived from different cell lines. The most frequent are those arising from the surface epithelium, the **epithelial tumors,** which account for over 90% of all ovarian malignancies. **Germ cell tumors** constitute 2% of ovarian cancers and include dysgerminomas, embryonal carcinomas, endodermal sinus tumors, malignant teratomas, and choriocarcinomas. The **sex cord-stromal** group of tumors accounts for another 2% and includes granulosa cell tumors and the Sertoli-Leydig cell tumors. Other primary tumors of the ovary include sarcomas and lymphomas and make up less than 1% of the malignancies of the ovary.

The common **epithelial tumors** include the serous, mucinous, endometrioid, and clear cell adenocarcinomas. As they are the most frequent of the ovarian malignancies, subsequent discussion will be based on the data relative to these epithelial tumors. Epithelial tumors probably arise as ovarian surface epithelial inclusions that develop into cystic structures lined by specific epithelia that designate the lesion (i.e., serous or mucinous cystadenomas). There is very little information about precancerous lesions of the ovary. The average age of women with benign cystadenomas is at least 10 years less than that of patients with malignant cystadenocarcinomas, and the presence of malignant foci in benign cystadenomas would suggest that there is a precursor lesion [1]. Malignancies enlarge, invade the adjacent ovarian stroma, and grow and spill into the peritoneal cavity to be disseminated throughout the intraperitoneal space, implanting on all peritoneal surfaces; they may obstruct subdiaphramatic lymphatics, contributing to ascites. In the early stages of growth, the patient experiences little if any symptoms and becomes symptomatic after there is extensive tumor spread and palpable masses and ascites.

There is not a clearly definable, clinically detectable precursor state with a long latent period, the therapy of which would modify mortality from this disease. In addition, the ovary is not an accessible organ in terms of screening, and present methods of evaluation have limited sensitivity and specificity and are complex and invasive. These characteristics, therefore, make ovarian cancer an unfavorable entity for significant screening.

B. Epidemiology. Ovarian cancer is the fourth most frequent fatal cancer in women and is the third most frequent, but the most lethal, of all genital cancers. An estimated 11,600 deaths occur annually; the incidence and deaths from ovarian cancer have shown little change over the past 2 decades, and, if anything, have increased slightly in both parameters [2]. These poor statistics reflect the insidious clinical course and consequent delayed or late diagnosis of ovarian cancer, and the lack of an adequate screening mechanism to establish early diagnosis. About 60–70% of cancers, at diagnosis, are quite advanced and widely disseminated. The overall 5-year survival rate is only 15–25%.

Risk factors [1, 3–6] associated with ovarian cancers include:

1. **Age.** Epithelial cancers are rare before menarche but increase in frequency thereafter with the greater incidence occurring in perimenopausal and menopausal women.
2. **Nulligravidity.** Women of low parity who experience difficulty in conceiving or conceive at a later age are at increased risk for developing ovarian epithelial cancers. Nuns, for example, experience more cancers of the ovary (and breast, endometrium, and colon) and fewer cervical cancers than a group of comparable secular women.
3. **Familial ovarian cancer.** Several reports of similar neoplasms of the ovaries in succeeding generations have been described. Maternal or sibling history, especially of serous cystadenocarcinoma, identifies a high-risk patient.
4. **Abnormalities in hormonal function** may be contributory. Epithelial tumors are rare before menarche, and they increase during perimenopause and menopause.

Epithelial tumors share host characteristics with those of breast cancer; indeed, women with breast cancer have twice the expected rate of subsequently developing primary cancer of the ovary.

5. **Genetic factors**
   a. Peutz-Jeghers syndrome patients are at higher risk for developing ovarian lesions, especially a distinctive sex-cord tumor (sex-cord tumor with annular tubules), as well as cystadenomas.
   b. Basal cell nevus syndrome patients are prone to develop benign fibromas and, less likely, other ovarian neoplasms.
   c. Dysgenetic gonads in patients with Turner's syndrome, with an XO/XY mosaicism, are prone to develop dysgerminomas and gonadoblastomas.
6. **History of pelvic irradiation** has been found to be associated with a small excess of ovarian cancers.
7. An as yet unclear association between ovarian cancer and childhood viral diseases, especially mumps, which has an affinity for gonadal complication, has been identified.

II. Primary prevention. Although not yet to the level of general recommendation, some considerations in this area include:

A. **Oral contraceptives** may be protective and contribute to a decrease in incidence of ovarian carcinoma in the older woman. A relative risk of 0.11 is noted in women age 40–59 but not in women under 40 [7, 8]. Weiss, however, found a decreased risk in women age 35–55, especially if oral contraceptives had been used for more than 3 years [9].

B. **Postmenopausal estrogen therapy,** because of its suppression of gonadotropins, the elevation of which may have some association with the development of epithelial tumors [6], may also reduce the risk of ovarian carcinoma and should be a consideration when deciding estrogen replacement therapy.

C. **Oophorectomy** at the time of hysterectomy should be considered when there is no longer any ovarian function, since specific incidence rates for ovarian cancer increase with age. What constitutes absence of ovarian function is not clear, and different ages at which ovaries should be removed have been advocated, with consensus settling on age 40 or older.

III. Assessment

A. **Risk assessment.** There is not, at present, a specific, sensitive marker for ovarian cancer screening. Instead, a high-risk group of women (see Section **I. B.**) should be identified and considered for periodic examination and ultrasonography.

B. **Detection techniques.** As there is not at present an effective method of screening asymptomatic patients to detect a "precursor," clinical parameters in detection should include:

1. **Pelvic examination.** A palpable ovarian lesion can, by clinical characteristics, be separated into functional, nonneoplastic lesions and neoplastic lesions that require surgical intervention. In a high-risk patient, at a minimum, yearly periodic health care examinations including pelvic examination is **reasonable.** Unfortunately, small ovarian masses, which may contain substantial numbers of malignant cells, may not be palpable. Lack of sensitivity in a thin, cooperative patient is even more exaggerated in the bimanual examination of an obese patient who finds it difficult to relax completely.

   Palpation of a normal-sized ovary in a postmenopausal woman may represent an ovarian neoplasm [10] and deserves work-up. With newer imaging techniques to confirm palpatory findings, and serum determinations of tumor markers such as Ca 125 and carcinoembryonic antigen (CEA), women in this group may be found to have earlier lesions, and thereby improved survival.

2. **Ultrasonography (USG).** Ultrasonographic visualization of the ovaries, especially with high-resolution techniques, would detect small ovarian enlargements and would also define solid and cystic lesions. Routine use of USG as a screening technique, however, is impractical but may be justifiable to complement the periodic pelvic examination in high-risk patients.

   With the availability of transvaginal ultrasonic probes, a less tedious and simpler office type of imaging of the ovaries is possible and may become a more important technique in early diagnosis.

3. **Papanicolaou smears** have limited value in detecting ovarian carcinoma and depend on cells being shed from the ovarian lesions, a property that probably does not occur until a later stage of disease progression. Similarly, culdocentesis and cytologic examination of the cul-de-sac aspirate for malignant cells, if positive, would be indicative of intraperitoneal pathology and, therefore, of advanced disease.

4. **Laparoscopy** is definitive in detecting ovarian neoplasms, but is not practical as a routine screening technique as indeed, in addition to its expense, it has the considerable risks of an invasive surgical procedure, with or without anesthesia.
5. **Tumor markers.** The most promising technique for ovarian cancer screening may come from the identification and isolation of tumor-specific ovarian cancer antigens. Extensive investigations into enzymatic, hormonal, embryonic, and other markers are ongoing and have identified several antigenic determinants, but the most successful to date are the ovarian cancer associated antigens, notably Ca 125 [11, 12]. There is a greater than 90% correlation with the clinical course of epithelial tumors, but there are significant numbers of false-positives. In addition, the test lacks sensitivity, as a critical tumor mass must be attained before Ca 125 antigen levels become abnormal. Its greatest use is in following patients undergoing treatment and in detecting recurrent disease.

IV. **Intervention.** Therapy of ovarian carcinoma is not currently very successful. However, as with most cancers, the earlier the disease can be detected, the more successful new therapies are likely to be.

V. **Recommendations**

A. **Primary prevention**

1. No specific recommendations are made.
2. The potential value of oral contraceptives and postmenopausal estrogen therapy are noted and look promising.
3. Oophorectomy at the time of hysterectomy, when there is no longer ovarian function, should be considered.

B. **Assessment.** No general screening recommendations are made since there are no acceptable, available, screening tests or early intervention.

1. **Risk assessment.** Individuals at highest risk include:
   a. A perimenopausal or menopausal woman with vague lower abdominal and pelvic complaints, especially if associated with urinary and rectal symptoms, who:
      (1) Is nulliparous or of low parity.
      (2) Has a family history of ovarian cancer, especially if it is in her mother or sister, and the cancer was a serous cystadenocarcinoma.
      (3) Has had a previous breast cancer.
      (4) Has had a history of pelvic irradiation.
      (5) Has had a diagnosis of endometriosis or other ovarian cystic diseases.
   b. An individual with congenital or developmental abnormalities such as a Turner mosaic with an XO/XY karyotype, or who has multiple neoplastic syndromes such as Puetz-Jeghers or basal cell nevus syndrome.
   c. Postmenopausal patients with a palpable ovarian mass.
2. **Detection techniques** for ovarian cancer to be utilized in such individuals include:
   a. Careful abdominopelvic examinations.
   b. Papanicolaou smears, especially obtaining a specimen from the endocervical canal.
   c. High-resolution ultrasonography or other imaging techniques.
   d. Tumor marker determinations (Ca 125, CEA).

References

1. McGowan, L., et al. The woman at risk for developing ovarian cancer. *Gynecol. Oncol.* 7(3):325, 1979. *Three-year case control study identifying risk factors of presumed etiologic and diagnostic significance in primary epithelial ovarian cancers.*
2. Silverberg, E., anud Lubera, J. Cancer statistics, 1986. *CA* 36(1):9, 1986. *Survey of all cancers as tabulated by the Centers for Disease Control.*
3. Scully, R. E. Definition of precursors in gynecologic cancer. *Cancer* 48(2 suppl):531, 1981. *Review of the precursor lesions identified with gynecologic cancers; their pathobiology and significance related to malignant transformation.*
4. Berg, J. W., and Lampe, J. G. High-risk factors in gynecologic cancer. *Cancer* 48(2 suppl):429, 1981. *Epidemiologic survey of risk factors associated with gynecologic cancers.*
5. Casagrande, J. T., et al. "Incessant ovulation" and ovarian cancer. *Lancet* 2(8135):170, 1979. *A case control study indicating a decreased risk of ovarian cancer with increasing numbers of live births and oral contraceptives, and relating this decrease to periods of anovulation.*

6. Lingeman, C. H. Etiology of cancer of the human ovary. A review *J. Natl. Cancer Instit.* 53(6):1603, 1974. *An extensive review of known or suspected factors associated with cancers of the human ovary.*
7. Child, M., et al. Oral contraceptives and cancer risk. *M. M. W. R.* 31:393, 1982. *Multicenter case control study indicating a decreased risk of ovarian and endometrial cancer in oral contraceptive pill users.*
8. Cramer, D. W., et al. Factors affecting the association of oral contraceptives and ovarian cancer. *N. Engl. J. Med.* 307(17):1047, 1982. *Case control study of the relation between epithelial ovarian cancer and oral contraceptive use, indicating a decreased risk especially in older parous women.*
9. Weiss, N. S., et al. Incidence of ovarian cancer in relation to the use of oral contraceptives. *Int. J. Cancer* 28(6):669, 1981. *Case control study indicating that oral contraceptive use offers a measure of protection against the development of ovarian epithelial cancers.*
10. Barber, H. R., and Graber, E. A. The PMPO syndrome (postmenopausal palpable ovary syndrome). *Obstet. Gynecol.* 38:921, 1971. *Editorial suggesting that palpation of a normal-sized ovary in a patient 3–5 years postmenopausal is indicative of ovarian neoplasia and should be investigated promptly.*
11. Bast, R. C. Jr., et al. A radioimmunoassay using a monoclonal antibody to monitor the course of epithelial ovarian cancer. *N. Engl. J. Med.* 309(15):883, 1983. *Study of serum Ca 125 in patients with ovarian carcinoma indicating that Ca 125 levels may be useful in monitoring treatment responses.*
12. Krebs, H. B., et al. Role of Ca 125 as tumor marker in ovarian carcinoma. *Obstet. Gynecol.* 67(4):473, 1986. *Study of the ovarian cancer antigen Ca 125 as an immunodiagnostic screening device for ovarian carcinoma, indicating its usefulness in detection of persistent and recurrent disease.*

80 Testicular Carcinoma

Ernest L. Lewis

I. The problem

A. Description. Testicular carcinoma is divided into four primary cell types: seminoma, embryonal cell carcinoma, teratocarcinoma, and choriocarcinoma. It spreads from the cells of origin in the testicle to the structures of the spermatic cord, and then to the lymph nodes of the pelvis and paraaortic regions. Survival rates, while dependent on the stage of the disease, have increased significantly in recent years with the advent of effective chemotherapeutic agents and combinations of agents.

B. Epidemiology. While overall an uncommon disease, about 5300 cases in the United States annually, testicular carcinoma is the most common neoplasm in men between ages 15 and 34 and is the fifth most common cause of death in this age group. It accounts for approximately 1% of all malignancies in the male and is more common in whites than blacks by a factor of 4 or 5:1. There is some evidence that its incidence is increasing, especially in whites in the younger age group (15–19). While specific occupational factors have not been identified, testicular carcinoma is more common in higher socioeconomic groups.

The association of testicular cancer with cryptorchidism has been established. While the clinical literature suggests that patients with cryptorchidism have a 20- to 40-fold risk of developing testicular carcinoma, epidemiologic studies seem to indicate a risk factor more in the range of 10-fold. It would appear that while orchiopexy does not remove the risk, it significantly lowers it, especially if performed before the age of 6. There is some evidence that the incidence of cryptorchidism is increasing in the United States since the 1940s. Undescended testicles show some degree of dysgenesis, as do other normally descended members of the pair, and this seems to be gaining strength as an etiologically significant factor of the condition, rather than increasing temperature. This would correlate with the reports that as high as 20% of cryptorchid-associated testicular carcinomas occur in the normally descended organ of the pair.

Also of particular interest is the reported increased incidence of cryptorchidism and related testicular dysgenesis and infertility in males exposed to exogenous maternal estrogens during pregnancy. Since use of these agents was rather common practice in the period from 1940–1960 for various complications of pregnancy, the suggestion is raised that this may correlate with the increased incidence of cryptorchidism and testicular carcinoma in patients born during this period. An interesting extension of the testicular dysgenesis/cryptorchid data is the observation that as many as 25% of patients with gonadal dysgenesis, a rare genetic disorder that includes cryptorchidism and incomplete masculinization of the external genitalia, develop testicular carcinoma.

A history of testicular trauma, postviral orchitic atrophy, and radiation exposure have also been reported as being associated with testicular carcinoma, but the exact relationship remains obscure.

II. Secondary prevention

A. Early detection

1. Methods

a. Testicular self-exam. All males from puberty at least through 35 years should be instructed to examine the testicles from time to time while bathing or showering. Brochures on testicular self-examination can be obtained from the American Cancer Society. Patients should be instructed to report to a physician any lump on a testis.

b. Health care provider testicular examinations. The most common presentation of testicular carcinoma is that of a young man who seeks evaluation of a painless mass in the scrotum, which he has detected while showering or upon self-examination following some trivial injury. This mass has commonly been present anywhere from 2 weeks to 6 months. The other common presentation is of a similar patient who has been previously diagnosed as having "orchitis" or "epididymitis" and treated with antibiotic medication without resolution, and who seeks another opinion because of this lack of improvement. In both of these instances, suspicion and adequate examination lead to proper diagnosis.

The patient should be examined, if possible, in the standing position with the examiner seated before him The testicles and scrotum with the cord structures and epididymes should be gently palpated and compared from side to side. The presence of a firm, often nontender, mass within the testicle itself alerts the examiner to the possible presence of testicular carcinoma. Transillumination will differentiate between a solid mass (tumor) and a fluid-filled (cystic) lesion. Since physican misdiagnosis, principally of orchitis or epididymitis, is a factor in delaying appropriate therapy, the presence of a suspicious mass should result in referral of the patient to an appropriate practitioner. Needle biopsy or aspiration is to be condemned because of poor prognosis in patients who have had this procedure and who were found to have carcinoma.

2. **Justification.** No good studies of the value of testicular self-examination have been done, but it would seem prudent to encourage its widespread acceptance since testicular cancer is often quite treatable when detected early. Since suspicion of the presence of testicular carcinoma is based on physical examination alone, there are no risks or side effects to the examination alone. Follow-up risks and costs can obviously occur. If health care providers make a careful examination of testicles, including transillumination, a routine part of their physical examination, patients should accept responsibility for self-examination.

B. Early intervention

1. **Methods.** Surgical intervention with high ligation of the spermatic cord and removal of the entire cord and testicle is the early treatment of choice. Prior to this procedure, blood should be drawn for determination of alpha fetoprotein and chorionic gonadotrophin levels. Again, it should be stressed that in no case should an attempt at needle aspiration be carried out.
2. **Justification.** It has been clearly demonstrated that prognosis in cases of testicular carcinoma is related to early detection and appropriate therapy. In no case where testicular carcinoma is suspected should early surgical therapy be postponed awaiting either the efficacy of other therapeutic modalities or the return of laboratory values.

III. Recommendations

A. Early detection

1. All men 18–35 years should be instructed in the proper technique of periodic self-examination of the testes.
2. Examination of the testicle, including transillumination, should be part of the routine physical examination on any male patient.
3. Particular care should be taken in patients who have a history of undescended testicle, old testicular trauma, or orchitis associated with mumps.

B. Intervention/treatment

1. Surgical consultation should be obtained immediately when a testicular mass is discovered.
2. At the time of referral, blood for alpha fetoprotein and human chorionic gonadotrophin levels should be drawn.
3. In no case should continued observation, antibiotic therapy, or needle aspiration be attempted.

Suggested Readings

Borski, A. A. Proceedings: Diagnosis, staging, and natural history of testicular tumors. *Cancer* 32:1202, 1973. *An interesting review of various aspects of the disease, especially the natural history and reasons for delay.*

Fraley, E. E. Symposium on testicular tumors: Foreword. *Urol. Clin. North Am.* 4(3):343, 1977; and Fraley, E. E., Markland, C., and Lange, P. H. Surgical treatment of stage I and stage II nonseminomatous testicular cancer in adults. *Urol. Clin. North Am.* 4(3):453, 1977. *A thorough review of all aspects of this disease.*

Lewis, E. L., and Palmer, J. M. Office diagnosis of epididymitis, epididymoorchitis, and orchitis. *West. J. Med.* 133(3):270, 1980. *A discussion of proper techniques of examination of the scrotum and its contents.*

Mostofi, F. K., Theiss, E. A., and Ashley, D. J. Tumors of specialized gonadal stroma in human male patients. Androblastoma, sertoli cell tumor, granulosa-thecal cell tumor of the testis, and gonadal stromal tumor. *Cancer* 12:944, 1959. *A detailed discussion of the pathophysiology of testicular tumors.*

Patton, J. F., Hewitt, C. B., and Mallis, N. Diagnosis and treatment of tumors of the testis. *J. A. M. A.* 171:2194, 1959. *A good review of a large series of cases.*

Skinner, D. G., and DeKernion, J. B. (eds.). *Genitourinary Cancer.* Philadelphia: Saunders, 1978. *A good general reference.*

Teter, J., and Boczkowski, K. Occurrence of tumors in dysgenetic gonads. *Cancer* 20:1301, 1967. *A discussion of this rare but interesting entity.*

81 Colorectal Cancer

James E. Crutcher

I. The problem

A. Description. Speculation about the etiology of colonic neoplasia centers around genetics and environment. The genetic link is fostered by the increased incidence of this disease in individuals with a family history of colorectal cancer or polyps, but this finding could be a secondary association with environmental factors. Other studies incriminate factors in the environment, the most important being diet. Arguments focus on the role of bulk, fiber, bile acids, and meats, but most of the evidence rests on international epidemiologic studies or animal models [1].

Regardless of these theories, certain polyps are probably precursors of malignancy. The adenomatous polyp, the juvenile polyp, and the Peutz-Jeghers polyp all have documented malignant potential. The common hyperplastic polyp carries very little, if any, risk for degeneration [2].

B. Epidemiology. According to the American Cancer Society (ACS), colorectal cancer accounts for 15% of all malignancies and is second only to lung cancer in new cases of deaths. It will strike approximately 145,000 persons/year and will kill one half of those stricken. More people in this country may have died of cancer of the colon in the past 50 years than of any other malignancy, but unfortunately there has been little change in its outcome; the overall 5-year survival rate of 50% remains little changed since the 1950s [3].

The pattern of bowel cancer is changing and making early detection more difficult. Lesions of the sigmoid colon, which are easier to detect and have better prognosis (greater than 90% Duke's A), have decreased from more than 90% of all bowel cancers in 1933 to 50% in 1973. At the same time, lesions of the ascending colon, which are harder to detect and have a poor prognosis (less than 25% Duke's A), have increased from less than 10% to greater than 30% of all bowel malignancies. Right-sided lesions predominate in women, while left-sided lesions predominate in men [4]. Current data do not show a statistically significant sexual predominance in incidence or deaths [3], but this may change as lesions shift.

Because the disease is relatively common, a search for colonic neoplasia is frequently rewarded. Sixteen separate, uncontrolled screening trials with various methods found from 1–2 colorectal cancers per 1000 screened patients, with lesions skewed toward earlier Duke's classification [5]; some found as many as 80% of the lesions in Duke's A or B [6], compared to 40% Duke's A or B in nonscreened groups [7]. Furthermore, current evidence suggests asymptomatic people may benefit most from screening. Screened asymptomatic patients had a much higher percentage of Duke's A than screened symptomatic patients (80% versus 15%); and a 15-year survival rate as high as 90% has been reported in screened asymptomatic patients when colorectal malignancy was found. However, symptomatic individuals with localized disease had only a 71% 5-year survival rate [8].

Regardless of these impediments, early detection can be improved by careful attention to certain conditions that put individuals into a high-risk group (Table 81-1). Of all of these factors, polyps are probably the most common and may be found in one-third of a screened population [6]. Colonic cancer is five times more common among patients with polyps than in a normal population [9]. Investigators note a marked decline in cancer in patients who had polypectomies, but these findings may be due to statistical influences and not to the disease process itself [10]. A knowledge of these risk factors, along with a sound screening protocol, can go a long way in meeting the goal of early detection.

However, prospective controlled studies have yet to demonstrate a decrease in mortality in screened populations when compared to control groups. A screening procedure may pick up the disease earlier in its course; therefore, the patient may appear to live

Table 81-1. Colorectal cancer high-risk groups

Age 50 or greater
Prior-treated colorectal cancer
Prior colon adenomas
Ulcerative colitis, lasting more than 7 years and involving entire colon
History of female genital cancer
Family history of polyposis or nonpolyposis syndromes
Anal intercourse
Multiple cancers
Female genital (endometrial) cancer, breast and bladder cancer
Peutz-Jeghers syndrome

Source: H. P. Stelling, et al. New screening method for occult gastrointestinal bleeding: Immunologic and guaiac slide tests. *J. Fam. Pract.* 19(6):757, 1984; and L. S. Leffall, Jr. Colorectal cancer prevention and detection. *Cancer* 47(5 Suppl):1170, 1981.

longer between diagnosis and death without actually altering the time of death. Controlled cohort studies are still needed before early detection can claim a decrease in mortality. Since research is inconclusive, the clinical benefit in the detection and treatment of asymptomatic colorectal cancer is still unquestionable [10], and a healthy controversy about the value, safety, and cost-effectiveness of routine screening in asymptomatic individuals rages in the literature [11]. The recommendations set forth in this chapter are reasonable and are promoted by the American Cancer Society, but they are not entirely proved by research. Until these controversies are settled, the physician needs to follow his or her clinical judgment. Certainly, the highest yield from screening asymptomatic patients will come to those in the high-risk profile (see Table 81-1).

II. Secondary prevention

A. Early detection. Secondary prevention depends on using three commonly accepted tools: the guaiac impregnated slide, sigmoidoscopy, and digital rectal exam.

1. Methods

a. Guaiac impregnated slide

(1) Description. Guaiac is impregnated into special test paper, and when hydrogen peroxide is added, the guaiac is oxidized in the presence of blood to a blue color. In this chemical reaction, hemoglobin has peroxidase-like activity that varies considerably in the clinical situation. The better commercial products also have test indicators that give a positive and negative reading for each slide. These indicators serve as controls to minimize reading errors and to test the potency of the developing solution (stabilized hydrogen peroxide). In addition, Table 81-2 lists the common causes for false-positive and false-negative slides. Newer procedures that claim to be more sensitive (i.e., Hemo-Quant, which depends on fluorescence of heme pigment) or better accepted (i.e., Coloscreen, which places the chemically treated paper directly into the toilet bowl) are being investigated, but large-scale clinical trials are lacking [12, 13]. Radial immunodiffusion (RID) also makes superior claims but needs further testing [14].

(2) Performance. There are numerous brand names of guaiac paper on the market, but the Hemoccult II (SKF-Diagnostics) has been extensively studied, and most of the comments refer to this slide. The American Cancer Society [15] recommends the following procedure, even though controlled clinical trials are lacking:

(a) A meat-free, vitamin C-free, high-fiber diet, should begin at least 48 hours before preparing the first slide. The dietary addition of fiber aids in scraping the lesion and promoting bleeding if the tendency is present. Since bleeding may be intermittent, additional fiber may decrease false-negative slide results. These fibers may come from fresh or cooked vegetables (especially lettuce, spinach, corn), fruit (especially prunes, grapes, plums, apples), and bran from cereal. Some investigators also restrict beets, horseradish, vitamins, and aspirin as well [5, 16, 17]. The dietary restrictions may well be the most critical, in that better than 70% of positive slides may become negative with the above diet changes

Table 81-2. Common causes for false-positive and false-negative slides

Factors producing false-positive[a] guaiac
Iron preparations
Aspirin
Povidone-iodine
Exogenous hemoglobin (red meats, fish)
Natural peroxidases (horseradish, beets)
Factors producing false-negative[b] guaiac
Lack of dietary residue
Prolonged storage of slide (> 4 days)
Vitamin C
Factors producing no effect on guaiac
Cimetidine (false-positive gastric aspirate only)
Barium sulfate
Glyceryl guaiacolate

[a]False-positive means the slide is reacting with either exogenous hemoglobin or dietary peroxidases, and the positive reading is not due to neoplasia.

[b]False-negative means blood from neoplasia is present in the stool but not detected.

Source: J. B. Simon. Occult blood screening for colorectal carcinoma: A critical review. *Gastroenterology* 88(3):820, 1985; and B. F. Overholt. *Colonoscopy and Colon Cancer: Current Clinical Practice.* New York: American Cancer Society, 1981.

[18], but studies with dietary modification do not show a difference in cancer detection [10]. A breakdown of the dietary and other factors that may give false-negative or false-positive readings is presented in Table 81-2, and Fig. 81-1 summarizes a protocol for screening that adjusts for the dietary protocol.

(b) **No rehydration of the slides.** Rehydration renders the chemicals too sensitive, lowering specificity and increasing false-positives from 0.5% to between 4.5% and 20.0% [10].

(c) **Obtaining two separate samples on a single stool on each of 3 consecutive days.** Multiple slides of the same specimen and of consecutive specimens are important. Different slides taken from the same specimen may be positive or negative [19], and a single slide has a sensitivity of only 40% [20]. Although statistical arguments against multiple slides seem relevant [21], the practical point remains—bleeding is intermittent and multiple slides are critical.

(d) **Handling of a single positive slide as if all slides are positive.** There is no correlation between the number of positive slides and neoplasia.

(e) **Storage of specimens for less than 4 days before testing.** A strongly positive slide will remain positive for at least 10 days, while a weakly positive result may be equivocal after only 2–4 days [20].

(3) **Interpretation.** Record all results as positive or negative. Doubtful readings should be recorded as negative and trace readings as positive. Only the blue color change should be called positive; all green discoloration should be ignored. All positive tests need to be investigated by thorough radiologic and/or endoscopic evaluation.

(4) **Timing.** Although no good studies have demonstrated the ideal interval, the ACS recommends that the test be performed once every year.

(5) **Population.** See Table 81-1 for age and risk groups for screening. Since the disease is distributed between both sexes, these recommendations apply to all men and women.

b. Flexible fiberoptic sigmoidoscopy (FFS)

(1) **Description.** The FFS is a 30- or 60-cm flexible tube that moves up/down and right/left by rotary controls. Multiple light-conducting filaments allow the flexibility and are attached to an intense light source for clear, bright fields. The tube is also equipped with multiple ports for rinsing the tip, suction, and biopsy. Since the tube is significantly more narrow than the rigid scope, it is claimed to be more comfortable.

(2) **Interpretation.** Deviation from the normal, healthy, pink mucosa or any growth from the colonic wall needs further investigation and possible biopsy.

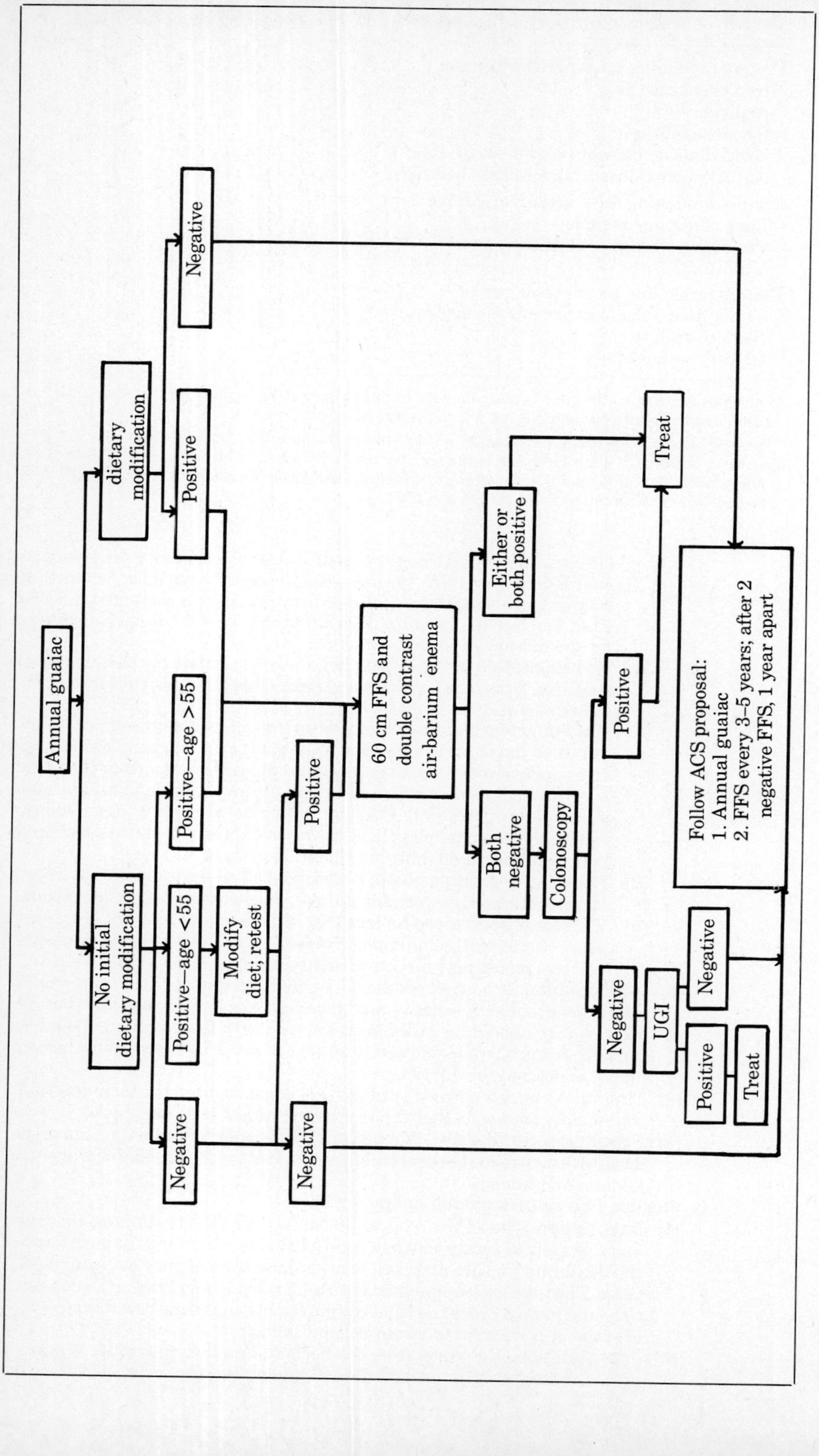

Fig. 81-1. Colorectal cancer screening for average-risk individuals starting at age 50.

Special attention needs to be paid to areas behind mucosal folds or under feces and mucus. Usually, some type of formal training and practice experience is necssary before proficiency develops; the smaller, granular field and increased manual dexterity make FFS more difficult to master than rigid sigmoidoscopy.

(3) **Timing.** The American Cancer Society suggests that sigmoidoscopies be done yearly for two consecutive exams; all polyps should be removed and suspicious lesions biopsied. After two negative examinations occurring 1 year apart, follow-up every 3–5 years depending on risk factors is appropriate. These recommendations are based on several clinical observations: There is evidence that adenomas go through a cycle, degenerating into carcinoma in situ and on to invasive malignancy [2]. Since adenomas may be found in 2–17% of the population initially [10], removal would interrupt progression to cancer. Therefore, follow-up exams are less frequent because the incidence of polyps decreases with repeated examinations [22], and the doubling time of tumors is probably greater than 500 days [9].

(4) **Population.** Routine screening needs to be performed on all patients over the age of 50, regardless of sex. A special effort is needed to evaluate all patients in the high-risk category (see Table 81-1). Since the incidence of colorectal cancer increases with increasing age, there is no theoretical age to stop proctosigmoidoscopy. Practical considerations may cause problems in the elderly, but the FFS will be less limiting than rigid sigmoidoscopy.

c. **Rigid sigmoidoscopy**

(1) **Description.** The rigid sigmoidoscope is a 25-cm tube of plastic (disposable) or metal (reusable) with a light source/magnifier at the proximal end and an obturator to ease insertion at the distal end. The large-bore scope, light, and magnification provide excellent visualization of the anal canal and rectum that many examiners feel is superior to the flexible fiberoptic scopes. Although FFS is a superior screening instrument in many regards, the rigid scope is far cheaper and easier to use.

(2) **Interpretation** is the same as for FFS.

(3) **Timing** is the same as for FFS.

(4) **Population** is the same as for FFS.

d. **Digital rectal exam**

(1) **Description.** A gloved and lubricated finger is inserted into the anus with the patient either leaning over an examination table, in the knee-to-chest position, or in the lithotomy position during pelvic evaluation. Careful attention is paid to the entire wall for 360°; the rectal shelf above the coccyx in both sexes and the pouch of Douglas in the female need special attention.

(2) **Interpretation.** Any palpable mass needs further exploration.

(3) **Interval.** The exam should be performed yearly.

(4) **Population.** Individuals of both sexes after the age of 40 should have the examination.

2. **Justification**

a. **Guaiac impregnated slide**

(1) **Test characteristics.** Two to six percent of an asymptomatic population will have at least one positive slide. Of these, false-positives (positive slides but no malignancy) can be very high, and only 5% of positive slides will be due to cancer. However, the predictive value of a positive slide may be as high as 50% in older patients [23]. Another 20% will be due to adenomas. False-negatives (negative slides but subsequent cancer found) will be in the 5–9% range and are a real clinical concern; these are cases of neoplasia that are missed. At least part of the false-negative rate may be explained by the small size and lack of ulceration in the tumor. Many investigators have commented on the lack of sensitivity of the slides to polyps, and false-negative rates in polyps alone may be as high as 75% [10].

(2) **Risks.** There are no risks for the test itself, but false-positives may subject patients to a risky and unnecessary evaluation.

(3) **Cost.** Several studies give actual costs around $2500 for each cancer found. These figures may be optimistically low because of indirect and "hidden" costs [2, 10]. Of course, the real cost and safety depends on how many people get needless barium enemas or colonoscopies with or without complications because of false-positive results, or how many tumors are missed because of false-negative tests.

(4) **Acceptability.** Investigators report a 50–75% compliance rate for the slides in well-motivated patients. However, in unmotivated populations, compliance can be as low as 15% [10].

b. **Flexible fiberoptic sigmoidoscopy**

(1) **Test characteristics.** Skilled endoscopists using the 60-cm scope report a gain in diagnostic yield of neoplastic pathology of at least 100% over the conventional rigid scope and report as much as a six-fold increase in pathology. In one study, the FFS detected lesions in 27% of patients that were in reach of but were missed by the rigid scope [24]. There is no doubt that greater skills are needed to master the FFS, but several recent studies show that these skills are easily within the province of the primary care physician [25, 26].

(2) **Risks.** Experience has proven the FFS safe and acceptable. One author reports 11 complications in 10,000 examinations for trained physicians [24]. However, these risks may dramatically increase when a population that required biopsy or polypectomy is analyzed separately and when populations are rescreened following a protocol, but fewer neoplasias are found [2].

(3) **Costs.** The charges for FFS vary widely. In 1985, average costs for the 35-cm scope were $80–100 and were approximately $120–150 for the 60-cm scope. If the fees are standardized to that of the rigid sigmoidoscope and the procedure is at least twice as effective, then the FFS will be the screening procedure of choice providing the lowest cost-lesion ratio.

(4) **Acceptability.** Patient acceptance is generally greater than rigid endoscopy. One author recently marked a sustained increase in FFS when compared to rigid sigmoidoscopy in an asymptomatic population undergoing routine investigation. FFS seems better accepted by physician and patient alike [26].

c. **Rigid sigmoidoscopy**

(1) **Test characteristics.** The results are adversely affected by the limitations of the instrument. Only 15–30% of all colonic neoplasms are within the 20-cm reach of the scope [4], and the sigmoidoscope is reliable only under 16 cm. Therefore, up to 65% of colorectal cancer or polyps may be missed by sigmoidoscopy alone [9].

(2) **Risks.** The safety of the procedure is well established. The most significant complication of sigmoidoscopy is bowel perforation. Larger studies show perforations occurred from 8 out of 9150 studies to 5 in over 103,000 procedures [9, 27]. These numbers translate into a ratio that may vary from one perforation for every 2–100 cancers found in an asymptomatic population; the real complication rate probably rests between these two extremes.

(3) **Costs.** Based on the cost of $50 per procedure and one cancer per 1000 procedures, approximately $50,000 dollars in sigmoidoscopy costs alone (not including barium enemas, biopsy and pathology reports, or colonoscopy) would be incurred for each colorectal cancer found. One estimate placed the cost of a "curable" lesion (greater than 5-year survival) at about $15,000 in 1978 dollars [9]; this would probably be considerably more in current dollars.

(4) **Acceptability.** Patient acceptability of the procedure is a real problem. Healthy people are concerned about the test and question the discomfort involved. Doctors as well may have some aversion that limits its usefulness as a screening procedure. Despite these real disadvantages, rigid sigmoidoscopies still have a role to play. When combined with fecal occult blood testing, sigmoidoscopy, and polypectomy, new cancers in an asymptomatic, screened population were reduced by almost 80% over the expected incidence for the community, and those malignancies detected on follow-up were all localized [23].

d. **Digital rectal exam**

(1) **Characteristics.** The digital rectal exam is a time-honored test with very little known about its effectiveness. As a screening test for colorectal cancer, only 10–13% of malignancies are within reach of a finger [4].

(2) **Risks.** The risks are minimal to none.

(3) **Costs** vary with the office charge. Few, if any, health care providers have a separate charge for this procedure.

(4) **Acceptability.** The digital rectal exam is barely tolerated.

B. Early intervention

1. **Methods.** The double contrast barium enema and flexible colonoscopy are not screening procedures, but they do play a key role in follow-up of positive fecal occult blood and sigmoidoscopies, or in evaluation of high-risk patients (i.e., those with ulcerative colitis). It is essential that all follow-up be done with double contrast air/barium studies to more clearly outline mucosal lesions. Fig. 81-1 outlines a reasonable procedure for follow-up when doing routine occult blood testing on asymptomatic patients.

   During colonoscopy, all lesions need to be biopsied and all polyps removed. Because some polyps have little malignant potential and polypectomy or biopsy increases risks, some authors challenge this recommendation. Although early malignant polyps can sometimes be removed through the colonoscope [24], surgery is the preferred method for treatment.

   Patients with a higher risk of colorectal malignancy (see Table 81-1) need to be screened more vigorously. These patients should have a colonoscopy done annually for 2 consecutive years, followed by air/contrast barium enema and colonoscopy every 3–5 years. Fecal occult blood testing should also be done annually unless periodic bleeding is a part of the disease process (i.e., ulcerative colitis).

2. **Justification**

   a. **Effectiveness.** Neither the double contrast barium enema nor the colonoscope is completely valid alone for follow-up of a positive screen: barium enemas may miss 25% or more of colon cancers and over two thirds of colon polyps found by colonoscopy [28]. Colonoscopy alone may miss 5–8% of adenomas over 1 cm [24]. Together, the two procedures complement each other; the barium enema is best at flexures and in the detection of right-sided lesions, while the colonoscope is best on the upper sigmoid and descending colon beyond the sigmoidoscope.

      Although clinical trials that show increased longevity from aggressive, early screening are missing, early intervention and the possibility of Duke's A and B type lesions strongly suggest that screening of asymptomatic patients in primary care is reasonable. When colorectal cancer is detected and treated in early, localized stages, the 5-year survival rate is better than 70%. If the disease has spread to other parts of the body, this rate drops to 28% [3].

   b. **Costs.** Although prices vary considerably, in 1985 double air contrast barium enema costs were around $150. Fees vary even more for colonoscopy. Without biopsy or polypectomy, which of course cost considerably more, basic colonoscopy charges were around $450, with approximately $50–100 additionally as a room charge.

III. Recommendations

A. Early detection

1. **Digital rectal exam** should be performed annually after age 40.
2. **Stool occult blood slide** should be performed annually after age 50.
3. **Proctosigmoidoscopy** should be performed annually for the first two examinations starting at age 50, then every 3–5 years.

B. Intervention

1. Fig. 81-1 summarizes the evaluation of colorectal disease with fecal occult blood screening [28, 29].
2. Patients with a higher risk of colorectal malignancy (see Table 81-1) may need to be screened more vigorously.

References

1. Wynder, E. L. Dietary habits and cancer epidemiology. *Cancer* 43(5 Suppl):1955, 1979. *A short, concise discussion on dietary habits and bowel neoplasia.*
2. Fenoglio-Preiser, C. M., and Hutter, R. V. Colorectal polyps: Pathologic diagnosis and clinical significance. *CA* 35(6):322, 1985. *A clear delineation of polyp types and characteristics.*
3. Silverberg, E., and Lubera, J. Cancer statistics, 1987. *CA* 37(1):2, 1987. *The annual compilation of cancer statistics and demographics.*
4. Abrams, J. S., and Reines, H. D. Increasing incidence of right-sided lesions in colorectal cancer. *Am. J. Surg.* 137(4):522, 1979. *A discussion on changing epidemiology of bowel cancer and the problems that these changes create for screening.*

5. Diehl, A. K. Screening for colorectal cancer. *J. Fam. Pract.* 12(4):625, 1981. *A good, general review but slightly dated.*
6. Gilbertsen, V. A., et al. The earlier detection of colorectal cancers: A preliminary report of the Occult Blood Study. *Cancer* 45(11):2899, 1980. *A report on a general population arguing for routine asymptomatic screening.*
7. Winawer, S. J., et al. Progress report on controlled trial of fecal occult blood testing for the detection of colorectal neoplasia. *Cancer* 45(12):2959, 1980. *Another asymptomatic population with favorable outcomes from screening.*
8. Winawer, S. J., et al. Screening for colorectal cancer with fecal occult blood testing. *Front. Gastrointest. Res.* 5:28, 1979. *Excellent review of fecal occult blood screening.*
9. Dutton, J. J. Sigmoidoscopy as a periodic screening test. *J. Fam. Pract.* 7(5):1041, 1978. *A somewhat dated discussion of rigid sigmoidoscopies.*
10. Simon, J. B. Occult blood screening for colorectal carcinoma: A critical review. *Gastroenterology* 88(3):820, 1985. *An excellent review of all the issues of routine occult blood screening.*
11. Frank, J. W. Occult-blood screening for colorectal carcinoma: The benefits. *Am. J. Prev. Med.* 1(3):3, 1985. *Good arguments against routine occult blood screening.*
12. Rodney, W. M., and Ruggiero, C. The coloscreen self-test for detection of fecal occult blood. *J. Fam. Pract.* 21(3):200, 1985. *One of the first literature reports on a new method of screening that has yet to be verified.*
13. Ahlquist, D. A., et al. Fecal blood levels in health and disease. A study using HemoQuant. *N. Engl. J. Med.* 312(22):1422, 1985. *General discussion of "normal" blood loss through the bowel from exogenous and endogenous sources.*
14. Stelling, H. P., et al. New screening method for occult gastrointestinal bleeding: Immunologic and guaiac slide tests. *J. Fam. Pract.* 19(6):757, 1984. *Another new test that overcomes the limitations of guaiac; still needs further clinical trials.*
15. Cancer of the colon and rectum. *CA* 30(4):208, 1980. *A general but thorough discussion of neoplastic bowel disease.*
16. Leffall, L. S. Jr. Colorectal cancer prevention and detection. *Cancer* 47(5 Suppl):1170, 1981. *The official viewpoint on colorectal cancer and its causes from the American Cancer Society.*
17. Bolt, R. J. Evaluation of screening tests for colorectal cancer. *Primary Care* 7(4):683, 1980. *An excellent discussion on pros and cons of current, accepted screening methods.*
18. Hardcastle, J. D., Balfour, T. W., and Amar, S. S. Screening for symptomless colorectal cancer by testing for occult blood in general practice. *Lancet* 1(8172):791, 1980. *Article details the British system of bowel screening in an asymptomatic population, with a rigid but acceptable protocol.*
19. Screening for colorectal cancer (editorial). *Lancet* 2(8154):1222, 1979. *A short comment that shows the problems of interpretation, and implementation of screening an asymptomatic population.*
20. Winawer, S. J., et al. Current status of fecal occult blood testing in screening for colorectal cancer. *CA* 32(2):100, 1982. *Although the discussion is no longer "current," the strengths and weaknesses of the hemoccult screening tool presented here are timeless.*
21. Neuhauser, D., and Lweicki, A. M. What do we gain from the sixth stool guaiac? *N. Engl. J. Med.* 293(5):226, 1975. *A valid but "nit-picking" statistical discussion that revolves around how many guaiacs are enough.*
22. Gilbertsen, V. A., and Nelms, J. M. The prevention of invasive cancer of the rectum. *Cancer* 41(3):1137, 1978. *The original paper showing decreasing bowel neoplasia with subsequent screening. This observation serves as the basis for arguments showing screening not to be cost-effective.*
23. Goulston, K., and Davidson, P. Faecal occult blood testing in patients with colonic symptoms. *Med. J. Aust.* 2(12): 667, 1980. *This presentation deals with symptomatic Australians, but the pathology discovered is surprising.*
24. Crespi, M., et al. The role of proctosigmoidoscopy in screening for colorectal neoplasia. *CA* 34(3):158, 1984. *A good, current discussion of the strengths and weaknesses of the flexible sigmoidoscope.*
25. Semerdjian, G. Flexible sigmoidoscopy for screening in primary practice. A key to improved survival in colon cancer. *Postgrad. Med.* 78(3):47, 1985. *Defends FFS in the primary care office.*
26. Rodney, W. M. Screening flexible sigmoidoscopy: Is it worthwhile? *J. Fam. Pract.* 25(6):601, 1987. *Rodney defends screening FFS in the primary care office while Paul Frame opposes it in an adjacent article.*
27. Kiser, J. L., Spratt, J. S. Jr., and Johnson, C. A. Colon perforation occurring during sigmoidoscopic examinations and barium enemas. *Missouri Med.* 65:969, 1968. *Simply points out rate of complications of our follow-up procedures.*

28. Greegor, D. H. Colorectal cancer screening (letter). *J. A. M. A.* 243(2):119, 1980. *A rational argument for age-related screening protocol. There is no good research evidence that supports this view yet.*
29. Overholt, B. F. *Colonoscopy and Colon Cancer: Current Clinical Practice.* New York: American Cancer Society, 1981. *Good review of the role of colonoscopy in colorectal cancer.*

82 Cancer of the Prostate

Frederick J. Meyers

I. The problem

A. Description. At first glance, routine screening for cancer of the prostate seems a promising effort, since the organ can be palpated by an examiner and since only a defined subgroup of the population need be screened. Unfortunately, early detection has had limited impact on the outcome of the disease because of the biology of the tumor.

B. Epidemiology [1, 2, 3]. Adenocarcinoma of the prostate is the second most common cancer in the male and the third most frequent cause of death from cancer in men, after carcinoma of the lung and colon. In 1983, 73,000 new cases were discovered and 25,000 men died of prostatic cancer. The incidence by age groups (Table 82-1) is more useful than the crude rates above. Cancer of the prostate rarely occurs before age 40; screening will not be productive in these patients. Age is the only confirmed risk factor for the development of prostatic cancer. There is no clearly increased risk for prostatitis, degree of sexual activity, or benign prostatic hypertrophy.

C. Staging. Table 82-2 indicates a popular schema for staging prostatic cancer. At the time of diagnosis, 60–80% of patients have stage C or D disease. Most of these patients will succumb to prostatic carcinoma. However, stage is only one important factor in determining prognosis. One cannot conclude that detecting tumors at an earlier stage necessarily improves mortality rates. If metastases have occurred but are undetectable by standard radiographic methods, the patient will succumb to his disease at the same time as if he had not been entered into a screening program. This is known as lead-time bias.

A screening program must be evaluated not only on its crude ability to detect the tumors but also on its ability to detect the neoplasm at a time when its stage (extent) permits therapy to improve mortality rates.

II. Secondary prevention

A. Early detection

1. **Methods. Screening for prostate cancer with currently available methods is not justified.** The available screening tests are inaccurate, and early detection does not appear to alter prognosis. However, when a nodule is noted during a rectal exam done as part of ongoing care or when screening for colorectal carcinoma, it must be evaluated to rule out cancer of the prostate.

2. **Justification.** The rectal examination is the most accurate screening test available (Table 82-3), yet it is far from accurate enough for screening. In a study of patients referred to urologists for urologic symptoms, 23% were found to have prostatic cancer [4]. The rectal exam identified 70% of the cancers, but only 50% of palpable nodules were cancerous. This percentage rises to 70% if there is loss of anatomic margins and if the induration extends into the seminal vesicles.

   Like all screening tests, the rectal exam suffers considerably when the prevalence of the disease falls. With a prevalence of 23%, the chance that a nodule is cancer is 50%; when the prevalence is less than 1% (a frequency more representative of a primary physician's office with patients not presenting with urologic symptoms) [5], the chance that a nodule is cancer is only 6%. This means that for each cancer found, 17 older men will be subjected to the risk and expense of prostatic biopsy, an unacceptably high price to pay considering that an improved mortality rate has not been demonstrated.

   In addition, one cannot infer an improved prognosis merely by assessing the clinical stage of prostatic carcinoma [6, 7]. The digital rectal exam has been shown by subsequent suprapubic prostatectomy to understage established disease. Many patients with stage B disease in fact have stage C disease. In addition to the preoperative local extent being underestimated, retroperitoneal lymph node dissection has shown that unsuspected systemic spread is often present. The incidence of lymph

Table 82-1. Incidence of cancer of the prostate by age groups, United States, 1975

100,000 cases/year	Whites	Blacks
45–49	4.6	7.1
50–54	16.6	36.2
55–59	52.2	116.6
60–64	126.8	269.5
65–69	254.2	462.6
70–74	429.5	785.3
75–79	655.9	922.6
80–84	825.6	1274.6
85 +	882.4	865.8

Source: S. J. Cutler and J. L. Young (eds.), *Third National Cancer Survey: Incidence Data.* Bethesda, Md: National Cancer Institute, 1975.

Table 82-2. Staging of prostatic cancer

Stage	Definition	% lymph node involvement
A	No palpable nodule	
A_1	< 3 chips involved at transurethral prostatectomy, well-differentiation	0
A_2	> 3 chips, poorly differentiated	15–25
B	Confined to prostate—no penetration of capsule	
B_1	Limited to one lobe, not > 1.5 cm	8–20
B_2	> 1.5 cm, extends across midline	15–45
C	Penetration of capsule, extension to seminal vesicles or bladder	40–80
D_1	Involvement of draining lymph nodes without distant metastases	
D_2	Distant metastases—bone, lung, etc.	

node metastases (stage D) rises with the degree of local spread and with the histologic grade of the tumor. That is, the less well-differentiated a tumor, the greater the chance of lymph node metastases. The variation in the degree of differentiation between tumors accounts for the range in percent of lymph node involvement within any one stage (Table 82-2).

As can be seen in Table 82-3, other tests proposed for screening are even less accurate [4]. This includes various assays of acid phosphatase and urine cytology. Table 82-3 represents the study where the prevalence of cancer was 23%; a prevalence of less than 1% results in very low predictive values (column 4).

B. Early intervention

1. **Perspective.** The behavior of prostatic cancer prevents earlier detection from improving prognosis. A useful taxonomy can be constructed that demonstrates the difficulty in screening for prostatic cancer.
   a. **Group 1.** Well-differentiated, predominantly localized disease with little potential to inflict morbidity or mortality. These older patients usually succumb to an intercurrent illness, for example, heart disease. This group is far larger than clinical studies indicate. Autopsy examinations of prostatic tissue in men previously not suspected of having prostatic carcinoma have revealed a 10% and greater overall prevalence of localized carcinoma. As in the clinical series, the incidence rises dramatically with age, peaking in frequency in the mid-70s age group.
   b. **Group 2.** A small group (5–10%) with local disease by rigorous staging (B_1) but with a potential for dissemination. These patients **may** benefit from early detection followed by radical prostatectomy or vigorous radiation therapy.

Table 82-3. Results of screening tests for prostate cancer

			If prevalence		
	Sensitivity	Specificity	23% predictive value[a]	1% predictive value[a]	Cost[b]
Rectal examination	0.69	0.89	67	6	
Acid phosphatase enzyme	0.56	0.94	74	8	6
Acid phosphatase radioimmuno-assay	0.20	0.85	28	1	15
Urine cytology					
Before massage	0.17	0.98	72	8	15
After massage	0.22	0.98	77	10	15

[a]Percentage of patients correctly classified.
[b]Exclusive of physician time.
Source: Modified from P. Guinan, et al. The accuracy of the rectal examination in the diagnosis of prostate carcinoma. *N. Engl. J. Med.* 303(9):499, 1980.

c. **Group 3.** Poorly differentiated tumor, usually locally advanced and with lymph node involvement at the time of diagnosis. Only palliative therapy is available and these patients die of prostatic cancer. A subpopulation of cells within these tumors have an ability to metastasize early in development and to negate any efforts at early diagnosis. There is reason to think that many group 3 patients progress in an orderly fashion from low stage to advanced stage disease.

2. **Justification.** There is no need to screen for group 1 patients. The cost of the test and the cost of subsequent evaluation and therapy of these often incidental cancers is not justified. Group 3 patients have systemic disease early in their disease. If effective systemic therapy were available (e.g., adjuvant chemotherapy), then early detection would be valuable. Such systemic therapy is not available.

   No one has yet offered evidence that a screening routine can increase the rate of detection of group 2 patients. Only group 2 patients may benefit from early detection, but this group is quite small compared to groups 1 and 3. Any evaluation of screening and of definitive therapy must include a control group or the test group must at least be compared to a standardized, age-adjusted, actuarial survival curve.

III. Recommendations

A. There is no known primary prevention for prostatic cancer, as the only known risk factor is age.

B. Screening for prostatic cancer is not justified because:

1. There is presently no screening test available that has a positive predictive value greater than 10%.
2. The vast majority of prostatic cancer does not appear to be affected by early detection.

C. When a rectal exam is done as a part of ongoing care or when screening for colorectal carcinoma and a nodule is palpated, it must be evaluated to determine whether prostatic cancer is present.

References

1. Klein, L. A. Prostatic carcinoma. *N. Engl. J. Med.* 300(15):824, 1979. *A comprehensive review of prostatic carcinoma.*
2. Von Eschenback, A. C. Cancer of the prostate. *Curr. Probl. Cancer* 5(12):3, 1981. *Good review.*

3. Cutler, S. J., and Young, J. L. (eds.). *Third National Cancer Survey: Incidence Data.* Bethesda, Md: National Cancer Institute. 1975. *Good source on cancer epidemiology.*
4. Guinan, P., et al. The accuracy of the rectal examination in the diagnosis of prostate carcinoma. *N. Engl. J. Med.* 303(9):499, 1980. *Compares a variety of diagnostic tests for prostate cancer.*
5. Gleason, D. F. Histologic Grading and Clinical Staging of Prostatic Carcinoma. In M. Tannenbaum (ed.), *Urologic Pathology: The Prostate.* Philadelphia: Lea & Febiger, 1977. Pp.171–198. *Defines the pathophysiology of prostatic cancer.*
6. Byar, D. P. VACURG Studies on Prostatic Cancer and Its Treatment. In M. Tannenbaum (ed.), *Urologic Pathology: The Prostate.* Philadelphia: Lea & Febiger, 1977. Pp.241–267. *Defines the pathophysiology of prostatic cancer.*
7. Gilbertsen, V. A. Cancer of the prostate gland: Results of early diagnosis and therapy undertaken for the cure of the disease. *J. A. M. A.* 215:81, 1971. *Large screening program found prostatic cancers in 0.26% of rectal exams performed.*

83 Diethylstilbestrol Exposure

Duane Townsend

I. The problem

A. Description. Between the years 1945 to 1970, approximately 4 million pregnant women were given synthetic, nonsteroidal estrogens (diethylstilbestrol [DES]), or chemically similar dienestrol, for threatened abortions, habitual abortion history, diabetes, and a variety of other factors that may jeopardize pregnancy. This has resulted in a population of exposed individuals that is equally distributed between males and females with unique medical problems.

In utero exposure to DES produced developmental and structural changes that appear to increase cancer risks, negatively impact pregnancy, and have major psychological ramifications. Appropriate management of affected individuals will reduce the impact of DES exposure.

The effects noted in the exposed individuals are primarily on the reproductive systems.

1. **Male changes** initially included low sperm counts and minor abnormalities of the penis and scrotal contents. More recent studies have refuted these earlier findings. There is no known increased risk of cancer in the males, although case reports have raised this possibility.
2. The most significant effect in the **female** is an apparent increased risk for developing a very rare malignancy—clear cell carcinoma of the vagina and cervix. The tumor is most common in the vagina (two thirds of the cases). Over 500 cases are known to have occurred in the last 20 years. Peak age incidence is 19. It is rarely seen after the age of 30. Early detection is synonymous with high cure. The risk of an exposed female developing this malignancy is around 1/1000.
3. **A number of benign changes** are easily detectable in DES-exposed women. Adenosis (benign endocervical-type epithelium within the vagina) is detected about 35% of the time. This change, which appears red and granular to the naked eye, disappears spontaneously and does not need therapy. Women with adenosis may be at the highest risk for developing vaginal cancer.
4. **Cervical structural changes,** called collars or cock's combs, are noted in 25% of exposed women. These changes also disappear over time.
5. **The uterus** may have an abnormal cavity. This is found most commonly in women who have adenosis and/or cervical structural changes. Many women with uterine abnormalities have problems with reproductive function.
6. **The problems with reproduction** include an increased risk of spontaneous abortions, ectopic pregnancies, a slight increase in premature labor, and second trimester losses. Fertility rates are probably unaffected, but a rare case of DES-induced infertility probably occurs.
7. Recent reports suggest an **increased risk** for developing squamous cell neoplasia of the cervix and vagina. These data are still under investigation.
8. Women who took DES may have an **increased risk** of developing breast cancer. Other areas of concern include cancer of the uterine lining.

B. Epidemiology. About 2 million males and 2 million females born between 1945–1970 were exposed in utero to DES. Most women who were given DES lived in the major metropolitan areas of the United States, that is, Boston, New York, Philadelphia, Detroit, Houston, and Los Angeles, with the greatest concentration in the colonial states. Most of the women were white and were from the middle to upper middle class.

Studies point out that women exposed before 20 weeks, over a long period of time, and to a higher total dose, are most likely to exhibit DES changes. However, records are usually lacking in such individuals, and a careful examination is necessary to attempt to determine DES changes.

II. Secondary prevention

A. Early assessment methods

1. **History.** Although many will not know if their mother took DES, and half of those with physical evidence of DES will be unable to locate records documenting exposure, it is worth inquiring of all women born between 1945 and 1970 if their mother took DES.
2. **Examination.** Women thought to be exposed to DES in utero should have a thorough evaluation for DES changes. The findings of such changes is presumptive evidence of exposure, although efforts to obtain records to confirm the exposure should be sought from physicians' records, pharmacies, and hospitals. In half of the cases, such records are not available.
   a. **Performance and interpretation.** Examination of DES-exposed women is similar to a pelvic examination, except for some minor additions. Some patients may be virginal, and manual dilation of the hymen or the usage of tampons prior to the exam may be helpful. Initially, the vagina is palpated from the hymen to the cervix, noting nodularity that must be sampled subsequently. An appropriate size speculum is inserted. Excess vaginal discharge is removed. Vaginal and cervical Pap smears are obtained separately and placed on individual slides. The tissues are inspected grossly. Vaginal adenosis appears red and granular. Cervical columnar tissue has a red appearance as well. Cervical structural changes, such as collars and cock's combs, are noted. When available, colposcopy is performed at this time, with findings noted. If colposcopy is not available, the cervix and vagina should be stained with one-half strength aqueous Lugol's solution. Adenosis and the tissue that replaces it, that is, squamous metaplasia, will stain a light yellow. However, neoplasia also lacks glycogen and will stain a light yellow. Biopsies are taken of suspicious areas. After any tissue sampling, a bimanual examination, including rectovaginal, is performed to rule out adnexal masses or any obvious pelvis abnormalities. A baseline colposcopic examination is recommended.
   b. **Intervals.** Follow-up exams are based on changes found in the vagina. If the woman has nonstaining tissue in the vagina (vaginal epithelial change), which is benign, it is suggested that she be examined every 6 months, similar to the initial examination, but colposcopy is not necessary. Colposcopic assessment is appropriate every 3–4 years. If the patient does not have vaginal epithelial changes, the examination should be annual and identical to the standard gynecologic exam. If a woman has an abnormal Papanicolaou test (i.e., one suggestive of dysplasia or worse, or class II or worse), she should be referred to an individual who is experienced in colposcopic assessment of DES-exposed individuals.
   c. **Population.** DES examination should be performed on any woman who thinks she is a DES daughter or who is noted to have DES changes in a pelvic examination. DES examinations need not be done before the age of 17 because of the rare case of clear cell adenocarcinoma found before this age, unless there are specific symptoms suggesting problems.
   d. **Referral.** The subset of DES daughters with vaginal epithelial changes and cervical structural changes are the ones who require the greatest degree of attention, for their cancer risk may be higher and their reproductive problems are highest. Patients with squamous cell lesions need early and prompt referral. Individuals who have already demonstrated reproduction problems should be referred.

B. Justification

1. **Test characteristics**
   a. **History.** The accuracy of an individual reporting that she is a DES daughter is uncertain. The prevalence of DES daughters will vary in different practice settings.
   b. **Exam.** About 40–45% of DES-exposed women will have a definitive DES change. This includes evidence of adenosis, as well as cervical structural changes. In the remaining individuals, the examination findings will be similar to those noted examining nonexposed individuals.
2. **Risks.** Risks of examination are quite small except when the individual is virginal and has not been properly prepared for the exam. Psychological impact can be easily managed if the physician is well informed about DES and points out the low risk for cancer. The pelvic examination can be made less stressful through proper preexamination preparation and a methodical, carefully performed examination.
3. **Costs.** Examination costs are extremely variable. They involve the cost of the regu-

lar examination and in some cases colposcopy. Those individuals who have a history of reproductive dysfunction will require x rays, which include a hysterosalpingogram and possibly ultrasound.

4. **Acceptability.** Patient acceptance has been excellent. Negative reports occur because of painful examination and lack of physician knowledge about DES. There are many negative psychological impacts of DES because of misleading and inappropriate lay medical reports.

III. Early intervention

A. Methods

1. **Counseling.** Once proper identification of DES-exposed individuals has occurred, appropriate information regarding their exposure history can be offered. Many individuals will have no physical problems related to DES, and accurate information may be sufficient. Others may have concerns about the future or may already have physical problems, which should be handled through supportive individual or group counseling in addition to an understanding primary physician.
2. **Medical management of DES-related problems.** Therapy of structural genital tract changes (i.e., collars, cock's combs) as well as vaginal and cervical epithelial changes is not necessary, since virtually all of these changes will disappear over time. When a DES-exposed woman becomes pregnant, it is recommended that she be referred to a high-risk perinatal center. At the center, she may have an ultrasound performed to determine if she is developing an incompetent cervical os. The management of first trimester abortions has not been satisfactory. Premature labor responds to appropriate use of medication.

B. Justification

1. **Effectiveness**
   a. **Counseling.** Improvements in the psychological impact of being a DES daughter have been demonstrated on numerous occasions in large studies. Patients, when aware of their exposure to DES and accurately informed in a supportive way of what to expect, can deal with the problems on an appropriate basis.
   b. **Medical intervention.** The structural and epithelial changes due to DES exposure require no therapy since they are self-limited and will disappear over time. This information, when passed along to the DES-exposed individual, invariably lessens the psychological impact of the exposure.

   Those individuals who appear to have a pregnancy-related problem show marked psychological improvement and usually have fewer problems when care is given by an individual who is particularly experienced in dealing with the DES-exposed offspring.
2. **Risks and side effects**
   a. **Counseling.** The information provided to the patient can have a negative impact and has in a few cases. Counseling is sometimes necessary for these individuals when they have been informed of the impact of DES exposure.
   b. **Medical intervention.** When individuals are first informed of possible DES exposure because of a structural or an epithelial change noted during an examination, a negative impact can result unless the patient is also counseled as to the minimum impact of these changes. Moreover, DES-like changes are noted in about 4% of the population even though they have not been exposed. As a consequence, to sweepingly assume that all individuals with such changes have been exposed is not necessarily appropriate. This information also must be passed along to the patient. However, for management of pregnancy the treatment remains the same, whether they are exposed or not, if they have structural and vaginal epithelial changes.
3. **Costs**
   a. **Counseling.** These potentially include the costs of psychological and psychiatric care, which are rarely needed nowadays.
   b. **Medical intervention.** The costs of therapy for treating patients who have a neoplastic problem will vary depending on the findings but are not any higher than the usual costs for treating such problems.
4. **Acceptability.** Most patients are thankful when they have been properly counseled and examined regarding their DES exposure. Often the individual's fears are markedly alleviated.

IV. Recommendations

A. Early assessment

1. All women born between 1945 and 1970 should be queried to determine if there is a history of DES exposure.

2. All women exposed to DES should be carefully evaluated. This includes inspection of the vulva, palpation of the vagina, cytology of the cervix and/or vagina, depending on the presence or absence of the vaginal epithelial changes. Lugol's staining annually, and colposcopic examination every 3 years. Biopsies of any suspicious areas should be taken. A bimanual examination, including rectal examination, completes the examination.
3. Frequency of examinations is determined by findings: every 6 months if there is adenosis, past or present; otherwise, annually. Colposcopic assessment should be done initially, then every 3–4 years.

B. Early intervention

1. The impact of DES exposure on these individuals should be discussed with the patient as well as her family, and appropriate support and counseling offered as needed.
2. Literature regarding the impact of DES is available both from the federal government and from DES-action groups throughout the United States and is helpful to supplement information for the DES-exposed offspring.
3. If there is suggestion of a neoplastic problem, abnormal findings, or abnormal Pap smear, then the patient should be referred to a specialist who is experienced in dealing with these problems.
4. Women with structural DES changes or a history of DES-related reproductive dysfunction should also be referred to a specialist who is comfortable in dealing with their problems.
5. Contraceptive usage in DES-exposed offspring is at the patient's and physician's discretion. Birth control pills are not known to have a negative impact. Diaphragms can be difficult to use because of cervical structural changes. Intrauterine devices may be difficult to wear because of uterine abnormalities. Sponges and local spermicidal methods have no negative impact on DES-exposed women.
6. Less common problems of DES exposure include possible increased breast cancer in women who took the drug. These individuals should be carefully evaluated, including mammography on an appropriate basis.
7. DES-exposed males appear to have little problem and they need not be assessed at this time. However, in this ever-changing field, this could alter within the next decade.

Suggested Readings

Dieckmann, W. J., et al. Does the administration of diethylstilbestrol during pregnancy have therapeutic value? *Am. J. Obstet. Gynecol.* 66:1062, 1953. *Article from a Chicago lying-in hospital that questioned use of DES.*

Herbst, A. L., Ulfelder, H., and Poskanzer, D. C. Adenocarcinoma of the vagina. Association of maternal stibestrol therapy with tumor appearance in young women. *N. Engl. J. Med.* 284(15):878, 1971. *The article that brought DES problems to the attention of medicine.*

Kaufman, R. H., et al. Upper genital tract abnormalities and pregnancy outcome in diethylstilbestrol-exposed progeny. *Am. J. Obstet. Gynecol.* 148(7):973, 1984. *Study that relates genital tract changes and reproductive problems—excellent.*

Leary, F. J., et al. Males exposed in utero to diethylstilbestrol. *J. A. M. A.* 252(21):2984, 1984. *Male study from the Mayo Clinic pointing out the lack of changes in males.*

Noller, K. L. In Utero Exposure to Diethylstilbestrol. In *Novak's Textbook of Gynecology.* Baltimore, MD: Williams & Wilkins (in press). *Excellent review on the subject of DES exposure.*

Robboy, S. J., et al. Increased incidence of cervical and vaginal dysplasia in 3,980 diethylstilbestrol-exposed young women. Experience of the National Collaborative Diethylstilbestrol Adenosis Project. *J. A. M. A.* 252(21):2979, 1984. *A study that demonstrates possible increased risk of squamous cell changes.*

Shafer, M. A., et al. Self-concept in the diethylstilbestrol daughter. *Obstet. Gynecol.* 63(6):815, 1984. *Reports some of the psychological changes in DES-exposed women.*

Smith, O. W. Diethylstilbestrol in the prevention and treatment of complications of pregnancy. *Am. J. Obstet. Gynecol.* 56:821, 1948. *One of the original articles on the use of DES in pregnancy.*

84 Screening for Oropharyngeal Cancer

F. L. Don McClurg, Jr.

I. The problem

A. Description. The rich diversity of embryologic cell types found in the head and neck provides the potential for a vast array of tumor cell types to present in this region. Despite this diversity, the vast majority of malignant tumors arising in the head and neck are squamous cell carcinomas arising from the mucosa of the upper aerodigestive tract, followed in frequency by carcinoma of the thyroid.

The upper aerodigestive tract (UADT) anatomically consists of the **lips, oral mucosa, gingiva, tongue, tonsils, nose, nasopharynx, oropharynx, hypopharynx,** and **larynx.** Each of these areas can be accurately evaluated using basic techniques of visualization and palpation. Examination of the relatively more remote areas of the nasopharynx, hypopharynx, and larynx require skills in the use of a headlight, mirrors, and fiberoptic instrumentation. For screening purposes, we shall limit discussion to the lips, oral mucosa, gingiva, tongue, and tonsils: the mouth and oropharynx (MOP). The early detection of these cancers, leading to early intervention, enhances the cure rate. When one analyzes the risk factors, one will be able to identify the population at risk for squamous cell carcinoma (SCC) arising from the epithelium of the UADT. Applying techniques of screening for early detection to this population will produce a significant increase in the effectiveness of such efforts, because SCC arising from UADT has known predisposing factors and is frequently preceded by identifiable premalignant changes of the mucosa.

B. Epidemiology. Approximately 3% of all new cancers in the United States will fall into the category of SCC of the MOP.

C. Risk factors of UADT cancer are well studied and include the following:

1. **Age.** Although these tumors (SCC) have been reported to occur as early as the second decade, the most prevalent incidence is from 50–70 years of age. Recent observations, however, indicate a rapid onset of oral carcinoma in **teenagers** heavily using snuff.
2. **Sex.** Most studies indicate a high (3:1, 5:1) ratio of men to women. Whether this is really sex-related or habit-related (as noted in cancer of the lung) is unclear. Since the 1940s, however, the ratio of male-female incidence has been decreasing, suggesting the latter interpretation.
3. **Tobacco.** There is a very clear and well-defined relationship between tobacco use and the occurrence of SCC of the MOP [1].
   a. **Cigarettes.** There is a dose-related risk and mortality in smokers, with a smoker-nonsmoker mortality ratio of 13. A linear correlation exists between the number of cigarettes smoked daily and the occurrence of, as well as the mortality from, SCC of the MOP [2].
   b. **Pipe and cigars.** There appears to be no difference between the methods of smoking and the occurrence of oral cancer.
   c. **Snuff dipping and chewing smokeless tobacco.** There is a 4:1 incidence of oral cancer in women who dip snuff, compared to a control group of nonusers. The relative risk for long-term snuff users for oral SCC is 50. The relationship between teenage snuff users and the early presentation of oral SCC appears to be a direct one; however, the shortened time between exposure and presentation is as yet unexplained.
4. **Ethanol use.** There is an increase in the incidence of MOP SCC in nonsmoking drinkers. The carcinogenic potential is much lower than tobacco; however, combined use of tobacco and alcohol has a potentiating effect [2].
5. **Sun exposure** pertains to the lips only, this region being affected by solar exposure in the same manner as the skin, producing actinic changes of the epithelium. Tobacco use is an additive factor.

6. **Prior diagnosis of MOP SCC.** Twelve percent of patients who had been treated for SCC of the UADT will, over time, develop a new primary carcinoma. Forty percent will occur within the first year [3]. The period at risk is 5–10 years. The risk is lessened if the patient ceases tobacco and alcohol use but does not return to the control population risk for 16 years [2]. Two thirds of the second primary carcinomas will be within the region of the aerodigestive tract; one third will be at remote sites such as colon or bladder.

II. Secondary prevention

A. Early detection. The detection of high-risk patients afforts the opportunity to counsel the patient. Periodic screening by the patient, as well as the examiner, will identify premalignant (leukoplakia, erythroplasia) as well as carcinomatous lesions. Early identification of premalignant of small (T-1) [1] lesions will improve survival as well as decrease posttherapeutic morbidity.

1. Methods

a. History

(1) Routine questioning regarding risk factors should be included in one's questionnaire or interview, allowing population, age, geography, social, and industrial factors to identify individuals who are at risk.

(2) The at-risk population should be questioned regarding specifics, such as the types and duration of exposures, that is, pack-years of smoking, average daily alcohol consumption, and occupation. These facts need to be documented not only for the current period but also for the prior 15 years for use in follow-up.

(3) Specific symptoms that may be related to SCC of the MOP include rough, sore, or irritated areas; bleeding; nonhealing ulcers or sores; and poorly fitting dentures.

b. Physical examination. Although the head and neck exam is included in all routine physical examinations, at-risk individuals require a more intense and thorough examination. This serves not only to identify individual variation and to document areas of suspicion but to psychologically reinforce the importance of counseling regarding risk factors and toxic exposures.

(1) Inspection. Inspection of the lips, mouth, and throat requires only a light, a tongue blade, and an organized attention to all of the regions within the anatomic area.

(2) Palpation. Visualization is directly supplemented by palpation of the head and neck. Palpation identifies the important qualities of suppleness of the tissues, tenderness, integrity of the mucosa (easy bleeding, friability), and induration. Bimanual palpation is the only way to accurately identify these qualities as well as the size and location of lymph nodes, the usual site of early metastases.

c. Performance

(1) History. The use of a printed questionnaire versus a direct interview technique depends on the examiner's skills and the time available for person-to-person contact. A succinct questionnaire has the advantage of avoiding omission, as well as possibly lowering the cost of the screening method by decreasing direct labor cost.

(2) Examination. Performing a thorough examination of the MOP is essential [4]:

(a) Careful, detailed, and organized normal examinations will educate the finger and the eye to the benign normal findings, as well as benign normal variants. Examples of such findings include prominent circumvallate papillae, fissured tongue, geographic tongue, and mandibular or palatal tori.

(b) The examination should be performed in the same sequence each time, thus training the examiner to carefully assess each area.

(c) A suggested sequence is as follows: lips, buccal mucosa, gingiva (buccal, lingual), teeth, floor of mouth (the examiner will have to make a special effort to see the posterior-most region where the tongue obscures the junction of the floor of the mouth, posterior mandible, anterior pillar, and lateral tongue), palate, tonsils, and oropharynx.

(d) Using a gloved hand, one or two fingers are placed into the mouth, and the tissues are individually palpated. The cheeks and floor of the mouth are then felt in a "bimanual" fashion by simultaneously feeling the tissues between the intraoral fingers with the other hand placed on the overlying skin.

(e) The neck is then palpated, again using two hands to allow the examiner to feel the integumentary tissue between the major structures, the larynx, sternomastoid muscle, carotid sheath, cervical spine, and trapezius muscle. Abnormal findings of unusual tenderness, decreased mobility, or of mass lesion should be noted.

d. Documentation is of the utmost importance not only for medicolegal reasons but particularly for longitudinal follow-up as well as for observation of response to counseling or therapy.

(1) Line drawings are easy to do and require no specialized technique or equipment. The prime requirements are accurate location and accurate measurement of size. Both the apparent size and the palpated size or surrounding induration should be recorded. A verbal description of color and texture is also helpful.

(2) Commercially prepared diagrams of the head and neck and contained structures are available, if desired.

(3) Photography is helpful, but the expense of the equipment requires justification. If photography is used, a back-up drawing is helpful if the photos do not develop clearly.

e. Interpretation

(1) History identifies those individuals in whom initial screening is appropriate and suggests those in whom regular interval follow-up examinations are appropriate.

(2) Physical examination data determine the assessment of the overall health of the mucosa of the MOP. Irritation, tenderness, excessive gagging, or erythema are usually present in all or in part in the patient with heavy tobacco and alcohol use. These findings stress the need for counseling and follow-up, although tumors may occur in patients without these findings. The following physical findings are especially important:

(a) Premalignant lesions. Leukoplakia is a white, raised, nontender lesion of mucosa. The more dangerous, dysplastic leukoplakia may be ulcerated before becoming carcinoma in situ. Erythroplasia of the otal mucosa is usually a circumscribed area of erythema, which may be tender or friable and may be indistinguishable from carcinoma in situ by physical examination alone.

(b) Malignant lesions may be any size or location. They may or may not be tender or painful. Pain usually indicates deep involvement of nerves or periosteum, frequently with fixation of the tissue to an underlying structure. They may be superficial or have surrounding induration. The surface, however, is usually quite different in appearance from surrounding mucosa and frequently is friable. The examiner may have to wipe the surface with gauze to appreciate these changes.

(c) Lymphadenopathy. SCC metastasizes initially to regional lymph nodes. In some instances, the metastasis may be more apparent than the primary lesion. Knowledge of the lymphatic drainage of the head and neck is requisite to analyze the meaning of an enlarged lymph node. A neck mass requires explanation [5].

f. Interval evaluations. When to initiate care and how frequently one follows the patient at risk is a matter of judgment based on the risk profile developed during the initial encounter. The patient should be educated as to self-examination and should be advised to report all changes in his or her symptoms or examination immediately.

(1) Monthly reexaminations may be indicated for a 2- to 3-month period if inflammation or local trauma is suspected or if the examiner treats the suspected cause and reexamines the patient to determine response.

(2) Three-month follow-up may be appropriate for patients with identified premalignant lesions, in conjunction with appropriate therapy.

(3) Twelve-month follow-up may be appropriate in patients with identified risk factors but normal examinations.

2. Justification. Screening for SCC of the MOP is a low-cost, low-risk procedure utilizing the basic techniques of history-taking and physical examination. With the skill developed through directed and purposeful examination technique, prebiopsy diagnoses can be made with a high degree of accuracy. The reliability of the examination and, therefore, the cost per patient, is directly related to the skill of the examiner.

B. Early intervention

1. Methods

a. Counseling. High-risk patients must be made aware of the need to modify their habits, as well as the probable sequelae of failure to make such modifications.

(1) If the patient stops tobacco and alcohol use, the mucosa often gradually returns to normal and nondysplastic leukoplakia usually disappears.

(2) The decision to remove or observe leukoplakia depends on the pathologic description, location, extensiveness, and response to removal of irritant effects of tobacco or alcohol.

(3) Continued tobacco and alcohol abuse may result in frank malignant degeneration. A patient who continues to use tobacco after the treatment of SCC of the MOP stands a tenfold greater probability of developing a second primary than a similar patient who stops smoking.

b. Biopsy defines the nature of the lesion in question and determines the steps in management. The biopsy technique itself may influence the management techniques, as well as survival (5-year survival rate).

(1) Prior to biopsy, **document** size, location, surrounding induration, and regional lymph node enlargement.

(2) Incisional and excisional techniques depend on the size and location of the lesion.

(3) Fine-needle aspiration biopsy should be directly applied for suspicious neck or thyroid masses.

c. Consultation

(1) For completion of the screening exam. Any at-risk patient who has suspicious findings in the oropharynx or who has symptoms must have a complete otolaryngologic examination.

(2) For confirmation of the clinical diagnosis. If in doubt regarding the significance of your findings, obtain consultation.

(3) For biopsy. The biopsy is best performed by an individual who will continue to be intimately involved in the therapeutic decisionmaking and long-term follow-up.

2. Justification

a. Effectiveness

(1) Through **identification** of the risk factors, populations needing interventional counseling can be identified and the patient informed. This applies to all ages but especially to the younger patient in whom the risk can be significantly reduced.

(2) Premalignant lesions can be identified and treated with minimum morbidity and high probability of cure.

(3) Malignant lesions. Only through early identification and biopsy can small lesions be identified and treated. Curative treatment of small lesions can be implemented with either radiation or surgery alone, often decreasing the morbidity of combined therapy with a high probability of cure. The cure rates for small MOP lesions (< 2 cm) of the UADT should be 90% or greater, depending on location and degree of differentiation.

b. Risks and side effects

(1) Incisional and excisional biopsy should have minimal morbidity. The greatest risk is of inaccurately staging the lesion. Since staging is the primary factor in determining treatment, this may affect the survival rate if the lesion is understaged.

(2) Fine-needle aspiration biopsy is a highly reliable method for diagnosis of subcutaneous masses. The results are reproducible. The chance of seeding either benign or malignant tumors is exceedingly low, especially compared to older methods of needle biopsy or incisional/excisional biopsy of suspicious masses.

c. Costs

(1) Labor cost for the initial screening should be minimal, especially if included in a routine health examination.

(2) Procedures in Northern California in 1988:

(a) Otolaryngologic examination: $45–65.

(b) Office biopsy: $55–95.

(c) Pathologic interpretation: $80–150.
(d) Fine-needle aspiration: $150.

d. **Acceptability.** Most procedures can be performed under local anesthetic in an office setting.

III. Recommendations

A. Early detection

1. Patients at risk must be identified using history and physical exam and evaluated accordingly.
2. Cancer suspects should be triaged as to the probability of:
   a. Suspicious benign.
   b. Premalignant.
   c. Suspicious malignant.

B. Early intervention

1. Based on triage, patient management and follow-up is determined.
   a. **Suspicious benign.** Treatment of suspected cause; biopsy if the lesion does not resolve.
   b. **Premalignant.** Biopsy, removal of irritant factor.
   c. **Suspicious malignant.** Biopsy.
2. Consultation and/or biopsy is indicated based on:
   a. Degree of risk determined by data analysis.
   b. Probability of premalignant or suspicious malignant category.
   c. Need to complete the head and neck examination:
      (1) Nasopharyngoscopy.
      (2) Indirect laryngoscopy.
      (3) Fiberoptic examination.
   d. Need for second opinion.
   e. Need to evaluate a cervical mass.
   f. Consideration for ancillary studies. A complete and thorough head and neck examination (otolaryngologic, ear, nose, and throat examination) should be accomplished prior to serious consideration of other ancillary diagnostic techniques such as computerized tomography (CT scanning) or magnetic resonance imaging (MRI), if at all possible. The indications and implications of these studies are beyond the scope of this text.

References

1. American Joint Committee on Cancer. *Staging of Cancer of Head and Neck Sites and of Melanoma, 1980.* Chicago: American Joint Committee on Cancer, 1980. *Available without charge on request at 55 East Erie Street, Chicago, IL.*
2. Fielding, J. E. Smoking: Health effects and control (1) *N. Engl. J. Med.* 313(8):491, 1985. *Excellent summary review of health-related effects of tobacco use. This data must be reviewed by health professionals.*
3. Vrabec, D. P. Multiple primary malignancies of the upper aerodigestive system. *Ann. Otol. Rhinol. Laryngol.* 88(Part 1):846, 1979. *Excellent review of problem of multiple malignancies in patients having demonstrated tobacco-use associated cancer. Paper based on personal review of 1500 cases.*
4. Montgomery, W. W. *Surgery of the Upper Respiratory System.* Philadelphia: Lea & Febiger, 1971. *Photographs and text clearly outline the topical anatomy and examination techniques pertinent to the head and neck region.*
5. Jacques, D. A. Management of Metastatic Nodes in the Neck from an Unknown Primary. In M. M. Paparella and D. A. Shumrick (eds.), *Otolaryngology.* Philadelphia: Saunders, 1980. Pp.2298–3003. *Basic otolaryngology text, detailed and referenced to give primary care as well as specialty care practitioners sound information pertaining to otolaryngology.*

85 Thyroid Cancer

Lindy Kumagai

I. The problem

A. Description. Although benign thyroid nodules are very common, clinically detectable thyroid cancer is relatively rare. Therefore, the problem of managing thyroid nodules is important so that the majority of patients with nodules will not be subjected to unnecessary surgery. Thyroid carcinoma consists of a group of tumors ranging from well-differentiated, slowly growing neoplasms (which ordinarily have an excellent prognosis) to the poorly differentiated, rapidly growing anaplastic type (which are associated with a very poor outcome). The well-differentiated types, papillary and follicular, constitute the large majority (approximately 80%) and occur at any age with peak incidences between the third and fifth decades. However, because of their natural prolonged history, mortality due to the carcinoma is very uncommon under the age of 40, even in the presence of distant metastases. The major determinants regarding prognosis are age of the patient, tumor size (< 1.5 cm is benign), and the presence or absence of distant metastases or invasiveness. The natural history of both papillary and follicular carcinomas related to survivorship, when patients are compared to normals of comparable age and sex, have demonstrated that survival is the same as normals if the cancers are intrathyroidal or noninvasive at the time of operation [1]. However, when distant metastases or invasiveness are found at the initial time of diagnosis, survivorship is significantly decreased. After 10–15 years, approximately 50% of patients with papillary carcinomas with distant metastases, and 20–25% of invasive follicular carcinomas, continue to survive. Medullary carcinoma, which constitutes approximately 5% or less of thyroid cancers, tends to follow a course similar to follicular carcinoma. On the other hand, anaplastic or undifferentiated carcinoma, which is rare under the age of 40 and comprises approximately 10% of all thyroid cancers, follows a very rapid downhill course and survival beyond 1–2 years after operation is extremely rare [2]. Therefore, although the large majority of thyroid cancers are well differentiated and follow a very prolonged course, early detection and treatment are important.

The etiology and pathogenesis of thyroid cancer is not clearly understood. In animal models, chronic thyroid-stimulating hormone (TSH) stimulation produced by partial thyroidectomy, thyroid radiation, iodine deficiency, and chronic antithyroid drug administration caused tumor development. In humans, the only known cause of thyroid cancer is ionizing irradiation. Irradiation of the head and neck regions during childhood was related to thyroid cancers in children, as reported by Duffy and Fitzgerald in 1950 [3] and Clark in 1955 [4]. In the 1970s, it was clearly recognized that irradiation in childhood could predispose to cancer development in adults occurring 20 years or later [5–11]. The large majority of irradiation-associated cancers have been papillary or mixed papillary-follicular.

B. Epidemiology. The incidence of clinically palpable nodules (> 1 cm) varies with a number of factors, for example, age, sex, dietary iodine, and geographic areas. The incidence of a palpable thyroid nodule (or nodules) and subsequent follow-up of a large, middle-aged adult population (35–59 years) in Framingham, Massachusetts, was reported to be 4%, with one half of the subjects having solitary nodules and the other half having multinodular glands. New nodules appeared with an incidence of 0.1%/year [8]. Although thyroid nodules are quite common, thyroid cancer is very uncommon. The incidence of thyroid cancer was reported to be 3.7/100,000 in the Third National Cancer Survey in 1969–1971 [9], which was slightly increased over the Second National Cancer Survey (2.9/100,000), and was attributed to the occurrence of radiation-associated neoplasms [10]. The incidence of thyroid cancer in patients exposed to irradiation is at least 7%. The annual death rate from thyroid cancer is about 0.9/100,000, or about 0.3% of all cancer deaths.

II. Secondary prevention

A. Early detection

1. Methods

a. Palpation. Inspection and palpation of the thyroid and neck are performed and provide useful information. The presence of a scar might indicate previous surgery; identification of a nodule or goiter from surrounding structures may be observed during the act of swallowing. Since deglutition is very important in examining the thyroid, water should be made available to the patient. In addition to observing possible enlargement, abnormal fixation should be noted. Palpation will confirm and amplify the findings of inspection. It can be performed by either facing the patient or standing behind the patient and palpating the neck. Relaxation of the sternocleidomastoid muscle is essential; and, if the gland is low lying (partially substernal), as is frequently the case in the elderly, slight hyperextension of the neck may be helpful. Preliminary palpation with the fingertips will indicate the gland's size, contour, symmetry, consistency, and tenderness. Since the lobes may normally be asymmetric or located differently, the cricoid cartilage and isthmus, which is always found within 1 cm below the cricoid, are used as landmarks. Normally, the lobes are barely palpable: their total weight is approximately 15–20 gm. With deglutition, the majority can be palpated. Therefore, the presence of nodules of 0.5–1.0 cm or larger is usually detectable. As alluded to earlier, clinically significant carcinomas are usually greater than 1.5 cm. After preliminary palpation, minimal medially directed pressure on one lobe with the fingertips will force the contralateral lobe outward slightly so that it can be readily palpated. Each lobe can then be carefully palpated separately. Most carcinomas are firm and not hard as is often thought and are quite discrete. If a nodule or goiter is palpated, attempts should be made to measure or quantitate the size during the initial and follow-up exams. After the lobes are defined, pre- and paratracheal areas should be palpated for lymph nodes, because thyroid cancer spreads beyond the gland to adjacent lymph nodes, as well as elsewhere. Occasionally, if a substernal goiter is suspected, percussion over the upper sternum may reveal a widened area of dullness. In hyperthyroid patients, auscultation over the lobes, especially the superior portions, may reveal a thyroidal bruit.

b. Risk assessment. Because of the poor predictive value of palpation, health care providers should, through clinical features and further tests, select out a high-risk group before referring them. Several clinical features should raise the suspicion of carcinoma: nodules in children or young adults, especially males, are associated with a higher incidence of malignancy; recent occurrence of the nodule (within weeks to a few months); the history of head or neck irradiation, especially during childhood; the history of dysphagia or dysphonia; recent onset of persistent pain; and family history of thyroid malignancies or multiple endocrine adenomata. Certain physical findings are important: a solitary nodule that is especially firm or hard and discrete; fixation of the nodule to strap muscles or trachea; or a nodule associated with pretracheal or paratracheal lymphadenopathy or with dysphagia or hoarseness.

2. Justification. There are no studies on the sensitivity of palpation. However, thyroid cancer grows so slowly that periodic palpation has a very good chance of picking up significant lesions. On the other hand, the majority of nodules detected will not prove to be malignant. The likelihood that a palpable solitary nodule is malignant is about 10%.

Screening for thyroid cancer by palpation of the neck does not fully meet all the criteria for periodic screening but can be justified if done when patients are being seen for other reasons. Thyroid palpation is quick, easy, acceptable, reasonably accurate, and inexpensive if done while patients are already in the health care setting.

B. Further evaluation

1. Methods. The judicious use of a combination of clinical features and improved technical procedures, including thyroid imaging, ultrasonography, and needle biopsies, has improved selectivity of patients, resulting in 50% malignancy in surgically removed thyroid nodules [11]. A rational approach to selecting patients for operation in whom a palpable nodule is found is as follows: in a euthyroid patient with a past history of head or neck irradiation and the presence of a clinically palpable thyroid nodule, surgery should be recommended without further diagnostic testing. The same would also be the case if there is clinical evidence of fixation of the nodule to adjacent tissues. In ruling out a history of irradiation, it is advisable to have patients check with their parents or older siblings, if possible, because irradiation may have occurred during infancy or young childhood. In all of the patients with thyroid nodules, unless multiple and of very long standing without change, the following procedures may be used:

a. **Thyroid imaging** (approximate cost $190). Thyroid scanning is of relatively little discriminating value in the diagnosis of thyroid cancer, even though the large majority of cancers are associated with "cold" areas [5, 12]. Most cold or hypofunctional areas (about 80%) are benign nodules. The main diagnostic value is in identifying the "hot" or autonomously functioning nodule, which is rarely malignant. When performed, it should be done with ^{99}mTc pertechnetate or ^{123}I (preferred by the author), which delivers much less irradiation to the gland than ^{131}I. If the nodule is relatively small (< 1.5 cm), oblique views should be obtained in addition to the anterior views, so that the actual functional capacity of the nodule itself can be accurately ascertained.
b. **Thyroid ultrasonography** (cost $150). Echo-imaging using ultrasound can usually resolve lesions that are 1.5 cm or greater and can ascertain whether they are cystic, solid, or mixed. About 15–20% of all solitary nodules are cystic and are rarely malignant [13], and will appear as "cold" areas on scintiscan. Of the solid lesions, the majority are benign, and thyroid cancers constitute about 20% [14]. If needle aspirations or biopsies are routinely used, the echogram is probably unnecessary.
c. **Thyroid needle biopsy** (fine-needle aspiration [FNA] costs $190). Large needle biopsy has not been extensively used in the United States because of the potential complications in utilizing a large-bore, cutting needle for adequate tissue sample. Wang has reported a correct interpretation of 85–90% of biopsy specimens with about 5% false-positive or false-negative readings [15]. More recently, FNA is being utilized and is reported to be essentially free of complications and to have an accuracy of approximately 90% [16]. There is virtually no information on false-negatives because of the lack of long follow-up studies of unoperated cases. The major diagnostic problem with the FNAs are follicular lesions because of the inability to reliably distinguish follicular adenoma from carcinoma, so any regions with a follicular pattern should be considered suspicious. The most limiting aspect of the FNA technique is variability of expertise in reading thyroid cytologic smears.
d. **Diagnostic hormonal therapy.** If the nodule is considered to be functioning normally on scan or reported to be benign cytologically, thyroid suppression with exogenous thyroxin administration may be used. Approximately 65% of benign nodules will decrease significantly; however, this should not be considered absolute because, occasionally, malignant nodules may initially shrink on thyroid therapy [10]. The usual suppressive doses of thyroxine are about 0.2–0.25 mg/day; however, subsequent serum TSHs should be followed occasionally to ascertain adequate suppression. If there is no change after 6 months of T_4 suppression, a repeat FNA can be performed. If growth occurs, however, at any time while on suppression, surgery should be performed.
e. **Blood tests.** Thyroid cancer is not associated with altered thyroid status, so in the initial examination in patients with a thyroid nodule, blood tests (T_4, T_3-U, free T_4 indices [$25], and TSH [$40]) are usually not necessary unless there is clinical evidence of hyperthyroidism or hypothyroidism or reason to suspect the possibility of medullary carcinoma, in which event a serum calcitonin level may be helpful. Despite the fact that thyroglobulin (Tg) levels are increased in most patients with thyroid carcinoma, they are not recommended in the preoperative identification of thyroid malignancies because they may be elevated in a variety of thyroid disorders, including Graves' disease, thyroiditis, and others [17]. The same is true of thyroid antibodies.

2. **Justification.** Thyroid cancer can be easily diagnosed in the majority of cases during the long asymptomatic phase.

C. Early intervention

1. **Methods.** The extent of surgery in the management of thyroid carcinoma remains highly controversial; however, there is general agreement that radical neck surgery is rarely necessary. At the time of surgery, if the frozen section is papillary carcinoma and the tumor is less than 1.5 cm and without evidence of enlarged adjacent lymph nodes, lobectomy and isthmusectomy are sufficient in most instances. In

the case of follicular cancer (with capsular or blood vessel invasion), a near total thyroidectomy followed by ^{131}I therapy is recommended. In both instances, patients should be placed on thyroid hormone suppression following surgery.

2. **Justification.** Treatment during the asymptomatic period is effective and more simple than subsequently, when symptoms appear. In experienced hands, the major risks of thyroid surgery—for example, vocal card paralysis and hypoparathyroidism—are less than 1% if only lobectomy and isthmusectomy are performed. Even if a near total thyroidectomy is done, the risks remain small, so early intervention is justified. The total costs for hospitalization and fees would be approximately $6,000–8,000.

IV. Recommendations

A. Early detection

1. Palpation of the neck for thyroid nodules is not routinely indicated as a stand-alone periodic health exam test in the absence of risk factors.
2. However, if individuals have risk factors or are being seen in a medical setting anyway, palpation of the neck for thyroid nodules is indicated.

B. Evaluation. Patients with nodules and no history of head or neck irradiation or evidence of fixation to surrounding tissues should be evaluated using the modalities described in the text.

C. Early intervention

1. Patients with nodules and a history of head or neck irradiation, or evidence of fixation to surrounding tissues, should be sent to surgery.
2. Assuming that expert cytopathology is available, all patients in whom carcinoma is identified by fine-needle aspiration biopsy (FNAB) should have surgery. In most instances, if the dominant pattern is follicular, the lesion should be regarded as suspicious and the patient should be referred to surgery.

References

1. Woolner, L. B., et al. Thyroid carcinoma: General Consideration and Follow-up Data in 1181 Cases. In S. Young and D. R. Inman (eds.), *Thyroid Neoplasia*. London: Academic, 1968. Pp. 51–79. *Excellent review and long-term follow-up; a real classic.*
2. Werner, S. C. Medical (Suppressive) Surgical Therapy of the Thyroid Nodule; The Problem of Radiation Exposure of the Thyroid in Youth. In S. C. Werner and S. H. Ingbar (eds.), *The Thyroid* (4th ed.). Hagerstown, MD: Harper & Row, 1978. Pp. 573–583. *A very good, concise review of medical versus surgical management.*
3. Duffy, B. J. Jr, and Fitzgerald, P. J. Thyroid in children and adolescence: Report of 28 cases. *J. Clin. Endocrinol.* 10:1296, 1950.
4. Clark, D. E. Association of irradiation with cancer of the thyroid in children and adolescents. *J.A.M.A.* 159:1007, 1955.
5. DeGroot, L. J. Thyroid Neoplasia. In L. J. DeGroot, et al. (eds.), *Endocrinology*. New York: Grune & Stratton, 1979. Pp. 509–521. *Excellent, concise review.*
6. Favus, M. J., et al. Thyroid cancer occurring as a late consequence of head-and-neck irradiation. Evaluation of 1056 patients. *N. Engl. J. Med.* 294(19):1019, 1976.
7. Hempelmann, L. H., et al. Neoplasms in persons treated with X-rays in infancy: Fourth survey in 20 years. *J. Natl. Cancer Inst.* 55(3):519, 1975. *Survey of neoplasms developing in people treated with X-rays as infants.*
8. Vander, J. B., Gaston, E. A., and Dawber, T. R. The significance of nontoxic thyroid nodules. Final report of a 15-year study of the incidence of thyroid malignancy. *Ann. Intern Med.* 69:537, 1968. *Excellent study of the incidence in a large population with long-term follow-up.*
9. Cutler, S. J., and Young, J. L. (eds.) *Third National Cancer Survey: Incidence Data.* Bethesda, MD: National Cancer Institute, 1975. P. 25.
10. Mazzaferri, E. L. Papillary and follicular thyroid cancer: A selective approach to diagnosis and treatment. *Annu. Rev. Med.* 32:73, 1981. *Excellent review of papillary and follicular cancer in diagnosis and treatment.*
11. Blum, M., Rothschild, N. Improved nonoperative diagnosis of the solitary "cold" thyroid nodule. Surgical selection based on risk factors and three months of suppression. *J.A.M.A.* 243(3):242, 1980.
12. Mazzaferri, E. L., et al. Papillary thyroid carcinoma: The impact of therapy in 576 patients. *Medicine* 56(3):171, 1977. *Excellent review of therapy and the course of the disease.*

13. Clark, O.H., et al. Diagnosis and treatment of thyroid, parathyroid and thyroglossal duct cyst. *J. Clin. Endocrinol. Metab.* 48(6):983, 1979. *Excellent article regarding various cysts.*
14. Miskin, M., Rosen, I. B., and Walfish, P. G. B-mode ultrasonography in the assessment of thyroid gland lesions. *Ann. Intern. Med.* 79(4):505, 1973. *Use of ultrasound in evaluation of thyroid nodules.*
15. Wang, C. A., and Vickery, A. L. The role of needle biopsy in evaluating solitary cold thyroid nodules. *International Congress Series* (361):43, 1975. *Use of needle biopsy in assessment of cold nodules.*
16. Lowhagen, T., et al. Aspiration biopsy cytology (ABC) in nodules of the thyroid gland suspected to be malignant. *Surg. Clin. North Am.* 59(1):3, 1979. *Excellent article regarding fine needle aspiration biopsies.*
17. Ashcraft, M. W., and Van Herle, A. J. The comparative value of serum thyroglobulin measurements and iodine. 131 total body scans in the follow-up study of patients with treated differentiated thyroid cancer. *Am. J. Med.* 71(5):806, 1981. *Excellent review of the status of serum Tg and thyroid cancer.*

86 Skin Cancer

Elizabeth Kubiak

I. The problem

A. Nonmelanoma skin cancer

1. **Definition.** The spectrum of nonmelanoma skin cancers includes precancerous lesions (actinic keratoses), in-situ carcinomas (Bowen's disease), and the most common forms of skin cancer (basal cell epitheliomas and squamous cell carcinomas).
2. **Description.** Nonmelanoma skin cancers may appear as persistent, scaling, nodular, or ulcerated lesions, and they are found primarily on sun-exposed skin. The greatest single factor responsible for the development of nonmelanoma skin cancers is ultraviolet (UV) light, suggested both by the inverse relationship between the incidence of skin cancers and geographic latitude and by the predilection that these malignancies have for sun-exposed skin. Within the United States, there is a 15% increase in the incidence of skin cancers among Caucasians for each degree of latitude south [1]. Experimentally, ultraviolet light has both induced and promoted tumor formation [2]. Nonmelanoma skin cancers have a tendency to gradually enlarge and remain localized. However, squamous cell carcinomas, especially those found on mucous membranes, the lips, and covered portions of the body, are more likely to metastasize.
3. **Epidemiology.** The current estaimated incidence of nonmelanoma cutaneous malignancies is greater than 400,000 new cases per year, accounting for approximately one third of all malignancies [3]. Basal cell epitheliomas represent roughly 85% of these cases. The estimated mortality for skin cancers in 1986, exclusive of malignant melanoma, is 1900, or 0 4% of all cancer deaths [3].

   The primary risk factor is ultraviolet light, which causes cumulative damage to the skin. This encompasses both natural sunlight and artificial UV light. Both the shorter wavelengths (UVB) and the longer wavelengths (UVA—commonly used in tanning booths) are responsible for tumor formation. Individuals with a history of extensive, unprotected sun exposure and those who burn easily and tan poorly are most prone to develop premalignant and malignant skin lesions. In addition, patients on long-term immunosuppressive therapy are more susceptible to sun-induced skin cancers.

   Another risk factor is exposure to certain chemicals, primarily arsenic and polycyclic aromatic hydrocarbons. Inhalation or ingestion of trivalent inorganic arsenic predisposes an individual to develop Bowen's disease, squamous cell carcinomas, and basal cell epitheliomas after a lag period of 20 or more years. Inorganic arsenic exposure may have occurred secondary to medical therapy in the form of Fowler's solution, Donovan's solution, or Asiatic pills; these treatments were employed in times past for psoriasis, nervous disorders, and asthma [4]. Furthermore, arsenic exposure is incurred by persons smelting copper and lead in the metallurgic industry and by those involved in the manufacture and use of certain insecticides and fungicides [4,5]. Finally, well water in some regions contains high concentrations of arsenic, placing users of such water at risk for nonmelanoma skin cancer [4].

   Polycyclic aromatic hydrocarbon exposure may occur in tar distilling and coal gas manufacturing and in those occupations involving the fractionation and distillation of oil products or the use of creosote [5,6].

   Ionizing radiation is another known risk factor for the development of cutaneous malignancies. There is usually a lag period of 25–30 years between exposure and the appearance of skin cancer.

B. Malignant melanoma

1. **Description.** Primary malignant melanoma can develop de novo or within a preexisting mole. Clinically, it can be distinguished by one or more of the following features: asymmetry, irregular or notched borders, variegate coloration, diameter

greater than 6 mm, and ulceration. The diagnosis of malignant melanoma should be considered if an existing mole changes or becomes symptomatic or if a new pigmented lesion develops after the age of 40.

The exact etiology of melanoma remains uncertain, but sunlight has been strongly implicated as a significant factor for several reasons [2,7]. In general, an inverse relationship exists between the incidence of melanoma and geographic latitude. For example, within the continental United States there is a significantly higher incidence of melanoma in the southern states as compared with the northern states [8]. The risk of developing melanoma is also directly proportional to the duration of time spent in a sunny climate [8]. Typically, those individuals with fair skin, blonde-to-reddish hair, blue eyes, and poor tanning capability are at greater risk for developing melanoma. Recently, it has been found that individuals with a history of painful, blistering sunburns in childhood have a higher incidence of melanoma [9]. Moreover, blacks, due to their natural photoprotection, have a much lower incidence of melanoma than do Caucasians.

2. **Epidemiology.** The incidence of malignant melanoma has been rising dramatically in the United States and throughout the world. In the past 50 years, there has been a 600% increase in its incidence in the United States—a rate of progression exceeded only by lung cancer [10]. If the current trend continues, the estimated incidence of melanoma in this country will double every 10–15 years [7]. In 1986, it was estimated that there would be 23,000 new cases of malignant melanoma in this country [3]. It accounts for 2–3% of all malignancies, excluding nonmelanoma skin cancers [3].

   The mortality rate for malignant melanoma is also increasing throughout the world by approximately 3%/year [1]. In the United States, the mortality rate has doubled over the past 30 years [7]. The projected mortality rate for malignant melanoma in the United States for 1986 is 5600, which accounts for approximately 1.2% of all cancer deaths [3]. The prognosis for patients with melanoma is excellent if the lesions are surgically removed when they are still very superficial. Survival rates diminish with increasing thickness of the tumor, hence the importance of recognizing and removing these lesions at an early stage.

   Risk factors for the development of melanoma include the following:

   a. Poor tanning capability
   b. A history of painful sunburns in childhood
   c. Indoor occupation combined with outdoor recreational habits
   d. Dysplastic nevi
   e. Congenital nevi
   f. Past history of melanoma

II. **Primary prevention.** By including the skin as part of the routine physical exam and by learning to identify those individuals who are at particular risk for the development of skin cancer, the primary care physician can select those individuals in whom it is most critical to use sunscreens and to avoid excessive sun exposure.

A. **Methods**

1. **Sun protection**

   a. **Clothing.** Advise the use of protective clothing such as hats, long-sleeved shirts, and long pants. Bear in mind that loose-weave fabrics do not adequately protect the skin.

   b. **Sunscreens.** The use of a sunscreen, preferably one with a sun protective factor (SPF) of 15 or more, should be recommended. There are two principal varieties: physical sunscreens and chemical sunscreens. The physical agents, such as zinc oxide, contain particulate matter that reflects and scatters the ultraviolet radiation as well as visible light. Their chief disadvantage is cosmetic. The chemical sunscreens comprise the majority of products for sun protection currently available. The agents utilized for this purpose are PABA, PABA esters, cinnamates, and benzophenones. By absorbing ultraviolet radiation, these agents effectively screen out the wavelengths primarily responsible for sunburn [11,12,13].

2. **Sun avoidance.** One should minimize sun exposure between the hours of 10 A.M. and 3 P.M., the peak hours of solar intensity.

B. **Justification**

1. **Effectiveness.** Minimizing sun exposure by the above measures is effective in preventing, or at least lessening, the amount of actinic damage to the skin. Research indicates that sunscreens reduce the incidence of tumor formation.

2. **Side effects**

   a. **Allergic reactions** to sunscreens occur most often with PABA, some PABA esters, cinnamates, and benzophenones. Reactions may take the form of contact dermatitis or photo contact dermatitis. In addition, patients who are allergic to sulfonamides and benzocaine may also be allergic to PABA.

b. **Staining of clothing** may develop with PABA after exposure to ultraviolet light.

3. **Cost.** Sunscreens are sold over-the-counter, and the average price is $4–6 per tube or bottle.

4. **Acceptance.** Most patients who are at special risk for developing skin cancer comply with both the use of sunscreens and avoidance of excessive sun exposure.

III. Secondary prevention

A. Early detection

1. Methods: skin inspection

a. **Self-examination.** Each patient should learn to examine his or her own skin and to do so with each change of season—more often if he or she is at high risk for developing a cutaneous malignancy. It is easiest to do this after a bath or shower in a well-lit room. Equipment needed includes a full-length mirror, a hand-held mirror, a chair or stool, and a hand-held hair dryer (to examine the scalp). One should check all portions of the cutaneous surface, including the palms, soles, interdigital areas, groin, and scalp. Each individual should become familiar with his or her existing lesions and should have any new or changing lesions checked by a physician.

b. **Provider exam.** Inspection of the skin is an often neglected portion of the routine physical exam. It is a very simple and quick process that enables the primary care physician to identify patients with cutaneous malignancies and those who are at high risk for developing skin cancer.

For proper inspection of the skin, the patient should be completely undressed and the room should be equipped with good lighting. In addition, the physician must be familiar with the appearance of the more common premalignant and malignant skin lesions. A description of these follows:

(1) **Actinic keratoses** are typically confined to sun-exposed skin. They appear as rough, well-circumscribed lesions that range in color from tan to yellow to red. They are occasionally pigmented.

(2) **Bowen's disease** may be found on either sun-exposed or sun-protected skin. It appears as a chronic scaling erythematous plaque.

(3) **Basal cell epitheliomas** are located most frequently on sun-exposed skin, especially on the head and neck. There are three types of basal cell epitheliomas: noduloulcerative, superficial multicentric, and sclerosing. The noduloulcerative variety is the most prevalent, and it appears as a translucent papule with overlying telangiectases. With progression, a central ulceration may develop. Occasionally this type is pigmented, making it difficult to distinguish from malignant melanoma.

The superficial multicentric basal cell epithelioma is located primarily on the trunk. It appears as a well-defined, erythematous, scaling plaque with a threadlike, pearly border.

The sclerosing form of basal cell epithelioma usually is found on the face and it presents as a yellowish-white depressed area or as a spontaneously appearing scar.

(4) **Squamous cell carcinomas** arise primarily on sun-exposed skin, typically evolving from preexisting actinic keratoses or Bowen's disease. However, they may also develop at sites of previous radiation therapy, chronic trauma, or chronic inflammation, and they may arise de novo.

Squamous cell carcinomas appear as solitary, opaque papules, nodules, or plaques, the surface of which may be verrucous, scaly, or ulcerated. The base is often inflamed.

(5) **Dysplastic nevus syndrome** is characterized by the development of multiple nevi, often greater than 100, found primarily on the trunk and upper extremities. Dysplastic nevi can be distinguished from normal nevi by their larger size, irregular borders, and variegate pigmentation [14,15]. Although most dysplastic nevi are thought to be inherited in an autosomal dominant fashion, sporadic cases have been reported. Since patients with dysplastic nevus syndrome have a greater tendency to develop melanomas, it is imperative that they be identified early and followed closely [16].

(6) **Superficial spreading melanomas** may occur on any cutaneous surface, but they most frequently develop on the trunk, upper extremity, head and neck of males, and on the back, lower leg, upper extremity, and head and

neck of females. They begin as macular lesions that display a variety of colors, including shades of brown, black, blue, red, and white. The borders are usually irregular or notched. As the vertical growth phase ensues, one or more papules or nodules may develop within the lesion, and these, too, may vary in color. Ulceration may be present.

(7) **Nodular melanomas** have no predilection for specific sites. As the name implies, they appear as nodular lesions that exhibit very little, if any, radial growth. Their color varies, ranging from shades of blue to gray/black, brown, or red. A small percentage are amelanotic.

(8) **Lentigo maligna melanomas** are found on sun-exposed skin, most often on the face. They initially appear as slowly enlarging tan/brown macules, which then develop irregular borders and either slight elevations or dark brown to black nodules within them.

(9) **Acral lentiginous melanomas** develop on the palms, soles, terminal phalanges, and mucous membranes. They are the most common form of melanoma in blacks and Asians, although they also occur in a small percentage of Caucasians. These tumors appear as brown or black macules that become nodular as the vertical growth phase evolves. Eventually, ulceration may occur. Subungual melanomas may appear as a dark streak in the nail plate or as a distortion of the nail plate. Subsequent development of pigmentation in the proximal nail fold is a late clue to the diagnosis.

2. Justification

a. Test characteristics. Because most early cutaneous malignancies are asymptomatic, medical attention often is postponed until lesions are advanced. Patients are generally unfamiliar with the appearance of skin cancers and these lesions frequently occur at sites not easily inspected by the patient. Regular self-examination by patients and periodic cutaneous inspection by physicians will allow for the detection and proper treatment of early and hence smaller lesions. This, in turn, should result in decreased morbidity, mortality, and medical expenditures for persons with nonmelanoma skin cancer and those with malignant melanoma.

b. Risks. None are inherent in the exam itself, but false-negatives and false-positives, as well as follow-up tests such as biopsies, have well-known though minor risks.

c. Cost. The cost is that of a routine office visit, or it may be included in the fee charged for a general physical exam.

d. Acceptability. Acceptance by both patients and physicians should be excellent but has not been well studied.

B. Early intervention

1. Methods

a. Liquid nitrogen or topical 5-fluorouracil may be used to treat actinic keratoses.

b. Biopsy. When a cutaneous malignancy is suspected, a biopsy should follow to confirm the diagnosis. Either a shave biopsy or a punch biopsy is adequate in most instances for nonmelanoma skin cancers. However, if a malignant melanoma is suspected, the procedure of choice is an excisional biopsy. Appropriate treatment depends on verification of the diagnosis.

2. Justification

a. Effectiveness. Biopsy and appropriate treatment of nonmelanoma skin cancers results in a cure rate exceeding 92%. Long-term lesions generally are larger and technically more difficult to remove. In addition, the usual low rate of metastasis of nonmelanoma cutaneous malignancies increases with more advanced lesions, and with those developing on mucous membranes and at sites of damage imposed by chronic trauma, ionizing radiation, and burns.

The cure rate for excision of early melanomas is 98%. Those that are not detected at an early stage metastasize more readily and carry a poorer prognosis.

b. Risks. The risks from performing a skin biopsy are those associated with any minor surgical procedure: bleeding, wound infection, and scar formation. The incidence of these side effects is very low.

c. Cost. The total cost for performing a biopsy of a malignant lesion, including the fee for reviewing the histopathology, is approximately $150. Treatment cost depends on the modality chosen.

d. Acceptability. Both patient and provider acceptance has been excellent.

87

Tetanus

Chinh Le and Robert S. Chang

I. The problem

A. Definition. Tetanus is an acute intoxication caused by the fixation in the central nervous system of a neurotoxin (tetanusspasmin) secreted by the anaerobic bacillus, *Clostridium tetani.* It is a deadly disease with a case-fatality ratio of 26–60% [1]. Clinically, it is characterized primarily by painful spasm of the voluntary muscle. Death is usually due to asphyxiation during muscle spasms or complicating infections such as bacterial pneumonias. The toxin is elaborated in wounds contaminated by *C. tetani.* A wound is any injury that causes a skin break. Tetanus can be readily prevented by tetanus immunization.

B. Epidemiology [2]. Tetanus is now rare in the United States; approximately 70–100 cases are reported annually. Seventy percent of the cases are among persons 50 years of age or older, with a 52% case-fatality ratio for patients 60 years of age and older. This preponderance of cases among persons 50 years of age or older may be due to inadequate immunization coverage against tetanus among this segment of the United States population.

An epidemiologic analysis of tetanus cases during 1985–1986 identified an acute injury in over 70% (most frequently puncture wounds and laceration, frostbites, intravenous drug abuse; abortions can also be predisposing factors). About 20% of cases have a chronic wound such as a cutaneous ulcer. Thus, it appears that no wound is too minor to be immune from contamination by the tetanus bacilli.

Indoor injuries accounted for 41% of all tetanus cases associated with acute wounds; and garden- and outdoor-associated injuries for 39%. One must therefore assume that *C. tetani* is a ubiquitous microbe found also in the home environment.

II. Primary prevention

A. Method. Tetanus toxoid, a toxin modified by formaldehyde, is a highly effective immunogen that, after a primary series of immunization, induces protective levels of serum antitoxin lasting for at least 10 years. All persons, except when contraindicated, should have a primary series of tetanus immunization followed by a booster every 10 years after the last dose [3, 4].

Tetanus toxoid is marketed in combination with the following immunogens: (1) diphtheria and tetanus toxoids, and pertussis vaccine adsorbed (DTP); (2) diphtheria and tetanus toxoids adsorbed (for pediatric use) (DT); (3) tetanus and diphtheria toxoids adsorbed (for adult use) (Td); and (4) tetanus toxoid adsorbed (T) (rarely used). DTP and DT are combinations recommended for use during infancy and early childhood. In persons 7 years or older, the recommended vaccine is Td.

Primary immunization against tetanus is generally given during infancy or early childhood (see Chap. 56). In adults who have not received the primary immunization or are uncertain of their immunization histories, a series of three doses of Td should be recommended. The Td should be given intramuscularly, with the second dose 4–8 weeks after the first, and the third dose 6–12 months after the second.

Side effects and adverse reactions of tetanus immunization, mild local reactions, generally erythema and induration with or without tenderness, are common after the administration of DT or Td.

Arthus-type hypersensitivity reactions characterized by severe local reactions (generally starting 2–8 hours after an injection) may occur, particularly in persons who have received multiple prior boosters.

Rarely, severe systemic reactions such as generalized urticaria, anaphylaxis, or neurologic complications have been reported after receiving diphtheria, tetanus, and pertussis antigens. A few cases of peripheral neuropathy have been reported following tetanus toxoid administration, although a causal relationship has not been established.

The only **contraindication** to tetanus and diphtheria toxoids is a history of neurologic or severe hypersensitivity reaction following a previous dose. Local side effects alone

Table 87-1. Summary guide to tetanus prophylaxis in routine wound management, United States, 1985

History of adsorbed tetanus toxoid (doses)	Clean, minor wounds		All other wounds[a]	
	Td[b]	TIG[c]	Td[b]	TIG[c]
Unknown or < 3	Yes	No	Yes	Yes
≥ 3[d]	No[e]	No	No[f]	No

[a]Such as, but not limited to, wounds contaminated with dirt, feces, soil, saliva, etc.; puncture wounds; avulsions; and wounds resulting from missiles, crushing, burns, and frostbite.
[b]For children under 7 years old, DTP (DT if pertussis vaccine is contraindicated) is preferred to tetanus toxoid alone. For persons 7 years old and older, Td is preferred to tetanus toxoid alone.
[c]Human tetanus immune globulin—250–500 units IM at separated site from Td injection.
[d]If only three doses of *fluid* toxoid have been received, a fourth dose of toxoid, preferably an adsorbed toxoid, should be given.
[e]Yes, if more than 10 years since last dose.
[f]Yes, if more than 5 years since last dose. (More frequent boosters are not needed and can accentuate side effects.)
Source: Immunization Practices Advisory Committee. Diphtheria, tetanus, and pertussis: Guidelines for vaccine prophylaxis and other preventive measures. *M. M. W. R.* 34(27):405, 1985.

do not preclude continued use. If a systemic reaction is suspected to represent allergic hypersensitivity, appropriate skin testing or measurement of antitoxin antibody level may be useful before discontinuing tetanus toxoid immunization altogether. This would be helpful in documenting immediate hypersensitivity, although mild, nonspecific skin-test reactivity to tetanus toxoid appears to be fairly common. Most individuals who have been vaccinated develop cutaneous delayed hypersensitivity to the toxoid.

Major **local reactions** generally beginining 2–8 hours after injection have been reported in some adults, particularly those who have received frequent (e.g., annual) doses of tetanus toxoid. Persons experiencing these severe reactions usually have very high serum tetanus antitoxin levels. They should not be given further routine or emergency booster doses of Td more frequently than every 10 years.

B. Justification. Ninety-five percent of tetanus patients had not received a full 3-dose primary series of tetanus toxoid. Serosurveys done since 1977 indicated that from 49–66% of persons 60 years of age or older lacked protective levels of circulating antitoxin antibody against tetanus. Although tetanus toxoid is one of the most effective immunizing agents, it does not provide absolute protection. The failure rate is, however, exceedingly small (estimated at 3.8 cases of tetanus/10^8 immunized persons/year).

III. Recommendations [3–5]

A. All persons should have adequate immunity against tetanus. Adequate immunity is achieved by a primary series of immunization using a vaccine that contains tetanus toxoid and is maintained by a booster dose once every 10 years therafter. An adult who has not received the primary immunization or who is unsure of his or her immunization history should receive without delay a series of three doses of tetanus toxoid. The preferred vaccine for adults is Td. Td should be injected intramuscularly with the second dose 4–8 weeks after the first, and the third dose 6–12 months after the second.

B. Tetanus prophylaxis in routine wound management. Wound cleaning and debridement, when indicated, are important. Table 87-1 provides a summary guide for the use of Td and TIG.

C. Use of Td is not contraindicated in pregnancy. Unimmunized or incompletely immunized pregnant women should receive appropriate Td doses, preferably starting during the second trimester. This is very important to prevent tetanus neonatorum.

References

1. LaForce, F. M., Young, L. S., and Bennett, J. V. Tetanus in the United States (1965–1966): Epidemiologic and clinical features. *N. Engl. J. Med.* 280:569, 1969. *A classic review of tetanus in the United States.*

2. Tetanus—United States, 1985–1986. *M. M. W. R.* 36(41):477, 1987. *A more recent review of the epidemiology of tetanus in the United States.*
3. Immunization Practices Advisory Committee. Diphtheria, tetanus, and pertussis: Guidelines for vaccine prophylaxis and other preventive measures. *M. M. W. R.* 34(27):405, 1985. *Current Centers for Disease Control recommendations for diphtheria, tetanus, and pertussis immunizations.*
4. Immunization Practices Advisory Committee. Adult immunization. *M. M. W. R.* 33(Suppl 1s):105, 1984. *CDC general guidelines for adult immunizations.*
5. Schofield, F. Selective primary health care: Strategies for control of disease in the developing world XXII. Tetanus: A preventable problem. *Rev. Inf. Dis.* 8:144, 1986. *Excellent article on tetanus control.*

88 Diphtheria

Chinh Le and Robert S. Chang

I. The problem

A. Definition. Toxigenic strains of *Corynebacterium diphtheriae* have the capability of colonizing some parts of the upper respiratory tract or surface wound. In persons not immune to diphtheria, toxins secreted by the bacterium damage tissue at the site of colonization and may also damage organs at distant sites such as the myocardium, peripheral nerves, and kidneys. In persons immune against diphtheria, the bacterial toxin is neutralized by antibodies and tissue damage is prevented. Immunity against diphtheria is acquired through prior infection or immunization. Immunity prevents diphtheria but does not prevent colonization by *C. diphtheriae*.

B. Epidemiology. Diphtheria is now an uncommon disease in the United States. In 1980, there were only three reported cases, two of which were in adults over 40 years old [1]. The case-fatality ratio of diphtheria remains at 5–10%; the ratio is said to be the highest among the very young and the elderly. Among unimmunized household contacts of a diphtheria patient, the secondary attack rate of clinical diphtheria among adults is about 10%.

II. Primary prevention

A. Method. Formaldehyde treatment of diphtheria toxin converts the toxin into toxoid, which is no longer toxic to tissue but retains its immunogenicity. Diphtheria toxoid is generally adsorbed onto aluminum salt to enhance its immunogenicity. Diphtheria toxoid is available in the following combinations:

1. Diphtheria and tetanus toxoids and pertussis vaccine adsorbed (DTP). Recommended for persons 7 years old or younger.
2. Diphtheria and tetanus toxoids adsorbed (DT). DT is also recommended for persons 7 years old or younger in whom pertussis vaccine is contraindicated.
3. Tetanus and diphtheria toxoids adsorbed (Td). Td contains lesser amounts of diphtheria toxoid than DT and is intended for use in persons 7 years old or older ("lesser" means 2 Lf of diphtheria toxoid/dose, compared to 7–25 Lf in DPT). With the reduced amount of diphtheria toxoid, the frequency and severity of local reaction is also reduced, while adequate antibody response is retained.

Side effects and adverse reactions to the above preparations are usually local and mild (erythema and induration with or without tenderness). Fever and other systemic symptoms are much less common following administration of preparations not containing pertussis vaccine. Arthus-type hypersensitivity reactions characterized by severe local reactions (generally starting 2–8 hours after an injection) may occur, particularly in persons who have received multiple prior boosters. Rarely, severe systemic reactions such as generalized urticaria, anaphylaxis, or neurologic complications have been reported after receiving diphtheria, tetanus, and pertussis antigens.

B. Justification. Diphtheria is a severe disease for which the efficacy of chemoprophylaxis has not been established, and the case-fatality ratio is high. Serosurveys in the United States population in the 1970s revealed that 40–80% of adults lacked protective levels of circulating antitoxin against diphtheria. From 1977 through 1982, 56% of the 34 reported cases occurred in adults. Complete and appropriately timed immunization and booster doses are at least 95% effective in preventing diphtheria.

III. Recommendations. All persons, except when contraindicated, should have a primary series of diphtheria immunizations followed by a booster every 10 years after the last dose. Primary immunization is generally given during infancy or early childhood (see Chap. 54). In adults who have not received the primary immunization or who are uncertain of their immunization histories, a series of three doses of Td should be recommended. The Td should be given intramuscularly, with the second dose 4–8 weeks after the first, and the third dose 6–12 months after the second. Pregnancy is not a contraindication to administration of Td, although it is a reasonable precaution to wait until the second trimester.

The only **contraindication** to diphtheria toxoids is a history of neurologic or severe hypersensitivity reaction following a previous dose. Local side effects alone do not preclude continued use. If a systemic reaction is suspected to represent allergic hypersensitivity, appropriate skin testing may be useful before discontinuing diphtheria toxoid immunization altogether. This would be helpful in documenting immediate hypersensitivity, although mild, nonspecific skin test reactivity to diphtheria toxoid appears to be fairly common. Most vaccinated individuals develop cutaneous delayed hypersensitivity to the toxoid. Major local reactions, generally beginning 2–8 hours after injection, have reported in some adults, particularly those who have received frequent (e.g, annual) doses of Td. Persons experiencing these severe reactions usually have very high serum antitoxin levels. They should not be given further routine or emergency booster doses of Td more frequently than every 10 years.

Prophylaxis for household contacts. All household contacts of patients with respiratory diphtheria should promptly receive a dose of diphtheria toxoid-containing preparation appropriate for their age (Td for all adults) and should be examined for 7 days for evidence of diphtheria. Previously unimmunized or inadequately immunized adult contacts should have prompt chemoprophylaxis, such as a single intramuscular dose of 1.2 million units of benzathine penicillin, or a 7-day course of erythromycin orally. In these same persons, the primary series of Td immunization should also be completed according to schedule (i.e., second dose 4–8 weeks after the first, and third dose 6–12 months after the second).

References

1. Immunization Practices Advisory Committee. Diphtheria, tetanus, and pertussis: Guidelines for vaccine prophylaxis and other preventive measures. *M. M. W.R.* 34(27):405, 1985. *Centers for Disease Control recommendations.*

89 Poliomyelitis

Chinh Le and Robert S. Chang

I. The problem

A. Definition [1]. Polioviruses infect primarily the upper respiratory and the intestinal tracts causing mild, transient, febrile illnesses that generally are not recognized clinically. On rare occasions, the virus may invade the meninges and the nervous system, resulting in aseptic meningitis and paralysis. There are three serologic types of polioviruses; for practical purposes, immunity induced by infection or vaccination is type-specific.

B. Epidemiology. Poliovaccines, widely used since 1955, have drastically reduced the incidence of poliomyelitis in the United States; there are now only 5–10 cases reported yearly in the United States [2].

Vaccine-associated poliomyelitis has become the predominant form of poliomyelitis contracted in the United States. From 1973–1984, 274.1 million doses were given, resulting in 104 cases of vaccine-associated poliomyelitis in the United States [2]: 30 were among vaccine recipients, and 41 among contacts of vaccinated individuals. Ninety-two percent of vaccinated persons who developed poliomyelitis were preschool-age children, while 73% of persons who acquired poliomyelitis after contacts with vaccinated individuals were adults. Incidences of vaccine-associated poliomyelitis among vaccinated persons and contacts are estimated at 1/2.64 million doses of vaccine distributed in the United States. Despite the very low incidence, vaccine-associated poliomyelitis has become a major issue in the choice of poliovaccine.

II. Primary prevention

A. Method (the vaccines). Two types of vaccine are currently in use in the United States: oral polio vaccine (OPV) and inactivated polio vaccine (IPV).

1. **OPV** contains the three types of polioviruses in live attenuated form. After being taken orally, one or more of the viruses establish a mild, transient intestinal infection, thereby inducing in the vaccinated individual both systemic and local immunity against the serotype that successfully established the infection. Ninety percent of persons vaccinated are immune after the first dose of OPV. However, not all three types of polioviruses may simultaneously establish infections in the vaccinated individual after the first dose; and active infections by nonpolioviruses can also prevent infection by vaccine polioviruses. It is because of this interference that multiple doses of OPV are recommended in primary vaccination.

   OPV is a very effective vaccine. After completion of the primary series, virtually all vaccinated individuals acquire solid and presumably lifelong immunity against the polioviruses.

   OPV does not cause local side effects, but it may cause polio paralytic disease in an occasional vaccinated person or contact. This can occur in both immunodeficient or otherwise healthy individuals. The incidence of vaccine-associated poliomyelitis is exceedingly low; the estimates are 1/8 million for those vaccinated and 1/6 million for household contacts.

2. **IPV** contains purified polioviruses that have been inactivated by formalin. All three types of viruses are represented. After a series of primary vaccination by injection according to instructions of the manufacturer, over 95% of vaccinated individuals develop immunity to all three types of polioviruses. The immunity of the newly licensed IPV with enhanced potency has been demonstrated to be greater than 5 years. Since IPV does not contain live viruses, vaccine-associated poliomyelitis does not occur following its use. Administration of IPV to persons with any form of immunologic defects does not result in progressive infection. Indeed, serious adverse reactions are not anticipated with the current IPV product.

3. **Relative advantage of the two vaccines.** OPV is easier to administer (oral rather than parenteral), is less costly, does not require boosters after the primary series

to maintain immunity, induces both systemic and intestinal immunity, is more expeditious in conferring immunity, results in immunization of some contacts of vaccinated persons, and has a record of having essentially eliminated poliomyelitis from the United States. The sole disadvantage of OPV is its potential for inducing vaccine-associated poliomyelitis in an occasional vaccinated individual or contacts, and of causing progressive infection in persons with immunologic defects.

B. Justification. Although the risk of poliomyelitis is very small in the United States, epidemics could occur if the high immunity level of the general population is not maintained by immunizing children routinely, or if wild poliovirus is introduced into susceptible populations with low immunization levels.

III. Recommendations [3]. Recommendations for infants, children, and teenagers have already been described (see Chaps. 52 and 57). For adults 18 years old and older in the United States, routine primary vaccination against poliomyelitis is unnecessary because most adults are already immune and have only a very small risk of exposure to poliovirus. For certain adults who are at higher risk of exposure to wild polioviruses than the general population, immunization is recommended. These include travelers to countries where poliomyelitis is endemic or epidemic, members of communities in which poliomyelitis caused by wild poliovirus has been reported, laboratory workers who handle specimens that may contain polioviruses, and health care workers in close contact with patients who may be excreting polioviruses.

For those adults who have no previous polio vaccination and who are at increased risk of exposure to poliomyelitis, primary immunization with IPV is preferred (because the risk of vaccine-associated paralysis following OPV is slightly higher in adults than in children). The first two doses should be given at intervals of 1–2 months, followed by a third dose 6–12 months after the second. The need for routine boosters with the new IPV is unknown at this time [4]. For those who have previously received less than a full primary course (i.e., three doses of IPV or OPV), the remaining required doses should be given regardless of the interval since the last dose and the type of vaccine previously received.

In circumstances where time will not allow at least three doses of IPV before protection is required, it is recommended that: (1) If less than 4 weeks are available, a single dose of OPV be given, and (2) If less than 8 weeks are available, two doses of IPV be given 4 weeks apart. In both situations, the remaining doses required in primary immunization should be given while in the high-risk situations.

Adults who have not been adequately immunized are at a very small risk of developing vaccine-associated poliomyelitis when children in the household are given OPV. About four such cases have occurred annually in the United States. Because of the overriding importance of ensuring prompt immunization of the child and the extreme rarity of vaccine-associated poliomyelitis among contacts, it is usual practice in the United States to give OPV to the child regardless of the polio immunity status of household adults. The responsible adult should be informed of the small risk involved. An acceptable alternative is to complete the primary immunization of the adult before giving OPV to the child.

OPV is **contraindicated** in persons who are or may be immunocompromised as the result of immune deficiency or immunosuppression. Nor should it be used for immunizing household contacts of such persons. IPV should be used instead.

Pregnancy is not a contraindication to polio immunization with either IPV or OPV, although it is prudent on theoretical grounds to avoid vaccinating pregnant women. However, if the pregnant woman is at increased risk of exposure to wild polioviruses, and immediate protection is needed, OPV is recommended.

References

1. Hortsman, D. M., Quinn, T. C., and Robbins, F. C. (guest eds.). International symposium on poliomyelitis control. *Rev. Infect. Dis.* 6(Suppl 2):301s, 1984 *Excellent review.*
2. Poliomyelitis — United States, 1975–1984. *M.M.W.R.* 35(11):180, 1986. *Recent epidemiology of polio in the United States.*
3. Immunization Practices Advisory Committee. Adult immunization. *M.M.W.R.* 33(Suppl 1s):205, 1984. *Centers for Disease Control recommendations on adult immunizations.*
4. Immunization Practices Advisory Committee. Poliomyelitis prevention: Enhanced potency inactivated poliomyelitis vaccine—supplementary statement. *M. M. W. R.* 36:795, 1987. *CDC recommendations on new IPV.*

90 Measles

Chinh Le and Robert S. Chang

I. The problem

A. Definition. Measles is usually a childhood disease characterized by a severe febrile upper respiratory tract infection followed by the appearance of a generalized exanthematous eruption, which appears first on the face around the fourth day of illness and spreads downward to the lower extremities in about 48 hours. Otitis media and bronchopneumonia are frequent complications. Encephalitis occurs about once in 2000 cases. One of approximately 3000 reported cases ends in death. Measles can be very severe.

Persons who have been immunized with inactivated measles vaccine, available from 1963–1967, may develop atypical measles after exposure to natural measles or, rarely, after reimmunization with live measles vaccine [1]. The skin rash in atypical measles is vasculitic and differs from that in measles in that the rash starts on the extremities and spreads up the trunk to the face, and is a polymorphic mixture of papules, blisters, wheals, and pinpoint hemorrhages. Koplik's spots, a pathognomonic sign of measles, are absent in atypical measles. Atypical measles can be severe, with high fever and pneumonia. There is only one immunologic type of measles virus. Infection induces lifelong immunity.

B. Epidemiology. Since the licensing of measles vaccine in 1963, there has been a dramatic (99%) decrease in the incidence of measles [2]. The annual incidence in the United States nowadays is about 2000–6000 cases, with 30–40% of cases occurring in persons older than 15 years of age. Recent outbreaks in colleges underscore the persistent susceptibility of young adults to measles. In 1986, over 70% of cases in persons older than 20 years of age were preventable.

The most effective means of preventing measles is to induce immunity through immunization.

II. Primary prevention

A. Method (the vaccine). Three major types of measles vaccines have been in general use over the past 29 years: inactivated, live attenuated, and live further attenuated. Since the inactivated vaccine provides incomplete protection that may result in atypical measles upon infection by wild measles virus, and since live attenuated vaccine produces a high frequency of side effects, the live further attenuated vaccine is the one currently available for use in the United States. Its official name is measles virus vaccine, live, attenuated. The vaccine virus is grown in chick embryo cell culture. The vaccine, in addition to the measles virus, contains a trace amount of chicken protein and neomycin.

Although measles vaccine is considered a highly effective vaccine, failures have been encountered [3, 4, 5]. In 1986, 39% of measles cases had been adequately vaccinated. Vaccine efficacy has been variously estimated at 81–97%. Measles vaccine failures are believed to be due to the use of inactivated vaccine, vaccination before 1 year of age, and errors in vaccine handling.

Side effects associated with measles vaccine are relatively common. About 5–15% of vaccinated individuals may develop fever (up to 103 °F) about 6 days after vaccination and lasting for up to 5 days. Transient rashes have been reported in about 5% of vaccinated persons, and involvement in the central nervous system in 1/million doses administered. There is no evidence that side effects are more frequent or more severe in vaccinated persons who had previously received live measles vaccine or who had measles.

B. Justification. Continuous efforts must be made to maintain a high level of immunity to measles in the community for the following reasons: (1) Measles is a severe infection with a 0.5–2.0% mortality rate that is totally preventable by immunization; the benefit-risk of measles vaccination has been proved beyond doubt. (2) Gaps in immunization in various segments of the population create conditions for continuous outbreaks (in schools, colleges, and medical settings), which are costly to control. (3)

Importation of measles by international travelling can constitute a persistent source of reintroduction of measles in the United States if high immunity levels are not maintained.

III. Recommendation. Measles vaccine is recommended for all persons who are susceptible to measles and who were born after 1957 (unless contraindicated).

Susceptibility is defined as the lack of documentation of physician-diagnosed measles or of laboratory evidence of measles immunity (hemagglutination inhibition titer of $\geq 1:4$), or lack of written proof of adequate immunization with live measles vaccine on or after the first birthday.

In adults, ongoing programs immunizing or requiring proof of measles immunity for college entry and medical personnel would greatly enhance the degree of immunity in the general population. Furthermore, because measles is highly endemic in developing countries and the measles vaccine is not 100% effective, international travelers born after 1956 should be considered for a one-time booster dose of measles vaccine [6].

Contraindications are pregnancy, immunodeficiency, anaphylactoid allergies to egg proteins or neomycin, and administration of immune globulins within the last 3 months.

One single dose given subcutaneously to anyone who is 15 months old or older generally confers lifelong immunity. Combined measles/mumps/rubella vaccine (MMR) is the vaccine of choice if recipients are likely to be susceptible to rubella and mumps, as well as measles. There is no evidence that the live measles vaccine exacerbates tuberculosis. If a TB skin testing is needed, it can be done on the day of vaccination. For a recently vaccinated individual, it is prudent to wait 4–6 weeks after receipt of measles vaccine before administration of tubercular skin testing, since measles vaccine may temporarily suppress tuberculin reactivity.

Measles vaccine should be given 14 days before, or deferred for at least 6–12 weeks after, a person has received IG or blood products containing antibodies.

Because measles vaccine contains live measles virus, which is a relatively unstable virus, it is of utmost importance to adhere to the manufacturer's instructions concerning handling of the vaccine.

References

1. Atypical measles—California, 1974–1975. *M. M. W. R.* 25(31):245, 1976. *Epidemiology of atypical measles from killed vaccine in California.*
2. Centers for Disease Control. Measles—United States, 1986. *M. M. W. R.* 36(20):301, 1987. *Update on measles in the United States.*
3. McCormick, J. B., Halsey, N., and Rosenberg, R. Measles vaccine efficacy determined from secondary attack rates during a severe epidemic. *J. Pediatr.* 90(1):13, 1977. *Study of measles vaccine efficacy looking at an epidemic.*
4. Measles vaccine efficacy—United States. *M. M. W. R.* 29(39):470, 1980. *Review of measles vaccine efficacy.*
5. Hayden, G. F. Measles vaccine failure. A survey of causes and means of prevention. *Clin. Pediatr.* (Phila) 18(3):155, 1979. *Good review of measles vaccine failures.*
6. Immunization Practices Advisory Committee. Measles prevention. *M. M. W. R.* 36(26):409, 1987. *Centers for Disease Control recommendations for measles immunization.*

91 Mumps

Chinh Le and Robert S. Chang

I. The problem

A. Description. Mumps is an acute systemic infection with parotitis as its predominant sign. It is generally self-limiting but moderately debilitating. Meningoencephalitis occurs at a frequency of 2.6/1000 patients with mumps [1], and orchitis, 1/5 postpubertal males with mumps, but sterility is rare [2]. The case-fatality ratio is estimated at 1.8/10,000 reported cases. There is only one serologic type of mumps virus, and infection by the virus (natural or through immunization) confers long-lasting immunity. Approximately 30% of the naturally acquired infections are subclinical.

B. Epidemiology. Since the licensing of mumps vaccine in 1967, the annual incidence of reported cases has steadily decreased from about 90/100,000 in 1968 to about 5/100,000 in the 1980s [3–4], with 3000–6000 reported cases a year. Although mumps is considered a childhood disease, 24% of cases occurred in persons 15 years old and older [4].

II. Primary prevention

A. Methods (the vaccine). Mumps vaccine contains live attenuated mumps virus, which confers a long-lasting immunity in the vaccinated individual through a subclinical, noncommunicable infection. Over 90% of persons susceptible to mumps develop specific antibodies after vaccination, and the antibody persists for at least 12 years [3]. The vaccine virus is propagated in chicken embryo culture; therefore, the vaccine may also contain a trace amount of chick protein and neomycin.

B. Justification. Side effects after mumps vaccination are rare. Parotitis has been rarely reported. Allergic reactions (rash, pruritus, and purpura) have been associated temporally with mumps vaccination, but they are uncommon and usually mild. Very rarely, central nervous system involvement (febrile seizures, deafness, and encephalitis) has occurred within 30 days of mumps vaccination. There is no proof that mumps vaccination is responsible for these CNS involvements. Indeed, the incidence of CNS involvement among vaccinated persons within 30 days after mumps vaccination is lower than CNS illness among children 1–9 years old/30 days' period (0.9/million doses of mumps vaccine vs. 2.5/million children/30-day duration) [1].

There is no evidence that persons immune to mumps are at enhanced risk from receiving mumps vaccine [2].

III. Recommendations

A. General recommendations. All persons susceptible to mumps should be vaccinated against mumps unless contraindicated. Persons born before 1957 are generally considered immune due to prior natural infection by mumps virus. Persons born after 1957 are considered susceptible unless they have documentation of physician-diagnosed mumps, serum antibody against mumps, or immunization with mumps vaccine at the age of 12 months or older.

Skin testing or routine antibody determination for susceptibility to mumps is not dependable or cost effective. Since persons immune to mumps are not at enhanced risk from mumps vaccination, it is more beneficial to vaccinate persons without proper documentation of mumps immunity rather than to test for immunity and vaccinate if found negative.

B. Specific recommendations. Contraindications to mumps vaccination are pregnancy, immunodeficiency conditions, and anaphylactic reaction to neomycin (see package insert accompanying the vaccine). In persons who have received immune globulins, vaccination should be postponed for at least 3 months after the administration of immune globulins.

To persons who are susceptible to mumps and who have no contraindication to mumps vaccination, a single dose of vaccine in the volume specified by the manufacturer should be administered subcutaneously.

References

1. Hayden, G. F., et al. Current status of mumps and mumps vaccine in the United States. *Pediatrics* 62(6):965, 1978. *Good review of mumps and mumps vaccination.*
2. Immunization Practices Advisory Committee. Mumps vaccine. *M. M. W. R.* 31(46):617, 1982. *CDC recommendations on mumps immunization.*
3. *Mumps Surveillance, January 1977–December 1982.* Atlanta, GA: Centers for Disease Control, September 1984. *CDC mumps surveillance report.*
4. Mumps—United States, 1985–1986. *M. M. W. R.* 36:151, 1987. *Update on epidemiology of mumps in the United States.*

92 Rubella

Chinh Le and Robert S. Chang

I. The problem

A. Definition. Rubella is a mild, febrile illness usually accompanied by a generalized maculopapular rash. It is an innocuous disease except when it involves the fetus. The virus exits and enters the human body through the upper respiratory tract, and the infection is frequently accompanied by a transient viremia during which the virus may reach the fetus [1, 2].

1. Maternal rubella during the first trimester of pregnancy is almost always accompanied by fetal infection. Fetal infections result in congenital anomalies or growth retardation or both; an estimated 20% of the anomalies are sufficiently severe to be recognizable at birth, but other sequelae such as hearing loss or autoimmune endocrine disorders may not be detected until later in life.
2. The probability of fetal malformation is considerably lower if rubella occurs during the second or third trimesters. Preventing congenital rubella is the main reason for assessing rubella immunity in adults.

B. Epidemiology. The introduction of an effective rubella vaccine in 1969 has dramatically reduced the incidence of rubella. In the 1980s in the United States, there were about 600–2000 rubella cases and 5–10 cases of congenital rubella syndrome reported annually. The actual incidence may be higher since rubella is frequently overlooked, misdiagnosed, and unreported. About 10–20% of adolescents and young adults were still susceptible. Recent outbreaks in colleges and hospital personnel underscore the importance of achieving and maintaining a high level of immunity in adults as well as children.

II. Primary prevention

A. Method (rubella vaccine). The rubella vaccine contains a live attenuated rubella virus known as RA 27/3. Inoculated into a susceptible person, the vaccine virus undergoes a limited multiplication sufficient to induce immunity but not disease. At least 95% of susceptible adults can be expected to acquire long-term (probably lifelong) protection against clinical rubella and viremia after a single dose of rubella vaccine [3].

Side effects of rubella vaccination in adults consist primarily of arthralgia, not of sufficient intensity to disrupt daily activity [4]. Arthralgia usually begins 1–3 weeks after vaccination and lasts for several days. It may occur in up to 40% of vaccinated individuals. Frank arthritis may also occur, but in no more than 1% of vaccinated persons. Transient peripheral neuritic complaints such as paresthesias and pain are rare.

B. Justification. There is no treatment for rubella and its sequelae. Control of the disease and eradication of the congenital rubella syndrome rests on a high immunity level in the population. Gaps in immunization will allow continuous outbreaks, which can be costly to control.

III. Recommendations

A. Rubella vaccination is recommended for all susceptible women of childbearing age unless contraindicated. For the purpose of vaccination, the absence of rubella antibody or the lack of documented evidence for past rubella vaccination are accepted as evidence of susceptibility.

B. Vaccination is **contraindicated** in immunodeficient patients and pregnant women. In immunodeficient patients, regardless of the cause of immunodeficiencies (congenital, acquired, drug-induced, or secondary or leukemia/lymphoma), there is the potential danger of the progressive multiplication of the vaccine virus. Vaccination during pregnancy introduces the theoretical danger of fetal infection. However, the risk is extremely low [5]. Precautions to take before vaccinating women of childbearing age include: (1) asking women if they are pregnant; (2) excluding those who say they are; and (3) explaining the theoretical risks of the vaccine and counselling them not to become pregnant for 3 months after vaccination. The only known potential allergen in the vaccine is neomycin in trace amounts; hence, vaccination should be avoided in persons known to have an anaphylactic reaction to neomycin.

C. Requirements for proof of rubella immunity or mandatory vaccination, unless contraindicated, in population groups such as colleges, military bases and hospital employees (for both sexes) would certainly reduce the chance of epidemics and protect them against rubella. It is more cost-effective to recommend rubella vaccination to persons who do not have documented evidence of past rubella vaccination than to routinely do serologic testing to determine immunity status and only vaccinate seronegative persons [6]. Side effects of rubella vaccination in immune persons are uncommon.

References

1. Vesikari, T. Immune response to rubella infection. *Scand. J. Infect. Dis.* (Suppl 4), 1972. *A comprehensive virologic and serologic study of maternal rubella.*
2. Centers for Disease Control. Rubella and congenital rubella—United States, 1984–1986. *M. M. W. R.* 36(40):664, 1987. *Surveillance report on congenital rubella in the United States.*
3. Hinman, A.R. Special report: Prevention of congenital rubella infection: Symposium summary. *Pediatrics* 75(6):1162, 1985. *Excellent review.*
4. Immunization Practices Advisory Committee. Rubella prevention *M. M. W. R.* 33(22):301, 1984. *CDC recommendations for rubella immunization.*
5. Centers for Disease Control. Rubella vaccination during pregnancy—United States, 1971–1986. 36(28):457, 1987. *Review of risks to fetus with rubella vaccination during pregnancy.*
6. Preblud, S.R. Some current issues relating to rubella vaccine. *J. A. M. A.* 254(2):253, 1985. *Good review of some controversial issues.*

93 Hepatitis B

Chinh Le and Robert S. Chang

I. The problem

A. Definition. Hepatitis B is an acute infection of the liver by the hepatitis B virus (HBV). Varying degrees of hepatocellular degeneration are its basic pathology. In Table 93-1, the nomenclature used for various antigens and antibodies associated with HBV is defined. Although HBsAg can be detected in serum 30–60 days after exposure to HBV, typically the disease is characterized by a long incubation (45–160 days) and insidious onset of low-grade fever, anorexia, nausea, abdominal discomfort, and malaise, which may be followed by jaundice. Clinical manifestations (such as skin rashes and arthralgia) believed to be due to intravascular immune complex deposition may occur during incubation or acute phase of hepatitis B. Serum aminotransferase levels are markedly elevated. Clinically, hepatitis B is indistinguishable from hepatitis A or non-A non-B hepatitis. Differentiation from these two other varieties of viral hepatitis is best achieved by specific serology testing. HBV infection is also a prerequisite for hepatitis caused by the delta-hepatitis agent.

Hepatitis B infections vary in severity from subclinical to fulminating. Approximately 50% are subclinical, 30% and 25% result in anicteric and icteric hepatitis respectively, and only 0.1% are fulminating [1]. Among patients with nonfulminating hepatitis, 90% can expect complete resolution with solid immunity to reinfection, while 5–10% become chronic HBV carriers (defined as persons who are positive for HBsAg on two or more occasions at least 6 months apart). The majority of HBV carriers are asymptomatic, one third have chronic persistent hepatitis, and one fifth have chronic active hepatitis [1]. Chronic active hepatitis may progress to cirrhosis.

There is a strong association between hepatitis B and hepatocellular carcinoma [2]. The risk of developing this cancer is 12 to 300 times higher in HBV carriers than in the general population. The estimated lifetime risk for hepatocellular carcinoma for Asian male carriers of HBV is 40%.

B. Epidemiology. The sources of HBV are the blood and secretions of persons incubating or suffering from hepatitis B and of HBV carriers. HBV has not been shown to be transmitted via fecal/oral route or by contamination of food or water. Chronic carriers are by far the most important source of HBV, since there are approximately 0.5–1.0 million carriers in the United States, and over 200 million worldwide (areas of high endemicity are China, Southeast Asia, subSaharan Africa, most Pacific islands, the Amazon Basin, and some Mediterranean countries). Susceptible persons become infected through percutaneous or permucosal exposure to blood or secretions containing HBV. This mode of transmission generally requires intense exposure such as contact through the birth process resulting in perinatal infection, prolonged and intimate contacts (between sexual partners), inadvertent exposure to infected materials (health care personnel dealing with blood) [3], or intravenous drug abuse. Transmission of infection by transfusion of contaminated blood or blood products has been greatly reduced since the advent of routine screening for HBsAg. It is estimated that 200,000 persons, primarily young adults, are infected each year in the United States [4].

Varying risk of infection is reflected in the differing rates of HBV serologic evidence (Table 93-2) in different groups. Based on numerous studies (mostly survey type) of HBV antibody and antigens, Mulley, et al., have provided estimates of the prevalence of prior HBV infections and annual infection rates of 21 population groups in the United States [1]. Their estimates are summarized in Table 93-3.

II. Primary prevention

A. Methods (the vaccines)

1. **Content.** Two HBV vaccines are available. The first, licensed in 1982, is a suspension of HBsAg collected from the plasma of HBV carriers [4], and purified by a combination of biophysical (double ultra-centrifugation) and biochemical processes to

Table 93-1. Nomenclature for Hepatitis B

HBV	Hepatitis B virus	Etiologic agent of "serum" or "long-incubation" hepatitis; also known as Dane particle.
HBsAg	Hepatitis B surface antigen	Surface antigen(s) of HBV detectable in large quantity in serum; several subtypes identified.
HBeAg	Hepatitis B e antigen	Soluble antigen; correlates with HBV replication, high-titer HBV in serum, and infectivity of serum.
HBcAG	Hepatitis B core antigen	No commercial test available.
Anti-HBs	Antibody to HBsAg	Indicates past infection with and immunity to HBV, passive antibody from HBIG, or immune response from HBV vaccine.
Anti-HBe	Antibody to HBeAg	Presence in serum of HBsAg carrier suggests lower titer of HBV.
Anti-HBc	Antibody to HBcAg	Indicates past infection with HBV at some undefined time.
IgM anti-HBc	IgM class antibody to HBcAg	Indicates recent infection with HBV; positive for 4–6 months after infection.

Source: Immunization Practices Advisory Committee. Recommendations for protection against viral hepatitis. *M. M. W. R.* 34(22):313, 1985.

inactivate HBV and any known infectious agents in human blood, including HIV, the causative agent of AIDS. The second, licensed in 1986, is a recombinant DNA HBV vaccine produced by a common yeast onto which a plasmid containing the gene of HBsAg has been inserted. The HBsAg is then harvested, filtered, and treated to contain no detectable yeast DNA in the vaccine.

2. **Effectiveness.** After three doses of either vaccine, over 90% of healthy adults developed protective antibody. Actual field trials have shown an 85–95% efficacy in preventing infection or hepatitis among susceptible persons (but only up to 60% in hemodialysis patients). Used in combination with HBIG, the HBV vaccine series is also effective in preventing perinatal HBV infection. The duration of protection after a primary course of vaccination is not yet defined. However, only 10–15% of persons who develop adequate antibody after three doses lose antibody within 4 years, but still seem protected from viremic infection.

   Persons who failed to respond to the primary series have a one-third chance of developing protective antibody upon revaccination [4].

3. **Side effects and adverse reactions.** Side effects are essentially soreness and erythema at the site of inoculation [4]. More serious side effects temporally associated with but not proved to be caused by the vaccine have been reported in 1/7500 doses (arthralgia, neurologic disorders). Vaccination of immune persons does not result in adverse effect [4]. The vaccine produces neither therapeutic nor adverse effects in HBV carriers. No known cases of hepatitis B, non-A non-B hepatitis, or AIDS have been transmitted by the vaccine [6].

Table 93-2. Prevalence of hepatitis B serologic markers in various population groups

Population group	Prevalence of serologic markers of HBV infection	
	HBsAg (%)	All markers (%)
High risk		
Immigrants/refugees from areas of high HBV endemicity	13	70–85
Clients in institutions for the mentally retarded	10–20	35-80
Users of illicit parenteral drugs	7	60–80
Homosexually active men	6	35–80
Household contacts of HBV carriers	3–6	30–60
Patients in hemodialysis units	3–10	20–80
Intermediate risk		
Health-care workers with frequent blood contact	1–2	15–30
Prisoners (male)	1–8	10–80
Staff of institutions for the mentally retarded	1	10–25
Low risk		
Health-care workers with no or infrequent blood contact	0.3	3–10
Healthy adults (first-time volunteer blood donors)	0.3	3–5

4. **Vaccine storage.** Vaccine should be stored at 2–8 °C (36–46 °F) but **not** frozen—freezing destroys the potency of the vaccine.

B. **Justification.** Approximately 25,000 cases of HBV are reported each year in the United States (and many more cases are not reported), with significant morbidity and lifetime risks of sequelae. At the present time, HBV infection is not treatable. Eight to ten percent of persons exposed to HBV via accidental inoculation will develop clinical or subclinical HBV infection despite receipt of recommended IG regimens (standard or HBIG). Infected individuals become sources of secondary infections through sexual and perinatal transmission, and through accidental and occupational exposure. Administration of HBV vaccine to persons at high risk for HBV offers the major control of this infection. It is clear that HBV vaccine is currently underused because of anxiety and fear for vaccine safety. It is important to educate vaccine candidates about the benefits and the safety of the present HBV vaccines.

III. Recommendations

A. **HBV vaccine is recommended** for persons who are at substantial risk of HBV infection and who are (or judged likely to be) susceptible [4]. They include the following groups:

1. Homosexually active males and heterosexually active persons with multiple partners.
2. Illicit, intravenous drug users.
3. Persons who have blood-clotting disorder and are receiving factor VIII or IX concentrates.
4. Patients on hemodialysis.
5. Clients and staff of institutions for the mentally retarded.
6. Sexual and household contacts of HBV carriers.
7. Health care personnel. Risks of exposure to HBV for health care workers depend on their jobs and may vary among hospitals and geographic locations. Those with frequent exposure to blood and those in the professional training period are at the highest risk of acquiring HBV and should receive the highest priority in protection through vaccination (preferably during training).
8. **Special high-risk populations.** Depending on specific epidemiology and public health considerations, vaccination programs should be considered for certain eth-

Table 93-3. Prevalence of prior HBV infection and annual HBV attack rates in representative population groups

Population group	Prevalence of HBV prior infection (%)	Annual attack rate (%)
Health-care workers		
Dialysis staff	34–39	3–11
Oral surgeons	30	5
Staff of custodial institutions	22–33	13–20
Surgeons	23–28	5
Nurses in high-risk units	7–47	1–11
Blood bank workers	6–26	1–2
Laboratory technicians	11–26	1–3
Physicians (general)	12–19	2
Dentists (general)	14–15	2
Surgical house officers	10–17	4–10
Nurses (general)	5–21	1
High-risk patients		
Dialysis patients	42–59	3–14
Hemophiliacs	76–96	13–20
Institutionalized persons		
Mentally retarded	50–90	1–10
Prisoners	42	5–10
Other groups		
Homosexual men	60–68	12–19
Intravenous drug users	50–71	4–33
Household contacts of HBsAg carriers	26–61	2–5
Promiscuous homosexuals	15–31	2–5
Military personnel	7–20	0.5–12
General US population	5–10	0.1

Source: A. G. Mulley, M. D. Silverstein, and J. L. Dienstag. Indications for use of hepatitis B vaccine, based on cost-effectiveness analysis. Reprinted, by permission of the *New England Journal of Medicine* (307[1]:644, 1982).

nic groups (Eskimos, native Pacific Islanders, eastern Asians, and subSaharan Africans), and international travellers to areas with high endemic levels of HBV.

9. Inmates of long-term correctional facilities.

B. Vaccination schedule. A primary course consists of three doses IM: initial dose and 1 and 6 month doses. The dose is double the usual dose (see Table 93-5) for hemodialysis patients, for whom only the plasma-derived HBV should be used. The deltoid area should be used in adults (immunogenicity is low when injections are given in the buttock). Serologic confirmation of postvaccination immunity is usually unnecessary, and booster doses are not routinely recommended, except for hemodialysis patients [5]. The immunogenicity and efficacy of the intradermal route have not been firmly established at this time.

C. Prevaccination serologic screening for susceptibility. Persons who have HBV antibody from previous infection need not be vaccinated, while HBV carriers would not derive benefit from vaccination. The decision to screen potential vaccinees in order to exclude the immune and carriers is essentially an economic one. This economic decision depends on the cost of vaccination, the cost of screening, and the prevalence of immune individuals in the group. Based on the assumption that the cost of a primary series of vaccination is at least $100, the Centers for Disease Control has constructed a linear relation (Figure 93-1) between the expected prevalence of HBV serologic markers and screening cost per person [4]. From this figure, one may estimate whether prevaccination screening is cost-effective. For example, in a population group with an expected immunity rate of 20%, prevaccination screening to identify susceptible individuals would be cost-effective if the screening cost per person is less than $30.

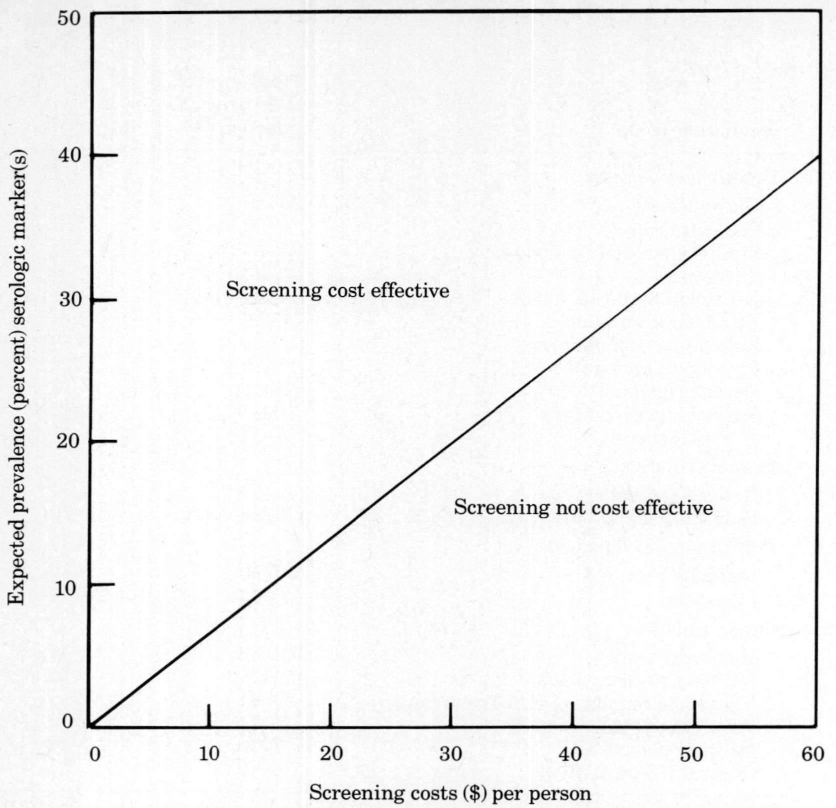

Fig. 93.1. Cost effectiveness of prevaccination screening of hepatitis B vaccine candidates. (From Hepatitis B virus vaccine safety: Report of an inter-agency group. *M. M. W. R.* 31(34):465, 1982.)

If prevaccination screening is to be done, either anti-Hbc or anti-Hbs may be used. Anti-HBc identifies all prior infections including carriers, while anti-HBs identifies all immune individuals. It is recommended that a minimum of ten- rather than two-radioimmunoassay sample ratio units of anti-HBs be used to designate immunity [4].

More recent data supports HBsAg screening of all pregnant women, regardless of stated absence of risk factors [7].

D. Postexposure recommendations for HBV. Prophylactic treatment with immune globulins should not be substituted for vaccination of high-risk groups. However, in case of significant HBV exposure in a previously unimmunized person, the recommendation for simultaneous administration of immune globulin and HBV vaccine is given in Tables 93-4 and 93-5 [4].

Table 93-4. Hepatitis B virus postexposure recommendations

	HBIG		Vaccine	
Exposure	Dose	Recommended timing	Dose	Recommended timing
Perinatal	0.5 ml IM	Within 12 hr	0.5 ml IM	Within 12 hr of birth,[a] repeat at 1 and 6 months
Sexual	0.06 ml/kg IM	Single dose within 14 days of sexual contact	1.0 ml IM	[b]

[a]The first dose can be given at the same time as the HBIG dose, but at a different site.

[b]Vaccine is recommended for homosexual men and for regular sexual contacts of HBV carriers, and is optional in initial treatment of heterosexual contacts of persons with acute HBV.

Source: Immunization Practices Advisory Committee. Recommendations for protection against viral hepatitis. *M. M. W. R.* 34(22):313, 1985.

Table 93-5. Recommendations for hepatitis B prophylaxis following percutaneous exposure

	Exposed person	
Source	Unvaccinated	Vaccinated
HBsAg-positive	HBIG x 1 immediately[a] Initiate HB vaccine[b] series	Test exposed person for anti-Hbs If inadequate antibody,[c] HBIG x 1 immediately, plus HB vaccine booster dose
Known source		
High-risk, HBsAg-positive	Initiate HB vaccine series Test source for HBsAg; if positive, HBIG x 1	Test source for HBsAg only if exposed individual is vaccine-nonresponder; if source is HBsAg-positive, give HBIG x 1 immediately, plus HB vaccine booster dose
Low-risk, HBsAg-positive	Initiate HB vaccine series	Nothing required
Unknown source	Initiate HB vaccine series	Nothing required

[a]HBIG dose 0.06 ml/kg IM.

[b]Plasma-derived HB vaccine dose 20 μg IM for adults; 10 μg IM for infants or children under 10 years of age. Recombinant HBV vaccine dose 10 μg IM for adults and 5 μg IM for infants and children under 10 years. First dose within 1 week; second and third doses, 1 and 6 months later.

[c]Less than 10 SRU by RIA, negative by EIA.

Source: Immunization Practices Advisory Committee. Recommendations for protection against viral hepatitis. *M. M. W. R.* 34(22):313, 1985.

References

1. Mulley, A. G., Silverstein, M. D., and Dienstag, J. L. Indications for use of hepatitis B vaccine, based on cost-effectiveness analysis. *N. Engl. J. Med.* 307(1):644, 1982. *An excellent article dealing with the cost-effectiveness of hepatitis B vaccine*

2. Maupas, P., and Melnick, J. L. Hepatitis B infection and primary liver cancer. *Prog. Med. Virol.* 27:1, 1981. *An excellent review on the association between hepatitis B and hepatocellular carcinoma.*
3. Dienstag, J. L., and Ryan, D. M. Occupational exposure to hepatitis B virus in hospital personnel: Infection or immunization. *Am J. Epidemiol.* 115(1):26, 1982. *Study of HBV infection rates in hospital personnel.*
4. Immunization Practices Advisory Committee. Recommendations for protection against viral hepatitis. *M. M. W. R.* 34(22):313, 1985. *CDC recommendations on hepatitis immunization.*
5. Immunization Practices Advisory Committee: Update on hepatitis B prevention. *M. M. W. R.* 39(23):353, 1987. *CDC analysis of the impact of HBV vaccination on disease incidence, description of the new recombinant HBV vaccine, and update on recommendations.*
6. Francis, D. P., et al. The safety of hepatitis B vaccine: Inactivation of the AIDS virus during routine vaccine manufacture. *J. A. M. A.* 256(7):869, 1986. *Study demonstrating the inactivation of HIV during HBV vaccine manufacture.*
7. Stevens, C. E. Perinatal hepatitis B virus infection: Screening of pregnant women and protection of the infant. *Ann. Int. Med.* 107:412, 1987. *Editorial reviewing recent studies supporting routine perinatal HBsAg screening.*

94 Influenza

Chinh Le and Robert S. Chang

I. The problem

A. Description. Influenza is an acute respiratory tract infection caused by influenza virus. The infection is generally accompanied by prominent constitutional symptoms such as fever, headache, generalized myalgia, and prostration, and by frequent dry hacking cough with retrosternal pain. During the infection, there is a reduction in respiratory functions, which can be significant for persons with prior impairment of respiratory reserve. Influenza damages the respiratory mucosa, thereby lowering resistance to secondary bacterial invaders; hence, secondary bacterial pneumonias constitute the major cause of morbidity and mortality among patients with influenza.

B. Epidemiology [1, 2, 3]. Influenza tends to occur in winter in major worldwide epidemics every 10–12 years, and in minor regional epidemics every 2–3 years. During an epidemic, 30–50% of the population can be expected to develop influenza. About 40% of those are seen by a physician, and 3% of those seen by physicians are subsequently hospitalized.

II. Primary prevention

A. The vaccine

1. Antigenic characteristics of influenza viruses. To understand why influenza is difficult to prevent despite the availability of a reasonably effective vaccine, familiarity with the antigenic characteristics of the influenza virus is helpful.

There are three key antigens: two surface antigens (hemaglutinin, or H, and neuraminidase, or N) and a protein inside the virion. H is the most important component regarding immunity against influenza. It is through the H component that an influenza virus attaches onto and then infects a susceptible cell. Antibody against H will form complexes with the H component and thereby prevents the virus from attaching onto a susceptible cell. N is an enzyme that hydrolyzes neuraminic acid (an important component of mucus), and thereby thins the mucus, allowing the local spreading of the virus; hence, adequate immunity against N reduces severity of the disease. The internal protein is believed to be responsible for the "toxic" manifestations (e.g., myalgia and prostration) of influenza; antibody against this protein plays no significant role in preventing infection.

Influenza viruses are typed into A, B, and C, according to the antigenicity of the internal component. Most epidemics of influenza are caused by type A viruses, some by type B, and none by type C. Immunity to influenza is type-specific.

Type A viruses are further classified into subtypes on the basis of their H and N antigens: H1, H2, and H3; and N1 and N2. Immunity to influenza type A virus is subtype-specific; a person immune to H1 virus is still susceptible to H2 or H3 viruses. Similar antigenic analysis of isolates of type B reveals only one H and one N antigen.

The H and N antigens of types A and B have the propensity of undergoing partial variations known as antigenic drifts. Because of this antigenic drift, immunity acquired against one strain may be only partially protective against other strains of the same subtype. The bigger the antigenic drift, the less cross-protective the immunity.

An isolate of the influenza virus is designated by its serotype, H and N components, and the place and year first isolated. For example, an A/Brazil/78(H1N1) virus is a type A virus with the H1 and N1 components, and was first isolated in Brazil in 1978. However, this designation does not tell the extent of antigenic drifting between two viruses of the same subtype.

The existence of three types of influenza viruses, of numerous subtypes of type A virus, and the antigenic drifting of types A and B, provide the biological basis for recurring major and minor epidemics, the susceptibility of a person during each of the epidemics, the necessity of frequent vaccination against influenza, and the changing composition of vaccines.

2. **Vaccine content.** Influenza vaccine contains inactivated influenza virions grown in chick embryos. Influenza vaccine may be mono-, bi-, or trivalent, depending on its content of one, two, or three types or subtypes of virions. Influenza vaccine may be whole-virion or subvirion (split-virus) preparations. The subviron preparation contains only the protective antigens (H and N) and is less toxic but also may be less immunogenic than the whole-virion preparation.

   The content of influenza vaccine may vary from year to year. Generally, those influenza viruses that prevailed in the preceding winter are incorporated into the vaccine for the succeeding winter. The types and subtypes of viruses are specified on the vaccine package insert for each yearly vaccine product.

3. **Risks and side effects of vaccine.** Pain, redness, and induration at vaccination site, lasting for 1 or 2 days, occur in about one third of vaccines. In some individuals, especially children, local reaction is accompanied by fever, malaise, and myalgia. By using subvirion instead of whole-virion vaccine, the frequency of febrile reaction among vaccinated children has been reduced to 2%. Persons with a history of anaphylactic reactions to egg proteins may develop immediate allergic reactions (e.g., flare, wheal, and asthma).

B. **Justification.** No other respiratory viruses possess influenza's potential for high attack rates, acute morbidity, and pulmonary compromise, nor for its community-wide impact, even in nonpandemic years. Rates of hospitalization for adults with high-risk medical conditions increase by two- to five-fold during major epidemics, reaching about 800/100,000 population, with a pneumonia mortality of about 250/1 million. Excess mortality averages about 10,000 every epidemic year in the United States [4]; about 90% of these excess deaths occur among persons 65 years of age or older. Recent influenza outbreaks in nursing homes have claimed attack rates as high as 60%, and case-fatality ratios of 30% or more. Since the proportion of elderly persons and patients with chronic diseases is increasing in the United States, the toll of influenza may also increase unless control measures are used more vigorously than in the past.

1. **Vaccine efficacy.** Nearly all vaccinated young adults develop protective antibodies to vaccine strains. However, the elderly, the very young, and patients with certain chronic diseases (cancer, hemodialysis) may develop lower and less-sustained antibody response. Nevertheless, studies have shown that vaccination can yield a 37% reduction in illnesses, a 72% reduction in hospitalization, and a 79–87% reduction in mortality in elderly people during influenza outbreaks.
2. **Vaccine cost-benefits.** Calculated for 1970 health care dollars, vaccination of an elderly person 65 years of age or older saved net medical care costs while improving health. Even with medical costs in extended years of life, the cost-effectiveness ratios are reasonable—about $2000 for an extra year of healthy life for an average person aged 65 years and older, and about $4000 for an elderly high-risk person [5].
3. **Alternative measures.** Prophylaxis with amantadine (only for influenza A) and treatment with amantadine or ribavirin are 70–90% effective for individual patients, but do not have the preventive value of influenza vaccine at community or public health levels.

III. **Recommendations** [6]

A. **Vaccine indications.** Influenza vaccine should be given to the following groups in order of priority:

1. **Highest priority.** Adults and children with chronic cardiovascular and pulmonary disease severe enough to have required regular medical follow-ups or hospitalization during the preceding year; residents of nursing homes or chronic care facilities.
2. **Second priority.** Otherwise healthy adults over 65 years of age; adults and children with chronic metabolic diseases (diabetes, renal dysfunction, anemia, immunosuppression, asthma, or children and adolescents on long-term aspirin therapy).
3. **Third priority.** Physicians, nurses, and other personnel and household members who have extensive contact with high-risk patients; persons providing essential community service.

B. **Vaccine dose and timing of administration.** Influenza vaccine should be given in the fall. Doses are given according to age and previous influenza vaccinations. Yearly public health recommendations and package inserts should be reviewed and followed. For patients receiving immunosuppression, it is best to receive the vaccine at the time of the least immunosuppressive effect of their therapy.

C. **Cautions.** Influenza vaccine is considered safe for pregnant women. Nonetheless, waiting until after the third trimester is a reasonable precaution to minimize any concern over adverse effects of the vaccine on the pregnancy.

Influenza vaccine should not be given to persons who have an anaphylactic sensitivity to eggs.

Influenza vaccine has been reported to decrease elimination of some drugs metabolized by the hepatic cytochrome p450 system, specifically **theophylline** and **warfarin**. However, further studies have failed to show any adverse effects of influenza vaccine among patients taking these drugs.

D. Patients who are candidates for the influenza vaccines are also candidates for the **pneumococcal vaccine** (the latter should be given only once, however). These two vaccines can be given simultaneously (see Chap. 95).

E. **Amantadine and rimantidine** can prevent influenza A or be used therapeutically to reduce symptoms of influenza A infections. It is not effective against influenza B and C, and is **not** a substitute for vaccine.

References

1. Centers for Disease Control. *Influenza Surveillance* July, 1979–June, 1981. HHS Publication No. (CDC) 84-8295, June 1984. [Report No. 94.] *CDC surveillance report on influenza in the United States.*
2. Kilbourne, E. D. Influenza pandemics in perspective. *J. A. M. A* 237(12):1225, 1977. *Good review of influenza epidemiology.*
3. Couch, R. B., et al. Influenza: Its control in persons and populations. *J. Infect. Dis.* 153(3):431, 1986. *A thorough look at the subject.*
4. Gregg, M. B., et al. Influenza-related mortality. *J. A. M. A.* 239(2):115, 1978. *Study of the mortality attributable to influenza.*
5. Riddiough, M. A., Sisk, J. E., and Bell, J. C. Influenza vaccination: Cost effectiveness and public policy. J. A. M. A. 249(23):3189, 1983. *Examination of the issue of cost savings and influenza vaccination.*
6. Immunization Practices Advisory Committee. Prevention and control of influenza. *M. M. W. R.* 36(24):373, 1987. *CDC recommendations on influenza immunization.*

95 Pneumococcal Diseases

Chinh Le and Robert S. Chang

I. The problem [1]

A. Description of the organism and related diseases. The pneumococcus *(Streptococcus pneumoniae)* is a common human pathogen, causing pneumonia, meningitis, otitis, sinusitis, and primary bacteremia. About 35–60% of normal, healthy persons harbor pneumococci in the nasopharynx. Pathogenicity of the organism is mainly related to the presence of the capsule that interferes with phagocytosis. Host factors that predispose to local or systemic infections include the inability to produce protective antibodies against the capsular polysaccharide, defects in the reticular and hematopoietic system, genetic predisposition, and other ill-defined risk factors.

B. Epidemiology. Data on the precise occurrence of pneumococcal diseases are not available, but estimates from surveys and research reports are summarized in Table 95-1 [2].

Although the pneumococcus causes less than 25% of all pneumonia, its incidence increases with age, with a twofold increase among those over 60 years of age.

II. Primary prevention

A. Method: the pneumococcal vaccine. The present vaccine consists of a mixture of purified capsular polysaccharides from the 23 most prevalent or invasive pneumococcal types accounting for about 90% of pneumococcal serotypes isolated from blood or other sterile body sources (CSF, middle ear, pleural effusions, etc.). Each 0.5 ml dose of vaccine contains 25 μg of each polysaccharide (compared to 50 μg in the previous 14-valent pneumococcal vaccine).

Antibody rise following immunization may vary among serotypes, and it also depends on various host factors. Immunity against capsular polysaccharides is usually serotype-specific, except on rare occasions (i.e., 6A and 6B serotypes). The duration of protection is unknown at this time.

Adverse reactions. About 50% of vaccines develop mild pain and erythema at the injection site. Severe reactions are very rare (fever, 1%; anaphylaxis, 1/5 million doses).

B. Justification. Morbidity and mortality of pneumococcal infection remain high (Table 95-1), despite early treatment and exquisite sensitivity of most (97%) clinically significant pneumococci to antibiotics. However, the problem of multiple-antibiotic resistance is a worldwide concern of increasing importance.

Vaccine efficacy. There is unequivocal evidence from three randomized, controlled trials that pneumococcal vaccines are effective among selected populations: in young South African miners and in Papua, New Guinea, there was an 80–90% reduction in pneumococcal pneumonia and bacteremia, with a concurrent 44% reduction in mortality. However, demonstration of vaccine effectiveness in the United States rests on less secure ground. Two clinical trials (one of outpatients over 45 years old; the other of inpatients at a chronic care psychiatric facility) failed to show significant benefit. Five other studies designed to evaluate the efficacy of pneumococcal vaccine estimated a 0–70% reduction of bacteremic pneumococcal diseases in high-risk patients. Among patients with cirrhosis and renal failure, the estimated efficacy is lower, and no conclusive documentation of efficacy is shown for patients with chronic lung disease or immunosuppression [3–7].

The vaccine itself costs approximately $5 per dose (plus provider's fees). It is calculated that vaccination of a person age 65 or older could gain a year of healthy life for about $6000 in 1983 dollars [5].

III. Recommendations

A. Pneumococcal vaccine is recommended for selected high-risk groups [8, 9].

1. Adults with chronic illnesses, especially those with cardiovascular and chronic pulmonary disease.
2. Adults with chronic illnesses specifically associated with an increased risk of pneumococcal disease or its complications. These include splenic dysfunction or anatomic

Table 95-1. Estimated occurrence of serious pneumococcal diseases, United States, 1981

Pneumococcal disease	Estimated incidence (per 100,000 population/year)	Case-fatality ratio (%)	
		Overall	High-risk group
Pneumonia	68–280	5–7	25
Meningitis	1.2–2.8	32	55
Bacteremia	7–25	20	40

asplenia, Hodgkins' disease, multiple myeloma, cirrhosis, alcoholism, renal failure, chronic dialysis, CSF leaks, and conditions associated with immunosuppression.

3. Healthy adults over 65 years of age.

B. Vaccine precautions. The safety of pneumococcal polysaccharide vaccine in pregnant women has not been established. Women at high risk of pneumococcal disease ideally should be vaccinated when not pregnant. Booster doses of vaccines should not be given in adults because of increased incidence of adverse reactions.

C. Vaccine strategy. Like the influenza vaccine, the pneumococcal vaccine seems underutilized by health care providers. More effective programs are needed for giving vaccine in physicians' offices, nursing homes, and other chronic care facilities. Vaccine should be given to hospitalized patients in the high-risk groups before discharge. Pneumococcal vaccine and influenza vaccine can be given simultaneously at different sites without an increase in side effects.

References

1. Give, P. G., et al. The pneumococcus. *Rev. Infect. Dis.* 3:183, 1980.
2. Immunization Practices Advisory Committee. Pneumococcal polysaccharide vaccine. *M. M. W. R.* 30(33):410, 1981.
3. Austrian, R. A reassessment of pneumococcal vaccine [editorial]. *N. Engl. J. Med.* 310(10):651, 1984.
4. Bolan, G., et al. Pneumococcal vaccine efficacy in selected populations in the United States. *Ann. Intern. Med.* 104(1):1, 1986.
5. Sisk, J. E., and Riegelman, R. K. Cost effectiveness of vaccination against pneumococcal pneumonia: An update. *Ann. Intern. Med.* 104(1):79, 1986.
6. Forrester, H. L., et al. In efficacy of pneumococcal vaccine in a high-risk population. *Am. J. Med.* 83:425, 1987. *Case-control study showing lack of prevention of bacteremic disease in vaccinated high-risk patients.*
7. Simberkoff, M. S., et al. Efficacy of pneumococcal vaccine in high-risk patients. Results of the Veterans Administration cooperative study. *N. E. J. M.* 315:1318, 1986. *Placebo-control study demonstrating lack of efficacy of pneumococcal vaccine in preventing pneumonia or bronchitis.*
8. Immunization Practices Advisory Committee. Update: Pneumococcal polysaccharide vaccine usage—United States. *M. M. W. R.* 33(20):273, 1984.
9. American College of Physicians. Health and Public Policy Committee: Pneumococcal vaccine. *Ann. Intern. Med.* 104(1):118, 1986.

96 Tuberculosis

Neil Flynn

I. The problem

A. Definition. Tuberculosis is best defined as clinical or radiographic disease, either active or healed, resulting from progressive infection with *Mycobacterium tuberculosis*. In this chapter simple skin-test reactivity to purified protein derivative (PPD), without evidence of active or old disease by chest x-ray, history, or clinical examination, is referred to as tuberculous infection, not tuberculosis. Maintaining a distinction between simple latent **infection** and overt or latent **disease** is important for an understanding of preventive strategies in the management of tuberculosis.

B. Description. Tuberculosis results from the proliferation of, and subsequent host cell-mediated immunologic response to, *M. tuberculosis (M. tb.)* The complex interactions among the bacteria and their products, and host immune cells and their products, occur over many months to many years. The potential for clinically or radiographically evident tuberculous disease following infection with *M. tb.* is lifelong. Disease can occur at any time after infection, when the cell-mediated response becomes inadequate to the task of limiting local proliferation to small numbers of bacteria contained in a relatively few, small, well-organized foci of infection [1].

Following inhalation of aerosolized wet or inspissated droplets of sputum containing *M. tb.* that are of appropriate size to reach terminal bronchioles or alveoli, the organisms begin to grow. They grow relatively slowly, with a doubling time of 1–3 days (*E. coli* doubling time is in the range of 30–60 minutes). Initial host immune response to growth of the organism is indolent and ineffective in suppressing proliferation. However, as cell-mediated immunity develops over weeks to months following initial (primary) infection, with containment of organisms in discrete granulomas, proliferation ceases. If effective host immune response is delayed or inadequate, proliferation of organisms at the primary site of infection may lead to the migration of *M. tb.*-laden macrophages to regional and central lymph nodes, and then to the bloodstream, to be spread hematogenously throughout the body. This hematogenous spread accounts for disease occurring in extrapulmonary sites and in the apices of the lungs. Any of these pulmonary or extrapulmonary sites may subsequently become a focus for progressive primary disease; or, if the primary infection is controlled within a short time by host immunity as it is in the majority of *M. tb.* infections, these foci can become the sites of reactivation disease years later [1, 2].

Primary prevention of tuberculosis consists of reducing the likelihood of inhaling *M. tb.* by reducing exposure in the environment (identifying and treating potential sources of infection in the patient's environment), while secondary prevention centers around preventing disease in infected persons.

C. Epidemiology. There are approximately 10 million Americans infected with *M. tb.* Approximately 22,000 cases of active tuberculosis are reported annually in the United States and 1800 of these die as a result of tuberculous disease [3].

Several features of the epidemiology of tuberculous infection and disease are pertinent to this discussion of health promotion and disease prevention. These include identification of populations at higher risk of infection or of disease following infection, identification of individuals in these groups who are actually infected, and, finally, the impact of isoniazid (INH) on the epidemiology of disease.

Table 96-1 lists the prevalence of a positive skin test for *M. tb.* infection in various subgroups of the United States population [3, 4, 5]. Among those infected with *M. tb.* in these groups, certain individuals are at higher risk of developing active tuberculous disease than are others. Table 96-2 lists factors that increase the risk of active disease. Special attention has been focused on outbreaks of tuberculosis among nursing home residents due to reactivation of latent infection in an elderly resident [4].

Table 96-1. Prevalence of tuberculous infection in various risk groups, United States, 1980

Description	Positive PPD (%)
General adult population (age-related) [2]	< 3–30
Hispanic [14]	25
Southeast Asian [14]	35
≥ 65 years old [2]	10–30
Nursing home residents [4]	20–50
Patient-care hospital workers (physicians, nurses, etc.)	5–20

Table 96-2. Factors that increase risk of progressive (primary or reactivation) tuberculous disease following infection with *M. Tuberculosis**

Newly infected (< 2 yr) with *M. tb.*
Abnormal (scarring) stable chest x ray
Past clinical tuberculosis, inadequate or incomplete chemotherapy
Silicosis
Poorly controlled diabetes mellitus
High-dose, long-term corticosteroid therapy
Immunosuppressive therapy
Hematologic or reticuloendothelial malignancy
Gastrectomy
Alcoholism
End-stage renal disease
HIV infection (see Chap. 100)
Severe malnutrition

*INH prophylaxis is usually indicated in these individuals, as well as in younger (< 35 years of age) infected individuals lacking these risk factors.

Source: Adapted from W. W. Stead, et al. Tuberculosis as an endemic and nosocomial infection among the elderly in nursing homes. *N. Engl. J. Med.* 312(23):1483, 1985; J. B. Bass, et al. Treatment of tuberculosis and tuberculous infection in adults and children. *Am. Rev. Respir. Dis.* 134(2):355, 1986; and G. W. Comstock. Prevention of tuberculosis among tuberculin reactors: Maximizing benefits, minimizing risks. *J. A. M. A.* 256(19):2729, 1986.

An otherwise healthy individual who is not at the extremes of age, with a positive PPD as the only indication of past infection with *M. tb.* (>2 years since infection), is at low risk of developing tuberculous disease: less than 0.1%/year of life.

II. Primary prevention

A. Methods

1. Description

a. Prevention of exposure. Primary prevention of tuberculosis consists of applying the principles of case-finding, treatment, and contact-tracing of cases of active tuberculosis. Early identification of active disease can prevent infection of household contacts. In addition, probably even more effective in preventing primary infection in others is the identification and INH prophylaxis of *M. tb.*-infected individuals at high risk of developing active, communicable pulmonary tuberculosis in the future [4, 6, 7, 12, 13]. See Tables 96-1 and 96-2 for groups with a high prevalence of infection, and individuals at high risk for active, communicable disease who should be identified and evaluated for INH prophylaxis.

b. Bacille Calmette-Guérin (BCG) immunization is not recommended for use in United States populations for several reasons (see B.)

2. Performance. PPD testing should be carried out in each adult at least once, and then at appropriate intervals based on the probability of exposure to *M. tb.* and for clinical suspicion of illness compatible with tuberculosis. Positive reactors should be evaluated for INH prophylaxis according to guidelines set by the American

Thoracic Society (see Sec. **III.A.1.**) [7, 8, 12, 13]. This strategy is likely to reduce the number of primary infections in households and close contacts exposed to individuals with active, communicable disease. Public health departments are best equipped to evaluate and provide prophylaxis efficiently for persons infected with *M. tb.*

B. Justification

1. **Prevention of exposure.** Since primary prevention consists of prevention of exposure to active pulmonary tuberculosis, it is synonymous with detection and prophylaxis of individuals at risk for progressive primary or reactivation pulmonary disease, and with detection and treatment of individuals with active pulmonary disease.

   The risks of primary prevention are to the infected person given INH prophylaxis, not to those in whom infection is to be prevented.

2. **BCG.** Efficacy studies of recent BCG preparations have called into question their effectiveness [6]. The incidence rate of infection with *M. tb.* is so low in United States populations that BCG immunization is not cost-effective. Further, BCG immunization may convert the tuberculin skin test to reactive, reducing the utility of skin testing. Finally, treatment of active tuberculosis, early detection of infection, and INH prophylaxis when indicated are believed to be a more effective strategy for the control of tuberculosis in the United States.

III. Secondary prevention

A. Early detection. Early detection of latent infection with *M. tb.* depends on the proper application and interpretation of the tuberculin (PPD) skin test [8-11]. In persons found to be PPD-positive, a chest radiograph should be obtained to aid in the assessment of risk for development of active tuberculous disease. Persons at high risk for development of disease (see Table 96-2) or infected persons at normal risk for disease but below the age of 35, should be considered for INH prophylaxis [6, 12, 13].

Early detection of active tuberculosis and prevention of more severe disease requires a high index of suspicion in the presence of symptoms compatible with pulmonary or extrapulmonary tuberculous disease [1, 2]. Active tuberculosis will not be discussed here.

1. **Methods**

   a. **The tuberculin skin test**

      (1) **Performance.** The intradermal (Mantoux) route of administration of tuberculin is preferred [6]. A site for injection should be chosen on the forearm of the patient; it should have no cutaneous or subcutaneous tissue nodularity that might be mistaken for induration when reading the skin test. Once drawn up for injection, the PPD should be administered within a short time, since it declines in potency if left sitting in the syringe. One-tenth (0.1) ml of Tween 80 stabilized PPD containing 5 TU is injected between the layers of the skin with a 26- or 27-gauge needle, taking care not to inject subcutaneously. A wheal of approximately 5–8 mm in diameter, which disappears in minutes to hours, should be produced if injection is truly intradermal. A record should be made of the site of injection that is sufficiently precise to permit identifying the site for reading at 48–72 hours [11].

      (2) **Interpretation.** On the second or third day after injection, the site should be examined for induration. Measured induration 10 mm or greater is considered presumptive evidence of prior infection with *M. tb.* Induration between 5 and 9 mm is significant (suspicious for infection) in persons who have recently had close contact with someone whose sputum is positive for *M. tb.*, or in persons whose chest radiographs or clinical findings are compatible with past or present tuberculosis. Prior immunization with BCG may produce an intermediate or positive reaction, particularly if the immunization was recent (1–2 years). However, for purposes of evaluating patients for INH prophylaxis, most experts consider a definite positive to be an indication of actual infection with *M. tb.* and not merely secondary to BCG.

      The size of induration should always be recorded, even if it is less than 10 mm. Multiple puncture tests are not as accurate as intradermal injection, provided the injection and reading of the Mantoux test are performed properly (see Table 53-1).

      In persons over 50–55 years of age, an initial negative skin test should be followed by a repeat skin test administered within 1–2 weeks after the first, in order to detect individuals who have been previously infected with *M. tb.* but whose skin test reactivity has waned. These individuals will usually become positive on a repeat test given within 1–2 years of the first test (**booster phenomenon**). Failure to repeat the test soon after the initial test may lead to improperly designating the individual as a "converter" when the test is repeated a year or two later and found to be positive [6–10].

(3) **Interval/timing.** The skin test should be performed when there is suspicion of active or healed tuberculosis or if there is known exposure, and the individual is not known to be skin-test positive. Periodic testing is controversial. Most clinicians test low-risk individuals on admission to their practice if the individual has not been tested for several years and again at intervals of 2–5 years. Higher risk individuals such as health care personnel with direct patient contact, nursing home or institutional residents, or children of immigrants from areas highly endemic for tuberculosis, can be tested at intervals of 1–2 years. Testing is often performed at the place of employment or institutional residence.

(4) **Population.** The skin test should be performed in any individual who does not give a clear history of either a positive or negative skin test for tuberculosis. If the patient gives a clear history of a positive skin test or of tuberculosis, the skin test should not be repeated unless there is a specific reason for doing so, for example, the physician is considering the administration of INH prophylaxis and is not satisfied with the history of a positive test. If the prior skin test reaction was very large or vesicular, the 5 TU dose may produce a severe local reaction; 1 TU should be used in this setting if confirmation of reactivity is desired. If the patient gives a clear history of a negative skin test within the past 5 years, he has had no known contact with someone with active tuberculosis, and is not from a known high-risk group for infection with *M. tb.*, the skin test need not be repeated.

(5) **Evaluation**

(a) **Positive PPD.** A positive skin test should prompt the physician to ask two basic questions. First, is there any evidence that the patient has active tuberculosis? Second, if there is no evidence of active tuberculosis, is the patient a candidate for INH prophylaxis? The first question can usually be answered by the clinical examination and the chest radiograph. The answer to the second question is more complex, involving the integration of the patient's age, chest radiograph findings, underlying diseases that might increase the risk of developing active disease, and the patient's perception of risk of immediate disease from INH versus future disease from tuberculosis [12].

(b) **Contacts of cases.** A special circumstance arises in the evaluation of recent close or household contacts with a case of active pulmonary tuberculosis. These individuals are at risk for progressive primary disease and should receive close monitoring with frequent (initially and at 3 months following exposure) skin testing, symptom checks, and radiograph, when indicated by symptoms or positive skin test. In addition, young children should receive INH prophylaxis for 3 months even if the initial skin test is negative [6].

b. **Chest radiograph.** The chest radiograph is essential for the proper evaluation of individuals with a positive skin test for tuberculosis. It helps to identify those with active disease and those with old, healed disease of sufficient extent to place them at high risk of reactivation disease. Individuals with a positive skin test and a stable, abnormal chest radiograph (nonprogressive previous disease) should receive INH prophylaxis unless a contraindication exists, regardless of age [6, 13]. Those with abnormal radiographs and symptoms of active disease should be evaluated with sputum examination and culture and a follow-up radiograph in 3–6 months, and should be started on two or three antituberculosis agents pending culture and sensitivity data. Those with normal radiographs and no indications of active tuberculosis should be considered for prophylaxis if under the age of 35 years [6, 13]. Some authors suggest that INH prophylaxis is beneficial regardless of age, based on decision analysis of the age question [7, 13].

A single radiograph at the time of discovery of a positive skin test is sufficient for classification of extent of disease. Yearly chest radiography is no longer recommended for follow-up of the positive reactor, since it is not sensitive for detecting reactivation disease (most cases come to medical attention as a result of symptoms), and is very expensive when applied to large numbers of infected individuals.

2. Justification

a. The skin test

(1) Test characteristics. The intermediate (5 tuberculin units, or TU PPD) intradermal skin test for tuberculosis is 85% or greater sensitive and specific for prior infection with *M. tb.* in otherwise healthy individuals [8–10]. False-positives ($\geq$ 10 mm induration) occur in some individuals who have had prior infection with nontuberculous mycobacteria or who have received BCG [8]. False-negatives occur for a variety of reasons, including improper application of the test, decreased potency of the tuberculin used, improper reading of the test, and patient factors including *M. tb.* infection many years prior to skin testing, recent viral infections, metabolic and nutritional derangements, immunosuppression, and malignancies [8, 10].

(2) Risks. Injection of PPD may cause a large (> 5 cm) area of induration, or may produce vesiculation of the skin. Such large reactions resolve slowly, especially the discoloration [11]. Patients should be warned to return immediately if the reaction appears to be very large or is beginning to vesiculate. Immediate application of a concentrated fluorinated corticosteroid cream topically to the site may help to limit the reaction. An individual who has had a severe reaction to PPD in the past is likely to have a similar reaction if PPD is applied again.

(3) Costs. The PPD skin test costs approximately $10 to administer and to interpret in office settings when included as part of a routine visit or evaluation for possible tuberculosis. Costs are lower when mass screening is done.

(4) Acceptability. The skin test is a benign procedure that is readily accepted by most patients. Multiple puncture techniques are somewhat easier to administer and can be read at home, but are less sensitive and specific than intradermal testing. An experienced individual can administer the PPD quickly and with minimal discomfort.

b. Chest radiograph

(1) Test characteristics. The chest radiograph is a sensitive method for detection of persons at higher risk of reactivation disease. The presence of visible scarring compatible with tuberculosis in an individual with a positive skin test defines a population 5–10 times more likely to develop clinical tuberculosis in the future than a skin test-positive individual with a normal radiograph [3, 6]. Radiographic abnormalities are not specific for granulomatous disease due to tuberculosis, however. Tumors, scarring from other causes, acute bacterial or viral infections, and other entities may resemble tuberculosis changes closely.

(2) Risks. A single chest radiograph is essentially without medical risk. Even in the pregnant woman, the dose of radiation received by the fetus, using modern equipment and film and abdominal shielding, is exceedingly small.

(3) Costs. The radiograph costs approximately $75–100 for performance and interpretation.

(4) Acceptability. The radiograph is noninvasive, painless, and carries virtually no risk, so is acceptable to the majority of patients and physicians. Misunderstandings regarding the radiation dose received are due to unfamiliarity with modern methods.

B. Early intervention

1. Methods

a. Isoniazid prophylaxis. All persons previously infected with *M. tb.* (by definition those with a significant tuberculosis skin test reaction) are at risk of developing tuberculosis at some time during their lives—either progressive primary (occurring within 1-2 years of infection) or reactivation tuberculosis (occurring years after infection). The degree of risk is related to factors that decrease the ability of cell-mediated immunity to contain the growth of the organism within well-organized granulomata [6] (see Table 96-2).

Isoniazid (INH) prophylaxis should be considered for infected individuals having one or more of the risk factors listed in Table 96-2 **or** who are less than 35 years of age.

A history of prior antituberculosis drug treatment or prophylaxis should be sought and, when elicited, evaluated for adequacy. If adequate, no further therapy is needed. Adequate treatment for active disease must have included at least two drugs (INH should be one of them) for 18 months, or INH plus rifampin for at least 9–12 months. If INH prophylaxis was given, it should have consisted of a daily or twice weekly regimen for at least 6 months for persons with a normal radiograph or 9–12 months for those with stable granulomatous changes on radiograph.

The decision to recommend INH prophylaxis involves five major considerations. First, is the patient at appreciable risk for disease [7, 13]? Second, if the patient is given INH is it likely that he or she will reliably recognize and report symptoms of serious hepatitis and return immediately for evaluation? Third, does the patient have risk factors for developing severe hepatitis? Fourth, if INH prophylaxis was not given, electing instead to monitor for symptoms of tuberculous disease, would the patient be able to recognize such symptoms and seek medical evaluation? Finally, does the patient have active tuberculosis? "Yes" answers to the first two questions favor giving prophylaxis. "Yes" answers to any of the last three questions weigh against giving prophylaxis in patients at low risk of developing active disease.

Active tuberculosis must be ruled out because failure to administer at least two drugs to which the patient's *M. tb.* isolate is susceptible frequently leads to INH resistance and failure of therapy.

If the decision is made to give INH prophylaxis, it should be given at a dosage of 300 mg/day in adults. Pyridoxine 50 mg can be given concomitantly to persons at risk for neurotoxicity or who complain of paresthesias or hypesthesia during therapy. Patients with a normal chest roentgenogram are probably adequately treated with a 6-month course. Those with stable abnormalities on chest roentgenogram should receive INH for 12 months [14]. INH should be dispensed on a monthly basis and persons receiving INH should be questioned monthly, either in person or by telephone, to elicit symptoms of hepatitis. These include unexplained anorexia, nausea, vomiting, fatigue, weakness, fever or epigastric or right upper quadrant pain and tenderness exceeding 3 days in duration, dark urine, or icterus. The patient should be given a written list of the symptoms and signs of hepatitis, and it should be posted where he or she stores the INH, for quick reference. Additionally, symptoms of frequent headache, paresthesias of hands and feet, irritability, drowsiness, and confusion should be sought. If symptoms of hepatitis are elicited, the INH should be stopped and liver function tests should be obtained immediately. An elevation in SGOT of 3 to 5 times normal should prompt discontinuation of INH. Additionally, in monitoring patients over the age of 35, baseline and periodic SGOT determinations (e.g., monthly) should be obtained. An SGOT elevation 3 to 5 times above baseline probably warrants discontinuation of INH. Finally, patients should report symptoms of hepatitis immediately if they occur between monthly evaluations, and the patient should be assessed as above for INH-induced hepatitis [6].

b. BCG. Immunization with live bacille Calmette-Guérin is not recommended in the United States [6].

2. Justification

a. INH

(1) Effectiveness of INH prophylaxis. INH taken regularly for 6–12 months appears to reduce the incidence of disease in infected persons by 60–80% [4, 6–7, 13, 14]. In addition, by preventing reactivation it prevents subsequent tuberculous infection in individuals who would be exposed when reactivation occurs [7].

(2) Risks and side effects. With careful monitoring, the benefits of INH prophylaxis clearly outweigh the risks in most infected individuals [7, 13]. Side effects are relatively common with INH, but are usually mild and can be ameliorated by adjustments in the timing of the dose (for nausea, CNS side effects of drowsiness, confusion) or by adding pyridoxine (for peripheral neuropathy). Toxicities of a serious nature from INH are relatively rare. These include severe hepatitis, arthritis, and seizures, among others. The risk of severe or fatal hepatitis may have been overestimated [7].

Some individuals are at increased risk for INH toxicities and either should not be given it or should be given it with very close supervision: those with active liver disease (elevated serum liver enzymes), heavy alcohol use, or age of 35 years or older, which predispose to INH hepatitis; or those with conditions that might predispose to peripheral neuropathy, such as diabetes mellitus or alcoholism. Possible drug interactions should be evaluated prior to beginning prophylaxis [6]. Women at risk for pregnancy should be counseled against becoming pregnant during INH prophylaxis even though the drug has not been shown to be teratogenic or to increase the risk of spontaneous abortion.

(3) **Costs.** The cost of INH prophylaxis is appreciable. INH itself is inexpensive ($15/year), but evaluation of the positive skin test with a chest roentgenogram ($75–100), monthly monitoring ($5–20/month), evaluating possible hepatitis ($20), and other side effects of INH add greatly to the cost of evaluation and prophylaxis. For these reasons, it is usually preferable to refer the patient to the local county health department for roentgenogram, evaluation, prophylaxis, and monitoring whenever possible.

(4) **Acceptability.** Approximately 20–50% of individuals who are begun on INH prophylaxis fail to complete it, either because of side effects or noncompliance. Careful explanation of the reasons for prophylaxis and the expected benefits, and a willingness to work with the patient to minimize bothersome side effects help to reduce this failure rate. Public health departments are usually more successful in getting a patient through a course of INH prophylaxis than is the general practitioner.

b. **BCG.** BCG is not recommended in the United States. There are several strains of varying potency and effectiveness, and immunization may interfere with subsequent interpretation of PPD skin tests, an important tool in the strategy for containment of tuberculosis in the United States [1, 2, 6].

IV. Recommendations

A. Primary prevention

1. Detect infected individuals and evaluate for INH prophylaxis.
2. Maintain a high index of suspicion for active pulmonary tuberculosis in the presence of a compatible clinical picture.
3. BCG is not recommended for use in United States populations.

B. Secondary prevention

1. Early detection

a. Skin test all adults without definite history of positive or negative skin test in the previous 5 years. Use two-step skin test procedure in individuals over age 50.

b. Perform chest radiograph on individuals found to be positive on skin testing or who have had recent household or close contact exposure to active pulmonary disease.

c. Perform repeat skin testing at appropriate intervals (1–2 years at a routine visit) on individuals at high risk for tuberculous infection. These include direct patient care hospital personnel and residents of nursing homes or institutions.

2. Early intervention

a. Evaluate tuberculin reactors for INH prophylaxis—indications versus risks of toxicity.

b. Refer to county health department for INH therapy if it is indicated.

c. Administer INH 300 mg PO qd for 6 months to tuberculin reactors with normal chest radiograph and no history of clinical tuberculosis.

d. Administer INH 300 mg PO qd for 12 months to individuals with abnormal chest radiograph (quiescent disease) or history of clinical tuberculosis.

e. Give pyridoxine concomitantly to patients with risk factors for peripheral neuropathy or who develop symptoms of neuropathy during therapy with INH.

f. Assess the patient monthly for symptoms of hepatitis. Obtain SGOT if symptoms develop.

g. On persons over age 35 or persons with chronic liver disease or alcoholism who receive INH prophylaxis, also obtain baseline and periodic SGOT determinations for the duration of therapy.

h. Discontinue INH if the SGOT value in recommendation **f.** or **g.** above exceeds 3–5 times the normal/baseline or if worsening symptoms of hepatitis occur.

i. In recently infected young children or others at extremely high risk of disease, use alternative prophylactic regimen if INH is too toxic (serious hepatitis) or intolerable.

References

1. Des Prez, R. M. and Goodwin, R. A. Jr. Mycobacterium Tuberculosis. In G. L. Mandell, R. G. Douglas, Jr., and J. E. Bennett (eds.), *Principles and Practice of Infectious Diseases* (2nd ed.). New York: Wiley, 1985, Pp.1383–1406. *General review of tuberculosis.*
2. Harris, H. W., and McClement, J. H. Pulmonary Tuberculosis. In P.D. Hoeprich (ed.), *Infectious Diseases* (3rd ed.). Philadelphia Harper & Row, 1983. Pp.378–404. *General review of clinically relevant information.*
3. US Public Health Service, Centers for Disease Control, Tuberculosis Control Division. Tuberculosis, final data—United States, 1986. *M. M. W. R.* 36(50, 51):817, 1988. *Statistics on incidence, prevalence, demographics, etc., of tuberculous infection and disease. Except for a slowing in the rate of decline due to an influx of Southeast Asian refugees to the United States, and now an increase due to reactivation TB among HIV-infected persons, there has been a steady decline in the incidence of tuberculous disease in the United States for decades.*
4. Stead, W. W., et al. Tuberculosis as an endemic and nosocomial infection among the elderly in nursing homes. *N. Eng. J. Med.* 312(23):1483, 1985. *Documents a high incidence of new infection and reactivation disease in nursing home patients.*
5. Tuberculosis among migrant farm workers—Virginia. *M. M. W. R.* 35(29):467, 1986. *MMWR often has updates on clinically and epidemiologically important features of tuberculosis.*
6. Bass, J. B., et al. Treatment of tuberculosis and tuberculous infection in adults and children. *Am. Rev. Respir. Dis.* 134(2):355, 1986. *ATS official statement. Concise recommendations for prophylaxis of tuberculous infections in adults.*
7. Comstock, G. W. Prevention of tuberculosis among tuberculin reactors: Maximizing benefits, minimizing risks. *J. A. M. A.* 256(19):2729, 1986. *An excellent discussion of the philosophic and scientific basis of prophylaxis.*
8. Comstock, G. W., et al. The tuberculin skin test. *Am. Rev. Respir. Dis.* 124:356, 1981. *ATS official statement. The most recent statement of the ATS on the use of tuberculin skin testing.*
9. Chaparas, S. D., et al. Tuberculin test. Variability with the Mantoux procedure. *Am. Rev. Respir. Dis.* 132(1):175, 1985. *Sensitivity, specificity, and reproducibility of the Mantoux skin test. Accompanying editorial by J. Sbarbaro.*
10. Snider, D. E. Jr. The tuberculin skin test. *Am. Rev. Respir. Dis.* 125(3:2):108, 1982. *A more in-depth discussion of TB skin testing and its history.*
11. Caplin, M. *The Tuberculin Test in Clinical Practice: An Illustrated Guide.* London: Bailliere-Tindall, 1980. *Practical information on the application and interpretation of the PPD skin test.*
12. Taylor, W. C., Aronson, M. D., and Delbanco, T. L. Should young adults with a positive tuberculin test take isoniazid? *Ann. Intern. Med.* 94(6):808, 1981. *Disagrees with ATS recommendation for INH prophylaxis in young adults with a positive PPD skin test as the only manifestation of TB infection.*
13. Rose, D. N., Schechter, C. B., and Silver, A. L. The age threshold for isoniazid chemoprophylaxis. A decision analysis for low-risk tuberculin reactors. *J. A. M. A.* 256(19):2709, 1986. *A reaffirmation of the utility of prophylaxis in low-risk adults. Accompanying editorial by G. W. Comstock (ref. 7) makes several important points.*
14. Snider, D. E., Caras, G. J., and Koplan, J. P. Preventive therapy with isoniazid. Cost-effectiveness of different durations of therapy. *J. A. M. A.* 255(12):1579, 1986. *Courses of prophylaxis of 6–12 months measurably reduce the incidence of active tuberculosis after infection.*

97 Gonorrhea

Dewey Sandberg

I. The problem

A. Description. The spectrum of disease caused by *Neisseria gonorrhoeae* ranges from asymptomatic infections of the urogenital tract, rectum, or pharynx to acute, symptomatic infections of these same sites, with or without local complications. Disseminated gonococcal infection can give rise to arthritis, meningitis, endocarditis, and septicemia.

Infection with gonococcus requires that a viable inoculum of this relatively fragile organism come into contact with a mucous membrane where adherance, mediated by pili and surface proteins, is followed by tissue invasion and, usually, a rather brisk inflammatory response. The course of the disease varies, depending on both host and pathogen, from a self-limiting to a devastating systemic infection [1].

B. Epidemiology [2, 3]. The incidence of gonorrhea in the United States has increased rapidly from 1960, when about 260,000 cases were reported, to its peak in 1979 of over a million reported cases, or about 460/100,000. The incidence has declined slowly since then to its present level of about 900,000 cases annually; a rate of 375/100,000. It is important to note, also, that it is estimated that fewer than half of all cases treated are reported. There is a slight male preponderance, with about 60% of infections reported in men.

Gonococcal infections can occur in anyone, at any age, in a number of sites, but a few clinical patterns account for most of the cases. In men, acute anterior urethritis is the most common manifestation. Complicated, ascending infections of the male genital tract are uncommon since the advent of antibiotics. In heterosexual men, anorectal infections rarely, if ever, occur, and pharyngeal infections can be found in 3–7% of cases. Homosexual men have the same penile manifestations, but higher rates of anorectal (35–50%) and pharyngeal (10–25%) infections contributing to the total number of cases.

In women, the endocervical canal is the primary site of infection, though the urethra will also usually be colonized. Unlike males, in which ascending infection is rare, pelvic inflammatory disease (PID) accounts for about 10% of the cases of gonorrhea in females. Nearly 70% of these are under 24 years of age; hence the profound consequences for future fertility [4]. Anorectal infections occur in about 35–50% of women with gonorrhea—this does not seem to be due to anal intercourse but rather to perineal contamination. Pharyngeal infection, usually asymptomatic, occurs in as many as 20% of women with gonorrhea and is attributed to fellatio.

Pregnancy does not seem to change the risk of infection, but reduces the risk of PID and increases the risk of pharyngeal infection. Urogenital tract infection in pregnancy can profoundly complicate the course and outcome of pregnancy [1] (see Chap. 16).

Gonorrhea in children is indicative of sexual abuse until proved otherwise, is not a screening issue, and so is beyond the scope of this discussion.

There is disagreement in the literature on the percentage of cases that are asymptomatic. It is estimated that 20–60% of males with urethral colonization are asymptomatic, 40–60% of females with urogenital tract infections, and 40–90% of anorectal infections in women and homosexual men. These estimates of asymptomatic carrier rates suggest a large reservoir of infection [1,5].

Mortality due to gonorrhea is rare. Fewer than 10 deaths/year are attributed to gonorrhea in the United States [2].

High risk groups for gonorrhea infection include individuals who are young (16–24 years old), poor, single, urban dwellers, with early experience with sex, or prior history of gonorrhea or other sexually transmitted disease. Male homosexuals are also at high risk [3].

II. Primary prevention.

Primary prevention. Primary prevention is a consideration in gonorrhea. While abstinence is the only entirely effective way to prevent gonorrhea, risk can be reduced by observing such precautions as avoidance of multiple partners, anonymous partners, prostitutes, and others with multiple sex partners or with genital discharge or lesions [6]. Use of condoms and diaphragms, in combination with vaginal spermicides, has been studied and may be effective in preventing sexually transmitted diseases [7, 8].

III. Secondary prevention

A. Early detection

1. Methods

a. Description. The diagnosis of gonorrhea is made by culture on a selective medium. Modified Thayer-Martin is the generally accepted medium.

b. Performance. Urethral cultures from men are obtained by inserting a fine calcium alginate swab approximately 2 cm into the anterior urethra and inoculating on culture medium.

Endocervical cultures are obtained by exposing the cervix with a bivalve speculum, without the use of commercial lubricants, cleansing the cervix of adherent mucus, and inserting a sterile cotton-tipped swab into the endocervical canal. The swab is twirled for several seconds within the canal and then inoculated on culture medium.

Rectal cultures are performed by inserting a cotton-tipped applicator 2.5 cm into the anal canal, taking care to avoid contamination with feces, and inoculating on culture medium.

Pharyngeal cultures may be performed by swabbing the tonsils and posterior pharynx [9].

c. Interpretation. Growth of small, mucoid colonies of oxidase-positive, gram-negative diplococci on gonococcus-selective media is reported as positive for *N. gonorrhoeae.* While this is correct in 97% of urogenital specimens, several other *Neisseria* species, notably *N. meningitidis,* grow from specimens collected from other sites. Therefore, specimens collected from the rectum or oropharynx, or from any site in children, must have confirmatory tests that they are indeed gonococcus [10].

d. Interval/timing. Except in pregnancy, there is no routine screening schedule for gonorrhea.

e. Population. Routine screening for gonorrhea in the general population is not indicated [11]. There are groups of patients, however, that do merit special attention.

There is general consensus that expectant mothers must have a screening endocervical culture for gonorrhea at the first prenatal visit. Women at high risk for sexually transmitted disease should have a repeat culture late in the third trimester [12] (see Chap. 16).

There is less agreement on screening other groups. It has become common practice to test asymptomatic patients in the high-risk groups mentioned above, sexually active individuals with multiple partners, and those seeking care in public sexually transmitted disease (STD) clinics. It has been proposed that the asymptomatic male represents the most important reservoir in the population, and that rather than emphasizing only treatment of symptomatic men and detection of asymptomatic women, more effort should be concentrated on finding and culturing asymptomatic male contacts of women at high risk—women with frequent repeated infections or with pelvic inflammatory disease [5]. This and other approaches to screening have not been investigated to the point where recommendations can be made. An important distinction to make at this point is that individuals exposed to known cases of gonorrhea within the past 30 days should be examined, cultured, and treated prophylactically [6]. Treatment is given before culture results are known.

In summary, testing contacts of high-risk individuals is a reasonable practice, but pregnant women remain the only group clearly requiring routine screening.

2. Justification

a. Test characteristics. Cultures done with selective media, from most anatomic sites, have sensitivities of 80–95%, a predictive value positive of 95–100%, and remain the standard for screening.

Gram-stained smears, while very sensitive and specific in men with symptomatic urethritis, are inadequate for any screening exam [1].

Gonozyme, a solid-phase enzyme immunoassay, with sensitivity of 85–100% and specificity of over 90% (based on a standard of modified Thayer-Martin, a 80–90% sensitive test) compares favorably with culture. The predictive value positive is over 80% in a high-prevalence population, but in an asymptomatic, low-prevalence population is as low as 31.9% [13]. Gonozyme has not been advanced as a substitute for culture in asymptomatic individuals.

b. **Cost, risks, and acceptability.** The screening culture is generally accepted by the patient and physicians, cost approximately $18–43 (average $32, Sacramento, 1986), and risks are negligible.

B. Early intervention

1. Methods [6]

a. **Treatment** of uncomplicated gonococcal infections of the urethra, endocervix, and rectum also includes treatment for coexisting chlamydial infection, which may be assumed to be present, except in homosexual men.

Use amoxicillin (3.0 gm) or ampicillin (3.5 gm) PO, or aqueous procaine penicillin G (4.8 million U IM), or ceftriaxone (250 mg IM) as a single dose. Except when ceftriaxone is used, probenecid (1.0 gm PO) should accompany the antibiotic.

In addition, tetracycline HCl (500 mg PO) qid for 7 daysx, or doxycycline (100 mg PO) bid for 7 days is given for coverage for chlamydia infection, regardless of whether such infection was sought or found. In pregnancy and lactation (see Chap. 16), and for other patients in whom tetracyclines are contraindicated or not tolerated, erythromycin base (500 mg) or erythromycin ethylsuccinate (800 mg) PO qid for 7 days should be given for chlamydia coverage. Chlamydia infection has been documented in up to 45% of gonorrhea cases, except in homosexual men where the rate is much lower (see Chap. 99). Therefore, homosexual men do not require presumptive coverage for chlamydia.

Spectinomycin (2.0 gm IM) may be used in patients allergic to penicillin.

Regarding rectal infection, although these regimens are effective in women, homosexual men with rectal gonorrhea should receive aqueous procaine penicillin G (4.8 million units IM) plus probenecid (1.0 gm PO) or ceftriaxone (250 mg IM), or, in penicillin-allergic patients, spectinomycin (2.0 gm IM).

b. **Follow-up.** When a diagnosis of gonorrhea is made, every effort should be made to identify, locate, and promptly evaluate the patient's sex partners. Most local health departments offer STD patient referral and follow-up services through disease intervention specialists who are trained to deal with this often sensitive situation. Anyone exposed to gonorrhea within the past 30 days should be examined, cultured, and treated prophylactically with a regimen to cover gonorrhea and chlamydial infections. Individuals being treated for gonorrhea should be urged to abstain from sexual contact until a posttreatment culture confirms a cure [4].

Syphilis serology should be tested in all patients who are treated for gonorrhea (see Chap. 98, Syphilis, for further recommendations).

Gonococcal infections are notifiable diseases in many states. In such states, reporting is required by law. It may be done by phone, letter, or with pre-prepared postcards.

A test-of-cure, or repeat culture, should be obtained from the infected sites 3–7 days after completion of treatment, or 4–7 days if the patient received doxycycline. Rectal cultures should be obtained from all women (including pregnant women) after treatment for gonorrhea, regardless of whether rectal infection was sought or found prior to therapy.

Treatment failures require further treatment. If gonorrhea persists after treatment, spectinomycin (2.0 gm IM) should be used. If spectinomycin was used initially, ceftriaxone (250 mg IM) is recommended. Recurrent infection is commonly due to failure to find and treat the patient's partners. Two forms of penicillin resistance have been described: penicillinase-producing *N. gonorrhoeae* and chromosomally mediated resistant *N. gonorrhoeae*. All posttreatment isolates should be tested for antimicrobial sensitivity; lack of beta-lactamase production does not ensure penicillin sensitivity.

Culture and treatment of victims of rape and incest are certainly vital to their care, but are beyond the scope of this discussion.

2. Justification

a. **Effectiveness.** There is little information on the effectiveness of screening and treatment of asymptomatic infection in pregnancy; but one study [14] estimated that about 28% of prenatal patients with untreated gonorrhea developed complications of pregnancy, compared with 5.8% of treated cases, and 4% of patients with negative cultures. No study has shown that screening for gonorrhea reduces the incidence of complication in other categories of patients [11].

Table 97-1. Costs of antibiotics for treatment of gonorrhea*

Antibiotic	Dosage	Cost ($)
Amoxicillin	3.0 gm (PO)	7.00
Ampicillin	3.5 gm (PO)	5.50
Ceftriaxone	250 mg (IM)	13.50
Aqueous procaine penicillin G	4.8 million U (IM)	16.00
Spectinomycin	2.0 gm (IM)	15.00
Erythromycin base	250 mg #56 (7-day course) (PO)	11.00
EES	400 mg #56 (7-day course) (PO)	16.50

*Average costs in Sacramento, CA, 1986.

b. **Risks.** Assuming that antibiotic allergies are taken into account, the risk of new allergic reactions, gastrointestinal upset, and other mild intolerances of antibiotics are the same as for any application of antimicrobial and are generally accepted as outweighed by the benefits of treatment. Although the manufacturers of these medications note that safety for use in pregnancy has not been established, many organizations, including the Centers for Disease Control and American College of Obstetricians and Gynecologists, recommend their use as outlined above.

c. **Costs.** The costs of the recommended dosages of antibiotics are included in Table 97-1 (average costs in Sacramento, California, 1986).

d. **Acceptability.** The single-dose treatment of gonorrhea is particularly acceptable by most patients and physicians. The pain and greater allergic risks caused by the intramuscular injection of aqueous procaine penicillin G makes it less desirable in some instances. The 7 days of treatment required for presumed chlamydia infection creates a compliance problem for some patients.

IV. Recommendations

A. Primary prevention. Abstinence and, more realistically, reduced-risk sexual practices are the options for prevention of gonorrhea infection. Use of vaginal spermicides in combination with a barrier method has been suggested as possibly effective in preventing sexually transmitted diseases.

B. Secondary prevention

1. Early detection

a. All pregnant women should have an endocervical culture for *N. gonorrhoeae* during the first prenatal visit.

b. A second culture should be done late in the third trimester on all women at high risk.

c. Consideration may be given to the common practice of screening of high-risk individuals and contacts of high-risk individuals, but it does not meet the criteria for an effective screening test and is therefore nor clearly indicated.

2. Early intervention

a. Uncomplicated gonococcal infections of the urethra, endocervix, or rectum should be treated with oral amoxicillin or ampicillin PO, or IM aqueous procaine penicillin G, with probenecid, or with ceftriaxone, in a single dose.

b. Tetracycline or doxycycline should be given by mouth for a 7-day course to cover chlamydia infection, which may be assumed to be present in all adults treated for gonorrhea, except homosexual men.

c. Spectinomycin may be used in patients allergic to penicillin.

d. Erythromycin should be used for chlamydia coverage in pregnant women and other patients in whom tetracyclines are contraindicated or not tolerated. Tetracycline and doxycycline should not be used in women who are pregnant or nursing.

e. Homosexual men with rectal gonococcal infection should receive IM aqueous procaine penicillin G with probenecid PO, or IM ceftriaxone. No chlamydia coverage is needed.

f. Trace and treat prophylactically all sexual contacts of known cases of gonorrhea. The local health department may be very helpful in this task.

g. Advise patients being treated for gonorrhea to abstain from sexual contact until a repeat culture proves a cure.

h. Test syphilis serology in all patients being treated for gonorrhea.
i. Confirmatory tests should be done on all positive cultures from nonurogenital sites.
j. Report gonorrhea cases if required by state law.
k. Obtain posttreatment culture of the infected site 3–7 days after completion of treatment; 4–7 days if doxycycline was used.
l. Rectal cultures should be obtained from all women in the follow-up exam, even if no rectal infection was initially suspected or confirmed.
m. Gonorrhea persisting after treatment should be treated with spectinomycin or ceftriaxone.
n. All posttreatment isolates of gonococcus should be tested for antimicrobial sensitivity.
o. Recurrent gonorrhea should prompt increased efforts to trace sexual contacts and to ensure patient education about sexually transmitted disease.

References

1. Handsfield, H. H. Gonorrhea and Uncomplicated Gonococcal Infection. In K. K. Holmes, et al. (eds.), *Sexually Transmitted Diseases.* New York: McGraw-Hill, 1984. Pp.205-220. *A thorough text that includes detailed discussions of all aspects of gonococcal infections.*
2. 1984 annual summary. Reported morbidity and mortality in the United States. *M. M. W. R.* 33(54):1, 1986. *Contains statistics on gonorrhea infections since 1945.*
3. Hook, E. W. 3d, and Holmes, K. K. Gonococcal infections. *Ann. Intern. Med.* 102(2):229, 1985. *A broad-scoped review of clinical aspects of gonococcal infection.*
4. State of California, Department of Health Services. Pelvic inflammatory disease in California. *Calif. Morbidity* No.8, 1983. *A brief discussion of epidemiology of pelvic inflammatory disease.*
5. Potterat, J. J. and King, R. D. A new approach to gonorrhea control. *J. A. M. A.* 245(6):578, 1981. *Results of a public health intervention employing a control strategy based on removing asymptomatic men from the disease reservoir.*
6. 1985 STD (Sexually Transmitted Disease). Treatment guidelines. *M. M. W. R.* 34(4s Suppl):75s, 1985. *CDC guidelines for treatment of sexually transmitted disease. A very useful reference, frequently updated. Contains a short discussion of public health considerations.*
7. Jick, H., et al. Vaginal spermicides and gonorrhea. *J. A. M. A.* 248(13):1619, 1982. *A study suggesting a protective effect of vaginal spermicides against gonorrhea.*
8. Cates, W. Jr, Weisner, P. J., and Curran, J. W. Sex and spermicides; Preventing unintended pregnancy and infection. (editorial) *J. A. M. A.* 248(13):1636, 1982. *An editorial by noted authorities on the use of spermicides and their potential for preventing sexually transmitted diseases.*
9. Riccardi, N. B., and Felman, Y. M. Laboratory diagnosis in the problem of suspected gonococcal infection. *J. A. M. A.* 242(24):2703, 1979. *A review of the various techniques, culture media, and culture systems available for laboratory diagnosis.*
10. State of California, Department of Health Services. Reliability of presumptive-positive reports on culture of genito-urinary tract specimens for gonorrhea. *Calif. Morbidity* No. 48, 1983. *A clarification of the significance of nongonococcal* Neisseria *species, and the circumstances under which confirmatory tests are needed.*
11. Frame, P. S. A critical review of adult health maintenance. Part 2. Prevention of infectious diseases. *J. Fam. Pract.* 22(5):417, 1986. *An update of the landmark series published in 1975. Vitally important reading for all primary care physicians.*
12. *Gonorrhea and Chlamydial Infections.* Chicago: ACOG Technical Bulletin No. 89, November 1985. *American College of Obstetricians and Gynecologists recommendation for screening and management of gonorrhea and chlamydial infections.*
13. Bronken, T. P., Dyke, J. W., and Andruszewski, M. H. A solid-phase enzyme immunoassay in detection of cervical gonorrhea in a low-prevalence population. *J. Fam. Pract.* 20(1):43, 1985. *A comparison of Gonozyme with culture on modified Thayer-Martin medium in diagnosing cervical gonorrhea in a population with low prevalence of gonorrhea.*
14. Charles, A.G., et al. Asymptomatic gonorrhea in prenatal patients. *Am. J. Obstet. Gynecol.* 108(4):595, 1970. *A study of asymptomatic gonorrhea in pregnant women.*

98 Syphilis

Neil Flynn

I. The problem

A. Definition. Syphilis is a "disease of many faces," the "great imitator." Infection with *Treponema pallidum* produces a plethora of signs, symptoms, and organ dysfunctions collectively referred to as syphilis. Tissue injury is produced both by the proliferation of the organism and by the tissue and immune reactions to it [1].

B. Description. The current system of classification of syphilis is based on the duration of infection and the organ system manifesting disease [2–4, 6, 7] (Table 98-1). Ten days to 3 months after inoculation of *T. pallidum* onto genital mucosa or adjacent skin, or oral or rectal mucosa, a painless, indurated, primary chancre develops at the site of entry of the organism. The base of the chancre is teeming with spirochetes. Half of chancres may be atypical in some way, particularly if extragenital [7]. Over the ensuing weeks to months, the infection disseminates to regional lymph nodes, leading to enlargement, and then systemically, producing the manifestations of secondary syphilis in varying combinations: anorexia, malaise, sore throat, headache, rashes and a wide variety of skin lesions, fever, night sweats, generalized adenopathy, nephrotic syndrome, hepatitis, or alopecia [3, 4, 7]. A significant fraction of infected individuals have no discernible secondary phase.

The secondary phase may last up to several months and then gradually subsides. Any organ system may become infected, setting the stage for later tertiary manifestations in that organ. The infection then enters the so-called early latent phase, which is usually defined as the first 1–2 years after infection. Secondary signs and symptoms may recur occasionally during the early latent phase [3]. Infection may remain clinically silent for life (latent), or may manifest as organ dysfunction (secondary or tertiary syphilis). In the preantibiotic era, approximately 15–40% of untreated patients developed late (tertiary) complications of syphilis [8, 9].

C. Epidemiology. The incidence of tertiary disease is low and declining. The use of antibiotics active against *T. pallidum* for intercurrent infections (e.g., cellulitis, pharyngitis) as well as widespread screening of high-risk populations with nontreponemal tests for syphilis (NTTSs), has probably resulted in a decrease in the late (tertiary) manifestations of syphilis [2]. Transmission of syphilis occurs almost exclusively through unprotected sexual exposure to an individual in the primary, secondary, or early latent phase of infection. CDC estimates that more than 30,000 Americans become infected with *T. pallidum* yearly [10]. In recent decades, at least one-third of infections occurred among gay men, but the incidence has recently fallen dramatically in this group as a result of precautions taken to avoid AIDS [11, 12] (see Chap. 100). Most cases of primary and secondary syphilis occur in sexually active adolescents and young adults (ages 15–30 years).

II. Primary prevention methods and justification

A. Education. Health education of adolescents, sexually active adults, and persons at particularly high risk of acquiring syphilis (e.g., promiscuous homosexual men and heterosexual men and women), emphasizing use of condoms and reduction in the number of sexual partners, is an effective method for the prevention of infection with *T. pallidum.* However, it is considered offensive by a vocal and influential minority who believe that discussion and education promote promiscuous behavior, and so education has not been used to full advantage. The rate of sexually transmitted diseases (STD), including syphilis, has declined dramatically in the gay male population, presumably the result of vigorous educational campaigns to educate gay men about AIDS, but is increasing among heterosexuals [10–12].

The primary care practitioner should ascertain the sexual habits of his or her patients and counsel them accordingly on the use of condoms for prevention of transmission of all STDs, including syphilis.

B. Detection and treatment of infectious persons. Detection and treatment of individuals

Table 98-1. Various classifications and treatment of infection with *T. Pallidum* [2, 3, 5, 9, 10, 14]

Stage	Definition	Lab test results	Organ systems involved	Recommended Rx	Comments
Primary syphilis[a]	From infection to appearance of secondary signs and symptoms or disappearance of primary chancre. Usually < 3 months.	Darkfield exam positive in nearly all patients if repeated 3 times. NTTS may be negative for up to 40 days, or longer if concomitantly infected with HIV.	Integument at site of inoculation, regional lymph nodes.	2.4 million units benzathine penicillin G IM x 1 **or** tetracycline **or** erythromycin 500 mg PO qid for 15 days. Doxycycline 100 mg bid following meals, for 15 days, may be better tolerated than tetracycline.	Darkfield exam should be performed by experienced technician. Oral lesions may contain nonsyphilis treponemes (false positive darkfield).
Secondary syphilis[a]	Presence of signs and symptoms usually associated with secondary syphilis; variation extremely wide.	NTTS uniformly positive (96–100%) in high titer. MHA-TP and FTA-ABS positive. Specific organ function tests may be abnormal.	Virtually any [15].	Same as for primary syphilis if infection <1 year. Same as for syphilis of >1 year duration if infection >1 year.	Secondary syphilis relapses may occur up to 3–5 years after infection (rare).
Early syphilis[b]	Syphilis of <1 year duration (primary, secondary, or latent infection of <1 year duration).	NTTS & confirmatory tests positive, except very early in primary syphilis.	See above.	Same as for primary syphilis. Persons concomitantly infected with HIV may require more aggressive treatment for cure.	May be difficult to determine elapsed time since infection. If doubt exists, use 3-week regimen below.
Early latent syphilis[a]	Historic or serologic evidence for syphilis, without clinical manifestations, **and** less than 2–4 years since infection, depending on author.	Usually reactive NTTS, reactive treponemal test, normal CSF examination.	No clinical or laboratory evidence of organ dysfunction or injury.	As for early syphilis above, if <1 year after infection. As for syphilis of >1 year duration below, if >1 year or indeterminate time since infection.	Do not confuse with CDC early syphilis classification for treatment.

Late latent syphilis[a]	Historic or serologic evidence for syphilis, without clinical manifestations and >2–4 years since infection, depending on author.	25% negative NTTS, usually reactive treponemal test, normal CSF exam, if done.	No clinical or laboratory evidence of organ dysfunction or injury.	2.4 million units benzathine penicillin G IM weekly x 3 successive weeks **or** tetracycline **or** erythromycin 500 mg PO qid for 30 days. Doxycycline 100 mg PO bid after food may be better tolerated.	Tolerance of tetracycline and erythromycin regimens is poor and compliance must be monitored very closely.
Tertiary syphilis[a]	Clinical or pathological evidence of organ involvement by late syphilis.	May have negative NTTS, usually reactive treponemal test, abnormal tests of organs involved.	Skin, bone, CNS, cardiac valvular, vascular, other viscera.	Same as for "late latent syphilis," except if neurosyphilis is present.	Becoming rare, probably because of incidental treatment of syphilis during other antibiotic therapy.
Late syphilis (syphilis of >1 year duration)[b]	Syphilis of more than 1 year duration, except neurosyphilis.	Up to 25% negative NTTS directly proportional to longer duration of infection.	Same as latent or tertiary above.	As above for late latent syphilis.	LP to exclude neurosyphilis in asymptomatic individuals is controversial [4, 5, 15].
Neurosyphilis, secondary or tertiary[ab]	Evidence of prior syphilitic infection, with CSF abnormality or clinical response to treatment for neurosyphilis.	25% negative serum NTTS; 10% normal CSF (normal cells, protein, and negative VDRL).	Central and peripheral nervous systems—neurological or psychiatric dysfunction.	Aqueous crystalline penicillin G, 2–4 million U IV every 4 hrs for 10 days, followed by benzathine penicillin G IM weekly x 3 **or** aqueous procaine penicillin G, 2.4 million U IM daily **plus** probenecid 500 mg PO qid for 10 days, followed by benzathine penicillin G IM weekly x 3 **or** benzathine penicillin G 2.4 million U IM weekly x 3. Alternative regimens for penicillin allergy are same as for late latent, but failure rate may be high.	Elevated CSF cell count that responds to Rx is best indication of neurosyphilis. Alternative regimens must be closely monitored for effectiveness. Manifestations of neurosyphilis may include depression, psychosis, stroke, dementia, personality change, ataxia, sensorineural disturbances, ocular disturbances, deafness. Thus, careful examination is necessary to exclude neurosyphilis. When in doubt, perform lumbar puncture.

[a]Traditional classification.
[b]U.S. Public Health Service and CDC classification for treatment.

in the infectious stages of syphilis (primary, secondary, and early latent) prevents subsequent spread of syphilis. An infected person may transmit the infection sexually for up to 4 years after infection, though transmission is unlikely after 1–2 years. An infected person exposes, on the average, three partners sexually while in the infectious stages, of whom approximately half become infected themselves [4].

III. Secondary prevention

A. Early detection

1. **Methods.** Early detection of infection with *T. pallidum* is simple and inexpensive. The nontreponemal screening tests for syphilis (e.g., VDRL, RPR) can be performed on serum either as a separate test or, more commonly today, are included in the inexpensive screening panels offered by most clinical laboratories. These tests detect the presence of antibodies in the patient's serum to purified lipid antigens contained in the test mixture.

   Disorders other than syphilis can result in a false-positive test, so the nontreponemal test should be followed by a more confirmatory test for antibody to components of *T. pallidum* itself. Two tests are in common use: the fluorescent treponemal antibody-absorbed (FTA-ABS) test, and the microhemagglutination-*T. pallidum* (MHA-TP) test. In individuals born in the United States, positive reactions on both the nontreponemal antigen test and a treponemal antigen test are considered sufficiently diagnostic of past or present infection with *T. pallidum* to warrant evaluation for therapy [5]. In areas endemic for yaws or pinta, these infections may result in false-positive reactions on both tests. Persons concomitantly infected with HIV may have a negative NTTS despite active secondary syphilis.

   Distinguishing between past, adequately treated infection, and present, latent infection is often difficult. A history of adequate treatment with penicillin or an equivalent antibiotic should be sought. The details of treatment and the response of the VDRL or RPR titer should be evaluated for efficacy of the treatment. Ordinarily, the RPR or VDRL titer of the patient's serum is 1:8 or greater in untreated or inadequately treated early syphilis. There should be at least a four-fold decrease in titer within 6 months of treatment in primary or secondary syphilis (e.g., 1:16 going to 1:4), and eventual (1–2 year) decline in the titer to 1:2 or less. Failure of the titer to decline following treatment, or persistent high titer ($\geq$ 1:8), suggests failure of treatment or reinfection [13].

   In some patients who give no history of specific, adequate treatment for syphilis, the titer is low ($\leq$ 1:8). Most often this occurs in late, latent infection, many years after the initial infection. These patients should receive standard therapy for late, latent infection despite the low titer. Their low ($\leq$ 1:8) RPR or VDRL titer may not decline following therapy. This is not an indication for retreatment unless the NTTS remains reactive > 5 years after treatment. A rise in titer, however, suggests reinfection and the need for treatment [4].

   Screening for syphilis should be performed at intervals that take into account, to some degree, the patient's sexual history. At entry into the practice, most patients without a prior known negative serologic test (NTTS) for syphilis should be tested. Promiscuous individuals who do not routinely use a condom should be tested at least annually and whenever symptoms compatible with syphilis occur, or when another sexually transmitted disease, particularly gonorrhea, is found. Particularly promiscuous individuals, especially promiscuous gay men who do not practice "safe sex" or who have a prior history of syphilis, should be tested every 6–12 months. All recent sexual partners of an individual with early syphilis should be tested and treated. The local public health department is best equipped to do this "contact tracing" and treatment of contacts. Finally, hospitalized patients without a documented history of a prior negative STS should probably be tested [5, 14].

2. **Justification.** The nontreponemal tests for syphilis (NTTS) have an estimated sensitivity of 40% in primary syphilis of less than 30 days' duration, and 96% in syphilis of more than 40 days' duration. Sensitivity in secondary or early latent infection approaches 100%. It falls again in late latent infection to 75% [5, 13].

   Specificity of NTTS in otherwise healthy persons is 99.5% or greater, but in persons with underlying chronic diseases may be as low as 75–85%. The sensitivity of treponemal tests (MHA-TP and FTA-ABS) varies from 100% in secondary syphilis to 94–100% in late, latent infection. Their specificity varies from approximately 80% in ill patients with other underlying diseases to greater than 99% in otherwise healthy individuals [5]. Their predictive value varies with the prevalence of syphilis in the risk population of which the patient is a member. For example, a positive NTTS in a young, otherwise apparently healthy, sexually promiscuous individual is very likely to represent a true positive. A positive test in an older, apparently monogamous, chronically ill individual is more likely to represent a false-positive test related to age or underlying disease, such as a rheumatologic disorder [5]. However, in one study 50% of "false-positive" test results were subsequently considered to have been true positive results based on long-term follow-up of clinical and laboratory parameters [5]. All positive, nontreponemal tests should be confirmed with a specific treponemal test. Even if this is done some of the confirmed positive tests are actually false positive.

There are no risks associated with serologic testing other than the interpersonal problems that often arise from the finding of a confirmed positive test (some of which are false-positive) in an apparently monogamous individual, or in an "exclusive" sexual partnership.

The cost of a NTTS is approximately $15–30 if performed as a single test, but is often included in a screening panel of 20–30 tests available from most clinical laboratories, priced at $20–30. The confirmatory test costs approximately $15–30 from a private or hospital laboratory, but can usually be obtained from the county health department for $10–20.

Acceptability of the test can be problematic when it is ordered as a separate screening test in an individual who denies risk factors for syphilis. Some patients express resentment and embarrassment at the implication that they might have syphilis; hence, the popularity of the automated "screening panel" under such circumstances—the NTTS is seen as incidental by the patient, not as an accusation of promiscuity or infidelity.

B. Early intervention. Primary or secondary syphilis is communicable, so early intervention can prevent further spread of the infection to other sexual partners. Untreated, latent syphilis will eventually lead to serious disease in approximately 15–40% of individuals [8, 9]. Treatment appears to reduce these complications by 80–90%.

Table 98-1 also summarizes treatment of various stages of syphilitic infection as recommended by CDC. Treatment costs are approximately $5/injection of benzathine penicillin, plus the cost of the office visit for injection. Follow-up RPR costs are $15–30. In many United States counties, the local health department will provide treatment and follow-up at a reduced cost or free of charge.

The question often arises as to whether to perform lumbar puncture (LP) in order to examine cerebrospinal fluid for evidence of neurosyphilis. Recently, the technique of decision analysis has been applied to this problem [15]. Factors in favor of performing LP and determining whether CSF abnormalities exist are: (1) the long, asymptomatic incubation period of neurosyphilis; (2) the failure of standard therapy for latent syphilis to eradicate incubating neurosyphilis in up to 10% of cases; (3) the nonspecific and often subtle clinical findings of early neurosyphilis (depression or mild dementia, or neurosensory abnormalities); and (4) the ease and safety of LP. Factors against the routine performance of LP are cost, small but documented complication rates, its lack of sensitivity (< 80%), and the rarity of progression to symptomatic neurosyphilis after standard treatment of latent syphilis [5, 15]. LP should be performed in any patient with a confirmed positive NTTS (MHA-TP or FTA-ABS positive) who: (1) has any neuropsychiatric symptom or finding on examination, (2) may be lost to follow-up and/or who is a poor historian and seems unlikely to relate the history of syphilis to subsequent physicians, (3) is being evaluated for retreatment (presumed treatment failure), (4) is treated with a regimen other than penicillin, or (5) is an infant suspected of having congenital syphilis [5, 15]. LP may not be indicated in an individual with absolutely no neuropsychiatric findings and who will be available for long-term follow-up and/or can be relied on to inform subsequent physicians of his or her prior treatment for syphilis, indefinitely. LP in these patients has a low yield of individuals who will not be cured of neurosyphilis by standard regimens and who will develop neurosyphilis as a result. If the decision is made to perform LP, and the CSF is abnormal (increased cell count), repeat LP must be performed 6–12 months after therapy to determine whether treatment has been adequate [4, 5, 15].

IV. Recommendations

A. Primary prevention

1. Complete sexual history to assess risk (includes the sexual histories, if known to the patient, of the patient's partner(s)).
2. History of testing for syphilis, results, and treatment received.
3. Risk-reduction education: reduce number of partners, avoid high-risk partners (pick-ups, prostitutes), use condoms.

B. Early detection

1. Nontreponemal test for syphilis (RPR, VDRL) at entry into practice or hospital, if not previously performed, preferably as part of a screening panel, provided the

physician uses the screening panel in a cost-effective manner (see Chap. 70).

2. Repeat NTTS at 6–12 month intervals for promiscuous individuals, particularly gay men who are not **always** using a condom.
3. Repeat NTTS if patient shows signs or symptoms of syphilis or acquires any other sexually transmitted disease.
4. Perform NTTS in elderly patients being evaluated for dementia.
5. Always confirm a positive nontreponemal test with a specific treponemal test.

C. Intervention

1. See Table 98-1 for treatment based on presumed stage of infection and disease.
2. Perform follow-up RPR or VDRL to ensure adequacy of treatment.
3. Perform LP if any neuropsychiatric signs are present or if long-term follow-up or patient reliability is in question.

References

1. Musher, D. M. Biology of *Treponema pallidum*. In K. K. Holmes, et al. (eds.), *Sexually Transmitted Diseases*. New York: McGraw-Hill, 1984. Pp. 291–298. *An excellent review of pathophysiology as of 1980.*
2. Sparling, P. F. Natural History of Syphilis. In K. K. Holmes, et al. (eds.), *Sexually Transmitted Diseases*. New York: McGraw-Hill, 1984. Pp. 298–305. *A brief review of the stages and organs involved in syphilis.*
3. Knox, J. M., and Rudolph, A. H. Acquired Infectious Syphilis. In K.K. Holmes, et al. (eds.), *Sexually Transmitted Diseases*. New York: McGraw-Hill, 1984. Pp. 305–313. *A more detailed description of clinical manifestations of syphilis.*
4. Tramont, E. C. *Treponema pallidum* (Syphilis). In G.L. Mandell, R.G. Douglas Jr., and J.E. Bennett (eds.), *Principles and Practice of Infectious Diseases.* (2nd ed.). New York: Wiley, 1985. Pp. 1323–1333. *A concise review of syphilis.*
5. Hart, G. Syphilis tests in diagnostic and therapeutic decision making. *Ann. Intern. Med.* 104(3):368, 1986. *A thorough review of diagnostic testing for syphilis.*
6. The Medical Letter on Drugs and Therapeutics. Treatment of sexually transmitted diseases. 30(Issue 757):5, 1988. *Both the Medical Letter and the CDC STD treatment guidelines are updated periodically. Refer to* M. M. W. R. *for CDC updates.*
7. McPhee, S. J. Secondary syphilis: Uncommon manifestations of a common disease. *West. J. Med.* 140(1):35, 1984. *"Know syphilis in all its manifestations and relations, and all other things clinical will be added unto you" (Osler, 1897). The unusual or uncommon manifestations of syphilis continue to be reported and studied. In the aggregate, they occur more commonly than "usual" presentations of syphilis.*
8. Rockwell, D. H., Yobs, A. R., and Moore, M. B. Jr. The Tuskegee study of untreated syphilis; The 30th year of observation. *Arch. Intern. Med.* 114:792, 1964. *The ethics of this study have been soundly criticized, and rightly so. The information it contains pertains specifically to blacks, but is probably extrapolatable to other races. It describes neurological, cardiovascular, and other complications of untreated syphilis.*
9. Rosahn, P. D. Autopsy studies in syphilis. *J. Ven. Dis. Inform.* (supp. 21):1, 1947. *Almost 5% of 4000 autopsies showed anatomic lesions attributable to syphilis. The natural history of syphilis is changing in the antibiotic era, however.*
10. Centers for Disease Control. Continuing increase in infectious syphilis—United States. *M. M. W. R.* 37(3):35, 1988. *Syphilis is on the rise in heterosexuals. Does this mean HIV will follow?*
11. Centers for Disease Control. Declining rates of rectal and pharyngeal gonorrhea among males—New York City. *M. M. W. R.* 33(21):295, 1984. *An encouraging trend, probably due to fear of AIDS and increasing adherence to "safe sex" guidelines.*
12. Judson, F. N. Fear of AIDS and gonorrhoea rates in homosexual men. *Lancet* 2(8342):159, 1983. *Rates of gonorrhea and syphilis have fallen dramatically among gay men due to precautions taken to avoid AIDS.*
13. Brown, S. T., et al. Serological response to syphilis treatment. A new analysis of old data. *J. A. M. A.* 253(9):1296, 1985. *Early syphilis should respond to treatment with a titer fall to one quarter of the initial titer by 3–6 months.*
14. Tomecki, K. J., and Tomecki, E. C. Neglect of syphilis in hospitalized patients. *South. Med. J.* 77(9):1118, 1984. *Hospital admission, particularly to a public hospital, may provide an opportunity for serologic testing—it may be the point of entry for a patient into the health care system.*
15. Wiesel, J., et al. Lumbar puncture in asymptomatic late syphilis. An analysis of the benefits and risks. *Arch. Intern. Med.* 145(3):465, 1985. *This analysis questions the value of routine lumbar puncture.*

99 Chlamydia

Mark Lipman

I. The problem

A. Description. Chlamydiae are obligate intracellular organisms. Constituent analysis of their cell wall reveals that they are most closely related to gram-negative bacteria. They differ from other bacteria in that they require the host cell's metabolic machinery to survive. They inhabit columnar and pseudostratified columnar mucosal lining cells.

Within the chlamydia genus, there are only two species. *Chlamydia trachomatis* primarily infects humans and is transmitted by close physical contact. *C. psittaci* primarily infects birds, but occasionally may produce zoonotic infections in humans.

The chlamydia life cycle can be considered to consist of two distinct forms: the elementary body and the initial body. The elementary body is the infectious particle capable of entering uninfected cells. The initial body exists as an intracytoplasmic particle surrounded in a vacuole composed of host-cell membrane constituents. It multiples by binary fission and is capable of condensing to form new elementary bodies. These are liberated by cell rupture and are capable of infecting other cells.

Over the last decade, a large amount of data has accumulated about the epidemiology and treatment of chlamydial infections. In men, *C. trachomatis* is the leading cause of nongonococcal and postgonococcal urethritis [1], as well as a major cause of epididymitis. The primary focus of infection in women appears to be an asymptomatic mucopurulent cervicitis [2]. Infection may ascend to the upper genital tract, leading to acute pelvic inflammatory disease [3] and possible Fitz-High–Curtis syndrome [4]. Chlamydial upper genital tract infection contributes significantly to infertility and subfertility in women. *C. trachomatis* infection in the female may also present as an acute urethral syndrome in a manner similar to that seen in the male.

It has been known for some time that *C. trachomatis* is the etiologic agent of lymphogranuloma venereum. Inclusion conjunctivitis may occur in adults or infants after hand-to-eye transmission, or exposure during birth, respectively. Chlamydia has been associated with proctitis in men and women, and may contribute to the "gay bowel syndrome" [4]. *C. trachomatis* has also been shown to be a major cause of pneumonias within the first year of life [1].

B. Epidemiology. *C. trachomatis* is now recognized as the number one sexually transmitted disease in the United States [4]. There are an estimated 3 million chlamydial infections in the United States each year, compared to 2 million gonococcal infections [1]. The infection rate has been found to vary between 5.5% and 22.5% in women attending family planning clinics [5]. Frommell reported that 61% of infants born to women with chlamydial infections become colonized. A significant portion of these infants develop inclusion conjunctivitis and/or chlamydial pneumonias [6]. Chlamydial infection has been found in 26% of sexually active adolescents [7] and 12% of men visiting a sexually transmitted disease clinic [8]. It is estimated that 10–20% of the 1 million recognized PID cases in the United States each year are secondary to *C. trachomatis* and that the nationwide prevalence of chlamydial infection in general is 5% [9].

Because asymptomatic individuals form an important reservoir of infection and because culture and screening tests for *C. trachomatis* are expensive and have not been widely available, several studies have examined the clinical and epidemiologic factors associated with infection [5, 6, 7, 8]. When present, an endocervical polymorphonuclear leukocytic exudate (termed mucopurulent cervicitis), manifested either by visible yellow mucopus or by the presence of 10 or more polymorphonucleocytes per high-powered field of endocervical mucus, has been shown to correlate with culture of *C. trachomatis* [10]. Historical factors that have been shown to correlate with increased risk of infections include: a younger age group, black race, nulliparity, multiple sexual partners, and a history of previous sexually transmitted diseases. Women using barrier methods of contraception are less likely to be infected than those who used other forms, or no form, of contraception. In fact, chlamydial infection may be enhanced by oral contraception use [11]. Among men, the prevalence of *C. trachomatis* ureteral infection has been shown to be greater in heterosexual than homosexual men (14% versus 5%), men under 20 years of age, and blacks [8, 12].

II. Secondary prevention

A. Early detection

1. Method

a. Risk assessment. There is no single risk factor that is sufficient to determine who should be screened for chlamydial infection. Instead, local determinants of risk, as well as historical and clinical information, must be used to construct a composite of risk factors. The CDC recommends that all individuals attending facilities with a high prevalence of chlamydial infections, such as sexually transmitted disease clinics or family planning clinics, and who otherwise would not be offered anti-chlamydial therapy, be screened [13]. In this setting, asymptomatic, high-risk women should receive the highest priority, followed by heterosexual and then by homosexual men.

Asymptomatic persons attending low-risk, or undetermined risk, facilities (such as certain private practices or emergency rooms) should be screened for infection if they otherwise would be considered at high risk because of young age, multiple sex partners, etc. All symptomatic patients visiting such facilities should also be screened for chlamydial infection. Because of the high prevalence of asymptomatic infection, and the consequences of transmission to the newborn, screening of all pregnant women in high-risk groups should receive the highest priority (see Chap. 15).

b. Laboratory techniques

(1) Chlamydial culture is considered the gold standard for laboratory diagnosis. Its major disadvantages include high cost ($88 at our institution), stringent transport and storage requirements, and prolonged turnaround time (4–6 days).

(2) Direct fluorescent antibody tests utilize fluorescein-conjugated monoclonal antibodies directed against the chlamydial major outer membrane protein. In men, a genitourethral calcium alginate swab is inserted 2–3 cm into the urethra, rotated and withdrawn. It is then smeared on an 8–10 mm diameter area of slide. The slide is then allowed to air dry, fixed with acetone, and finally, incubated with the fluorescent antibody reagent. Under a fluorescent microscope, the slide is examined for 10 or more bright apple-green disks, consistent with *C. trachomatis* elementary bodies. In women, the procedure is similar except the exocervix is first cleaned with a cotton or Dacron swab to remove exudate and mucus. Then a Dacron or calcium alginate swab is inserted into the endocervical canal, rotated against the wall, and removed.

The turnaround time is typically less than 1 hour. Sensitivities of 70–100% and specificities of 94–99% have been reported. In high-risk populations, the positive and negative predictive values have been reported to be 84% and 95%, respectively [14].

(3) An **enzyme-linked immunoassay** that detects genus-specific *C. trachomatis* antigen is also available for screening. Swabs of the urethra or endocervix are obtained in a manner similar to the immunofluorescent antibody test. Once the specimen is obtained, it is placed in a transport tube containing storage reagent and is sent to the lab. There, eluent from the swab is serially incubated with rabbit antibody to *C. trachomatis* antigen, horseradish peroxidase-labeled goat anti-rabbit globulin, and finally, with a substrate indicator solution containing O-phenylenediamine and hydrogen peroxide. A spectrophotometer is then used to obtain the optical density of the solution. Processing time is approximately 4 hours.

Sensitivities from 67–90% and specificities from 92–97% have been reported. Positive and negative predictive values have ranged from 37–93% and 88–97%, respectively, depending on the population studied [13, 15].

Advantages of this method include uncomplicated transport and storage of specimens, the use of standard laboratory equipment, and the absence of a need for specially trained laboratory personnel.

2. Justification. See Table 15-2.

B. **Early intervention**

1. **Method.** The CDC recommends empiric antichlamydial therapy for adults considered to be at high risk for chlamydial infection and with the following chlamydial-associated syndromes: (1) mucopurulent cervicitis, (2) pelvic inflammatory disease, (3) epididymitis, and (4) nongonococcal urethritis.

   Treatment of the first three of the above syndromes should include antigonococcal therapy. Asymptomatic contacts of patients (contact within 30 days of the onset of their symptoms or clinical evaluation) should also be evaluated and treated for presumptive chlamydial infection. Patients in one of the previously described risk groups who have documented *Neisseria gonorrhoeae* infection of the endocervix or urethra, and their sexual contacts, should also receive antichlamydial treatment [13].

   The CDC recommends the following antichlamydial treatment for adults with uncomplicated urethral, endocervical, or rectal infections: tetracycline hydrochloride (HCl) 500 mg PO qid for 7 days, or doxycycline 100 mg PO bid for 7 days. Alternative regimens for patients in whom tetracyclines are contraindicated or not tolerated include: erythromycin base or stearate 500 mg PO qid for 7 days, or erythromycin ethylsuccinate 800 mg PO qid for 7 days.

   Sulfonamides may also be effective. The optimal dosage of sulfonamides for chlamydial infection has not been determined, but sulfamethoxazole 1.0 gm PO bid for 10 days is probably effective [13].

   A follow-up test of cure is advisable unless lab resources are limited. Since tetracycline-resistant isolates of *C. trachomatis* have not been reported, a positive follow-up test most likely represents patient noncompliance, failure to treat a sexual partner, or laboratory error. Therefore, if a follow-up test is positive, retreatment with one of the above regimens is advised.

2. **Justification**

   a. **Effectiveness.** When taken as directed, either the tetracycline or erythromycin regimens are felt to be more than 95% effective. Therefore, test-of-cure follow-up studies may be omitted if laboratory resources are limited.

   b. **Risk of antibiotics.** Tetracycline is fairly well tolerated. It is associated with gastrointestinal upset in approximately 4% of cases. Allergic reactions are rare. It should be avoided in pregnancy because of the possibility of discoloring the teeth in the fetus. Erythromycin is also fairly well tolerated, especially when given with meals.

   c. **Cost.** The cost to the pharmacist for a seven-day course of tetracycline is approximately $2.24 and for doxycycline is $5.74–$15.40. A seven-day course of erythromycin costs the pharmacist $3.36–$24.08.

   d. **Acceptability.** Once patients are informed of the potential risk of infertility in women with untreated chlamydial infections, acceptance appears to be high. As with any multiple dose, outpatient regimen compliance remains a major problem with therapy.

III. **Recommendations**

A. **Early detection**

1. Screen all high risk pregnant women for chlamydial infection.
2. Asymptomatic females seen at sexually transmitted disease or family planning clinics should receive the next highest priority for screening.
3. Patients seen in a low-risk setting, yet are considered to be in a high-risk group or have a chlamydial-associated syndrome, should be screened for chlamydial infection.
4. Screening with either the immunofluorescent antibody or enzyme-linked immunoassay is acceptable because of the high predictive value in high-risk groups.

B. **Early intervention**

1. For those patients with positive chlamydia screening tests, therapy with either tetracycline or erythromycin should be instituted.
2. Patients in high-risk groups with syndromes associated with chlamydial infection may be treated empirically, especially if lab resources are limited.
3. Sexual contacts (contact within 30 days) of either of the above groups should be evaluated for a sexually transmitted disease and treated.
4. Patients with gonococcal cervicitis or urethritis should also receive treatment directed against chlamydia.
5. Where financial resources permit, test-of-cure should be done, and if positive, patients should be retreated.

References

1. Schacter, J., and Grossman, M. Chlamydial infections. *Annu. Rev. Med.* 32:45, 1981. *A review of the spectrum of disease associated with* C. trachomatis, *with emphasis on infection in infants.*
2. Faro, S. Chlamydia trachomatis infection in women. *J. Reprod. Med.* 30 (3 Suppl):273, 1985. *A review of the epidemiology and pathophysiology of chlamydial infection in women.*
3. Mardh, P., et al. *Chlamydia trachomatis* infection in patients with acute salpingitis. *N. Engl. J. Med.* 296(24):1377, 1977. *Specimens for culture of chlamydia were obtained from the cervix and from the fallopian tubes during laparoscopy.*
4. Thompson, S. E., and Washington, A. E. Epidemiology of sexually transmitted *Chlamydia trachomatis* infections. *Epidemiol. Rev.* 5:96, 1983. *A complete review of the microbiology, pathophysiology, and epidemiology of chlamydial infections.*
5. Schacter, J., Stoner, E., and Moncada, J. Screening for chlamydial infections in women attending family planning clinics: Evaluation of presumptive indicators for therapy. *West. J. Med.* 138(3):375, 1983. *Data from a study looking at women attending five family planning clinics with regard to risk factor identification and efficacy of presumptive therapy.*
6. Frommell, G. T., et al. Chlamydial infection of mothers and their infants. *J. Pediatr.* 95(1):28, 1979. *A prospective study of infants born to chlamydia-culture positive and negative women for development of disease and disability.*
7. Chacko, M. R., and Lovchik, J. C. *Chlamydia trachomatis* infection in sexually active adolescents: Prevalence and risk factors. *Pediatrics* 73(6):836, 1984. *Data on the prevalence and risk factors for genital chlamydial infection in an urban population of adolescents are presented.*
8. Stamm, W. E., et al. *Chlamydia trachomatis* urethral infections in men: Prevalence, risk factors, and clinical manifestations. *Ann. Intern. Med.* 100(1):47, 1984. *An assessment of risk factors and a comparison of culture yields for* N. gonorrhoeae *and* C. trachomatis *in an unselected male patient population attending a sexually transmitted disease clinic.*
9. Schacter, J. Chlamydial infections. (First of three parts). *N. Engl. J. Med.* 298(8):428, 1978. *A three-part, all-encompassing review of chlamydial infection.*
10. Brunham, R. C., et al. Mucopurulent cervicitis—the ignored counterpart in women of urethritis in men. *N. Engl. J. Med.* 311(1):1, 1984. *A well-designed prospective study of the relation of cervicitis to cervical infection with* N. gonorrhoeae *and* C. trachomatis.
11. Washington, A. E., et al. Oral contraceptives, *chlamydia trachomatis* infection, and pelvic inflammatory disease: A word of caution about protection. *J. A. M. A.* 253(15):2246, 1985. *Epidemiologic data are reviewed to examine the relationships between PID, chlamydial infection, and oral contraceptive use.*
12. Judson, F. N. Epidemiology and control of nongonococcal urethritis and genital chlamydial infections: A review. *Sex. Transm. Dis.* 8(2 Suppl):117, 1981. *This paper reviews clinical and epidemiologic features of gonococcal and nongonococcal urethritis. Cost-benefit of alternative strategies for control are compared.*
13. *Chlamydia trachomatis* infections: Policy guidelines for prevention and control. *M. M. W. R.* 34(Suppl 3):53s, 1985. *The latest recommendations for risk assessment, management, and prevention of chlamydial genital infections.*
14. Lipkin. E. S., et al. Comparison of monoclonal antibody staining and culture in diagnosing cervical chlamydial infection. *J. Clin. Microbiol.* 23(1):114, 1986. *A large study of 1200 women from various population groups, comparing a fluorescein-conjugated monoclonal antibody system with tissue culture for diagnosing chlamydial infection.*
15. Howard, L. V., et al. Evaluation of chlamydiazyme for the detection of genital infections caused *chlamydia trachomatis. J. Clin. Microbiol.* 23(2):329, 1986. *A comparison of a commercial ELISA with culture results in a large group of patients from several different clinical settings.*

100

HIV Infection

Neil Flynn

I. The problem

A. Definition. The human immunodeficiency virus (HIV) (formerly called HTLV-III or LAV) has been identified as the underlying cause of the acquired immunodeficiency syndrome (AIDS). However, the reporting definition of AIDS is clinical, not virological. AIDS may be defined as the **presence** of a reliably diagnosed, life-threatening disease, at least moderately predictive of cellular immune deficiency, in the absence of other causes of immune deficiency, and usually in the presence of evidence of HIV infection [1, 2].

At the present time, the majority of cases of AIDS involve various combinations of: life-threatening or invasive infection with opportunistic pathogens (Table 100-1); Kaposi's sarcoma (KS); non-Hodgkin's B-cell lymphoma of high-grade pathologic type; chronic lymphoid interstitial pneumonitis in a child; and severe neurologic disease with or without other manifestations [1, 2].

In addition to AIDS itself, lesser degrees of illness involving combinations of clinical signs and symptoms and laboratory abnormalities are common following infection with HIV, but do not meet the CDC case definition requirements for full-blown AIDS. The CDC has recently proposed a simple classification scheme for HIV infection (Table 100-2) [3]. In addition, guidelines have been proposed for the definition of so-called AIDS-related conditions, or ARC, summarized in Table 100-3 [4].

Finally, many individuals remain completely asymptomatic for long periods of time following infection with HIV. Approximately one third of HIV-infected individuals remain symptom free at 5–7 years after infection.

B. Description. HIV is a member of the retrovirus group of single-stranded RNA viruses [5]. It appears to have a number of unusual properties, including frequent alteration in its genome, ability to insert its genome into the host-cell's genome, and tropism for several cell types. It infects human lymphocytes (of the T-helper subset), monocytes, and either infects or injures indirectly neurones in the central nervous system. Infection is followed by cell dysfunction and eventual destruction. In particular, T-helper lymphocytes may become so reduced in number and function that cell-mediated immunity, as well as other areas of immune function, are severely impaired [6].

The spectrum of clinical disease resulting from HIV infection is wide. A primary illness is described consisting of fever, lymphadenopathy, and fatigue, reminiscent of acute mononucleosis. This may be followed by complete resolution of signs and symptoms, or chronic signs and symptoms may develop as outlined in Table 100-3. Some of these may predict a high probability of development of full-blown AIDS within months to a few years: spontaneous oral candidosis; hairy leukoplakia of the tongue, a lesion peculiar to HIV infection; persistent and severe weight loss, fevers, night sweats, and fatigue; severe thrombocytopenia; markedly elevated erythrocyte sedimentation rate; or markedly reduced T-helper (T4) lymphocyte count ($\leq$400 T-helper cells) [7].

The development of opportunistic infections (see Table 100-1) or malignancies that meet CDC criteria for AIDS carries a poor prognosis. CDC-defined AIDS is usually fatal within 1–2 years, although some patients with Kaposi's sarcoma (KS) alone may survive considerably longer [8]. *Pneumocystis carinii* pneumonia (PCP) and KS are the most common presenting manifestations of AIDS. Neurologic and psychiatric dysfunction ranging from peripheral neuropathy to dementia and paralysis are becoming increasingly recognized as common manifestations of HIV infection [9].

C. Epidemiology. HIV is spread almost exclusively through sexual or blood-to-blood contact, in a manner similar to the transmission of hepatitis B. The virus is found regularly in the blood and semen of infected individuals, and less often in tears, saliva, and vaginal secretions [10]. The long latency period and infectious carrier state before disease develops are conducive to spread even though the modes of transmission are limited,

Table 100-1. Common opportunistic infections and malignancies that meet CDC case definition of AIDS

Opportunistic infections
- Viruses
  - [a]Disseminated, life-threatening CMV infection (pulmonary, GI, CNS)
  - [b]Mucocutaneous or disseminated varicella zoster or herpes simplex lasting longer than 1 month
  - Progressive multifocal leukoencephalopathy
- Bacteria
  - [a]Disseminated or pulmonary *Mycobacterium avium*-intracellular infection
  - Disseminated *Mycobacterium tuberculosis* in HIV antibody positive individual
- Fungi
  - [a]Invasive candidosis (GI, pulmonary, disseminated, biopsy-proven)
  - Cryptococcosis (usually involves CNS)
  - [b]Disseminated histoplasmosis
- Protozoal and helminthic infections
  - [a]*Pneumocystis carinii* pneumonia
  - [a]Central nercous system toxoplasmosis
  - [b]Severe, persistent cryptosporidial or isosporidial diarrhea (> 1 month)
  - Disseminated strongyloidiasis

Malignancies
- Kaposi's sarcoma (KS) in an individual under the age of 60 years or over 60 if HIV antibody-positive
  - [b]Non-Hodgkin's lymphoma of high-grade type, or B-cell lymphomas
  - Lymphoreticular malignancy diagnosed over >3 months after the diagnosis of an AIDS OI

Other
- Chronic lymphoid interstitial pneumonitis in a child (<13)
  - [b]Chronic lymphoid interstitial pneumonitis in an adult
  - Neurologic disease—dementia, severe neuropathy
  - HIV wasting syndrome

[a]Common.
[b]In the presence of a positive serologic or virologic test for HIV.

Table 100-2. Centers for Disease Control classification of HIV infection

Group I.	Acute infection		
Group II.	Asymptomatic infection[a]		
Group III.	Persistent generalized lymphadenopathy[a]		
Group IV.	Other disease		
	Subgroup A.	Constitutional disease	
	Subgroup B.	Neurologic disease	
	Subgroup C.	Secondary infectious diseases	
		Category C-1.	Specified secondary infectious diseases listed in the CDC surveillance definition for AIDS[b]
		Category C-2.	Other specified secondary infectious diseases
	Subgroup D.	Secondary cancers[b]	
	Subgroup E.	Other conditions	

[a]Patients in Groups II and III may be subclassified on the basis of a laboratory evaluation.
[b]Includes those patients whose clinical presentation fulfills the definition of AIDS used by CDC for national reporting.

Source: Classification system for human T-lymphotropic virus type III/lymphadenopathy-associated virus infections. *M. M. W. R.* 35(20):334, 1986.

Table 100-3. Definition of AIDS-related conditions (ARC) and associated disability scale: A proposal by the Scientific Affairs Committee of the Bay Area Physicians for Human Rights

This proposed definition assumes that other established causes of these abnormalities previously have been ruled out.

Requirements: Clinical — 2 major findings, or 1 major and 2 or more minor findings; **plus**
Immunologic — 1 or more findings; **plus**
Laboratory — 2 or more findings.

Check the appropriate findings for diagnostic assessment and place an "X" on the line following those primarily responsible for disability.

Clinical[a]

Major		Minor	
☐ Lymphadenopathy. Nodes must equal or exceed 1 cm at 2 or more extrainguinal sites for at least 6 months.	____	☐ Night sweats for at least 3 months.	____
☐ Oral thrush.	____	☐ Fatigue.	____
☐ Hairy leukoplakia.	____	☐ Pruritus for at least 1 month.	____
☐ Herpes zoster in persons under age 60.	____	☐ Bullous impetigo.	____
☐ Fever for at least 3 months.	____	☐ Refractory dermatophytosis.	____
☐ Diarrhea for at least 3 months.	____	☐ Extensive molluscum contagiosum.	____
☐ Weight loss of 10% or more of body weight, or at least 15 pounds.	____	☐ Extensive seborrheic dermatitis or eczema.	____
☐ Central or peripheral neurologic deficit.	____	☐ Unexplained, persistent sinusitis.	____

Laboratory	Immunologic
☐ HIV antibody positive.	☐ Helper T-cell count under 400/mm.*
☐ HIV virus culture positive.	☐ Helper-suppressor ratio < 1.0.
☐ Leukopenia (less than 4000/mm).*	☐ Cutaneous anergy (negative to 3 or more common skin tests).
☐ Anemia (hematocrit 35 or less).	
☐ Thrombocytopenia (< 100,000/mm).*	
☐ Serum globulins 3.5 gm/dl or greater.	
☐ Sedimentation rate 20 or greater.	
☐ Serum cholesterol < 135 mg%.	

*To be considered disabled, patient must have a Karnofsky score of 70 or less.[b] Refer to table below for descriptions.

Karnofsky Performance Status Scale

(circle)	
100	Normal, no complaints, no evidence of disease.
90	Able to carry on normal activity, minor disease signs, symptoms.
80	Normal activity with effort, some disease signs, symptoms.
70	Cares for self, but unable to carry on normal activity or to do active work.
60	Requires occasional assistance, able to care for most of own needs.
50	Requires considerable assistance and frequent medical care.
40	Disabled, requires special care and assistance.
30	Severely disabled, hospitalization indicated although death not imminent.
20	Hospitalization and active support treatment needed. Patient very sick.
10	Moribund, fatal processes progressing rapidly.

Although not part of the disease definition, the following factors sometimes associated with the disease also can be used in assessing disability:

nausea ____ malaise ____ dyspnea ____ headache ____ other(s) ________

Source: Reprinted with permission of Bay Area Association of Physicians for Human Rights.

[a]Most symptoms may be intermittent or continuous for the period and must occur in the absence of any identifiable cause.

[b]D. A. Karnofsky and J. H. Burchenal. The Clinical Evaluation of Chemotherapeutic Agents in Cancer. In C. M. MacLeod (ed.), *Evaluation of Chemotherapeutic Agents.* New York: Columbia University Press, 1949.

and the risk of transmission per sexual or IV needle-sharing exposure may be as low as 0.2-1.0% [11].

Between 1978 and 1986, as many as 2 million Americans became infected with HIV. Fifty thousand cases of AIDS were reported in the United States between 1981 and March 1988. This number is likely to double every 12–15 months for the next few years. The incidence of development of AIDS following HIV infection may be as high as 5–7% per year. The CDC estimates that there will have been over 200,000 cases of AIDS in the United States by 1991 [12, 13].

Table 100-4 lists high-risk groups for infection with HIV and subsequent development of AIDS. At the present time, the highest-risk groups for new infection are promiscuous gay and bisexual men, female sexual partners of bisexual men, IV drug users (IVDU) who share injection paraphernalia with other IVDU, and their sexual partners. Risk among heterosexually promiscuous men is currently low, but among promiscuous women will become significant in the next few years. Risk from blood transfusion has been greatly reduced by donor screening and HIV antibody screening [14]. Risk of infection to health care workers who provide bedside care for infected patients is quite low. It is less than 1/300 even after contaminated needle stick [15].

Spread from current high-risk groups to currently low-risk groups is occurring via bisexual men and needle-sharing among IVDU. Within the next decade, it is likely that all heterosexually promiscuous individuals will be at risk for infection with HIV.

II. Primary prevention methods

A. Education. Vigorous, visible educational programs must be developed that target individually the high-risk groups listed in Table 100-4. Content of the educational material must be specific with respect to activities that place individuals at risk, and the methods that the individual can use to reduce his or her risk. Education appears to have been moderately successful in decreasing high-risk activity among gay men, but probably not yet among IV drug users [12, 16-18]. Promiscuous, heterosexual women are currently at some risk through contact with bisexual or IV drug-abusing men, and must be targeted for education. Their risk will increase rapidly over the next decade. Table 100-5 lists specific high-risk activities and suggested goals of education. Explicit educational materials have been developed but are felt to be too explicit by some. This has resulted in limited distribution of such material to adolescents and IVDU, decreasing the effectiveness of education as a tool. Educational materials are available from regional AIDS foundations and the U.S. Public Health Service.

B. High-risk sexual contact. Table 100-5 lists specific sexual activities that are believed to be associated with transmission of HIV. Guidelines for so-called safe sex have been developed, which emphasize the following principles: (1) No anal, vaginal, or orogenital intercourse with an infected person or a person likely to be infected is preferable; (2) If these **are** engaged in, a condom should be worn throughout the activity, and probably provides a high degree of protection [19]; the addition of a nonoxanol-9-containing spermicide in vaginal intercourse may also assist in killing HIV if the condom ruptures; and (3) Activities that do not result in exchange of body secretions, such as mutual masturbation, are safest. Since the prevalence of infection is so high among certain risk groups such as gay men, IVDU, or hemophiliacs, even a single high-risk exposure, such as unprotected intercourse with a partner who is a member of a high-risk group, may be sufficient for transmission of the virus [10, 11].

C. IV drug use. Primary prevention of AIDS among IV drug users involves motivating users not to share their paraphernalia or to disinfect it between users, and to adhere to safe sex guidelines. There are many pressures among users to share paraphernalia, including sociability, laws that make possession of paraphernalia a criminal offense, unavailability of needles or syringes, the extreme impulsive nature of IV drug use, and an inability to translate knowledge into behavioral change [17, 18].

Education alone will probably be insufficient to change addict behavior. Consideration must be given to expanding drug treatment and maintenance programs, promoting effective, easy-to-perform techniques for disinfection of paraphernalia, and decriminalizing possession of paraphernalia [18]. Failure to prevent spread of the virus in IV drug users will result in creation of a large, new risk group—their sexual partners and infants born to infected women.

III. Secondary prevention

A. Early detection methods

1. Detection of HIV-infection risk. History of activities (or transfusion prior to institution of antibody screening) that carry risk of HIV infection should be solicited in the initial interview. HIV antibody testing should be discussed with individuals who have risk factors for HIV infection [20].

Table 100-4. Current and future high-risk groups for HIV infection[a]

Group	HIV positive (%)
Gay and bisexual men, large metropolitan area	20–30
Hemophiliacs	30–80[b]
Intravenous drug users	<5–80[c]
Regular sexual partner(s) of HIV-infected person (unprotected)	30
Infants born to HIV-infected mother	50
Heterosexually promiscuous persons	<0.01[d]
Recipients of blood transfusion 1980–1985	0.01[d]

[a]Prevalence of antibody to HIV (infection) in 1986.
[b]Dependent on age and severity of hemophilia.
[c]Dependent on area of residence and needle-sharing practices.
[d]Higher in areas of high AIDS incidence.

Table 100-5. High-risk activities and suggested interventions

	Inrervention	
Activity	Safe	Possibly safe
Male homosexual rectal intercourse	Avoid; mutual masturbation	Use condom
Promiscuous heterosexual oral, rectal, or vaginal intercourse	Avoid; mutual masturbation	Use condom
Sexual intercourse with known or suspected IV drug user	Avoid	Use condom
Sharing of IV drug-use paraphernalia	Avoid	High-level disinfection between persons (boil, clean in dilute bleach solution or other disinfectant)
Birth to infected mother	Pregnancy avoidance in infected mother	40–50% of infants of HIV-infected mothers escape infection. No breast-feeding.

2. **Physical examination** of HIV-infected individuals usually reveals palpable lymph nodes either in a region unusual for palpable nodes in adults in the absence of local infection (e.g., posterior cervical, occipital, or epitrochlear), or unusually large or numerous nodes (e.g., axillary). Discovery of such nodes should prompt the physician to inquire further about risk factors for HIV infection, remembering that patients often withhold such information if they detect a judgmental attitude in the physician. If a risk factor is elicited, HIV-antibody testing and a serologic test for syphilis should be discussed with the patient. Syphilis is a frequent cause of adenopathy in individuals at risk for HIV infection [18].
3. **Antibody testing.** Antibodies to HIV can be detected in the serum of most infected persons within 6 months of infection. The two most commonly used antibody detection tests are the enzyme-linked immunosorbent assay (ELISA) and the Western blot analysis. While the ELISA is undergoing continuous refinement, it has more false-positive results than the Western blot, as of this writing. The Western blot, on the other hand, has more false-negative results, which occur in the early phases of infection with HIV before all of the usual antibody responses have occurred.

   The ELISA is much less expensive to perform than is the Western blot. Thus, a combination of the ELISA for screening and the Western blot for confirmation of the positive ELISA is currently recommended [21]. A positive ELISA alone should never be used as definitive evidence of HIV infection, except, perhaps, in an individual with CDC-defined AIDS. There are numerous instances in which a falsely positive ELISA has led to much unnecessary psychological trauma to the patient, and embarrassment to the physician [20].

4. **Justification.** The ELISA test is between 95 and 99% sensitive, and false-positive results occur in less than 1–3% of tests, depending on the manufacturer of the test used and the ratio of patient serum reaction to control that is defined as a positive. The Western blot has an extremely low false-positive rate, but may have a false-negative rate of 1–5%, depending on the recency of infection (for possibly up to 6 months after infection) [21]. The ELISA test is readily available for about $25, but the Western blot is more difficult to obtain and costs $50–100 to the patient. The tests can be obtained in some states free of charge, and anonymously or confidentially in some states from local health departments.

   There is a major risk of serious social, economic, and personal consequences for the HIV antibody-positive individual if confidentiality of the test result is compromised or, in some cases, even if it becomes known to an employer or insurer that the person has sufficient risk factors to warrant testing for HIV antibody. Therefore, the physician must help the patient maintain confidentiality by counseling that the test be obtained anonymously at a so-called alternative testing site, or that the test not be billed to the patient's health insurance, etc. Patients should expect and receive every possible consideration for keeping knowledge of the performance of the test and its results strictly between themselves and their physicians. Undoubtedly, litigation will arise frequently when this trust is breached by the physician or his or her staff [20].

B. Early intervention. Once infection with HIV has occurred, early detection of infection may be useful for preventing further spread of the virus to new contacts, but prevention of disease in the infected individual is problematic. Some investigators postulate that prevention or early treatment of intercurrent infections in HIV-infected persons, such as shigellosis, hepatitis B, or syphilis, for example, may delay or prevent development of AIDS. Therefore, the primary physician should counsel the patient in ways to avoid new infections [19, 20, 22, 23]. Consideration should be given to treatment with zidovudine in patients with ARC symptoms or T-helper lymphocyte count < 400/mm^3.

Hepatitis B serology, syphilis serology, TB skin test, and stool examination and culture in patients with diarrhea, should be performed in HIV-infected persons.

III. Recommendations

A. Primary prevention

1. Identification of individuals with risk factors for acquisition of HIV.
2. Education of persons at risk of HIV infection through sexual or needle-sharing exposure. Give "safe sex" guidelines (preferably written materials) and "safe shooting" guidelines to appropriate individuals [19, 23].
3. Identification of infected persons, for counseling of them and their high-risk contacts.

B. Early detection

1. Encourage individuals in high-risk groups to have confidential or anonymous HIV antibody testing, to facilitate appropriate counseling.
2. Exercise extreme care to avoid breach of confidentiality.
3. Counsel antibody-positive individuals in methods of risk reduction for their sexual or needle-sharing partners.

C. Intervention and treatment

1. Counsel avoidance of new infections that might precipitate AIDS in HIV antibody-positive individuals (e.g., cytomegalovirus [CMV]).
2. Treat new or latent infections (e.g., syphilis) early.
3. Obtain T-helper lymphocyte count in antibody-positive individuals.
4. Consider zidovudine for symptoms of ARC or T-helper cell count < 400/mm^3.

References

1. Revision of the CDC surveillance case definition for acquired immunodeficiency syndrome. *M. M. W. R.* 36(Supp. 1):1S, 1987. *This revised definition expands the range of illness classified as AIDS.*
2. Revision of a case definition of acquired immunodeficiency syndrome for national reporting—United States. *M. M. W. R.* 34(25):373, 1985. *People died of HIV-related disease without meeting the CDC's reporting criteria for AIDS in this prior case definition.*

3. Classification system for human T-lymphotropic virus type III/lymphadenopathy-associated virus infections. *M. M. W. R.* 35(20):334, 1986. *ARC comes under groups IV A, B, C-2, and E.*
4. Bay Area Physicians for Human Rights: Definition of AIDS-related conditions (ARC) and associated disability scale. *AIDS Alert* 1(9):167, 1986. *Provides a framework for assessing illness related to HIV in persons who do not have "AIDS."*
5. Gallo, R. C., and Wong-Staal, F. A human T-lymphotropic retrovirus (HTLV-III) as the cause of the acquired immunodeficiency syndromes. *Ann. Intern. Med.* 103(5):679, 1985. *A description of the human immunodeficiency virus(es) and their relationships to other human retroviruses.*
6. Bowen, D. L., Lane, H. C., and Fauci, A. S. Immunopathogenesis of the acquired immunodeficiency syndrome. *Ann. Intern. Med.* 103(5):704, 1985. *Virtually all aspects of immune function are altered, directly or indirectly, by HIV infection.*
7. Curran, J. W., et al. The epidemiology of AIDS: Current status and future prospects. *Science* 229(4720):1352, 1985. *We can identify some HIV-infected patients who have a high probability of developing AIDS within 1–2 years.*
8. Fauci, A. S., et al. NIH conference. The acquired immunodeficiency syndrome: An update. *Ann. Intern. Med.* 102(6):800, 1985. *Twenty to 30% of patients with opportunistic infection die during the initial episode. For those who survive it, prognosis is 12–18 months.*
9. Levy, R. M., Bredesen, D. E., and Rosenblum, M. L. Neurological manifestations of the acquired immunodeficiency syndrome (AIDS): Experience at UCSF and review of the literature. *J. Neurosurg.* 62(4):475, 1985. *The dimensions of the problem of CNS injury may become staggering.*
10. Peterman, T. A., and Curran, J. W. Sexual transmission of human immunodeficiency virus. *J. A. M. A.* 256(16):2222, 1986. *It is unlikely that saliva is capable of transmitting infection or that oral ingestion of virus carries significant risk.*
11. DeGruttola, V., Mayer, K., and Bennett, W. AIDS: Has the problem been adequately assessed? *Rev. Infect. Dis.* 8(2):295, 1986. *Epidemiologically speaking, it takes many exposures to become infected; individually speaking, however, it may take only a single exposure. If the virus spreads heterosexually so easily, as it did homosexually, many more millions of Americans will become infected—unless, of course, condoms become much more popular.*
12. Morgan, W. M., and Curran, J. W. Acquired immunodeficiency syndrome: Current and future trends. *Public Health Rep.* 101(5):459, 1986. *Projections for the next 5 years are grim in the absence of a breakthrough in treatment for HIV infection itself.*
13. Goedert, J. J., et al. Three-year incidence of AIDS in five cohorts of HTLV-III-infected risk group members. *Science* 231:992, 1986. *The studies are consistent—whether or not almost all of the infected people will eventually develop AIDS remains to be seen but seems likely.*
14. Pindyck, J., et al. Measures to decrease the risk of acquired immunodeficiency syndrome transmission by blood transfusion. *Transfusion* 25(1):3, 1985. *Risk from transfusion if only screened (donor deferral program) volunteer blood donors are used, and each unit tested for HIV-Ab is probalby less than 1 in 40,000 units.*
15. McCray, E. Occupational risk of the acquired immunodeficiency syndrome among health care workers. *N. Engl. J. Med.* 314(17):1127, 1986. *By The Cooperative Needlestick Surveillance Group: the 95% confidence intervals for risk of HIV infection following contaminated needlestick are* **0.2%** to **4.4%**.
16. McKusick, L., Horstman, W., and Coates, I. J. AIDS and sexual behavior reported by gay men in San Francisco. *Am. J. Public Health* 75(5): 493, 1985. *Most older gay men have gotten the message. However, adolescent gay males have not, and must be reached.*
17. DeJarlais, D. C., Friedman, S. R., and Hopkins, W. Risk reduction for the acquired immunodeficiency syndrome among intravenous drug users. *Ann. Intern. Med.* 103(5):755, 1985. *IVDU have been considered unreachable by educational efforts in the past. This article documents their concern over AIDS, but also their ineffective behavior changes.*
18. Flynn, N., et al. Unpublished data, 1987. *Changing behavior among IVDU, especially in the current punitive social and political climate, will be extremely difficult, according to our survey work. Also, addict knowledge has not been translated into change in behavior, at least in our community.*
19. Chester, M. I., et al. *Hot'n Healthy Times.* San Francisco: Eroticus, 1986. *You can purchase this explicit "safe" sex material from the publisher: 333 Valencia St., #400, San Francisco, CA 94103. This is a "how-to," and ranks available condoms according to several parameters.*
20. Bayer, R., Levine, C., and Wolf, S. M. HIV antibody screening. An ethical framework for evaluating proposed programs. *J. A. M. A.* 256(13):1768, 1986. *There are a few concepts that a physician who attempts to counsel patients about HIV antibody testing should know. Other-*

wise, he or she can give bad advice that may harm the patient psychologically, economically, and socially.

21. Weiss, S. H., et al. Screening tests for HTLV-III (AIDS agent) antibodies. Specificity, sensitivity, and applications. *J. A. M. A.* 253(2):221, 1985. *The tests continue to improve in sensitivity and specificity. Remember that a test with 99% sensitivity and specificity, when applied to a population of 10,000 people with a prevalence rate of HIV infection of 0.5%, will detect all 50 true-positive and 100 false-positives.* Two thirds of the positives are false.
22. Wachter, H., et al. Who will get AIDS? *Lancet* 2(8517):1216, 1986. *Evidence suggesting that stimulation of T-cells may lead to expression of surface markers more attractive to HIV, and this, to infection and destruction, is all* in vitro.
23. Haight-Ashbury Free Medical Clinic. *Shooting Up and Your Health.* San Francisco AIDS Foundation, 333 Valencia St., San Francisco, CA 94103. *This brochure acknowledges the fact that most addicts will not stop shooting even though AIDS is a risk if they continue. Therefore, it emphasizes "safe" shooting.*
24. Karnofsky, D. A., and Burchenal, J. H. The Clinical Evaluation of Chemotherapeutic Agents in Cancer. In C. M. MacLeod (ed.), *Evaluation of Chemotherapeutic Agents.* New York: Columbia University Press, 1949. Pp.191–205.

Selected Reading

Centers for Disease Control. Human immunodeficiency virus infection in the United States: A review of current knowledge. *M. M. W. R.* 536(Suppl. S-6):1, 1987. *Excellent current review.*

101

Endocarditis

Neil Flynn

I. The problem

A. Definition. Infective endocarditis (IE) is a life-threatening condition arising from the growth of microorganisms on cardiac endothelium (usually damaged endothelium), aortic defects (patent ductus or coarctation), or surgically implanted prosthetic cardiac valves or foreign bodies.

B. Description. IE arises from attachment and growth of bloodborne chlamydia, rickettsiae, bacteria, or fungi to damaged cardiac endothelium, an intracardiac foreign body, or a lesion of the proximal aorta. Attachment appears to occur at areas of turbulent, high-pressure flow. A collection of fibrin and platelets on the damaged endothelium, termed nonbacterial thrombotic endocarditis, probably precedes, and sets the stage for, adherence and growth of organisms. Transient bacteremias are frequent in normal individuals and may be increased in frequency and bacterial concentration by untended gum disease, skin infection, colonic cancer, and certain medical and dental procedures. Nosocomial bacteremias contribute significantly to IE [1, 2]

Certain organisms are more likely than others to attach to and grow on cardiac lesions, partially accounting for the higher incidence of infection observed with these organisms. Once attached, the organisms become covered with a protective layer of fibrin and platelets. Growth of the organisms produces: (1) enzymatic and direct destruction of valvular or supporting structures, leading to valvular incompetence and functional compromise, and (2) macroscopic vegetations (often several centimeters in size) that release septic emboli that cause arterial obstruction, microabscess and aneurysm formation, and immune complex phenomena, accounting for many of the peripheral manifestations of IE.

Morbidity and mortality in IE are dependent on a number of factors including: the underlying valvular defect or other structure(s) involved, the organism and its virulence and antimicrobial susceptibility, the size and friability of the vegetations and embolic patterns, the general health of the individual, the speed of diagnosis of the condition and choice of antibiotics, the skill of the physician in assessing the need for early valve replacement, and the degree of patient cooperation, among others.

C. Epidemiology. Approximately 3,000 cases of bacterial endocarditis occur annually in the United States. About half of the cases of IE arise in persons with known preexisting cardiac lesions [3].

Only about 10% of cases of IE are preventable, that is, occur in persons who have a known lesion and who undergo a procedure for which prophylaxis has been recommended [3]. Table 101-1 lists various common cardiac lesions resulting in increased risk for IE, with estimates of the attendant lifetime risk of developing IE, risk as compared to a normal population (odds ratio), percentage of all individuals with IE who have that lesion, and references. These data are probably subject to a large selection bias. Table 101-2 is a more comprehensive listing of underlying conditions and estimated relative risk for development of IE.

While less than half of episodes of IE are preceded by a definable infection or procedure known to produce bacteremia, certain dental, medical, and surgical procedures are believed to pose significant risk of IE in susceptible individuals. Table 101-3 lists common procedures that result in bacteremia [1–3, 9, 10]. Dental, oropharyngeal, abscess drainage, and genitourinary procedures, especially in the presence of infection, appear to pose the highest risk of IE. Diagnostic procedures such as endoscopy, barium enema, and flexible bronchoscopy appear to pose little risk except, perhaps, in patients with prosthetic valves [1–3, 9–12].

Table 101-1. Risk of endocarditis with specified cardiac lesion

Lesion	Estimated % of population with condition	Lifetime risk of IE	Odds ratio	% of patients with IE	Comments
IHSS [4]	Rare	5%	8	<1	Greater incidence in persons with hemodynamically severe disease [4]
MVP [1, 5–14] without $\overline{M}$	5.0% [1, 4, 10]	Very low	1	≤1	No murmur at rest, prophylaxis is not indicated
MVP [1, 5–14] with $\overline{M}$	0.5%	5–8%	8.2	11–20	Murmur believed to indicate higher risk
Rheumatic [1, 6]		0.4%/year		37–76	Infrequent in younger U.S.–born individuals
Congenital [1, 6]	1.0%			6–24	
VSD [1, 6]	0.3%				
PVE [1, 7]		>1.5% 2.2% heterograft aortic 0.1% heterograft mitral 2.7% Starr-Edwards aortic 0.4% Starr-Edwards mitral		Increasing	Perhaps highest-risk lesion for IE

Key: IHSS = idiopathic hypertrophic subaortic stenosis; IE = infective endocarditis; MVP = mitral valve prolapse; VSD = ventricular septic defect; PVE = prosthetic valve endocarditis; M = cardiac murmur.

II. Prevention

A. Risk assessment

1. Methods

a. History. The physician should solicit information at the initial visit relative to risk factors for IE. These include a history of: an illness compatible with rheumatic fever (usually those with history of rheumatic fever are elderly or immigrants from underdeveloped countries); a heart murmur, defect, or surgery (particularly prosthetic valve surgery); congestive heart failure, which might reflect valvular disease; a history of previous endocarditis; or intravenous drug abuse.

b. Physical examination should include cardiac auscultation to determine the presence of significant cardiac murmurs, keeping in mind that innocuous "flow"-type murmurs are common in anemia, high cardiac output states (fever, thyrotoxicosis, Paget's disease), pregnancy, and thin-chested individuals and children, among others. These "flow" murmurs do not indicate a predisposition to endocarditis. If a murmur is detected that has features of a significant valvular abnormality or idiopathic hypertrophic subaortic stenosis (IHSS), in the absence of common causes of "flow"-type murmurs, its presence should be verified and its severity determined.

"Functional," "innocent," or "flow"-type murmurs occur in individuals with no history of prior cardiac disease and no symptoms compatible with reduced

Table 101-2. Estimated relative risk of developing infective endocarditis in various underlying cardiac conditions

Relatively high risk[a]	Intermediate risk[a]	Very low risk[c]
Prosthetic valves	Tricuspid valve disease	Arteriosclerotic plaques
Rheumatic valvular disease	Pulmonary valve disease	Coronary artery disease or bypass graft
MVP with murmur	IHSS(ASH), mild–moderate	MVP without murmur[b]
Mitral stenosis/ insufficiency	Nonvalvular intracardiac prosthetic implants	Atrial septal defects
Aortic valve disease	Right heart or pulmonary artery catheters[c]	Cardiac pacemakers
Ventricular septal defect	Calcific aortic sclerosis	Surgically corrected lesions (without prosthetic implants)
Coarctation of the aorta		
Patent ductus arteriosus		
Cyanotic congenital heart disease		
Arteriovenous fistulae		
Marfan's syndrome		
Intraatrial alimentation catheters		
Previous IE		
IHSS(ASH), severe		

[a]Prophylaxis recommended [10].
[b]Prophylaxis optional [3,5].
[c]Prophylaxis not indicated.
Key: MVP = mitral valve prolapse; IHSS(ASH) = idiopathic hypertrophic subaortic stenosis (assymetric septal hypertrophy).
Source: Adapted from D. T. Durack. Prophylaxis of Infective Endocarditis. In G. L. Mandell, R. G. Douglas Jr., and J. E. Bennett (eds.), *Principles and Practice of Infectious Diseases.* New York: Wiley, 1985; and D. T. Durack. Current issues in prevention of infective endocarditis. *Am. J. Med.* 28;78(6B):149, 1985.

Table 101-3. Percentage of patients developing bacteremia following various procedures

High risk	%	Intermediate risk	%	Low risk	%
Prostatectomy—infected urine*		Prostatectomy—sterile urine*		Sigmoidoscopy	2–10
Transurethral	58	Transurethral	11	Colonoscopy*	3–6
Retropubic	82	Retropubic	13	IUD insertion	0
Esophageal dilation, unsterile dilator*	100	Barium enema	11	Parturition	0.5
		Liver biopsy	3–13	Esophageal dilation,* sterile dilator	0
Tonsillectomy*	28–38	Rigid bronchoscopy*	15	Fiberoptic bronchoscopy*	0
Dental extraction*	18–85	Nasotracheal intubation	16	Orotracheal intubation	0
Periodontal surgery*	21–28	Nasotracheal suctioning, intensive care patients	16		
Burn surgery	46				
Surgery of infected areas*	54				

*Procedures for which endocarditis prophylaxis is recommended by the American Heart Association. Additional procedures include surgical procedures or biopsy involving respiratory mucosa, cystoscopy, urethral catheterization, urinary tract surgery, vaginal hysterectomy, gallbladder or colonic surgery, sclerotherapy of esophageal varices, upper gastrointestinal endoscopy, or sigmoidoscopy with biopsy.

Patient name: ______________________________ Date ________
Physician name: ____________ Address ____________ Phone ________
Diagnosis: ____

You have a condition known as ____________ that places you at a higher-than-normal risk for developing a heart infection called endocarditis. Your risk is still small, but you can reduce your risk further by following some simple guidelines.

1. Keep your teeth and gums in good condition. See your dentist regularly.
2. Tell (remind) your dentist that you have the above condition before each dental procedure. You may need an antibiotic to protect your heart during the procedure.
3. See a physician early for treatment of skin infections or other non-viral infections. (Colds and "flu" are viral and are not a risk.)
4. Tell any physician or nurse who is going to perform an operation or a procedure on you (such as urinary catheterization) that you have the above condition. You may need an antibiotic to protect your heart during the procedure.
5. Report fever, chills, and other symptoms of infection that do not go away in a week or so to your physician for evaluation.
6. If you change to a new physician or dentist alert them to the above condition.
7. Keep this information in your permanent household or medical files.

Fig. 101-1. Sample endocarditis patient information sheet.

exercise tolerance, angina, or congestive heart failure. They are usually crescendo/descrescendo, grade II/VI or less, do not radiate to axilla or carotids, and are associated with normal valvular opening and closing sounds (without a mid-systolic click), inspiratory splitting of the second sound, and normal apical impulse and carotid pulses.

c. **Further evaluation.** The presence and severity of the valvular lesion can be assessed by echocardiography, angiography, or through consultation with a cardiologist.

2. **Justification.** Clinical evaluation of murmurs is fraught with difficulty. The noninvasive and invasive cardiac tests developed over the past 2 decades have greatly improved our ability to define and quantitate the effects of valvular lesions. While such tests are relatively expensive (e.g., echocardiogram $400, cardiac cineangiography $3,000), they either confirm or deny our clinical diagnosis and quantitate the lesion's effects. The effects of incorrectly labeling an individual on the basis of clinical examination alone can be serious, affecting insurability, psychological stress, etc. Therefore, when the clinician believes that there is a significant valvular lesion present or probably present, an echocardiogram is in order. On the other hand, if the murmur has no features of a pathologic one, tests and prophylaxis should be avoided, since they are expensive, and the murmur should be followed at each periodic exam.

B. Primary prevention

1. **Methods.** Prevention of IE involves patient education (Fig. 101-1) and judicious use of antibiotic prophylaxis for high-risk procedures.

a. **Patient education** If the lesion is significant (see Tables 101-1 and 101-2—conditions that predispose to infectious endocarditis), the patient should be given instructions (preferably written materials) on the prevention of IE. Figures 101-1 is a sample instruction sheet. The patient's medical record should be flagged in some way to indicate risk for IE.

b. **Antibiotic prophylaxis.** The practitioner must integrate information on the relative propensity of a given cardiac lesion to become infected (see Tables 101-1 and 101-2), the relative risk of the procedure to produce a significant bacteremia with virulent organisms, and the risks of prophlaxis (penicillins and vancomycin carry risk of allergy or significant side effects), when deciding whether to give antibiotic prophylaxis [5, 8, 9].

If the physician decides that prophylaxis is warranted he or she should follow the guidelines of the American Heart Association [3, 10], the Medical Letter [11], or a well-known authority [3, 8, 9]. Table 101-4 lists regimens that meet the criteria of experimental efficacy, relatively low toxicity, and relatively low cost [3, 8–11].

2. **Justification**

a. **Effectiveness.** Models for the production of experimental endocarditis in animals have led to investigations of the efficacy of various antibiotic regimens in this setting. High-dose penicillin, penicillin plus an aminoglycoside, vancomycin, or amoxicillin is effective in preventing endocarditis in such a model. Durack has summarized these findings [8].

Failures of prophylaxis have been studied and reported [13]. They occurred in patients with mitral valve prolapse (33% of cases studied), cogenital abnormalities (29% of cases), rheumatic heart disease (21%), and prosthetic valves (19%). Ninety-two percent of cases followed a dental procedure. Sixty percent of the organisms were susceptible to the prophylaxis that had been used. Common errors in administering prophylaxis arise from failure to follow published guidelines closely, often because the patient has not received sufficiently clear instructions as to what time to take the antibiotic doses in relation to the procedure and how much antibiotic to take at each dose. Written instructions are best.

b. **Risks.** Frequently, regimens are used that do not even meet the theoretical requirements of effective prophylaxis established in animal studies. They are less likely to be effective and, therefore, may give a false sense of security and expose patients to antibiotic toxicity without even theoretical evidence of efficacy. Overuse of even recommended prophylaxis may expose a patient to unnecessary risks of side effects or allergy to antibiotics. For example, risk-benefit analysis suggests that using parenteral penicillin in patients with mitral valve prolapse, particularly prolapse without murmur, would result in net loss of life from fatal reactions as compared to no prophylaxis [14].

c. **Costs.** Table 101-4 lists currently recommended regimens and their approximate cost to the patient or third-party payer [8–11]. Cost-benefit analysis suggests that prevention of a single case of IE in patients with mitral valve prolapse may cost $2.6 million, or $1.5–4.7 million/year of life spared [14].

d. **Acceptability.** Patient acceptability of oral regimens is good. Rash is seen in less than 1% of patients receiving penicillin or ampicillin. Erythromycin frequently (10–20%) produces epigastric discomfort. Vancomycin produces a peculiar immediate flushing reaction or delayed rash in 1–5% of patients. These side effects should be sought for and evaluated for severity. Death from severe penicillin reactions is much higher in parenteral administration of the drug than in oral [14]. Acceptability of some regimens of prophylaxis by dentists may be low [15].

III. Recommendations

A. Risk assessment

1. Identify cardiac lesions by history and physical that place patients at increased risk for infective endocarditis.
2. If necessary, confirm presence and severity of lesion with echocardiography, angiography, or referral to a cardiologist.

B. Prevention. For patients with cardiac lesions that place them at increased risk for IE:

1. Educate about preventing conditions that lead to increased bacteremia (e.g., poor dental hygiene, chronic skin infection) [16].
2. Encourage prophylactic care of teeth in order to avoid gum disease, and dental treatment if gum disease is present [16].
3. Educate about high-risk dental, medical, and surgical procedures and the need for antibiotic prophylaxis.
4. Flag medical record of patients with risk factors for IE.
5. Treat any incidental bacterial infection (e.g. UTI, cellulitis, etc.) early and vigorously in patients with cardiac lesions that predispose them to endocarditis.
6. Administer appropriate prophylaxis to high-risk patients undergoing high-risk procedures (see Tables 101-1 through 101-4).

Table 101-4. Suggested regimens for prevention of infectious endocarditis related to dental, medical, or surgical procedures

Antiobiotic regimens for adults having dental or respiratory tract procedures	
Standard regimen* For dental procedures that cause gingival bleeding, and oral or respiratory tract surgery.	Penicillin V, 2.0 gm PO,† 1 hour before, then 1.0 gm 6 hours later. For patients unable to take oral medications, $2x10^6$ U of aqueous penicillin G IV or IM 30–60 minutes before a procedure and $1x10^6$ U 6 hours later may be substituted.
Special regimens Parenteral regimen for use when maximal protection is desired, for example, for patients with prosthetic valves.	Ampicillin, 1.0–2.0 gm IM or IV, plus gentamicin, 1.5 mg/kg body weight IM or IV, 0.5 hours before procedure, followed by 1.0 gm of oral penicillin V 6 hours later. Alternatively, the parenteral regimen may be repeated once every 8 hours later.
Oral regimen for patients allergic to penicillin.	Erythromycin, 1.0 gm PO 1 hour before, then 500 mg 6 hours later.
Parenteral regimen for patients allergic to penicillin.	Vancomycin, 1.0 gm IV, slowly over 1 hour, starting 1 hour before. No repeat dose is necessary.
Antibiotic regimens for adults having gastrointestinal or genitourinary tract procedures	
Standard regimen For genitourinary and gastrointestinal tract procedures listed in Table 101-3.	Ampicillin, 2.0 gm IM or IV, plus gentamicin, 1.5 mg/kg body wt IM or IV. One follow-up dose may be given 8 hours later.
Special regimens Oral regimen for minor or repetitive procedures in low-risk patients.	Amoxicillin 3.0 gm PO, 1 hour before procedure and 3.0 gm 6 hours later.†
Patients allergic to penicillin.	Vancomycin, 1.0 gm IV, given slowly over 1 hour, plus gentamicin, 1.5 gm/kg body weight IM or IV, given 1 hour before procedure. May be repeated once 8–12 hours later.

*Alternative: Amoxicillin 3 gm PO 1 hour before procedure. An additional 3-gm dose can be given 6 hours later if an extra margin of safety is desired. Gentamicin 1.5 gm/kg IM or IV can be added for high-risk GI or GU procedure where enterococcus is of concern. Cost of amoxicillin is approximately 1.5 times that of penicillin V.

†3 gm penicillin costs the pharmacists approximately $1.50; to the patient, cost is approximately $5–7; gentamicin is $0.65, and injection costs approximately $3.50.

Source: Adapted from D. Kaye. Prophylaxis for infective endocarditis: An update. *Ann. Intern. Med.* 104(3):419, 1986; and S. T. Shulman. Prevention of bacterial endocarditis. *Circulation* 70(6):1123A, 1984.

References

1. Scheld, W. M., and Sande, M. A. Endocarditis and Intravascular Infections. In G.L. Mandell, R.G. Douglas Jr., and J.E. Bennett (eds.), *Principles and Practice of Infectious Diseases.* New York: Wiley, 1985. Pp.504–530. *A good general review.*
2. Everett, E. D., and Hirschmann, J. V. Transient bacteremia and endocarditis prophylaxis. A review. *Medicine* 56(1):61, 1977. *Reviews the medical literature on the topic of bacteremia and endocarditis prophylaxis.*
3. Kaye, D. Prophylaxis for infective endocarditis: An update *Ann Intern. Med.* 104(3):419, 1986. *Excellent critical review of prophylaxis. Discussion of the use of oral amoxicillin to simplify and replace more complicated regimens for dental, respiratory GU, and GI procedures, except in highly susceptible individuals undergoing particularly high-risk procedures.*
4. Chagnac, A., et al. Infectious endocarditis in idiopathic hypertrophic subaortic stenosis: Report of three cases and review of the literature. *Chest* 81(3):346, 1982. *Distinguished high and low risk in IHSS.*
5. Hickey, A. J., MacMahon, S. W., and Wilcken, D. E. Mitral valve prolapse and bacterial endocarditis: When is antibiotic prophylaxis necessary? *Am. Heart J.* 109(3 Pt 1):431, 1985. *Distinguishes high and low risk MVP.*
6. Friedman, W. F. Congenital Heart Disease. In R. G. Petersdorf, et al. (eds.), *Harrison's Principles of Internal Medicine* (10th ed.). New York: McGraw-Hill, 1983, Pp.1383–97. *Frequency of occurrence of cardiac malformations at birth.*
7. Rossiter, S. J., et al. Prosthetic valve endocarditis. Comparison of heterograft tissue valves and mechanical valves. *J. Thorac. Cardiovasc. Surg.* 76(6):795, 1978. *Study of tissue and mechanical valve infectability.*
8. Durack, D. T. Prophylaxis of Infective Endocarditis. In G. L. Mandell, R.G. Douglas Jr., and J. E. Bennett (eds.), *Principles and Practice of Infectious Diseases.* New York: Wiley, 1985. Pp.539–44. *Efficacy, risks, and errors of prophylaxis discussed.*
9. Durack, D. T. Current issues in prevention of infective endocarditis. *Am. J. Med.* 28;78(6 B):149, 1985. *Emphasizes that risk of IE from procedure is dependent on at least two factors: the cardiac lesion present and the degree and type of bacteremia from the procedure.*
10. Shulman, S. T., et al. Prevention of bacterial endocarditis. A statement for health professionals by the Committee on Rheumatic Fever and Infective Endocarditis of the Council on Cardiovascular Disease in the Young. *Circulation* 70(6):1123A, 1984. *An "official" statement on prophylaxis.*
11. Prevention of bacterial endocarditis. *Med. Lett. Drugs Ther.* 29(754):109, 1987. *Current summary of recommended regimens.*
12. Flynn, N. M. Prevention of Infection in Surgical Patients. In R. J. Bolt (ed.), *Medical Evaluation of the Pre-Operative Patient.* Mt. Kisco, NY: Futura, 1987. Pp.195–240. *The second element in the equation determining who is likely to develop endocarditis following a procedure is the quantity and type of bacteria released into the bloodstream during the procedure. Viridans streptococci, enterococci, and staphylococci pose the greatest risk.*
13. Durack, D. T., Kaplan, E. L., and Bisno, A. L. Apparent failures of endocarditis prophylaxis. Analysis of 52 cases submitted to a national registry. *J. A. M. A.* 4;250(17):2318, 1983. *Review and commentary.*
14. Clemens, J. D., and Ransohoff, D. F. A quantitative assessment of pre-dental antibiotic prophylaxis for patients with mitral-valve prolapse. *J. Chronic Dis.* 37(7):531, 1984. *Risk-benefit and cost-benefit analysis of prophylaxis for this common clinical entity.*
15. Brooks, S. L. Survey of compliance with American Heart Association guidelines for prevention of bacterial endocarditis. *J. Am. Dent. Assoc.* 101(1):41, 1980. *Compliance was low, perhaps because of the complexity of the recommendations, unfamiliarity with them, or difficulty in identifying patients at risk.*
16. Guntheroth, W. G. How important are dental procedures as a cause of infective endocarditis? *Am. J. Cardiol.* 1;54(7):797, 1984. *Suggests that daily bacteremias from mastication, poor dental hygiene, and other conditions may far outweigh dental procedures as a cause of IE. Also suggests that scrupulous oral and dental hygiene is probably superior to chemoprophylaxis of dental procedures in prevention of IE.*

Appendixes

Prenatal Flow Sheets*

INITIAL HISTORY AND PHYSICAL

Age	Race	Religion	Marital status	Years married	Education	Occupation

Home address		Home tel.	Work tel.
Husband's name	Age	Husband's employer	Work tel.
Referring physician		Attending physician	

Medical History	Patient	Family	Check and detail positive findings including date and place of treatment. Precede findings by reference number.
1. Multiple births			
2. Diabetes mellitus			
3. Malignancies			
4. Hypertension			
5. Heart disease/R. Fever			
6. Pulmonary disease			
7. GI problems			
8. Renal disease/UTI			
9. Venereal disease			
10. Phlebitis, varicosities			
11. Nervous/mental disorders			
12. Anemia/hemoglobinopathy			
13. Blood dyscrasias			
14. Drug addiction			
15. Smoking/alcohol			
16. Infectious diseases			
17. Operations/accidents			
18. Blood transfusions			
19. Other hospitalizations			
Genetic diseases			
20. Congenital anomalies			
21. Age > 35			
22. Tay Sachs			
23. Sickle Cell/Thal			
24. Neural Tube			
25. Metabolic Disorders			
26. Other			

Menstrual History	Onset age	Cycle 8 days	Length days	Amount	LMP mo/day/yr quality

Pregnancy History	Grav	Term	Pret	Abort	Live	EDC mo/day/yr

No.	Month/year	Sex	Weight at birth	Wks gest	Hrs. in labor	Type of delivery	Anesth	Details of delivery: maternal or newborn complications
1								
2								
3								
4								
5								
6								
7								
8								

Sensitivities (detail positive findings)

27. ☐ None known
28. ☐ Antibiotics
29. ☐ Analgesics
30. ☐ Sedatives
31. ☐ Anesthesia
32. ☐ Other

Preexisting Risk Guide

Indicates pregnancy/outcome at risk

33. ☐ Age ≤ 15 or ≥ 35
34. ☐ < 8th grade education
35. ☐ Cardiac disease (class I or II)
36. ☐ Tuberculosis, active
37. ☐ Chronic pulmonary disease
38. ☐ Thrombophlebitis
39. ☐ Endocrinopathy
40. ☐ Epilepsy (on medication)
41. ☐ Infertility (treated)
42. ☐ 2 abortions (spontaneous/induced)
43. ☐ ≥ 7 deliveries
44. ☐ Previous preterm or SGA infants
45. ☐ Infants ≥ 4,000 gms
46. ☐ Isoimmunization (ABO, etc.)
47. ☐ Hemorrhage during previous preg.
48. ☐ Previous preeclampsia
49. ☐ Surgically scarred uterus
50. ☐ D.E.S. Exposure

Indicates pregnancy/outcome at high risk

51. ☐ Age ≥ 40
52. ☐ Diabetes mellitus
53. ☐ Hypertension
54. ☐ Cardiac disease (class III or IV)
55. ☐ Chronic renal disease
56. ☐ Congenital/chromosomal anomalies
57. ☐ Hemoglobinopathies
58. ☐ Isoimmunization (Rh)
59. ☐ Drug addiction/alcoholism
60. ☐ Habitual abortions
61. ☐ Incompetent cervix
62. ☐ Prior fetal or neonatal death
63. ☐ Prior neurologically damaged infant
64. ☐ ______

Initial Risk Assessment

65. ☐ No risk factors noted
66. ☐ At risk
67. ☐ At high risk

Signature

A. Health history summary.

*These flow sheets are intended for use in conjunction with the portions of the book that apply. They are examples, include partial information, and are not summaries of the book. The chapters must be read.

INITIAL HISTORY AND PHYSICAL

History Since LMP	Patient	Check and detail all positive findings below. Precede findings with symptom number.	15. Medications Since LMP
1. Headaches			(Rx, non-Rx, vitamins) ☐ None
2. Nausea/vomiting			Describe: ______
3. Abdominal pain			
4. Urinary complaints			
5. Vaginal discharge			
6. Vaginal bleeding			
7. Edema (specify area)			
8. Febrile episode			
9. Rubella exposure			**16. Nutritional Assessment**
10. Other viral exposure			☐ Adequate ☐ Inadequate
11. Drug exposure			
12. Radiation exposure			Remarks: ______
13. Other			
14. Last contraceptive ☐ None Type ______ Last used ______			

Initial Physical Examination	Height	Weight	Pregravid weight	B.P.	Pulse	OPTIONAL

System	Normal		Check and detail all positive findings below. Use system numbers.
17. Skin			
18. EENT			
19. Mouth			
20. Neck			
21. Chest			
22. Breast			
23. Heart			
24. Lungs			
25. Abdomen			
26. Musculoskeletal			
27. Extremities			
28. Neurologic			
Pelvic Examination			
29. Ext. genitalia			
30. Vagina			
31. Cervix			
32. Uterus (describe)			
33. Adnexa			
34. Rectum			
35. Other			

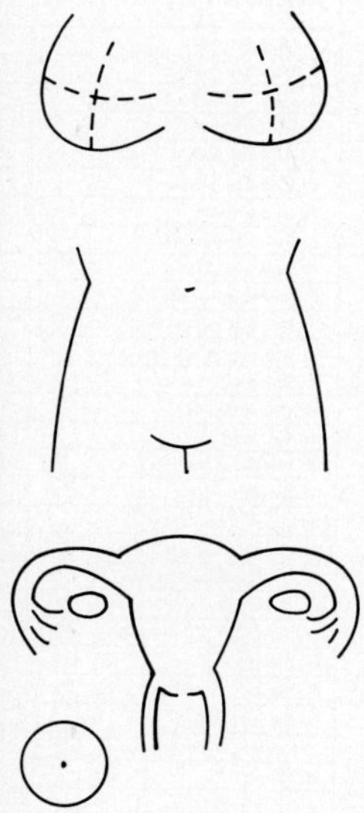

Bony Pelvis	36. Diag. conj.	37. Shape sacrum	38. S.S. notch	39. Ischial spines	44.
	40. Pubic arch	41. Trans. outlet	42. Post. sag. diam	43. Coccyx	45.

46. Classification: ☐ Gynecoid ☐ Android ☐ Anthropoid ☐ Platypelloid

47. Estimation: ☐ Adequate ☐ Borderline ☐ Contracted

Exam by:

B. Initial pregnancy profile.

INITIAL HISTORY AND PHYSICAL

Risk Guide for Pregnancy and Outcome

Preliminary Risk Assessment

- ☐ (0) No risk
- ☐ (1) At risk
- ☐ (2) High risk

Continuing Risk Guide (enter dates first noted and revise RISK STATUS)

Mo/day	Potential risk factors	Mo/day	High risk factors
/	3. Preg. without familial support	/	18. Diabetes mellitus
/	4. Second pregnancy in 12 months	/	19. Hypertension
/	5. Smoking (≥ 1 pack per day)	/	20. Thrombophlebitis
/	6. Rh negative (nonsensitized)	/	21. Herpes (type 2)
/	7. Uterine/cervical malformation	/	22. Rh sensitization
/	8. Inadequate pelvis	/	23. Uterine bleeding
/	9. Venereal disease esp. Herpes	/	24. Hydramnios
/	10. Anemia (Hct<30%: Hgb<10%)	/	25. Severe preeclampsia
/	11. Pyelonephritis/UTI	/	26. Fetal growth retardation
/	12. Failure to gain weight	/	27. Premature rupt. membranes
/	13. Multiple pregnancy (term)	/	28. Multiple pregnancy (preterm)
/	14. Abnormal presentation	/	29. Low/falling estriols
/	15. Postterm pregnancy	/	30. Significant social problems
/	16.	/	31.
/	17.	/	32.

Initial Prenatal Screen

Mo/day	Test	Result	Mo/day	Test	Result
/	Hct/Hgb		/	Int. PPD	
/	Patient's Blood Type and Rh		/	S.S. Screen	
/	Antibody Screen		/	Chlamydia Test	
/	STS		/	AFP	
/	Rubella titer		/	Postprandial glucose	
/	Urinalysis and Gm stain or culture		/	HBsAg	
/	Pap test		/	Herpes culture	
/	G.C.		/	HIV	

☐ Attends prenatal classes ☐ For sterilization

☐ Cesarean section ☐ Breast ☐ Bottle feeding

G	T	P	A	L	LMP mo/day/yr	EDC mo/day/yr

Flow Chart

Date	Weight this visit	Blood pressure	Urine: Protein	Urine: Sugar	Fundal height	Weeks by Dates	Fetal Movement	Fetal heart rate	OCT	NST	E3	HPL	B-Scan Results	Progress Notes (Include Lab Data)	M.D. Intl.
		/													
		/													
		/													
		/													
		/													
		/													
		/													
		/													
		/													
		/													
		/													
		/													

(Weight column header also includes: Year, Pre-gravid)

C. Prenatal flow record (page 1).

INITIAL HISTORY AND PHYSICAL

Flow Chart Date	Year / Weight this visit / Pre-gravid	Blood pressure	Urine Protein	Sugar	Fundal height	Weeks by Dates	Fetal Movement	Fetal heart rate	OCT	NST	E3	HPL	B-Scan Results	Progress Notes (Include Lab Data)	M.D. Intl.

C. Prenatal flow record (page 2).

PHYSICIANS PROGRESS RECORD

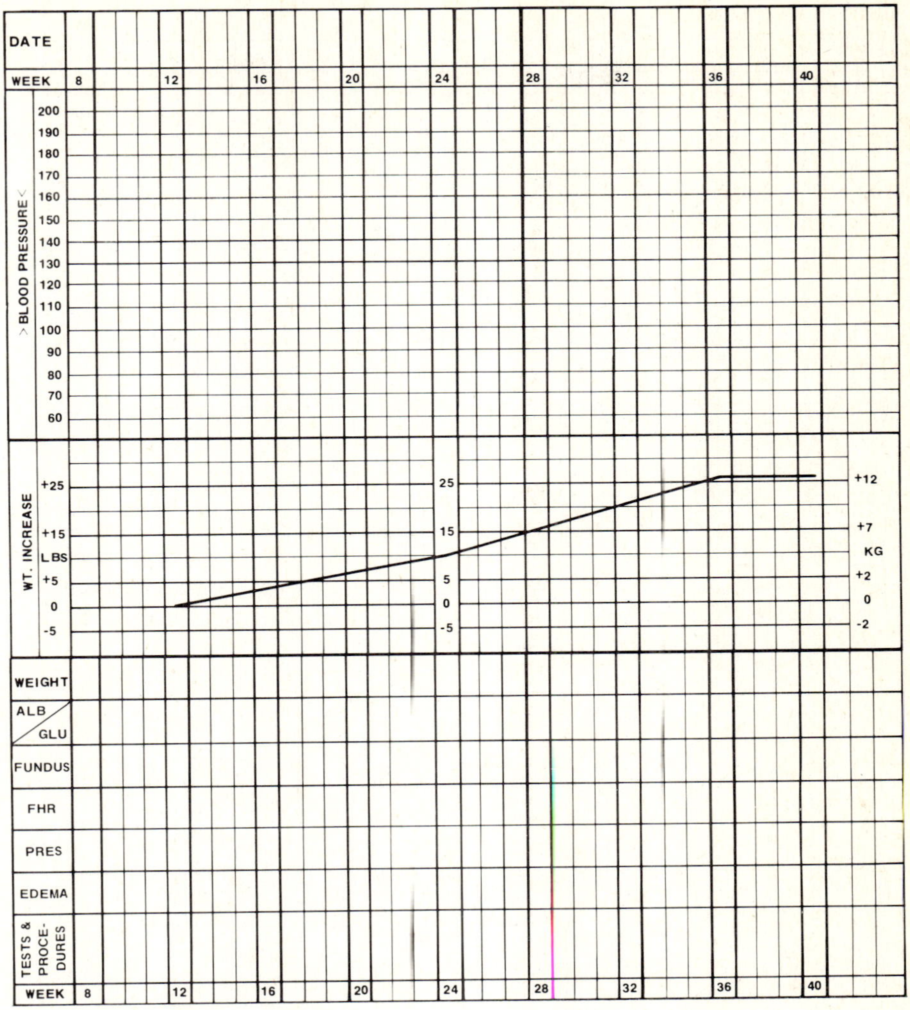

D. Prenatal graphics (page 1).

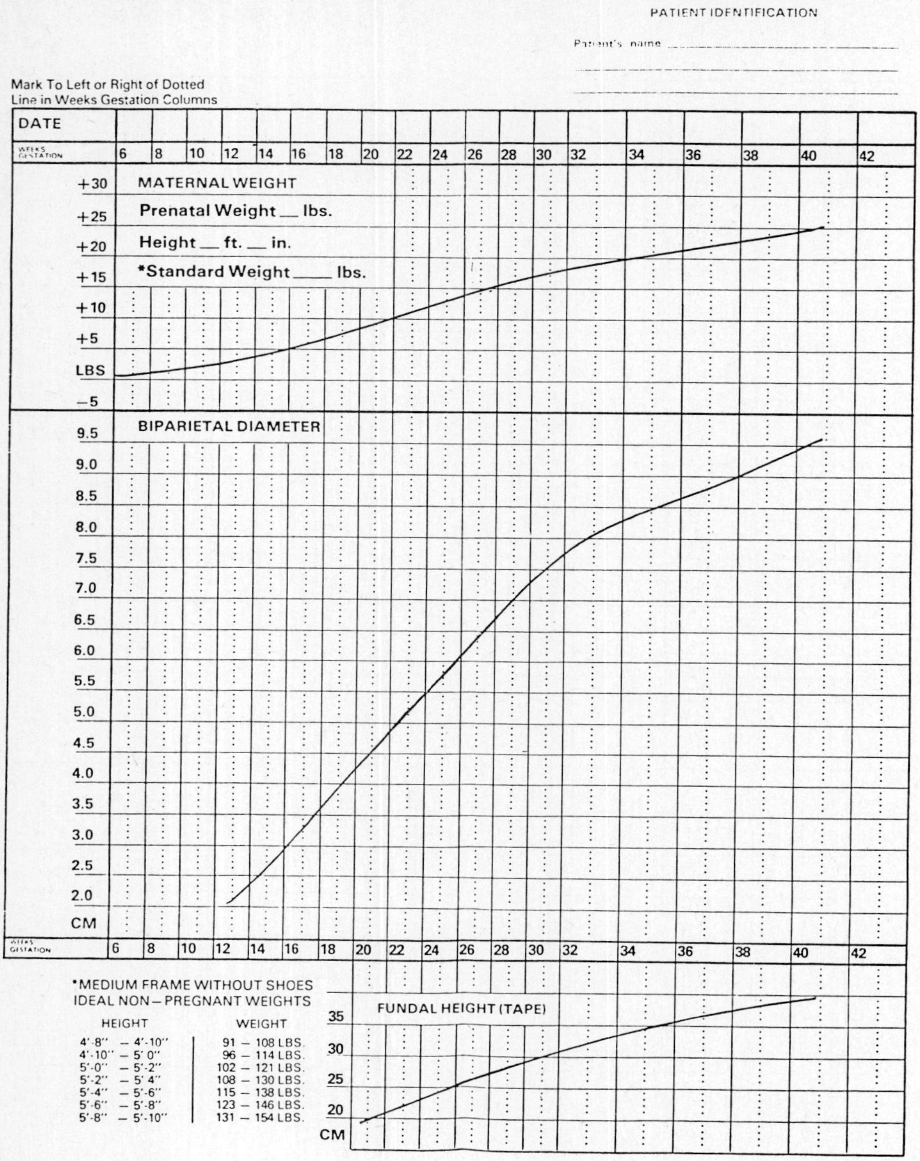

*MEDIUM FRAME WITHOUT SHOES
IDEAL NON–PREGNANT WEIGHTS

HEIGHT	WEIGHT
4'-8" – 4'-10"	91 – 108 LBS.
4'-10" – 5' 0"	96 – 114 LBS.
5'-0" – 5'-2"	102 – 121 LBS.
5'-2" – 5' 4"	108 – 130 LBS.
5'-4" – 5'-6"	115 – 138 LBS.
5'-6" – 5'-8"	123 – 146 LBS.
5'-8" – 5'-10"	131 – 154 LBS.

E. Prenatal graphics (page 2).

Pediatric Flow Sheets*

PHYSICIAN'S PROGRESS RECORD

RECORD DATES AND RESULTS — **HEALTH MAINTENANCE—PEDIATRIC (BIRTH—6 YEARS)**

Term ( ) AGA ( ) Pre ( ) SGA ( ) Post ( ) LGA ( )	Birth-24 hr	1-6 days	7-14 days	2 months	4 months	6 months	12 months	15 months	18 months	2 years	4 years	6 years
Exam Date / Actual Age												
Immunizations & TB												
DPT (DT)												
TOPV (Parents immunized?)												
MMR												
TB Skin Test	At 6 mo. to 15 mo. (prior to or simultaneous with MMR) then every 1-2yrs.											
Haemophilis Influenza												
Physical Exam												
Complete Exam				At least as often as immunizations								
Wt. (Birth)		At each examination and plot on growth curve										
Ht. (Birth)		At each examination and plot on growth curve										
OFC (Birth)		At each examination and plot on growth curve until 3 yrs.										
BP							At each visit from 3 yrs. on					
Hips	At well child visits until walking normally											
VISION: Media opacities - view retina & red reflex												
VISION: Strabismus					corneal light reflex and cover/alt. cover test							
VISION: Acuity											by age 4	
Hearing	High Risk Registry & ABR on registrants by 3 mo.					Speech/Noisemaker					Audiogram before school	
Development (Apgars)												
Laboratory												
PKU, T4, Galactosemia												
Hct. or Hgb.												
High Risk												
Lead (· E.P.)							Yearly E.P. for high risk children					

Patient Education Topics **

Topic	PRENATAL	
Nutrition		Fluoride ( ) Water Supply ( ) Fluoride Dose ( ) ( )
	Breast ( ) Formula ( )	Vits ( ) Iron ( ) Junk Food ( ) Solids ( ) Less Apetite ( ) Dental Care ( )
Accidents	Car seat ( ) Crib ( )	Roll/Falls ( ) Small Objects ( ) Ipecac ( ) Seat Belts ( ) Cabinets ( ) Stree ( ) Bike Safety ( ) H2O temp ( ) Elec. outlet ( ) Swimming ( )
Parenting	Bonding ( ) Sibs ( ) Abuse Risk ( )	Temperment ( ) Sleeping ( ) Read to Baby ( ) School Readiness ( ) Discipline ( ) Sharing ( ) Stooling ( ) Toilet Training ( ) Crying ( ) Sitter/Day Care ( )
Illness	Bulb Syringe ( ) Circ. ( )	Dehyd. ( ) Colds ( ) Fever ( ) When to call/come to MD/NP ( ) (**) Many of these topics should be discussed and reevaluated on an ongoing basis.

Annotation February 1988

A. Pediatric health maintenance (birth to 6 years).

*These flow sheets are intended for use in conjunction with the portions of the book that apply. They are examples, include partial information, have some added information, and are not summaries of the book. The chapters must be read.

PHYSICIAN'S PROGRESS RECORD

RECORD DATES AND RESULTS **HEALTH MAINTENANCE—PEDIATRIC (7—17 YEARS)**

	Services \ Age	7	8	9	10	11	12	13	14	15	16	17
	Exam Date											
Immunizations & TB	Td	Every 10 years if primary immunization complete										
	Rubella Titer or vaccine	Must have documented vaccine or documented titer										
	TB Skin Test	Every 1-2 years										
Physical Exam	Complete Exam	Every 1-2 years										
	Height	At every visit and plot on growth curve										
	Weight	At every visit and plot on growth curve										
	BP	At every visit										
	Scoliosis			♀ - at least once at 10-12 years		♂ once at 12-14 years						
	Visual Acuity											
Laboratory	Hematocrit ♀						With poor diet and heavy menses					
	PAP (from onset of sexual relations)						Annually once sexually active					
	Cholesterol	If family history of premature CHD, at entry to school & during adolescence										
High Risk												
Patient Education Topics**	Parenting	school ( ) peers ( ) family ( ) (**) Many of these topics should be discussed and reevaluated on an ongoing basis.										
	Accidents	seat/shoulder belts ( ) guns ( ) suicide risk ( )										
	Nutrition & Exercise	fluoride ( ) junk food ( ) exercise ( ) obesity ( ) menstruation anemia ( )										
	Sex Education	menstruation ( ) masturbation ( ) contraception ( ) STD's ( )										
	Substance Abuse	Parental: smoking ( ) alcohol ( ) drugs ( ) Childhood/ Adolescent: smoking ( ) alcohol ( ) drugs ( )										

Annotation February 1988

B. Pediatric health maintenance (7 to 17 years).

Adult Flow Sheets*

PHYSICIAN'S PROGRESS RECORD

RECORD DATES AND RESULTS **HEALTH MAINTENANCE — ADULT (18-40 YEARS)**

	Services / Age (Years)	18	19-20	21-22	23-24	25-26	27-28	29-30	31-32	33-34	35-36	37-38	39-40
	Exam Date / Actual Age												
Immunizations & PPD	Td	Every 10 years if primary immunization complete.											
	Rubella Titer or vaccine	Women and men working close to reproductive age women need vaccine or documented antibodies.											
	PPD	On entry to practice, then every 5 years and every 1-2 years in high risk individuals.											
		Hepatitis B, influenza or pneumococcal vaccine in high risk.											
Exam	Complete Exam	On entry to practice, then according to risk.											
	Wt. (Ht.)	Every 1-2 years.											
	BP	Every 1-2 years.											
	Provider Breast Exam	Every 3 years. Every year for high risk after 30.											
	Mammography	Baseline at 35. Baseline at 30 for high risk.											
	PAP Smear	Annually											
Laboratory	STS	Once on entry to practice; repeat every 6-12 months if high risk.											
	Cholesterol ♂	Every 3-5 years if low risk (< 200), more often if higher risk.											
High Risk	Note any high risk group not otherwise specified, such as DES, AIDS or skin cancer, etc.												

Patient Education Topics		
	Accidents	Safety belts ( ) Smoke alarm ( )
	Cancer	Testes self-exam ( ) Breast self-exam ( ) *These topics should be part of the initial assessment of all patients; follow-up and repeat inquiries usually required.
	Nutrition	Diet ( ) Menstruation anemia ( )
	Exercise	Coronary risk factors ( )
	Substance Abuse	Smoking ( ) Alcohol ( ) Drugs ( )
	Stress	School ( ) Family ( ) Job ( ) Sex ( )
	Contraception	

Annotation February 1988

A. Adult health maintenance (18 to 40 years).

*These flow sheets are intended for use in conjunction with the portions of the book that apply. They are examples, include partial information, and are not summaries of the book. The chapters must be read.

PHYSICIAN'S PROGRESS RECORD

RECORD DATES AND RESULTS — **HEALTH MAINTENANCE—ADULT (41 +YEARS)**

	Services / Age (Years)	41 Record age of patient here.
	EXAM DATE	Record exam date.
Immunizations & PPD	Td	Every 10 years if primary immunization complete.
	PPD	On entry to practice (2-step after age 50), then every 5 years; every 1-2 years in high risk individuals.
	Influenza	Every fall for high risk, and ≥ 65 years.
	Pneumococcal	Once only for high risk. Hepatitis B vaccine if high risk.
Exam	Complete Exam	Once on entry to practice; then according to risk.
	Wt. (Ht.)	Annually
	BP	Annually
	Tonometry	If pressure ≤ 20mm Hg; every 5 years to age 60, then every 2-3 years. Pressure > 20mm Hg, refer to ophthomologist.
	Digital Rectal	Annually
	Slide Guaiac	Annually
	Sigmoidoscopy	Every 3-5 years after 2 negatives one year apart starting at age 50.
	Provider Breast Exam	Annually, more often in high risk.
	Mammogram	3 yearly exams from 50, if negative, then every 2 years. Every 2 years from 40-50 for high risk, then annually.
	Pap Smear	Annually
Laboratory	STS	Once on entry to practice; repeat every 6-12 months if high risk.
	Cholesterol	Every 3-5 years if low risk (< 200); more often if higher risk.
High Risk	Note any high risk group not otherwise specified, such as osteoporosis, skin cancer, etc.	
Patient Education Topics	Nutrition & Exercise	*These topics should be part of all patient's initial assessment. Diet ( ) Exercise ( ) Calcium ( ) Follow-up and repeat inquiry
	Substance Abuse & Stress	Smoking ( ) Family ( ) Alcohol ( ) Sex ( ) Drugs ( ) Job ( ) Social Support ( ) Suicide ( ) usually required.
	Cancer	Breast self-exam ( ) Post-menopausal bleeding ( )
	Accidents	Safety belts ( ) Smoke Alarm ( ) Falls ( )

Annotation February 1988

B. Adult health maintenance (41 years and over).

Index

Index